Nurse's Handbook of
Combination
Drugs

Nurse's Handbook of
Combination
Drugs

Second Edition

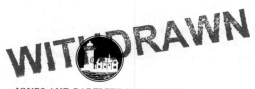

JONES AND BARTLETT PUBLISHERS
Sudbury, Massachusetts
BOSTON   TORONTO   LONDON   SINGAPORE

World Headquarters

Jones and Bartlett Publishers
40 Tall Pine Drive
Sudbury, MA 01776
978-443-5000
info@jbpub.com
www.jbpub.com

Jones and Bartlett Publishers
Canada
6339 Ormindale Way
Mississauga, Ontario L5V 1J2
Canada

Jones and Bartlett Publishers
International
Barb House, Barb Mews
London W6 7PA
United Kingdom

Jones and Bartlett's books and products are available through most bookstores and online book-sellers. To contact Jones and Bartlett Publishers directly, call 800-832-0034, fax 978-443-8000, or visit our website www.jbpub.com.

Substantial discounts on bulk quantities of Jones and Bartlett's publications are available to corporations, professional associations, and other qualified organizations. For details and specific discount information, contact the special sales department at Jones and Bartlett via the above contact information or send an email to specialsales@jbpub.com.

Production Credits

Publisher: Kevin Sullivan
Acquisitions Editor: Emily Ekle
Acquisitions Editor: Amy Sibley
Associate Editor: Patricia Donnelly
Editorial Assistant: Rachel Shuster
Senior Production Editor: Carolyn F. Rogers
Senior Marketing Manager: Barb Bartoszek

V. P., Manufacturing and Inventory Control: Therese Connell
Clinical Reviewer: Marlene Ciranowicz-Steenburg, RN, MSN, CDE
Composition: Catherine E. Harold
Cover Design: Kristin E. Parker
Cover Image: © ajt/ShutterStock, Inc.
Printing and Binding: Malloy, Inc.
Cover Printing: Malloy, Inc.

6048

Printed in the United States of America
13 12 11 10 09   10 9 8 7 6 5 4 3 2 1

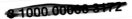

Contents

Reviewers and Clinical Consultants

Alison Calabrese, RPh.
Clinical Pharmacist
Lourdes Hospital
Binghamton, NY

Kimberly A. Couch, PharmD
Clinical Pharmacy Specialist,
 Infectious Diseases
Department of Pharmacy
Christiana Care Health System
Newark, DE

Thomas Forrest, RPh.
Clinical Pharmacist
Lourdes Hospital
Binghamton, NY

John P. Gatto, RPh.
Clinical Pharmacist
Eckerd Pharmacy
Owego, NY

Jeanne M. Hoff, RPh.
Clinical Pharmacist
Lourdes Hospital
Binghamton, NY

Mary Ann Klee, RPh.
Pharmacist
St. Joseph Hospital
Elmira, NY

Shannon M. Murray, PharmD, CGP
Clinical Pharmacy Specialist,
 Geriatrics
Christiana Care Health System
Newark, DE

Mirza E. Perez, PharmD, BCPS
Assistant Professor
Temple University, School of
 Pharmacy
Philadelphia, PA

How to Use This Book

Jones and Bartlett's *Nurse's Handbook of Combination Drugs, Second Edition,* provides what today's nurses and nursing students need: accurate, concise, and reliable drug facts when administering combination products, with their more complicated and more numerous interactions, adverse reactions, and nursing considerations. This book emphasizes the vital information you need to know before, during, and after combination drug administration. The information is presented in easy-to-understand language and organized alphabetically, so you can find what you need quickly.

What's Special

In addition to the detailed drug information you expect to find in each entry (see "Drug Entries," below, for details), the *Nurse's Handbook of Combination Drugs, Second Edition,* boasts these special features:

- **One concise, thorough drug entry for each combination** puts the information you need right at your fingertips, whether the combination contains two, three, or more drugs. No more having to look up the two or more drugs individually and then wonder if you have all the information you need for safe administration and care.

- **Practical trim size and good-size type** give you a book that's easy to carry, easy to read, and easy to handle. You can hold the book in one hand, see complete pages at a glance, and use your other hand to document or perform other activities.

- **No-nonsense writing style** that speaks everyday language and uses the terms and abbreviations you typically encounter in your practice and your studies—although a few abbreviations may not be used in certain facilities. (See *Abbreviations,* pages 827 to 830.) And to avoid sexist language, we alternate between male and female pronouns throughout the book.

- **Up-to-date drug information,** including the latest FDA-approved drugs, new and changed indications, new warnings, and newly reported adverse reactions.

- **Dosage adjustment,** highlighted in the text, alerts you to expected dosage changes for a patient with a specific condition or disorder, such as advanced age or renal impairment.

- **Warning,** highlighted in the text, calls attention to important facts that you need to know before, during, and after drug administration. For example, in the amplodipine and benazepril entry, this feature informs you that this drug combination may cause anaphylactoid reactions, including angioedema, especially after the first dose.

- **Useful appendices** give an overview of important drug facts and nursing considerations in antineoplastic combination drug therapy for selected common cancers and in combination oral contraceptives. You'll also find handy information you can use every day in your practice and studies, such as instructions for calculating drug dosages and checking which drugs are compatible in a syringe.

Drug Entries

Nurse's Handbook of Combination Drugs, Second Edition, clearly and concisely presents all the vital facts on the combination drugs that you'll typically administer. To help you find the information you need quickly, entries are grouped first according to their general classification, listed alphabetically:

- Anti-infective Drugs
- Cardiovascular Drugs
- Central Nervous System Drugs
- Dermatologic Drugs
- Endocrine Drugs
- Eye and Ear Drugs
- Gastrointestinal Drugs
- Genitourinary Drugs
- Respiratory Drugs

Generic Names

Each chapter lists its drugs alphabetically by generic name, making the first drug in the combination the one in the original FDA approval of the drug combination. For example, the combination drug glyburide and metformin hydrochloride is found in the chapter on Endocrine Drugs under the G listings, not the M listings. You can also find it in the index by looking up glyburide, metformin, or its trade name, Glucovance.

For consistency, details of the individual drug components within the entry present glyburide before metformin. In the dosage section of the entry, the combined dosage is given first but is followed in brackets, where appropriate, with the portion of the dosage for the first drug named in the combination generic name followed by the second drug.

Class, Category, and Schedule

Each entry lists the drug's chemical and therapeutic classes. With this information, you can compare drugs in the same chemical class but in different therapeutic classes—and vice versa.

The entry also lists the FDA's pregnancy risk category, which categorizes drugs based on their potential to cause birth defects. (For details, see *FDA pregnancy risk categories* on page x.)

Where appropriate, the entry also includes the drug's controlled substance schedule. (For details, see *Controlled substance schedules* on page xi.)

Indications and Dosages

This section lists FDA-approved therapeutic indications. For each indication, you'll find the applicable drug form or route, age-group (adults, adolescents, or children), and dosage (which includes amount per dose, timing, and duration).

Mechanism of Action

Set off by a box, this section concisely describes how a drug achieves its therapeutic effects at the cellular, tissue, or organ level, as appropriate.

Incompatibilities

You'll be alerted to drugs or solutions that are incompatible with the topic drug when mixed in a syringe or solution, or infused through the same I.V. line.

Contraindications

An alphabetical list details the conditions and disorders that preclude administration of the topic drug.

Interactions

This section presents the drugs, foods, and activities (such as alcohol use and smoking) that can cause important, problematic, or life-threatening interactions with the topic drug. For each interacting drug, food, or activity, you'll learn the effects of the interaction. Listed interactions begin with the combination agent; then, the interactions unique to each drug follow, as needed.

Adverse Reactions

Organized by body system, this section highlights common, serious, and life-threatening adverse reactions in alphabetical order.

Nursing Considerations

Warnings, precautions, and key information you must know be-

FDA PREGNANCY RISK CATEGORIES

Each drug may be placed in a pregnancy risk category based on the FDA's estimate of risk to the fetus. If the FDA hasn't provided a category, the *Nurse's Handbook of Combination Drugs, Second Edition,* notes that the drug is "Not rated." The categories range from A to X, signifying least to greatest fetal risk.

A Controlled studies show no risk

Adequate, well-controlled studies with pregnant women have failed to demonstrate a risk to the fetus in any trimester of pregnancy.

B No evidence of risk in humans

Adequate, well-controlled studies with pregnant women haven't shown increased risk of fetal abnormalities despite adverse findings in animals, or—in the absence of adequate human studies—animal studies show no fetal risk. The chance of fetal harm is remoate, but remains possible.

C Risk can't be ruled out

Adequate, well-controlled human studies are lacking, and animal studies have demonstrated a risk to the fetus or are lacking as well. A chance of fetal harm exists if the drug is administered during pregnancy, but the potential benefits may outweigh the risk.

D Positive evidence of risk

Studies in humans, or investigational or post-marketing data, have demonstrated fetal risk. Nevertheless, the drug's potential benefits may outweigh its risks. For example, the drug may be acceptable for use in a life-threatening situation or serious disease for which safer drugs can't be used or are ineffective.

X Contraindicated in pregnancy

Studies in animals or humans, or investigational or post-marketing reports, have demonstrated positive evidence of fetal abnormalities or risks; these risks clearly outweigh any possible benefit to the patient.

fore, during, and after drug administration appear in this section. Examples include whether or not a pill can be crushed and how to properly reconstitute, dilute, store, handle, or dispose of a drug.

CONTROLLED SUBSTANCE SCHEDULES

The Controlled Substances Act of 1970 mandated that certain pre-scription drugs be categorized in schedules based on their potential for abuse. The greater their abuse potential, the greater the restrictions on their prescription. The controlled substance schedules range from I to V, signifying highest to lowest abuse potential.

I High potential for abuse

No accepted medical use exists for Schedule I drugs, which include heroin and lysergic acid diethylamide (LSD).

II High potential for abuse

Use may lead to severe physical or psychological dependence. Prescriptions must be written in ink or typewritten and must be signed by the prescriber. Oral prescriptions must be confirmed in writing within 72 hours and may be given only in a genuine emergency. No renewals are permitted.

III Some potential for abuse

Use may lead to low-to-moderate physical dependence or high psychological dependence. Prescriptions may be oral or written. Up to five renewals are permitted within 6 months.

IV Low potential for abuse

Use may lead to limited physical or psychological dependence. Prescriptions may be oral or written. Up to five renewals are permitted within 6 months.

V Subject to state and local regulation

Abuse potential is low; a prescription may not be required.

Patient teaching information is also included in this section. You'll find important guidelines for patients, including how and when to take each prescribed drug, how to recognize and manage adverse reactions, which cautions to observe, when to contact the prescriber, and more. To save you time, however, this section doesn't repeat basic patient-teaching points. (For a summary of those, see *Teaching your patient about combination drug therapy* on pages xii and xiii.)

TEACHING YOUR PATIENT ABOUT COMBINATION DRUG THERAPY

Your teaching about combination drug therapy will vary with your patient's needs and your practice setting. To help guide your teaching, each drug entry provides key information that you must teach your patient about those combined drugs. For all patients, however, you should also:

☑ Teach the generic and trade names for each drug component in the prescribed combination drug that he'll take after discharge—even if he took the combination before admission.

☑ Clearly explain why each combination drug was prescribed, how it works, and what it's supposed to do. To help your patient understand the drug's therapeutic effects, relate its action to her disorder or condition.

☑ Review the drug form, dosage, and route with the patient. Tell him whether the drug is a tablet, suppository, spray, aerosol, or other form, and explain how to administer it correctly. Also, tell him how often to take the drug and for what length of time. Emphasize that he should take the drug exactly as prescribed.

☑ Describe the drug's appearance, and explain that scored tablets can be broken in half for safe, accurate dosing. Warn the patient not to break unscored tablets because doing so may alter the drug dosage. If your patient has difficulty swallowing capsules, explain that she can open ones that contain sprinkles and take them with food or a drink but that she shouldn't do this with capsules that contain powder. Also, warn her not to crush or chew enteric-coated, extended-release, sustained-release, or similar drug forms.

☑ Teach the patient about common adverse reactions that may occur. Advise him to notify the prescriber at once if a dangerous adverse reaction, such as syncope, occurs.

☑ Warn her not to suddenly stop taking a drug if she's bothered by mild, unpleasant adverse reactions. Instead, encourage her to discuss the reactions with her prescriber, who may adjust the dosage or substitute a drug that causes fewer adverse reactions.

☑ Warn the patient that some adverse reactions, such as dizziness and drowsiness, can impair his ability to operate machinery, drive a car, or perform other activities that require alertness. Help him develop a dosing schedule that prevents adverse reactions from interfering with such activities.

☑ Inform the patient which adverse reactions resolve with time.

☑ Teach the patient how to store the drug properly. Let him know if the drug is sensitive to light or temperature and how to protect it from these elements.

☑ Instruct the patient to store the drug in its original container, if possible, with the drug's name and dosage clearly printed on the label.

☑ Inform the patient which devices to use—and which ones to avoid—for drug storage or administration. For example, instruct him to use a calibrated device when measuring a dose of liquid brompheniramine and pseudoephedrine.

☑ Teach the patient what to do if she misses a dose. Generally, she should take a once-daily drug as soon as she remembers—provided that she remembers within the first 24 hours. If 24 hours have elapsed, she should take the next scheduled dose, but not double the dose. If she has questions or concerns about missed doses, tell her to contact the prescriber.

☑ Provide information that's specific to the prescribed drug. For example, if a patient takes amiloride and hydrochlorothiazide to manage hypertension or heart failure, instruct him to weigh himself daily at the same time of day, using the same scale and wearing the same amount of clothing. Or if the patient takes niacin extended-release and lovastatin to treat primary hypersholesterolemia, urge him to have periodic eye examinations during therapy.

☑ Advise the patient to refill prescriptions promptly, unless she no longer needs the drug. Also instruct her to discard expired drugs because they may become ineffective or even dangerous over time.

☑ Warn the patient to keep all drugs out of the reach of children at all times.

FOREWORD

Patients have always found taking one drug simpler to manage than taking several. A patient taking several medications confronts issues of timing doses, daily planning and organization, personal understanding and memory—among others; and nurses and prescribers struggle with patient confusion and compliance in such situations. One simplifier in this complex situation comes from combination drug products.

With this problem in mind, drug manufacturers have devised, the FDA has approved, and more and more prescribers have endorsed increasing numbers of combination drug formulations. With the convenience of needing only one formulation to take two or more medications simultaneously, a patient's drug regimen simplifies. Also, patient safety may improve when the number of daily pills to be taken declines, resulting in fewer potential medication errors.

For the nurse, however, the convenience of combination drugs is linked with the added responsibility to provide safe, effective drug therapy and complete patient teaching about the medications. The combination product may be simpler to take, but its potential for adverse reactions and drug and food interactions is, if anything, more complex—not less—than dosages of individual drugs. A medication error or adverse reaction involving a combination drug product becomes compounded because it poses not just the threat of adverse effects with one drug but with two or more.

Your Responsibilities in Combination Drug Therapy

Your basic responsibilities in administering a combination drug product are similar to those in administering any drug, including:
- administering the right combination drug in the right dose by the right route at the right time to the right patient
- knowing the therapeutic use, dosage, interactions, adverse reactions, and warnings of each administered combination drug
- being aware of newly approved combination drugs that may be prescribed
- knowing about changes to existing combination drugs, such as new indications and dosages and recently discovered adverse reactions and interactions

- concentrating fully when preparing and administering combination drugs
- responding promptly and appropriately to serious or life-threatening adverse reactions, interactions, and other complications
- instructing each patient about the combination drug, how it's administered, which effects the drugs together may cause, and which reactions to watch for and report to you or to the prescriber.

Beyond these basic responsibilities, however, you also need additional nursing knowledge to meet the demands of today's combination drug therapy, such as knowing how the two or more drugs contained in the drug formulation will affect your care of the patient and the things he needs to know to self-administer the combination drug safely at home.

Meeting Your Needs

Nurses and students need a reliable, accurate, easy-to-use, quick-reference drug book on combination drug therapy. The book in your hands, Jones and Bartlett's *Nurse's Handbook of Combination Drugs, Second Edition,* contains a wealth of reliable and easy-to-understand information on virtually all of the prescribed combination drug products you're likely to administer.

You can depend on the accuracy and reliability of the information contained in this Handbook because each entry has been written by nurses for nurses and reviewed by experts in nursing and pharmacology. What's more, every drug entry has been checked against the most respected drug references today, including the *American Hospital Formulary Service Drug Information, Drug Facts and Comparisons, Physician's Desk Reference,* and the *USP DI's Drug Information for the Health Care Professional.*

Jones and Bartlett's *Nurse's Handbook of Combination Drugs, Second Edition,* is practical and convenient, providing the information on the drugs included in each combination product in a single entry. It gives you the complete information you need and saves you from having to track down the information in any other handbook's two or more entries.

Organization

The *Handbook's* chapters are grouped by body system, giving you the advantage of finding all the combination drugs on cardiovascular disorders, for example, gathered together. Within each chapter, the entries are listed alphabetically by the generic name of the first drug in the combination—as defined by the manufacturer and approved by the FDA.

To speed you to each entry when you need it, the comprehensive index lists each generic drug, no matter whether it is the primary or a secondary drug in the combination, and no matter how many combinations it is part of. For example, neomycin sulfate appears in seven drug combinations in this book, and the index gets you to each one in a couple of seconds. Further, all trade names are indexed. So if you need to find Glucovance, you can do so whether or not you know it consists of glyburide and metformin. You can, of course, get to the Glucovance entry by looking up either glyburide or metformin in the index.

Two appendices cover combinations that do not receive entries in the main text: Antineoplastic Combination Drugs for Selected Cancers, and Combination Oral Contraceptives. Because drug regimens in cancer depend on the staging of the cancer, the absence or presence of metastasis, and the patient's physical status—among other important variables—coverage of this information is more efficiently presented in a table for your reference. Your relationship to patients taking oral combination contraceptives is probably advisory, and so the contraceptives table contains a good deal of patient teaching that is best concentrated in one place for your convenience.

Additional appendices include *Compatible Drugs in a Syringe*, *Drug Formulas and Calculations*, *Weights and Equivalents*, and *Abbreviations*.

Value in a Drug Reference

Whether you work in or are preparing to work in acute care, home care, long-term care, or another health care setting, you'll want your own copy of *Nurse's Handbook of Combination Drugs, Second Edition*. That's because this book will help you:

- reduce your risk of medication errors by giving you access to accurate, reliable drug information that's relevant to your practice
- stay current on the most up-to-date drug developments
- improve your drug administration skills and patient care during all stages of drug administration
- quickly detect and manage serious or life-threatening adverse reactions and complications—or prevent them from occurring
- save time because you won't have to sift through volumes of information or numerous web sites to find what you need, worry that the source you're using isn't timely, or juggle information from several sources on the component drugs in a combination

- increase your confidence about drug administration and enhance your professional interactions with other health care team members
- ensure the delivery of safe, effective care
- improve the depth and quality of your patient teaching.

Your Rewards

You deserve the latest and most beneficial resources to support you in delivering the safest and most informed care that you can to your patients. And today, you face greater challenges than ever: more patients who are acutely ill, tighter budgets and staffing, and more complex drug therapy. The reference you hold now adds to your armamentarium and, as such, is a must for your professional nursing library. Jones and Bartlett's *Nurse's Handbook of Combination Drugs, Second Edition,* is a one-of-a-kind reference you'll want to have at your fingertips. It's a resource you'll use often and confidently because of its accurate, clearly written, and essential information—a vital nursing tool.

Kathleen A. Dracup, RN, FNP, DNSc, FAAN
Dean of Nursing
University of California, San Francisco

Anti-Infective Drugs

abacavir sulfate and lamivudine
Epzicom

Class and Category
Chemical: Synthetic nucleoside analogues (abacavir, lamivudine)
Therapeutic: Antiretroviral (abacavir, lamivudine)
Pregnancy category: C

Indications and Dosages
▶ *To treat HIV-1 infection*
TABLETS
Adults. 600 mg abacavir and 300 mg lamivudine (1 tablet) daily with other antiretrovirals.

Mechanism of Action
Abacavir, a carbocyclic synthetic nucleoside analogue, becomes converted inside cells to carbovir triphosphate, an active metabolite. Carbovir triphosphate stops the activity of HIV-1 reverse transcriptase required in viral DNA synthesis by competing with the natural substrate dGTP and by becoming a part of the viral DNA. This action ends formation of the DNA chain.

Lamivudine, a synthetic nucleoside analogue, becomes phosphorylated inside cells to lamivudine triphosphate, an active metabolite. The metabolite stops the activity of HIV-1 reverse transcriptase by becoming part of the viral DNA, thus ending formation of the DNA chain.

Contraindications
Hepatic impairment; hypersensitivity to abacavir, lamivudine, or any of their components

Interactions
DRUGS
abacavir
methadone: Increased methadone clearance

lamivudine

interferon alfa, ribavirin: Possibly increased risk of toxicity, especially hepatic decompensation

trimethoprim and sulfamethoxazole: Increased lamivudine exposure

zalcitabine: Possibly inhibited intracellular phosphorylation, making both drugs ineffective

Adverse Reactions

CNS: Abnormal dreams, anxiety, depression, dizziness, fatigue, fever, headache, insomnia, malaise, paresthesia, peripheral neuropathy, seizures, vertigo, weakness

CV: Elevated triglycerides

EENT: Pharyngitis, stomatitis

ENDO: Hyperglycemia

GI: Abdominal pain, diarrhea, elevated liver enzymes, gastritis, hepatic steatosis, hepatomegaly, nausea, pancreatitis, posttreatment exacerbation of hepatitis B, vomiting

HEME: Anemia, aplastic anemia, neutropenia, splenomegaly, thrombocytopenia

MS: Elevated CK, muscle weakness, rhabdomyolysis

RESP: Cough, dyspnea, wheezing

SKIN: Alopecia, erythema multiforme, rash, Stevens-Johnson syndrome, toxic epidermal necrolysis, urticaria

Other: Anaphylaxis, fat accumulation or redistribution, immune reconstitution syndrome, lactic acidosis, lymphadenopathy

Nursing Considerations

- Because dosages of individual drugs can't be adjusted, the combination drug shouldn't be given to a patient who has a creatinine clearance less than 50 ml/min/1.73 m^2, hepatic impairment, or dose-limiting adverse reactions. If any of these problems develop during therapy, notify prescriber and expect the patient to be switched to a different medication.

- **WARNING** Notify prescriber immediately at first sign or symptom of hypersensitivity to abacavir and lamivudine, such as abdominal pain, cough, diarrhea, dyspnea, fatigue, fever, nausea, pharyngitis, rash, or vomiting. Stop drug immediately if hypersensitivity is suspected, and notify prescriber. The drug should not be restarted after hypersensitivity reaction resolves because more severe symptoms will recur within hours and may be fatal. The prescriber should register the hypersensitivity reaction with the abacavir hypersensitivity reaction registry by calling 1-800-270-0425.

- Monitor patient's liver function routinely, as ordered, and assess

patient for evidence of lactic acidosis and liver dysfunction that may result from abacavir and lamivudine therapy, especially in women and patients with a history of prolonged nucleoside exposure. In patients with a history of hepatitis B, expect to monitor liver function for several months after therapy stops.
- Monitor patient closely for opportunistic infections because combination antiretroviral therapy may cause an inflammatory response with these infections that could lead to immune reconstitution syndrome requiring additional therapy.

PATIENT TEACHING
- Advise patient that hypersensitivity reactions may occur with abacavir and lamivudine. Review the signs and symptoms listed on the warning card given with each prescription, and urge patient to stop the drug and seek immediate medical attention if hypersensitivity is even suspected. Warn patient never to take this or any abacavir-containing drug in the future if the drug is stopped because of hypersensitivity.
- Warn patient to take abacavir and lamivudine exactly as prescribed and not to interrupt therapy for any reason other than hypersensitivity because restarting the drug may cause a serious hypersensitivity reaction. Notify the prescriber immediately if interruption of therapy is unavoidable.
- Inform patients with a history of hepatitis B that it may worsen after abacavir and lamivudine therapy stops. Stress the need to monitor hepatic function for at least several months after therapy stops to detect an exacerbation that could warrant anti–hepatitis B therapy.
- Tell patient that abacavir and lamivudine may cause fat accumulation or redistribution. Advise patient to notify prescriber about central obesity, buffalo hump, limb or facial thinness, breast enlargement, or other signs of cushingoid appearance.
- Inform patient that taking abacavir and lamivudine won't cure HIV infection and won't reduce the risk of transmitting HIV to others.

abacavir sulfate, lamivudine, and zidovudine
Trizivir

Class and Category
Chemical: Synthetic nucleoside analogues (abacavir, lamivudine, zidovudine)

Therapeutic: Antiretroviral (abacavir, lamivudine, zidovudine)
Pregnancy category: C

Indications and Dosages

▶ *To treat HIV-1 infection*

TABLETS

Adults and adolescents weighing 40 kg or more. 300 mg
abacavir, 150 mg lamivudine, and 300 mg of zidovudine
(1 tablet) b.i.d.

Mechanism of Action

Abacavir sulfate, lamivudine, and zidovudine are nucleoside analogues and
are converted intracellularly to their respective active metabolites: abacavir
to carbovir triphosphate, lamivudine to lamivudine triphosphate, and zidovudine to zidovudine triphosphate. These active metobolites inhibit the activity
of HIV-1 reverse transcriptase by becoming incorporated into viral DNA. Carbovir triphosphate also inhibits the activity of HIV-1 reverse transcriptase by
competing with the natural substrate, dGTP. These activities prevent the formation of a linkage essential for the viral DNA chain to elongate, thereby
stopping viral DNA growth.

Contraindications

Hypersensitivity to abacavir, lamivudine, zidovudine, or their
components

Interactions

DRUGS

abacavir

methadone: Possibly increased methadone clearance

lamivudine

interferon alfa, ribavirin: Possibly increased risk of toxicity, especially hepatic decompensation

trimethoprim and sulfamethoxazole: Possibly increased lamivudine
exposure

zalcitabine: Possibly inhibited intracellular phosphorylation, making both drugs ineffective

zidovudine

doxorubicin, ribavirin, stavudine: Increased risk of antagonistic relationship between zidovudine and doxorubicin, ribavirin, or stavudine

*ganciclovir, interferon-alfa, and other bone marrow suppressive or cyto-
toxic agents:* Possibly increased hematologic toxicity

Adverse Reactions

CNS: Depression, dizziness, fatigue, fever, headache, insomnia, malaise, neuropathy, paresthesia, peripheral neuropathy, seizures
CV: Cardiomyopathy, hypotension
EENT: Conjunctivitis, nasal congestion, oral mucous membrane pigmentation or ulceration, pharyngitis, stomatitis
ENDO: Gynecomastia, mild hyperglycemia
GI: Abdominal cramps or pain, anorexia, diarrhea, elevated liver function tests, exacerbation of hepatitis B after treatment, hepatic failure or steatosis, nausea, pancreatitis, splenomegaly, vomiting
GU: Renal failure
HEME: Anemia, aplastic anemia, lymphopenia, neutropenia, pure red cell aplasia
MS: Arthralgia, muscle weakness, musculoskeletal pain, myalgia, myopathy, myositis, rhabdomyolysis
RESP: Acute respiratory distress syndrome, cough, dyspnea, respiratory failure, wheezing
SKIN: Alopecia, chills, erythema multiforme, rash, Stevens-Johnson syndrome, toxic epidermal necrolysis, urticaria
Other: Anaphylaxis, fat redistribution, hypersensitivity reactions, immune reconstitution syndrome, increased CK, lactic acidosis, lymphadenopathy

Nursing Considerations

- Use cautiously in patients with bone marrow suppression evidenced by a granulocyte count less than 1,000 cells/mm^3 or hemoglobin less than 9.5 g/dl because zidovudine can cause bone marrow suppression. Monitor patient's blood counts closely, as ordered.
- Be aware that because abacavir, lamivudine, and zidovudine are available only in a fixed-dose combination, patients who need a reduced dosage of lamivudine or zidovudine (such as those with a creatinine clearance less than 50 ml/min/1.73 m^2 and those who have impaired hepatic function of any degree) can't receive this drug combination. Likewise, patients weighing less than 40 kg (88 lb) shouldn't receive this drug combination because dosage adjustments can't be made.
- **WARNING** Notify prescriber immediately at first sign or symptom of hypersensitivity, such as abdominal pain, cough, diarrhea, dyspnea, fatigue, fever, nausea, pharyngitis, rash, or vomiting. Expect to stop abacavir, lamivudine, and zidovudine. The drug should not be restarted after a hypersensitivity reaction resolves because more severe symptoms will recur

within hours and may be fatal. The prescriber should register the hypersensitivity reaction with the abacavir hypersensitivity reaction registry by calling 1-800-270-0425.

- Monitor patient for fatigue or pallor because neutropenia and severe anemia have occurred with zidovudine use, especially in patients with advanced HIV disease. Notify prescriber if present.
- Monitor patient closely for opportunistic infections because combination antiretroviral therapy may cause an inflammatory response with these infections that could lead to immune reconstitution syndrome, requiring additional therapy.
- Monitor patient's hepatic function closely, including results of hepatic function studies, as ordered, because lactic acidosis and severe hepatomegaly have occurred with the use of nucleoside analogues such as abacavir, lamivudine, and zidovudine. Patients at risk include women, obese patients, and patients who have had prolonged exposure to nucleosides. Notify prescriber and expect to stop the drug combination if patient develops any signs or symptoms that suggest lactic acidosis or hepatic dysfunction, such as a change in level of consciousness, fatigue, jaundice, nausea, or vomiting.
- Monitor patients receiving abacavir, lamivudine, and zidovudine closely for myopathy and myositis that may occur with prolonged use of zidovudine.
- Monitor patients who have both hepatitis B virus and HIV closely when the combination drug is discontinued because severe acute exacerbations of hepatitis B may occur up to several months after stopping the combination drug.

PATIENT TEACHING
- Caution patient to take abacavir, lamivudine, and zidovudine exactly as prescribed and not to stop and then restart therapy without consulting prescriber because severe hypersensitivity reactions can occur with re-introduction of the drug.
- Review signs and symptoms of hypersensitivity with patient, and instruct him to notify prescriber immediately if any occur, such as abdominal pain, cough, diarrhea, dyspnea, fatigue, fever, nausea, skin rash, sore throat, or vomiting.
- Alert patient that this drug combination may cause fat redistribution.
- Advise patient that abacavi, lamivudine, and zidovudine therapy doesn't HIV infection and doesn't reduce the risk of transmitting the virus to others.
- Instruct patient to avoid people with infections because this combination drug may increase his risk of infections.

• Remind patient to have his blood counts monitored, as prescribed, so that adverse effects of the combination drug can be
detected early.

amoxicillin trihydrate and clavulanate potassium

Augmentin, Augmentin ES, Augmentin XR, Clavulin (CAN)

Class and Category

Chemical: Aminopenicillin, beta-lactamase inhibitor
Therapeutic: Antibiotic
Pregnancy category: B

Indications and Dosages

▶ *To treat otitis media, sinusitis, skin and soft-tissue infections, and
UTI caused by susceptible strains of gram-positive and gram-negative
organisms*

ORAL SUSPENSION, TABLETS

Adults and children weighing 40 kg (88 lb) or more. 500 mg
every 12 hr or 250 mg every 8 hr.

Children age 12 wk and over weighing less than 40 kg.
25 mg/kg/day in divided doses every 12 hr or 20 mg/kg/day in
divided doses every 8 hr.

Children under age 12 wk. 30 mg/kg/day every 12 hr.

▶ *To treat community-acquired pneumonia or acute bacterial sinusitis
caused by beta-lactamase–producing pathogens and* Streptococcus
pneumoniae *with reduced susceptibility to penicillin*

E.R. TABLETS

Adults. 4,000 mg in two divided doses daily at start of meals for
7 to 10 days for community-acquired pneumonia or 10 days for
acute bacterial sinusitis.

▶ *To treat respiratory tract infections and severe otitis media and
sinusitis caused by susceptible strains of gram-positive and gram-negative
organisms*

CHEWABLE TABLETS, ORAL SUSPENSION, TABLETS

Adults and children weighing 40 kg or more. 875 mg every
12 hr or 500 mg every 8 hr.

Children age 12 wk and over weighing less than 40 kg.
45 mg/kg/day in divided doses every 12 hr or 40 mg/kg every
8 hr.

Children under age 12 wk. 30 mg/kg/day in divided doses
every 12 hr.

DOSAGE ADJUSTMENT For a glomerular filtration rate (GFR) of 10 to 30 ml/min, dosage reduced to 250 or 500 mg every 12 hr, depending on the severity of the infection. For a GFR less than 10 ml/min, dosage reduced to 250 to 500 mg every 24 hr, depending on the severity of the infection. For hemodialysis patients, dosage reduced to 250 or 500 mg every 24 hr with another dose during and at the end of dialysis.

▶ *To treat acute otitis media caused by beta-lactamase–producing strains of* Haemophilus influenzae, Moraxella catarrhalis, *and* S. pneumoniae *(including penicillin-resistant strains)*

EXTRA-STRENGTH ORAL SUSPENSION
Children. 90 mg/kg/day in divided doses b.i.d. for 10 days.

Mechanism of Action

Amoxicillin trihydrate kills bacteria by binding to and inactivating penicillin-binding proteins on the inner bacterial cell wall, weakening the cell wall and causing lysis.

Clavulanic acid inactivates bacterial beta-lactamase enzymes, thus protecting amoxicillin from degradation by these enzymes and making the drug effective against many bacteria normally resistant to amoxicillin.

Contraindications

History of amoxicillin and clavulanate–induced cholestatic jaundice or hepatic dysfunction; hypersensitivity to amoxicillin, clavulanate, penicillin, or their components; phenylketonuria (chewable tablets); severe renal impairment (E.R. tablets)

Interactions

DRUGS

allopurinol: Increased risk of rash
aminoglycosides: Inactivation of both drugs
chloramphenicol, erythromycins, sulfonamides, tetracyclines: Reduced bactericidal effect of amoxicillin
heparin, oral anticoagulants: Possibly increased risk of bleeding with large doses of amoxicillin and clavulanate potassium
methotrexate: Risk of methotrexate toxicity
oral contraceptives with estrogen: Possibly reduced effectiveness of contraceptive
probenecid: Increased amoxicillin effects

Adverse Reactions

CNS: Agitation, anxiety, behavioral changes, confusion, dizziness, drowsiness, headache, insomnia, reversible hyperactivity

EENT: Black "hairy" tongue, glossitis, mucocutaneous candidiasis, stomatitis
GI: Diarrhea, enterocolitis, gastritis, hemorrhagic pseudo-membranous colitis, indigestion, nausea, vomiting
GU: Hematuria, interstitial nephritis, vaginal candidiasis, vaginal mycosis
HEME: Agranulocytosis, anemia, eosinophilia, leukopenia, neutropenia, thrombocytopenia, thrombocytopenic purpura
SKIN: Erythema multiforme, exfoliative dermatitis, pruritus, rash, Stevens-Johnson syndrome, urticaria
Other: Allergic reaction, anaphylaxis, angioedema, serum sickness–like reaction (such as arthralgia, arthritis, fever, myalgia, rash, and urticaria)

Nursing Considerations

- Use amoxicillin and clavulanate cautiously in patients with hepatic impairment. Monitor hepatic and renal function and CBC, as ordered, in patients receiving prolonged therapy. Also use cautiously in patients who are breast-feeding or elderly.
- For children under age 12 weeks, expect to use 125-mg amoxicillin/5-ml clavulanate suspension because experience with 200-mg/5-ml suspension is limited.
- WARNING If allergic reaction occurs, stop drug immediately. Expect to give antihistamine and I.V. corticosteroid. If anaphylaxis occurs, expect to manage airway and give epinephrine, oxygen, and I.V. corticosteroid.
- Monitor patient closely for diarrhea, which may indicate pseudomembranous colitis. If diarrhea occurs, notify prescriber and expect to withhold drug. Expect to treat pseudomembranous colitis with fluids, electrolytes, protein, and an antibiotic effective against *Clostridium difficile.*
- Be aware that Augmentin 250-mg regular tablets should not be substituted for chewable or E.R. tablets because they contain different amounts of clavulanic acid.
- For a child weighing less than 40 kg (88 lb), expect to give 250-mg chewable tablets because the ratio of amoxicillin to clavulanic acid differs from Augmentin 250-mg regular tablets.

PATIENT TEACHING
- Tell patient to take amoxicillin and clavulanate with food to reduce GI upset.
- Instruct patient to refrigerate reconstituted suspension.
- Tell patient to chew or crush chewable tablets and not to swallow them whole.

- Teach patient to recognize and report adverse reactions and to seek emergency care if signs of anaphylaxis occur.
- Tell patient to notify prescriber if infection continues or worsens after 72 hours.
- Urge patient to tell prescriber about diarrhea that's severe or lasts longer than 3 days. Remind patient that watery or bloody stools may occur 2 or more months after amoxicillin and clavulanate therapy, may be serious, and may need prompt treatment.

ampicillin sodium and sulbactam sodium
Unasyn

Class and Category
Chemical: Aminopenicillin, beta-lactamase inhibitor
Therapeutic: Antibiotic
Pregnancy category: B

Indications and Dosages
▶ *To treat skin and soft-tissue infections caused by beta-lactamase–producing strains of* Staphylococcus aureus, Escherichia coli, Klebsiella *species (including* K. pneumoniae*)*, Proteus mirabilis, Bacteroides fragilis, Enterobacter species, *and* Acinetobacter calcoaceticus; *intra-abdominal infections caused by beta-lactamase–producing strains of* E. coli, Klebsiella *species (including* K. pneumoniae*)*, Bacteroides *species (including* B. fragilis*)*, *and* Enterobacter *species; gynecologic infections caused by beta-lactamase–producing strains of* E. coli *and* Bacteroides *species (including* B. fragilis*)*
I.V. INFUSION, I.M. INJECTION
Adults and children age 12 and over weighing 40 kg (88 lb) or more. 1.5 (1 gram ampicillin and 0.5 grams sulbactam) to 3 grams (2 grams ampicillin and 1 gram sulbactam) every 6 hr, to a maximum of 8 grams ampicillin and 4 grams sulbactam daily.
Children age 1 and over weighing less than 40 kg.
300 mg/kg (200 mg of ampicillin and 100 mg of sulbactam) daily in divided doses every 6 hr.
DOSAGE ADJUSTMENT Dosing frequency reduced to every 6 to 8 hr for patients with creatinine clearance of 30 ml/min/ 1.73 m^2 or more. Dosing frequency reduced to every 12 hr for patients with creatinine clearance of 15 to 29 ml/min/1.73 m^2.

Frequency reduced to 1.5 to 3 grams every 24 hr for patients with creatinine clearance of 5 to 14 ml/min/1.73 m².

Mechanism of Action

Ampicillin inhibits bacterial cell wall synthesis. The rigid, cross-linked cell wall is assembled in several steps. The drug exerts its effects on susceptible bacteria in the final stage of the cross-linking process by binding with and inactivating penicillin-binding proteins (enzymes responsible for linking the cell wall strands). This action causes bacterial cell lysis and death. When ampicillin is given alone, beta-lactamases may degrade it, making it ineffective. When it's combined with sulbactam, degradation can't occur. So sulbactam extends ampicillin's bactericidal effects to beta-lactamase–producing bacteria.

Incompatibilities

Don't mix ampicillin sodium and sulbactam sodium with any aminoglycoside in the same I.V. bag, bottle, or tubing; otherwise, both drugs will be inactivated. If patient must receive both drugs, give them in separate sites at least 1 hour apart.

Contraindications

Hypersensitivity to ampicillin sodium, sulbactam sodium, their components, or any penicillin

Interactions

DRUGS

allopurinol: Increased risk of rash, particularly in hyperuricemic patient

aminoglycosides: Possibly inactivated action of aminoglycoside and ampicillin sodium and sulbactam sodium when given together

heparin, oral anticoagulants: Increased risk of bleeding

oral contraceptives: Possibly breakthrough bleeding and reduced contraceptive effectiveness

probenecid: Possibly increased serum ampicillin level and ampicillin toxicity

tetracyclines: Possibly impaired action of ampicillin sodium and sulbactam sodium

Adverse Reactions

CNS: Chills, fatigue, fever, headache, malaise
CV: Chest pain, edema, thrombophlebitis
EENT: Black "hairy" tongue, epistaxis, glossitis, laryngeal stridor, mucocutaneous candidiasis, stomatitis, throat tightness

GI: Abdominal distention, diarrhea, enterocolitis, flatulence, gastritis, nausea, pseudomembranous colitis, vomiting
GU: Dysuria, urine retention, vaginal candidiasis
HEME: Agranulocytosis, anemia, eosinophilia, leukopenia, thrombocytopenia, thrombocytopenic purpura
SKIN: Erythema multiforme; erythematous, mildly pruritic maculopapular rash or other rash; exfoliative dermatitis; mucosal bleeding; pruritus; urticaria
Other: Anaphylaxis, facial edema, injection site pain

Nursing Considerations

• Avoid giving ampicillin sodium and sulbactam sodium to patients with mononucleosis because of the increased risk of rash.
• Administer I.V. dose by slow injection over 10 to 15 minutes or by infusion over 15 to 30 minutes in greater dilutions with 50 to 100 ml of a compatible diluent.
• Reconstitute drug for I.M. use with sterile water for injection or 0.5% or 2% lidocaine hydrochloride injection. For a 1.5-g vial, add 3.2 ml of diluent; for a 3-g vial, add 6.4 ml of diluent. Let solution stand until foaming dissipates. Inspect vial before withdrawing drug to ensure dissolution. After reconstituting solution, inject it within 1 hour.
• Administer by deep I.M. injection.
• Monitor patient closely for anaphylaxis, which may be life-threatening. Patients at greatest risk are those with a history of hypersensitivity to penicillin, multiple allergies, hypersensitivity to cephalosporins, or a history of asthma, hay fever, or urticaria.
• **WARNING** If drug triggers an anaphylactic reaction, stop giving drug, notify prescriber immediately, and provide appropriate therapy. Anaphylaxis requires immediate treatment with epinephrine as well as airway management and administration of oxygen and I.V. corticosteroids, as needed.
• Monitor patient closely for diarrhea, which may herald pseudomembranous colitis. If diarrhea occurs, notify prescriber. If pseudomembranous colitis is diagnosed, expect to stop treatment and, possibly, administer fluids, electrolytes, protein, and antibiotic effective against *Clostridium difficile.*

PATIENT TEACHING
• Warn patient that I.M. injection of drug is likely to cause discomfort.
• Tell patient to report sudden or unusual symptoms immediately.
• Urge patient to tell prescriber about diarrhea that's severe or

lasts longer than 3 days. Remind patient that watery or bloody stools may occur 2 or more months after amoxicillin and clavulanate therapy, may be serious, and may need prompt treatment.

atovaquone and proguanil hydrochloride

Malarone

Class and Category

Chemical: Naphthalenedione (atovaquone), biguanide (proguanil)
Therapeutic: Antimalarial (atovaquone, proguanil)
Pregnancy category: C

Indications and Dosages

▶ *To treat acute, uncomplicated* Plasmodium falciparum *malaria when amodiaquine, chloroquine, halofantrine, or mefloquine resistance is suspected*

TABLETS, PEDIATRIC TABLETS

Adults and children weighing more than 40 kg (88 lb).
1 gram atovaquone and 400 mg proguanil (4 tablets) daily for 3 consecutive days.

Children weighing 31 to 40 kg (68 to 88 lb). 750 mg atovaquone and 300 mg proguanil (3 tablets) daily for 3 consecutive days.

Children weighing 21 to 30 kg (46 to 66 lb). 500 mg atovaquone and 200 mg proguanil (2 tablets) daily for 3 consecutive days.

Children weighing 11 to 20 kg (24 to 44 lb). 250 mg atovaquone and 100 mg proguanil (4 tablets) daily for 3 consecutive days.

Children weighing 9 to 10 kg (20 to 22 lb). 187.5 mg atovaquone and 75 mg proguanil (3 pediatric tablets) daily for 3 consecutive days.

Children weighing 5 to 8 kg (11 to 18 lb). 125 mg atovaquone and 50 mg proguanil (2 pediatric tablets) daily for 3 consecutive days.

▶ *To prevent P.* falciparum *malaria when patient is traveling to areas where chloroquine-resistant P.* falciparum *malaria has been reported*

TABLETS, PEDIATRIC TABLETS

Adults and children weighing more than 40 kg. 250 mg

atovaquone and 100 mg proguanil (1 tablet) daily starting 1 to 2 days before arrival in endemic area and continuing until 7 days after departure from endemic area.

Children weighing 31 to 40 kg. 187.5 mg atovaquone and 75 mg proguanil (3 pediatric tablets) daily starting 1 to 2 days before arrival in endemic area and continuing until 7 days after departure from endemic area.

Children weighing 21 to 30 kg. 125 mg atovaquone and 50 mg proguanil (2 pediatric tablets) daily starting 1 to 2 days before arrival in endemic area and continuing until 7 days after departure from endemic area.

Children weighing 11 to 20 kg. 62.5 mg atovaquone and 25 mg proguanil (1 tablet) daily starting 1 to 2 days before arrival in endemic area and continuing until 7 days after departure.

Mechanism of Action

Atovaquone selectively inhibits mitochrondial electron transport in the malarial parasite, which interferes with synthesis of pyrimidines needed for nucleic acid replication.

Proguanil mainly exerts its effects by inhibiting the enzyme dihydrofolate reductase, which disrupts deoxythymidylate synthesis in the malarial parasite. This action also interferes with synthesis of pyrimidines needed for nucleic acid replication, which prevents the malarial parasite from replicating.

Contraindications

Hypersensitivity to atovaquone, proguanil, or their components; severe renal impairment (creatinine clearance less than 30 ml/min/1.73 m^2).

Interactions

DRUGS

atovaquone

metoclopramide, rifabutin, rifampin, tetracycline: Reduced plasma levels of atovaquone

proguanil

oral coumarin-based anticoagulants, such as warfarin: Possibly potentiated anticoagulant effect

Adverse Reactions

CNS: Anxiety, asthenia, depression, dizziness, fever, headache, insomnia, vivid dreams

EENT: Oral ulcers, visual disturbances

GI: Abdominal pain, anorexia, diarrhea, dyspepsia, elevated liver enzyme levels, gastritis, hepatic failure, hepatitis, nausea, vomiting

HEME: Anemia, neutropenia, pancytopenia

MS: Back pain, myalgia

RESP: Cough, upper respiratory infection

SKIN: Erythema multiforme, photosensitivity, pruritus, rash, Stevens-Johnson syndrome, urticaria

Other: Anaphylaxis, angioedema, flu syndrome

Nursing Considerations

- Use cautiously in elderly patients and in patients with hepatic or renal impairment.
- Determine if patient diagnosed with recrudescent malaria has been treated in the past with a combination of atovaquone and proguanil. If so, alert prescriber because atovaquone and proguanil may not be effective in this situation.
- Monitor patient's renal and hepatic functions closely. Although rare, hepatitis and hepatic failure may occur with atovaquone and proguanil use.

PATIENT TEACHING

- Instruct patient to take atovaquone and proguanil combination at the same time every day with food or a milky drink because the rate and extent of absorption is greater than when the drug is taken on an empty stomach.
- Inform patient that drug may be crushed and mixed with condensed milk just before taking if he can't swallow them whole.
- Tell patient to notify prescriber if vomiting occurs because an antiemetic may be needed. In addition, tell patient to repeat the dose if vomiting occurs within 1 hour of ingesting dose.
- Advise patient to report any adverse effects, especially if severe or prolonged, to prescriber.

efavirenz, emtricitabine, and tenofovir disoproxil fumarate

Atripla

Class and Category

Chemical: Non-nucleoside reverse transcriptase inhibitor (efavirenz), synthetic nucleoside analog of cytidine (emtricitabine), acyclic nucleotide phosphonate analog of adenosine 5′-monophosphate (tenofovir)

Therapeutic: Antiretroviral (efavirenz, emtricitabine, tenofovir)
Pregnancy category: D

Indications and Dosages

▶ *To treat HIV-1 infection*

TABLETS

Adults. 600 mg efavirenz, 200 mg emtricitabine, and 300 mg
tenofovir (1 tablet) once daily, on an empty stomach, alone or
with other antiretrovirals.

Mechanism of Action

Efavirenz binds to reverse transcriptase, blocking RNA- and DNA-dependent
DNA polymerase actions needed for HIV-1 replication. This drug doesn't
need intracellular phosphrylation for its antiviral activity.

Emtricitabine and tenofovir disoproxil are phosphorylated by cellular enzymes to form emtricitabine 5'-triphosphate and tenofovir diphosphate respectively. These substances then compete with the natural substrate deoxycytidine 5'-triphosphate in the HIV-1 virus, becoming a part of the DNA. This
terminates the DNA chain, inhibiting viral replication.

Contraindications

Concurrent therapy with bepridil, cisapride, dihydroergotamine,
ergonovine, ergotamine, methylergonovine, midazolam, pimozide,
St. John's wort, triazolam, or voriconazole; hypersensitivity to
efavirenz, emtricitabine, tenofovir or any of their components;
moderate to severe renal impairment (creatinine clearance less
than 50 ml/min)

Interactions

DRUGS

efavirenz and tenofovir

atazanavir: Decreased effectiveness of atazanavir

emtricitabine and tenofovir

*nephrotoxic drugs such as acyclovir, adefovir dipivoxil, cidofovir, ganci-
clovir, valacyclovir, and valganciclovir; renal competitors for active tubular
secretion:* Increased serum levels of emtricitabine, tenofovir, and
other drugs eliminated via the kidneys

efavirenz

astemizole, bepridil, cisapride, pimozide: Increased risk of cardiac arrhythmias

ergot derivatives: Increased risk for acute ergot toxicity

amprenavir, carbamazepine, calcium channel blockers, clarithromycin, fosamprenavir, HMG-CoA reductase inhibitors, indinavir, itraconazole, ketoconazole, lopinavir, phenytoin, phenobarbital, rifabutin, saquinavir, sertraline: Decreased effectiveness of these drugs

carbamazepine, phenytoin, phenobarbital, rifampin, rifabutin, St. John's wort: Decreased effectiveness of efavirenz

methadone: Decreased plasma methadone level with signs of opioid withdrawal

midazolam, triazolam: Increased risk of prolonged or increased sedation or respiratory depression

ritonavir: Increased risk of dizziness, elevated liver enzyme levels, nausea, and paresthesia

voriconazole: Decreased voriconazole effectiveness; increased risk of efavirenz-induced adverse reactions

warfarin: Altered warfarin plasma level

emtricitabine

lamivudine: Increased emtricitabine effect

tenofovir

atazanavir, lopinavir, ritonavir: Increased serum tenofovir level, resulting in increased risk of adverse effects

didanosine: Increased serum didanosine level, resulting in increased risk of adverse effects

Adverse Reactions

CNS: Abnormal dreams or coordination, aggression, agitation, asthenia, ataxia, balance disturbances, delusions, depression, dizziness, emotional instability, fever, headache, hypoesthesia, insomnia, mania, neurosis, neuropathy, palpitations, paresthesia, paranoia, peripheral neuritis, psychosis, seizures, suicidal thoughts, tremor

CV: Chest pain, elevated cholesterol and triglyceride levels

EENT: Abnormal vision, rhinitis, tinnitus

ENDO: Gynecomastia, hyperglycemia, hypoglycemia, redistribution of body fat

GI: Abdominal pain, anorexia, constipation, diarrhea, dyspepsia, elevated bilirubin or liver or pancreatic enzyme levels, flatulence, hepatic failure, hepatitis B exacerbation, malabsorption, nausea, pancreatitis, vomiting

GU: Acute renal failure, acute tubular necrosis, Fanconi syndrome, interstitial nephritis, nephrogenic diabetes insipidus, polyuria, proteinuria, renal insufficiency

HEME: Decreased neutrophil count

MS: Arthralgia, back pain, decreased bone density, elevated creatine kinase level, myalgia, myopathy, osteomalacia

RESP: Cough, dyspnea, pneumonia

SKIN: Diaphoresis, erythema multiforme, flushing, hyperpigmentation on palms or soles, nail abnormalities, photoallergic dermatitis, pruritus, rash, skin discoloration, Stevens-Johnson syndrome, urticaria

Other: Allergic reaction, hypophosphatemia, immune reconstitution syndrome, lactic acidosis, weight loss

Nursing Considerations

- Be aware that because dosage adjustments can't be made to efavirenz, emtricitabine, and tenofovir combination, the drug shouldn't be given to a patient with a creatinine clearance less than 50 ml/min or a patient undergoing hemodialysis.
- Test patient for hepatitis B virus, as ordered, before starting efavirenz, emtricitabine, and tenofovir therapy. Expect to monitor liver function for several months after therapy stops because hepatitis B may worsen.
- Use cautiously in patients with a history of seizures because the drug may increase seizure activity.
- Give drug at bedtime if patient develops adverse neurologic reactions. These symptoms usually develop within 1 to 2 days after therapy starts and resolve in 2 to 4 weeks.
- Monitor patient's liver function throughout therapy, as ordered, and assess patient for evidence of lactic acidosis and liver dysfunction, especially in women, obese patients, and patients with a history of prolonged nucleoside exposure.
- Monitor patient's blood urea nitrogen and serum creatinine levels, as ordered, because drug may cause renal impairment.
- Monitor patient closely for changes in behavior because serious adverse psychiatric effects may occur with this combination drug. If changes develop, notify prescriber immediately.
- Assess patient for a rash. If present, notify prescriber and expect drug to be discontinued.
- Monitor patient closely for opportunistic infections because combination antiretroviral therapy may cause an inflammatory response to these infections and possible immune reconstitution syndrome, which requires additional therapy.
- Bone monitoring should be done in a patient with a history of pathologic bone fracture or a risk for osteopenia. Expect to give supplemental calcium and vitamin D, as ordered.

PATIENT TEACHING

- Inform patients with a history of hepatitis B that it may worsen after efavirenz, emtricitabine, and tenofovir therapy stops.

Stress the need to check hepatic function for at least several months after drug therapy stops to detect an exacerbation that may warrant anti–hepatitis B therapy.

• Tell patient that this combination drug may cause fat accumulation or redistribution. Advise him to notify prescriber about central obesity, buffalo hump, limb or facial thinness, breast enlargement, or other signs of cushingoid appearance.

• Inform patient that efavirenz, emtricitabine, and tenofovir therapy doesn't cure HIV infection and doesn't reduce the risk of transmitting HIV to others.

• For women of childbearing age, stress the need to notify the prescriber immediately about suspected pregnancy.

• Caution patient to consult prescriber before stopping therapy.

emtricitabine and tenofovir disoproxil fumarate
Truvada

Class and Category
Chemical: Synthetic nucleoside analog of cytidine (emtricitabine), acyclic nucleoside phosphonate analog of adenosine 5'-monophosphate (tenofovir)
Therapeutic: Antiretroviral (emtricitabine, tenofovir)
Pregnancy category: B

Indications and Dosages
▶ *To treat HIV-1 infection*
TABLETS
Adults. 200 mg emtricitabine and 300 mg tenofovir (1 tablet) daily with other antiretrovirals.
DOSAGE ADJUSTMENT For patients with a creatinine clearance between 30 and 49 ml/min/1.73 m², dosage interval increased to every 48 hours.

Mechanism of Action
Emtricitabine and tenofovir disoproxil are phosphorylated by cellular enzymes to form emtricitabine 5'-triphosphate and tenofovir diphosphatete respectively. These substances then compete with the natural substrate deoxycytidine 5'-triphosphate in the HIV-1 virus becoming a part of the DNA. This terminates the DNA chain resulting in viral death.

Contraindications

Concurrent or recent therapy with a nephrotoxic drug; hypersensitivity to emtricitabine, tenofovir, or any of their components; severe renal impairment (creatinine clearance less than 30 ml/min/1.73 m^2) including in patients receiving hemodialysis

Interactions

DRUGS

emtricitabine and tenofovir

nephrotoxic drugs such as acyclovir, adefovir dipivoxil, cidofovir, ganciclovir, valacyclovir, valganciclovir; renal competitors for active tubular secretion: Increased serum levels of emtricitabine, tenofovir, and other drugs eliminated via the kidneys

emtricitabine

lamivudine: Increased emtricitabine effect

tenofovir

atazanavir, lopinavir and ritonavir: Increased serum tenofovir level, resulting in increased risk of adverse effects

didanosine: Increased serum didanosine level, resulting in increased risk of adverse effects; suppression of CD4 cell counts

Adverse Reactions

CNS: Abnormal dreams, anxiety, asthenia, depression, dizziness, fever, headache, insomnia, neuropathy, paresthesia, peripheral neuritis, somnolence

CV: Chest pain, elevated cholesterol and triglyceride levels

EENT: Nasopharyngitis, rhinitis, sinusitis

ENDO: Hyperglycemia, hypoglycemia

GI: Abdominal pain, anorexia, diarrhea, dyspepsia, elevated bilirubin or liver or pancreatic enzymes, flatulence, hepatitis, nausea, pancreatitis, vomiting

GU: Fanconi syndrome, interstitial nephritis, nephrogenic diabetes insipidus, proximal renal tubulopathy, renal insufficiency or failure

HEME: Decreased neurtophils

MS: Arthralgia, back pain, decreased bone density, elevated creatine kinase, myalgia, osteomalacia

RESP: Cough, dyspnea, pneumonia

SKIN: Diaphoresis, hyperpigmentation on palms or soles, pruritus, rash, urticaria

Other: Allergic reaction, hypophosphatemia, immune reconstitution syndrome, lactic acidosis, weight loss

Nursing Considerations

- Be aware that because dosage adjustments can't be made to emtricitabine and tenofovir combination, the drug shouldn't be given to a patient with a creatinine clearance less than 30 ml/min/1.73 m² or a patient undergoing hemodialysis. For patients with a creatinine clearance of 30 ml/min/1.73 m² or higher, monitor creatinine and phosphorus levels routinely throughout therapy, and expect adjustments to the dosing interval.
- Test patient for the presence of hepatitis B virus, as ordered, before starting emtricitabine and tenofovir therapy. Expect to monitor the patient's liver function for several months after therapy stops because hepatitis B may worsen after emtricitabine and tenofovir are stopped.
- Monitor patient's liver function throughout therapy, as ordered, and assess patient for evidence of lactic acidosis and liver dysfunction that may occur as a result of emtricitabine and tenofovir therapy, especially in women, obese patients, and patients with a history of prolonged nucleoside exposure.
- Bone monitoring should be done in a patient with a history of pathologic bone fracture or who is at risk for osteopenia. Expect to give supplemental calcium and vitamin D, as ordered.
- Monitor patient closely for opportunistic infection because, if such infection occurs, combination antiretroviral therapy may cause an inflammatory response that could lead to immune reconstitution syndrome requiring additional therapy.

PATIENT TEACHING

- Inform patients with a history of hepatitis B that it may worsen after emtricitabine and tenofovir therapy stops. Stress the need to check hepatic function for at least several months after drug therapy stops to detect an exacerbation that may warrant anti–hepatitis B therapy.
- Tell patient that this combination drug may cause fat accumulation or redistribution. Advise him to notify prescriber about central obesity, buffalo hump, limb or facial thinness, breast enlargement, or other signs of cushingoid appearance.
- Inform patient that drug doesn't cure HIV infection and doesn't reduce trhe risk of transmitting HIV to others.

imipenem and cilastatin sodium

Primaxin (CAN), Primaxin ADD-Vantage, Primaxin IM, Primaxin IV

Class and Category
Chemical: Thienamycin derivative (imipenem), heptenoic acid derivative (cilastatin sodium)
Therapeutic: Antibiotic
Pregnancy category: C

Indications and Dosages
▶ *To treat severe or life-threatening bacterial infections (including endocarditis, pneumonia, and septicemia as well as bone, joint, intra-abdominal, skin, and soft-tissue infections) caused by gram-positive anaerobic organisms, such as most staphylococci and streptococci and some enterococci (including* Enterococcus faecalis*); most strains of* Enterobacteriaceae *(including* Citrobacter *species,* Enterobacter *species,* Escherichia coli, Klebsiella *species,* Morganella morganii, Proteus mirabilis, Providencia stuartii, *and* Serratia marcescens*); and many gram-negative aerobic and anaerobic species (including* Bacteroides *species,* Campylobacter *species,* Clostridium *species,* Haemophilus influenzae, Legionella *species,* Neisseria gonorrhoeae, *and* Pseudomonas aeruginosa)*

I.V. INFUSION (DOSAGES BASED ON IMIPENEM CONTENT)
Adults and adolescents. 500 mg every 6 hr to 1,000 mg every 6 to 8 hr. *Maximum:* the lower of 50 mg/kg or 4 grams daily.
Children age 3 months and over. 15 to 25 mg/kg every 6 hr. *Maximum:* 2,000 to 4,000 mg daily.
Infants ages 4 weeks to 3 months weighing 1,500 grams (3 lb, 3 oz) or more. 25 mg/kg every 6 hr. *Maximum:* 2,000 to 4,000 mg daily.
Neonates ages 1 to 4 weeks weighing 1,500 grams or more. 25 mg/kg every 8 hr. *Maximum:* 2,000 to 4,000 mg daily.
Neonates under age 1 week weighing 1,500 grams or more. 25 mg/kg every 12 hr. *Maximum:* 2,000 to 4,000 mg daily.
▶ *To treat moderate infections caused by the organisms listed above*
I.V. INFUSION (DOSAGES BASED ON IMIPENEM CONTENT)
Adults and adolescents. 500 mg every 6 to 8 hr up to 1,000 mg every 8 hr. *Maximum:* 50 mg/kg or 4 grams daily, whichever is lower.
Children age 3 months and over. 15 to 25 mg/kg every 6 hr. *Maximum:* 2,000 to 4,000 mg daily.
Infants ages 4 weeks to 3 months weighing 1,500 grams or more. 25 mg/kg every 6 hr. *Maximum:* 2,000 to 4,000 mg daily.
Neonates ages 1 to 4 weeks weighing 1,500 grams or more. 25 mg/kg every 8 hr. *Maximum:* 2,000 to 4,000 mg daily.

Neonates under age 1 week weighing 1,500 grams or more. 25 mg/kg every 12 hr. *Maximum:* 2,000 to 4,000 mg daily.

I.M. INJECTION (DOSAGES BASED ON IMIPENEM CONTENT)

Adults and adolescents. 500 to 750 mg every 12 hr. *Maximum:* 1,500 mg daily.

Children. 10 to 15 mg/kg every 6 hr.

▶ *To treat mild infections caused by the organisms listed above*

I.V. INFUSION (DOSAGES BASED ON IMIPENEM CONTENT)

Adults and adolescents. 250 to 500 mg every 6 hr. *Maximum:* 50 mg/kg or 4 grams daily, whichever is lower.

Children age 3 months and over. 15 to 25 mg/kg every 6 hr. *Maximum:* 2,000 mg (for fully susceptible organisms) to 4,000 mg (for moderately susceptible organisms) daily.

Infants ages 4 weeks to 3 months weighing 1,500 grams or more. 25 mg/kg every 6 hr. *Maximum:* 2,000 to 4,000 mg daily.

Neonates ages 1 to 4 weeks weighing 1,500 grams or more. 25 mg/kg every 8 hr. *Maximum:* 2,000 to 4,000 mg daily.

Neonates under age 1 week weighing 1,500 grams or more. 25 mg/kg every 12 hr. *Maximum:* 2,000 to 4,000 mg daily.

I.M. INJECTION (DOSAGES BASED ON IMIPENEM CONTENT)

Adults and adolescents. 500 to 750 mg every 12 hr. *Maximum:* 1,500 mg daily.

Children. 10 to 15 mg/kg every 6 hr.

▶ *To treat uncomplicated UTI caused by the organisms listed above*

I.V. INFUSION (DOSAGES BASED ON IMIPENEM CONTENT)

Adults and adolescents. 250 mg every 6 hr. *Maximum:* 50 mg/kg or 4 grams daily, whichever is lower.

▶ *To treat complicated UTI caused by the organisms listed above*

I.V. INFUSION (DOSAGES BASED ON IMIPENEM CONTENT)

Adults and adolescents. 500 mg every 6 hr. *Maximum:* 50 mg/kg or 4 grams daily, whichever is lower.

DOSAGE ADJUSTMENT Dosage reduced based on creatinine clearance for patients with impaired renal function.

Mechanism of Action

During bacterial cell wall synthesis, imipenem selectively binds to penicillin-binding proteins responsible for cell wall formation. This action causes bacterial cells to rapidly lyse and die.

Cilastatin sodium inhibits imipenem's breakdown in the kidneys, thus maintaining a high imipenem level in the urinary tract.

Incompatibilities
Don't give imipenem and cilastatin through the same I.V. line as beta-lactam antibiotics or aminoglycosides.

Contraindications
Hypersensitivity to imipenem, its components, other beta-lactam antibiotics, or amide-type local anesthetics (I.M.); meningitis (I.V.); severe heart block or shock (I.M.)

Interactions
DRUGS

cyclosporine: Increased adverse CNS effects of both drugs
ganciclovir: Increased risk of seizures
probenecid: Slightly increased blood level and half-life of imipenem
valproic acid: Increased risk of loss of seizure control

Adverse Reactions
CNS: Confusion, dizziness, fever, seizures, somnolence, tremor, weakness
CV: Hypotension
EENT: Oral candidiasis
GI: Diarrhea, hepatic failure, hepatitis, nausea, pseudomembranous colitis, vomiting
RESP: Wheezing
SKIN: Diaphoresis, pruritus, rash, urticaria
Other: Anaphylaxis, injection site thrombophlebitis

Nursing Considerations
- Obtain body fluid and tissue specimens for culture and sensitivity testing, as ordered, before giving first dose of imipenem and cilastatin. Expect to start drug before test results are available.
- For I.V. administration, add about 10 ml of diluent to each 250- or 500-mg vial and shake well. Transfer this reconstituted drug to at least 100 ml of prescribed I.V. solution. After the transfer, add another 10 ml of diluent to each vial, shake, and then transfer solution to infusion container. Shake infusion container until clear. To reconstitute piggyback bottles, add 100 ml of diluent to each 250- or 500-mg infusion bottle, and shake well.
- Give reconstituted drug within 4 to 10 hours, depending on diluent used (24 to 48 hours if refrigerated). Color may range from clear to yellow; don't give solution that contains particles.
- Infuse 500-mg or smaller dose over 20 to 30 minutes and 750- to 1,000-mg dose over 40 to 60 minutes.
- Inject I.M. form into a large muscle mass.
- Expect increased risk of imipenem-induced seizures in patients

with brain lesions, head trauma, or history of CNS disorders
and in those receiving more than 2 grams of drug daily.
- Assess patient for signs and symptoms of allergic reaction and
bacterial or fungal superinfection.
- Monitor patient closely for diarrhea, which may indicate
pseudomembranous colitis. If diarrhea occurs, notify prescriber
and expect to withhold drug. Expect to treat pseudomembranous colitis with fluids, electrolytes, protein, and an antibiotic
effective against *Clostridium difficile.*

PATIENT TEACHING
- Inform patient that imipenem and cilastatin must be given by
infusion or injection.
- Instruct patient to report discomfort at I.V. insertion site.
- Advise patient to report itching, signs of superinfection (such as
fever and sore mouth), and hives.
- Urge patient to notify prescriber about diarrhea that's severe or
lasts longer than 3 days. Remind patient that watery or bloody
stools may occur 2 months or more after imipenem and cilastatin therapy and can be serious, requiring prompt treatment.

lamivudine and zidovudine
Combivir

Class and Category
Chemical: Synthetic nucleoside analogues (lamivudine, zidovu-
dine)
Therapeutic: Antiretroviral (lamivudine, zidovudine)
Pregnancy category: C

Indications and Dosages
▶ *To treat HIV infection with other antiretrovirals*
TABLETS
Adults. 150 mg lamivudine and 300 mg zidovudine (1 tablet)
b.i.d.

Mechanism of Action
Lamivudine and zidovudine as nucleoside analogues are converted intracellularly to their respective active metabolites: lamivudine to lamivudine triphosphate and zidovudine to zidovudine triphosphate. These active metobolites
inhibit the activity of HIV-1 reverse transcriptase by becoming incorporated
into viral DNA. Once incorporated, they prevent formation of a linkage essential for the viral DNA chain to elongate, thereby stopping viral DNA growth.

Contraindications

Hepatic impairment; hypersensitivity to lamivudine, zidovudine or any of their components

Interactions

DRUGS

lamivudine

interferon alfa, ribavirin: Possibly increased risk of toxicity, especially hepatic decompensation

trimethoprim/sulfamethoxazole: Possibly increased lamivudine exposure

zalcitabine: Possibly inhibited intracellular phosphorylation of each other, making both drugs ineffective

zidovudine

doxorubicin, ribavirin, stavudine: Increased risk of antagonistic relationship between zidovudine and doxorubicin, ribavirin, or stavudine

ganciclovir, interferon-alfa, and other bone marrow suppressive or cytotoxic agent: Possibly increased hematologic toxicity

Adverse Reactions

CNS: Depression, dizziness, fatigue, fever, headache, insomnia, malaise, neuropathy, paresthesia, peripheral neuropathy, seizures, weakness

CV: Cardiomyopathy, hypotension, vasculitis

EENT: Conjunctivitis, nasal congestion, oral mucous membrane pigmentation or ulcerations, pharyngitis, stomatitis

ENDO: Gynecomastia, mild hyperglycemia

GI: Abdominal cramps or pain, anorexia, diarrhea, dyspepsia, elevated liver function tests, exacerbation of hepatitis B after treatment, hepatic failure or steatosis, nausea, pancreatitis, splenomegaly, vomiting

GU: Renal failure

HEME: Anemia, aplastic anemia, lymphopenia, neutropenia, pure red cell aplasia

MS: Arthralgia, muscle weakness, musculoskeletal pain, myalgia, myopathy, myositis, rhabdomyolysis

RESP: Acute respiratory distress syndrome, cough, dyspnea, respiratory failure, wheezing

SKIN: Alopecia, chills, erythema multiforme, rash, Stevens-Johnson syndrome, toxic epidermal necrolysis, urticaria

Other: Anaphylaxis, fat redistribution, hypersensitivity reactions, immune reconstitution syndrome, increased creatine phosphokinase, lactic acidosis, lymphadenopathy

Nursing Considerations

- Use cautiously in patients with bone marrow suppression evidenced by a granulocyte count less than 1,000 cells/mm^3 or hemoglobin less than 9.5 g/dl because zidovudine can cause bone marrow suppression. Monitor patient's blood counts closely, as ordered.
- Be aware that because lamivudine and zidovudine are available only in a fixed-dose combination, patients who need a reduced dosage of either one (such as those with a creatinine clearance less than 50 ml/min/1.73 m^2 and those who have impaired hepatic function of any degree) can't receive this drug combination. Likewise, patients weighing less than 40 kg (88 lb) shouldn't receive this combination because dosage adjustments can't be made.
- Monitor patient for fatigue or pallor because neutropenia and severe anemia may occur with zidovudine use, especially in patients with advanced HIV disease. Notify prescriber if present.
- Monitor patient's hepatic function studies, as ordered, because lactic acidosis and severe hepatomegaly have occurred with nucleoside analogues such as lamivudine and zidovudine. Those at risk include women, obese patients, and patients who have had prolonged exposure to nucleosides. Notify prescriber and expect to stop the drug combination if patient develops any signs or symptoms that suggest lactic acidosis or hepatic dysfunction, such as a change in level of consciousness, fatigue, jaundice, nausea, or vomiting.
- Monitor patients receiving this combination closely for myopathy and myositis, which may occur with prolonged use of zidovudine.
- Monitor patients infected with hepatitis B virus and HIV closely when lamivudine and zidovudine combination is stopped because severe exacerbations of hepatitis B may occur up to several months after therapy stops.
- Monitor patient closely for opportunistic infection because, if such infection occurs, combination antiretroviral therapy may cause an inflammatory response that could lead to immune reconstitution syndrome requiring additional therapy.

PATIENT TEACHING
- Caution patient to take lamivudine and zidovudine exactly as prescribed and not to stop and then restart therapy without consulting prescriber. Severe hypersensitivity reactions can occur when drug is restarted.

- Review signs and symptoms of hypersensitivity with patient and instruct him to notify prescriber immediately if any occur, such as abdominal pain, cough, diarrhea, dyspnea, fatigue, fever, nausea, skin rash, sore throat, or vomiting.
- Alert patient that this drug combination may cause fat redistribution.
- Advise patient that lamivudine and zidovudine therapy doesn't cure HIV infection and that he should continue taking precautions to reduce the risk of transmitting HIV to others.
- Instruct patient to avoid people with infections because the combination drug may increase his risk of infections.
- Remind patient to have his blood counts monitored as ordered so adverse effects of combinaiton drug can be detected early.

lopinavir and ritonavir
Kaletra

Class and Category
Chemical: Protease inhibitors (lopinavir, ritonavir)
Therapeutic: Antiretrovial (lopinavir, ritonavir)
Pregnancy category: C

Indications and Dosages
▶ *To treat HIV infection in patients who haven't received treatment previously and who won't be receiving efavirenz, fosamprenavir, maraviroc, nelfinavir, or nevirapine concurrently*
ORAL SOLUTION
Adults. 400 mg lopinavir and 100 mg ritonavir (5 ml) b.i.d. with food or 800 mg lopinavir and 200 mg ritonavir (10 ml) daily with food.
Children age 6 months to 18 years. 230 mg/m^2 lopinavir and 57.5 mg/m^2 ritonavir b.i.d. with food. Or, for children weighing less than 15 kg (33 lb), 12 mg/kg lopinavir and 3 mg/kg ritonavir b.i.d. with food. For children weighing 15 to 40 kg (33 to 88 lb), 10 mg/kg lopinavir and 2.5 mg/kg ritonavir b.i.d. with food.
Infants ages 14 days to 6 months. 300 mg/m^2 lopinavir and 75 mg/m^2 ritonavir b.i.d. with food. Or, 16 mg/kg lopinavir and 4 mg/kg ritonavir b.i.d. with food.
TABLETS
Adults. 400 mg lopinavir and 100 mg ritonavir (two 200/50-mg tablets) b.i.d. or 800 mg lopinavir and 200 mg ritonavir (four 200/50-mg tablets) daily.

Children ages 6 months to 18 years who have a body surface area of 1.4 m² or greater or who weigh more than 35 kg (77 lb) and can safely swallow tablets. 400 mg lopinavir and 100 mg ritonavir (four 100/25-mg tablets or two 200/50-mg tablets) b.i.d.

Children ages 6 months to 18 years who have a body surface area of 0.9 to 1.4 m² or who weigh 25 to 35 kg (55 to 77 lb) and can safely swallow tablets. 300 mg lopinavir and 75 mg ritonavir (three 100/25-mg tablets) b.i.d.

Children ages 6 months to 18 years who have a body surface area of 0.6 to 0.9 m² or who weigh 15 to 25 kg (33 to 55 lb) and can safely swallow tablets. 200 mg lopinavir and 50 mg ritonavir (two 100/25-mg tablets) b.i.d.

▶ *To treat HIV infection in patients who have been previously treated and are not currently receiving efavirenz, fosamprenavir, nelfinavir, or nevirapine*

ORAL SOLUTION

Adults. 400 mg lopinavir and 100 mg ritonavir (5 ml) b.i.d.

TABLETS

Adults. 400 mg lopinavir and 100 mg ritonavir (two 200/50-mg tablets) b.i.d.

▶ *To treat HIV infection in patients currently receiving efavirenz, fosamprenavir, nelfinavir, or nevirapine*

ORAL SOLUTION

Adults. 533 mg lopinavir and 133 mg ritonavir (6.5 ml) b.id. with food.

Children ages 6 months to 18 years. 300 mg/m² lopinavir and 75 mg/m² ritonavir b.i.d. with food Or, for children weighing less than 15 kg, 13 mg/kg lopinavir and 3.25 mg/kg ritonavir b.i.d. with food. For children weighing 15 to 45 kg (33 to 99 lb), 11 mg/kg lopinavir and 2.75 mg/kg ritonavir b.i.d. with food *Maximum:* Not to exceed adult dosage.

TABLETS

Adults and children who have a body surface area of 1.7 m² or greater or who weigh more than 45 kg. 500 mg lopinavir and 125 mg ritonavir (two 200/50-mg tablets and one 100/25-mg tablet) b.i.d.

Children ages 6 months to 18 years who have a body surface area of 1.2 to 1.7 m² or who weigh 30 to 45 kg (66 to 99 lb) and can safely swallow tablets. 400 mg lopinavir and 100 mg ritonavir (four 100/25-mg tablets or two 200/50-mg tablets) b.i.d.

Children ages 6 months to 18 years who have a body surface of 0.8 to 1.2 m² or who weigh 20 to 30 kg (44 to 66 lb) and can safely swallow tablets. 300 mg lopinavir and 75 mg ritonavir (three 100/25-mg tablets) b.i.d.

Children ages 6 months to 18 years who have a body surface area of 0.6 to 0.8 m² or who weigh 15 to 20 kg (33 to 44 lb) and can safely swallow tablets. 200 mg lopinavir and 50 mg ritonavir (two 100/25-mg tablets) b.i.d.

Mechanism of Action

Lopinavir inhibits the HIV protease by preventing cleavage of the Gag-Pol polyprotein. This causes production of immature, non-infectious viral particles, which abates replication of the HIV virus.

Ritonavir enhances lopinavir activity by inhibiting the CYP 3A–mediated metabolism of lopinavir, causing plasma lopinavir levels to increase.

Contraindications

Co-administration with astemizole, cisapride, dihydroergotamine, ergonovine, ergotamine, methylergonovine, midazolam, pimozide, terfenadine, or triazolam; hypersensitivity to lopinavir, ritonavir, or any of their components

Interactions

DRUGS

lopinavir and ritonavir

abacavir, atovaquone, ethinyl estradiol, methadone, voriconazole, zidovudine: Decreased plasma levels of these drugs

amiodarone, astemizole, bepridil, cisapride, flecainide, lidocaine, propafenone, pimozide, quinidine, terfenadine: Increased risk of life-threatening reactions, such as cardiac arrhythmias

amprenavir, atorvastatin, atovaquone, carbamazepine, clarithromycin, clonazepam, clorazepate, cyclosporine, desipramine, dexamethasone, diazepam, dihydropyridine calcium channel blockers, diltiazem, disopyramide, dronabinol, estazolam, ethosuximide, flurazepam, fluticasone, HMG-CoA reductase inhibitors, indinavir, ketoconazole, immunosuppressants, itraconazole, lidocaine, maraviroc, methamphetamine, metoprolol, mexilitine, nefazodone, nelfinavir, nifedipine, perphenazine, prednisone, propoxyphene, quinidine, rapamycin, rifabutin, risperidone, rosuvastatin, saquinavir, selective serotonin reuptake inhibitors, sildenafil, sirolimus, tacrolimus, tadalafil, tenofovir, thioridazine, timolol, tramadol, trazodone, tricyclics, vardenafil, verapamil, vinblastine, vincristine, zolpidem: Increased levels and adverse effects of these drugs* *atorvastatin, lovastatin, simvastatin, rosuvastatin:* Increased risk of my-opathy, including rhabdomyolysis

bupropion: Decreased antidepressant effects

dihydroergotamine, ergonovine, ergotamine, methylergonivine: Increased risk of acute ergot toxicity

disulfiram, metronidazole: Possibly disulfiram-like reactions with oral solution, which contains alcohol

midazolam, triazolam: Increased risk of prolonged or increased sedation or respiratory depression

St. John's wort: Decreased effectiveness of lopinavir and ritonavir, with possible future resistance to these drugs or to drugs of the protease inhibitor class

warfarin: Increased warfarin level and increased INR

lopinavir

amprenavir, fosamprenavir, carbamazepine, dexamethasone, efavirenz, nelfinavir, nevirapine, phenobarbital, phenytoin, rifamin, tipranavir: Decreased plasma lopinavir level

delavirdine: Increased lopinavir level

ritonavir

atovaquone, divalproex, ethinyl estradiol, lamotrigine, methadone, phenytoin, theophylline: Decreased levels and effectiveness of these drugs

fluticasone: Increased risk of adrenal suppression and Cushing's syndrome

meperidine: Increased analgesic activity and CNS stimulation

rifampin: Decreased ritonavir level

trazodone: Increased trazodone plasma level

Adverse Reactions

CNS: Asthenia, cerebral infarct, chills, depression, fever, headache, insomnia, paresthesia, seizures

CV: Atrial fibrillation, bradyarrhythmias, chest pain, hypertension, increased cholesterol and triglyceride levels, thrombophlebitis

EENT: Taste aversion

ENDO: Cushing's syndrome, fat redistribution, hyperglycemia, hypothyroidism

GI: Abdominal pain, anorexia, diarrhea, dyspepsia, dysphagia, flatulence, hepatotoxicity, increased liver enzymes, nausea, pancreatitis, vomiting

GU: Decreased libido, impotence, nephritis

HEME: Anemia, decreased platelet count, decreased neutrophil count, leukopenia, lymphadenopathy

MS: Myalgia

RESP: Asthma, bronchitis, pulmonary edema
SKIN: Erythema multiforme, rash, Stevens-Johnson syndrome
Other: Allergic reaction, facial angioedema, hypernatremia, hyponatremia, immune reconstitution syndrome, increased uric acid, lactic acidosis, weight loss

Nursing Considerations

- Use cautiously in a patient with hepatic impairment because lopinavir and ritonavir are metabolized by the liver.
- Assess a patient with advanced HIV infection for hepatic dysfunction and monitor liver enzymes, as ordered, for elevations, especially during the first several months of lopinavir and ritonavir therapy. Other patients at increased risk for hepatic dysfunction include those with underlying hepatitis B or C or who had marked elevations in transaminase before lopinavir and ritonavir therapy.
- Observe a hemophilic patient for bleeding tendencies. Although lopinavir and ritonavir haven't been known to increase bleeding risk, other drugs in their class (protease inhibitors) have.
- Determine patient's cholesterol and triglyceride levels, as ordered, before and periodically during therapy because these levels may rise markedly. Also, be aware that a patient with a markedly increased triglyceride level is at higher risk for pancreatitis during therapy. Notify prescriber if patient develops signs and symptoms of pancreatitis, such as nausea, vomiting, abdominal pain, or increased serum lipase or amylase values.
- Monitor the patient's blood glucose level, as ordered, because hyperglycemia may develop in a patient with no history of diabetes mellitus and blood glucose level may increase in patients with diabetes mellitus.
- Be aware that diarrhea may be more common in patients that take the combination drug only once a day.
- Monitor patient closely for opportunistic infection because, if such infection develops, combination antiretroviral therapy may cause an inflammatory response that could lead to immune reconstitution syndrome requiring additional therapy.

PATIENT TEACHING

- Emphasize the importance of the patient reporting all medications he takes, including OTC and herbal products, throughout lopinavir and ritonavir therapy because of the potential for drug interactions.
- Instruct patient to take lopinavir and ritonavir oral solution with food to decrease risk of stomach upset.

- Instruct patient prescribed tablet form that they may be taken with or without food but should be swallowed whole and not chewed, broken, or crushed.
- Inform patient that lopinavir and ritonavir therapy doesn't cure HIV infection or reduce the risk of transmitting HIV to others.
- Instruct a diabetic patient to monitor his blood glucose level closely because lopinavir and ritonavir can cause blood glucose levels to rise above normal.
- Tell a patient who takes didanosine to take it 1 hour before or 2 hours after taking lopinavir and ritonavir.
- Instruct female patients of childbearing age who take estrogen-based hormonal contraceptives to use additional or alternative contraceptive measures while taking lopinavir and ritonavir.
- Inform patient that he may notice a redistribution or accumulation of body fat after starting lopinavir and ritonavir therapy, and urge him to notify the prescriber if this occurs.
- Tell patient to keep tablets in original container and to avoid exposing them to high humidity.
- If patient will take oral solution, explain that drug must be refrigerated to remain stable until the expiration date on the label. If the drug is kept at room temperature, instruct patient to discard any remaining solution after 2 months.
- Caution patient to consult prescriber before stopping therapy.

penicillin G benzathine and penicillin G procaine
Bicillin C-R

Class and Category
Chemical: Penicillin (penicillin G benzathine, penicillin G procaine)
Therapeutic: Antibiotic (penicillin G benzathine, penicillin G procaine)
Pregnancy category: B

Indications and Dosages
▶ *To treat moderately severe streptococcal infections of the upper respiratory tract, scarlet fever, erysipelas, and skin and soft-tissue infections*
I.M. INJECTION
Adults and children weighing more than 27.5 kg (60 lb).
2.4 million units as a single injection. Alternatively, 1.2 million units given on day 1 and 1.2 million units given on day 3.

Children weighing 13.64 to 27.5 kg (30 to 60 lb). 900,000 to 1.2 million units as a single injection. Alternatively, 450,000 units given on day 1 and 450,000 units given on day 3.

Children weighing less than 13.64 kg (30 lb). 600,000 units as a single injection. Alternatively, 300,000 units given on day 1 and 300,000 units given on day 3.

▶ *To treat moderately severe pneumococcal infections (except pneumococcal meningitis)*

I.M. INJECTION

Adults. 1.2 million units every 2 or 3 days until body temperature is normal for 48 hours.

Children. 600,000 units every 2 or 3 days until body temperature is normal for 48 hours.

Mechanism of Action

Penicillin G benzathine and penicillin G procaine both inhibit the final stage of bacterial cell wall synthesis by competitively binding to penicillin-binding proteins inside the cell wall. Penicillin-binding proteins are responsible for various steps in bacterial cell wall synthesis. By binding to these proteins, penicillin leads to cell wall lysis.

Incompatibilities

Don't mix in the same syringe or container with aminoglycosides because aminoglycosides will become inactivated. Also, don't mix with drugs that may result in a pH below 5.5 or above 8.

Contraindications

Hypersensitivity to penicillin, procaine, or their components.

Interactions

DRUGS

penicillin G benzathine and penicillin G procaine

chloramphenicol, erythromycin, sulfonamides, tetracycline, thrombolytics: Possibly interference with penicillin's bactericidal effect

methotrexate: Decreased methotrexate clearance, increased risk of toxicity

probenecid: Increased blood penicillin level

Adverse Reactions

CNS: Anxiety, asthenia, chills, coma, confusion, dizziness, dysphasia, euphoria, fatigue, fever, hallucinations, headache, lethargy, myelitis, nervousness, neuropathy, neurovascular reaction, prostration, sciatic nerve irritation, seizures, somnolence, stroke, syncope, tremors

CV: Edema, labile blood pressure, palpitations, tachycardia, vasculitis, vasodilation, vasovagal reaction

EENT: Black "hairy" tongue, blindness, blurred vision, laryngeal edema, oral candidiasis, stomatitis, taste perversion

GI: Abdominal pain, blood in stool, diarrhea, elevated liver function test results (transient), indigestion, intestinal necrosis, nausea, pseudomembranous colitis, vomiting

GU: Elevated BUN and creatinine levels, hematuria, impotence, interstitial nephritis (acute), priapism, proteinuria, renal failure, vaginal candidiasis

HEME: Eosinophilia, hemolytic anemia, leukopenia, lymphadenopathy, thrombocytopenia

MS: Arthralgia, muscle twitching, rhabdomyolysis

RESP: Dyspnea, hypoxia, pulmonary hypertension or embolism

SKIN: Diaphoresis, exfoliative or maculopapular dermatitis, pruritus, rash, urticaria

Other: Anaphylaxis; electrolyte imbalances; elevated SGOT level; injection site necrosis, pain, or redness

Nursing Considerations

- Obtain body tissue and fluid samples for culture and sensitivity tests as ordered before giving first dose. Expect to start therapy before test results are known.
- Inject only deep into large muscle mass, such as the upper, outer quadrant of the buttock in an adult or the midlateral aspect of the thigh in small children.
- **WARNING** Don't inject intravenously because I.V. injection may be fatal and intra-arterial injection may cause extensive tissue and organ necrosis.
- Don't clear any air bubbles from the disposable syringe or needle because doing so may interfere with visualization of blood or discoloration during aspiration.
- Inject drug slowly and steadily; otherwise, the needle may be blocked by the high concentration of suspended material in the solution. Stop injection at once if patient reports sudden pain at the injection site or if a child shows signs of severe pain.
- Following injection, apply ice to the site for pain.
- Monitor patient closely for anaphylaxis, which may become life-threatening. Patients at greatest risk are those with a history of hypersensitivity to penicillin, cephalosporins, or multiple other allergies; those who have asthma or hay fever; and those who have developed urticaria in the past.

- **WARNING** If drug triggers an anaphylactic reaction, stop it immediately and notify prescriber. Provide appropriate therapy. Anaphylaxis requires immediate treatment with epinephrine and airway management. It may also require administration of oxygen and I.V. corticosteroids.
- Be aware that giving the combination drug I.M. slows its absorbtion, which may make allergic reactions difficult to treat.
- Monitor patient closely for diarrhea, which may herald pseudomembranous colitis. If diarrhea occurs, notify prescriber. If the patient has pseudomembranous colitis, expect to stop the drug and possibly administer fluids, electrolytes, protein, and an antibiotic effective against *Clostridium difficile*.

PATIENT TEACHING
- Instruct patient to report previous allergies to penicillins and cephalosporins and to notify prescriber immediately about adverse reactions, such as a fever, rash and hives.
- Warn patient that injection will be uncomfortable; advise keeping ice on site for pain relief for length of time prescribed.

piperacillin sodium and tazobactam sodium

Tazocin (CAN), Zosyn

Class and Category

Chemical: Piperazine derivative of ampicillin, acylureidopenicillin (piperacillin); penicillinate sulfone (tazobactam)
Therapeutic: Antibiotic
Pregnancy category: B

Indications and Dosages

▶ *To treat moderate to severe gram-negative or anaerobic infections, such as appendicitis, community-acquired pneumonia, diabetic foot ulcers, intra-abdominal infections, pelvic inflammatory disease, peritonitis, postpartum endometritis, and uncomplicated or complicated skin or soft-tissue infections caused by susceptible organisms, such as* Bacteroides species (including many strains of Bacteroides fragilis), Clostridium *species,* Enterobacter *species,* Enterococcus faecalis, Escherichia coli, Haemophilus influenzae, Klebsiella pneumoniae, Morganella morganii, Neisseria gonorrhoeae, Proteus mirabilis, Proteus vulgaris, Pseudomonas aeruginosa, *and* Serratia *species*

I.V. INFUSION
Adults and adolescents. 3.375 grams every 6 hr for 7 to

10 days. *Maximum:* 4.5 grams every 6 to 8 hr.
▶ *To treat nosocomial pneumonia caused by susceptible organisms*
I.V. INFUSION
Adults and adolescents. 4.5 grams every 6 hr in addition to aminoglycoside therapy for 7 to 14 days.
DOSAGE ADJUSTMENT Dosage possibly decreased to 2.25 grams every 6 hr for patients with creatinine clearance of 20 to 40 ml/min/1.73 m^2 or to 2.25 grams every 8 hr for those with creatinine clearance less than 20 ml/min/1.73 m^2. Decreased to 2.25 grams every 12 hr for patients receiving hemodialysis or continuous peritoneal dialysis.
▶ *To treat appendicitis or peritonitis caused by susceptible organisms in children with normal renal function*
I.V. INFUSION
Children weighing over 40 kg (88 lb). 3.375 grams every 6 hr for 7 to 10 days.
Children age 9 months and over weighing up to 40 kg. 100 mg/kg piperacillin and 12.5 mg/kg tazobactam every 8 hr for 7 to 10 days.
Children ages 2 to 9 months. 80 mg/kg piperacillin and 10 mg/kg tazobactam every 8 hr for 7 to 10 days.

Mechanism of Action

Piperacillin binds to specific penicillin-binding proteins and inhibits the third and final stage of bacterial cell wall synthesis. It does this by interfering with an autolysin inhibitor. Uninhibited autolytic enzymes destroy the cell wall and result in cell lysis.

Tazobactam doesn't change piperacillin's action, but it protects piperacillin against Richmond and Sykes types II, III, IV, and V beta-lactamases; staphylococcal beta-lactamases; and extended-spectrum beta-lactamases.

Incompatibilities

Don't mix piperacillin and tazobactam in same container with aminoglycosides because of chemical incompatibility (depending on concentrations, diluents, pH, and temperature). Also, don't give tobramycin with piperacillin and tazobactam via Y-site infusion because tobramycin may be inactivated.

Contraindications

Hypersensitivity to beta-lactamase inhibitors, cephalosporins, penicillins, piperacillin, tazobactam, or their components

Interactions

DRUGS

aminoglycosides: Additive or synergistic effects against some bacteria, possibly mutual inactivation

anti-inflammatory drugs (including aspirin and NSAIDs), heparin, oral anticoagulants, platelet aggregation inhibitors, sulfinpyrazone, thrombolytics: Increased risk of bleeding

hepatotoxic drugs (including labetalol and rifampin): Increased risk of hepatotoxicity

methotrexate: Increased blood methotrexate level and risk of toxicity

probenecid: Increased blood piperacillin level and risk of toxicity

vecuronium: Possibly prolonged neuromuscular blockade of vecuronium in perioperative period

Adverse Reactions

CNS: Chills, dizziness, fever, hallucinations, headache, lethargy, seizures, stroke

CV: Cardiac arrest, hypotension, palpitations, tachycardia, vasodilation, vasovagal reactions

EENT: Epistaxis, oral candidiasis, pharyngitis

GI: Cholestatic jaundice, diarrhea, elevated liver function test results, epigastric distress, hepatitis, intestinal necrosis, nausea, pseudomembranous colitis, vomiting

GU: Hematuria, impotence, nephritis, neurogenic bladder, priapism, proteinuria, renal failure, vaginal candidiasis

HEME: Agranulocytosis, eosinophilia, hemolytic anemia, leukopenia, neutropenia, pancytopenia, prolonged bleeding time, thrombocytopenia

MS: Arthralgia, prolonged muscle relaxation

RESP: Dyspnea, pulmonary embolism, pulmonary hypertension

SKIN: Erythema multiforme, exfoliative dermatitis, mottling, rash, Stevens-Johnson syndrome, toxic epidermal necrolysis, urticaria

Other: Anaphylaxis, facial edema, hypokalemia, hyponatremia

Nursing Considerations

- Obtain blood, sputum, or other samples for culture and sensitivity testing, as ordered, before giving piperacillin and tazobactam. Expect to begin therapy before the test results are available.
- Be aware that sunlight may darken powder for dilution but won't alter drug potency.

- Reconstitute with sterile water for injection, sodium chloride for injection, D_5W, or bacteriostatic water or normal saline solution that contains parabens or benzyl alcohol.
- For additional dilution (50 to 150 ml except as noted), use appropriate solution, such as sodium chloride for injection, sterile water for injection (no more than 50 ml), D_5W, or dextran 6% in normal saline solution.
- Shake vigorously after adding diluent to help drug dissolve, and inspect for particles and discoloration before administering.
- Administer over at least 30 minutes.
- Assess patient for bleeding or excessive bruising because drug can decrease platelet aggregation.
- Monitor serum potassium level to detect hypokalemia, which may result from urinary potassium loss.
- Monitor patient closely for diarrhea, which may indicate pseudomembranous colitis. If diarrhea occurs, notify prescriber and expect to withhold drug. Expect to treat pseudomembranous colitis with fluids, electrolytes, protein, and an antibiotic effective against *Clostridium difficile.*
- Administer aminoglycosides 1 hour before or after piperacillin and tazobactam, using a separate site, I.V. bag, and tubing.
- Watch for fluid retention and hypertension, especially in patients on restricted sodium intake, because piperacillin contains 64 mg of sodium per gram.
- Monitor patients with cystic fibrosis closely because piperacillin may increase the risk of fever and rash in these patients.

PATIENT TEACHING
- Advise patient to consult prescriber before using OTC drugs during treatment with piperacillin and tazobactam because of the risk of interactions.
- Inform patient that increased bruising may occur if she takes anti-inflammatory drugs, such as aspirin and NSAIDs, during piperacillin and tazobactam therapy.
- Advise patient to notify prescriber about signs of superinfection, such as white patches on tongue or in mouth.
- Urge patient to tell prescriber about diarrhea. Remind patient that watery or bloody stools can occur 2 or more months after piperacillin and tazobactam therapy and can be serious, requiring prompt treatment.
- Tell patient that combination drug contains 64 mg of sodium per gram and to consider this when monitoring daily sodium intake.

quinupristin and dalfopristin
Synercid

Class and Category
Chemical: Pristinamycin I and IIa derivative, streptogramin
Therapeutic: Antibiotic
Pregnancy category: B

Indications and Dosages
▶ *To treat serious or life-threatening infections, such as bacteremia caused by vancomycin-resistant* Enterococcus faecium
I.V. INFUSION
Adults and adolescents age 16 and over. 7.5 mg/kg every 8 hr.

▶ *To treat complicated skin and soft-tissue infections caused by methicillin-susceptible strains of* Staphylococcus aureus *or* Streptococcus pyogenes
I.V. INFUSION
Adults and adolescents age 16 and over. 7.5 mg/kg every 12 hr for at least 7 days.

Mechanism of Action
Quinupristin inhibits the late phase of protein synthesis by binding to the 50S ribosomal subunit.

Dalfopristin inhibits the early phase of protein synthesis by binding to the 70S or 50S ribosomal subunit.

Together, these drugs inhibit bacterial protein synthesis by irreversibly blocking ribosome function. Additionally, their combined activity inhibits transfer RNA (tRNA) synthetase activity, which decreases the amount of free tRNA in the cell. Without tRNA, bacterial cells can't incorporate amino acids into peptide chains, and the cells die.

Incompatibilities
Don't mix quinupristin and dalfopristin in saline solutions, including normal saline, half-normal (0.45%) saline, 3% sodium chloride, and 5% sodium chloride solutions, because drug is physically incompatible with these solutions.

Contraindications
Hypersensitivity to quinupristin or dalfopristin, other streptogramin antibiotics, or their components

Interactions

DRUGS

alfentanil, alprazolam, carbamazepine, delavirdine, diazepam, diltiazem, disopyramide, dofetilide, donepezil, erythromycin, ethinyl estradiol, felodipine, fexofenadine, indinavir, lidocaine, lovastatin, methylprednisolone, nevirapine, norethindrone, quinidine, ritonavir, saquinavir, simvastatin, tacrolimus, triazolam, trimetrexate, verapamil, vinblastine: Decreased elimination of these drugs, possibly resulting in toxicity
astemizole, cisapride, terfenadine: Decreased elimination of these drugs, possibly prolonged QT interval
cyclosporine, midazolam, nifedipine, terfenadine: Possibly increased blood levels of these drugs

Adverse Reactions

CNS: Anxiety, confusion, dizziness, fever, headache, hypertonia, insomnia, paresthesia
CV: Chest pain, palpitations, peripheral edema, thrombophlebitis, vasodilation
EENT: Oral candidiasis, stomatitis
GI: Abdominal pain, constipation, diarrhea, elevated liver function test results, indigestion, nausea, pancreatitis, pseudomembranous colitis, vomiting
GU: Hematuria, vaginitis
MS: Arthralgia, gout, muscle spasms, myalgia, myasthenia
RESP: Dyspnea, pleural effusion
SKIN: Diaphoresis, pruritus, rash, urticaria
Other: Injection site edema, inflammation, pain, or thrombophlebitis

Nursing Considerations

- Store unopened vials of quinupristin and dalfopristin in refrigerator.
- **WARNING** Reconstitute and further dilute with dextrose in water or sterile water for injection only. Don't use saline solutions because drug is physically incompatible with them.
- Dilute prescribed dose in 250 ml D₅W, and infuse over 1 hour through a peripheral I.V. line. If administered by central venous catheter, dilute prescribed dose in 100 ml of D₅W. Central venous administration may decrease risk of infusion site reaction. Use an infusion pump or device to control rate of infusion.
- Further dilute reconstituted solution within 30 minutes. Vials are for single use only. Discard any unused portion.

- Don't flush I.V. catheter with saline or heparin flush solution because of possible incompatibility. Flush I.V. catheter only with D₅W before and after drug administration.
- Monitor patient closely for diarrhea, which may indicate pseudomembranous colitis. If diarrhea occurs, notify prescriber and expect to withhold drug. Expect to treat pseudomembranous colitis with fluids, electrolytes, protein, and an antibiotic effective against *Clostridium difficile.*

PATIENT TEACHING
- Instruct patient to complete the full course of quinupristin and dalfopristin therapy, as prescribed.
- Inform patient that if he requires long-term therapy, drug will be given in hospital or clinic or by a home health care nurse.
- Urge patient to tell prescriber about diarrhea that's severe or lasts longer than 3 days. Remind patient that watery or bloody stools can occur 2 months or more after quinupristin and dalfopristin therapy and can be serious, requiring prompt treatment.

rifampin and isoniazid
Rifamate

Class and Category
Chemical: Semi-synthetic antibiotic derivative of rifamycin (rifampin), isonicotinic acid derivative (isoniazid)
Therapeutic: Antitubercular (rifampin, isoniazid)
Pregnancy category: C

Indications and Dosages
▶ *To treat pulmonary tuberculosis when initial therapy for tuberculosis has been ineffective*
CAPSULES
Adults. 600 mg rifampin and 300 mg isoniazid (2 capsules) daily.

Mechanism of Action
Rifampin inhibits bacterial and mycobacterial RNA synthesis by binding to DNA-dependent RNA polymerase, thereby blocking RNA transcription. Depending on the dose given, a bactericidal or bacteriostatic action results.

Isoniazid interferes with lipid and nucleic acid synthesis in actively growing tubercle bacilli cells. It also disrupts bacterial cell wall synthesis and may interfere with mycolic acid synthesis in mycobacterial cells, which halts the growth of tubercle bacilli.

Contraindications

Acute liver disease; concurrent use of nonnucleoside reverse transcriptase inhibitors or protease inhibitors (by patients with HIV); history of serious adverse reactions to isoniazid; hypersensitivity to rifampin, isoniazid, other rifamycins and their components

Interactions

DRUGS

rifampin and isoniazid

anesthetics (hydrocarbon inhalation, except isoflurane), hepatotoxic drugs: Increased risk of hepatotoxicity

ketoconazole: Possibly decreased blood ketoconazole level and resistance to antifungal treatment

rifampin

aminophylline, oxtriphylline, theophylline: Increased metabolism and clearance of these theophylline preparations

beta blockers, chloramphenicol, clofibrate, corticosteroids, cyclosporine, dapsone, digitalis glycosides, disopyramide, hexobarbital, itraconazole, mexiletine, oral anticoagulants, oral antidiabetic drugs, phenytoin, propafenone, quinidine, tocainide, verapamil (oral): Increased metabolism, resulting in lower blood levels of these drugs

bone marrow depressants: Increased leukopenic or thrombocytopenic effects

clofazimine: Decreased absorption of rifampin

diazepam: Increased elimination of diazepam, resulting in decreased effectiveness

estramustine, estrogens, oral contraceptives: Decreased estrogenic effects

methadone: Possibly impaired absorption of methadone, leading to withdrawal symptoms

probenecid: Increased blood level or prolonged duration of rifampin, increasing risk of toxicity

nonnucleoside reverse transcriptase inhibitors, protease inhibitors (indinavir, nelfinavir, ritonavir, saquinavir): Accelerated metabolism of these drugs by patients with HIV, resulting in subtherapeutic levels. Also delayed metabolism of rifampin, increasing the risk of toxicity

trimethoprim: Increased elimination and shortened elimination half-life of trimethoprim

isoniazid

acetaminophen: Increased risk of hepatotoxicity and possibly nephrotoxicity *alfentanil:* Decreased alfentanil clearance and increased duration of alfentanil effects

aluminum-containing antacids: Decreased isoniazid absorption

benzodiazepines: Decreased benzodiazepine clearance

carbamazepine: Increased blood carbamazepine level and toxicity; increased risk of isoniazid toxicity

corticosteroids: Decreased isoniazid effects

cycloserine: Increased risk of adverse CNS effects and CNS toxicity

disulfiram: Changes in behavior and coordination

enflurane: Increased risk of high-output renal failure

meperidine: Risk of hypotensive episodes or CNS depression

nephrotoxic drugs: Increased risk of nephrotoxicity

oral anticoagulants: Increased anticoagulant effects

phenytoin: Increased blood phenytoin level and risk of phenytoin toxicity

theophylline: Increased blood theophylline level

FOODS

isoniazid

tyramine-containing foods, such as cheese and fish: Increased responses to tyramine contained in foods, possibly resulting in chills, diaphoresis, headache, light-headedness, and red, itchy, clammy skin

ACTIVITIES

rifampin and isoniazid

alcohol use: Increased risk of hepatotoxicity

Adverse Reactions

CNS: Chills, clumsiness, confusion, dizziness, drowsiness, encephalopathy, fatigue, fever, hallucinations, headache, neurotoxicity, paresthesia, peripheral neuritis, psychosis, seizures, weakness

CV: Vasculitis

EENT: Discolored saliva, tears, and sputum; mouth or tongue soreness; optic neuritis; periorbital edema

ENDO: Gynecomastia, hyperglycemia

GI: Abdominal cramps, anorexia, diarrhea, discolored feces, elevated liver function test results, epigastric discomfort, flatulence, hearburn, hepatitis, heptotoxicity, jaundice, nausea, pseudomembranous colitis, vomiting

GU: Discolored urine

HEME: Agranulocytosis, aplastic anemia, eosinophilia, hemolytic anemia, sideroblastic anemia, thrombocytopenia

MS: Arthralgia, joint stiffness, myalgia

SKIN: Discolored skin and sweat, pruritus, rash

Other: Angioedema, flulike symptoms, hypocalcemia, hypophosphatemia

Nursing Considerations

- Expect to also give pyridoxine (vitamin B_6) to patients who are malnourished or predisposed to developing neuropathy, such as diabetics.
- Monitor results of patient's liver enzyme studies, which may be ordered monthly, because rifampin and isoniazid can cause hepatotoxicity. Monitor patient for evidence of hepatotoxicity, such as darkened urine, fever, jaundice, malaise, nausea, and vomiting.
- Be aware that about 50% of patients metabolize isoniazid slowly, which may lead to increased toxic effects of the combination drug. Monitor patient for such adverse reactions as peripheral neuritis; if they occur, notify prescriber and expect to decrease dosage.
- Be aware that patients with advanced HIV infection may experience more adverse reactions and in greater severity.

PATIENT TEACHING

- Instruct patient to take rifampin and isoniazid exactly as prescribed and not to stop taking it without consulting prescriber. Explain that interruptions in therapy can lead to increased adverse reactions. Remind patient that treatment may take months or years.
- Direct patient to take drug on an empty stomach 1 hour before or 2 hours after meals with a full glass of water. If GI distress occurs, instruct him to take drug with food or an antacid that doesn't contain aluminum.
- Advise patient to watch for and report signs of hepatic dysfunction, including darkened urine, decreased appetite, fatigue, and jaundice.
- Warn that drug may turn urine, feces, saliva, sputum, sweat, tears, and skin reddish orange to reddish brown.
- Caution patient against wearing soft contact lenses during therapy because drug may permanently stain them.
- Advise female patients who use an oral conceptive to use an additional form of birth control while taking this drug.
- Caution patient not to drink alcohol while taking drug because alcohol increases the risk of hepatotoxicity.
- Provide patient with a list of tyramine-containing foods to avoid when taking rifampin and isoniazid, such as cheese, fish, salami, red wine, and yeast extracts. Inform him that consum-

ing these foods during therapy may cause unpleasant adverse reactions, such as chills, pounding heartbeat, and sweating.

- Urge patient to keep appointments for periodic laboratory tests and physical examinations.
- Instruct patient to report fever, nausea, numbness and tingling in arms and legs, rash, vision changes, vomiting, and yellowing skin.

rifampin, isoniazid, and pyrazinamide
Rifater

Class and Category
Chemical: Semi-synthetic antibiotic derivative of rifamycin (rifampin), isonicotinic acid derivative (isoniazid), pyrazine analogue of nicotinamide (pyrazinamide)
Therapeutic: Antitubercular (rifampin, isoniazid, pyrazinamide)
Pregnancy category: C

Indications and Dosages
▶ *To treat pulmonary tuberculosis initially*
TABLETS
Adults weighing 55 kg (121 lb) or more. 720 mg rifampin, 300 mg isoniazid, and 1,800 mg pyrazinamide (6 tablets) daily.
Adults weighing 45 kg to 55 kg (99 to 121 lb). 600 mg rifampin, 250 mg isoniazid, and 1500 mg pyrazinamide (5 tablets) daily.
Adults weighing 44 kg (97 lb) or less. 480 mg rifampin, 200 mg isoniazid, and 1,200 mg pyrazinamide (4 tablets) daily.

Mechanism of Action
Rifampin inhibits bacterial and mycobacterial RNA synthesis by binding to DNA-dependent RNA polymerase, thereby blocking RNA transcription. Depending on the dose given, a bactericidal or bacteriostatic drug effect results.

Isoniazid interferes with lipid and nucleic acid synthesis in actively growing tubercle bacilli cells. It also disrupts bacterial cell wall synthesis and may interfere with mycolic acid synthesis in mycobacterial cells, which halts the growth of tubercle bacilli.

Pyrazinamide inhibits the growth of *Mycobacterium tuberculosis* organisms by decreasing the pH level. Depending on the blood pyrazinamide level, a bactericidal or bacteriostatic action results.

Contraindications

Acute gout or liver disease; concurrent use of nonnucleoside reverse transcriptase inhibitors or protease inhibitors (by patients with HIV); history of serious adverse reactions to isoniazid; hypersensitivity to rifampin, isoniazid, pyrazinamide, other rifamycins and their components

Interactions

DRUGS

rifampin and isoniazid

anesthetics (hydrocarbon inhalation, except isoflurane), hepatotoxic drugs: Increased risk of hepatotoxicity

ketoconazole: Possibly decreased blood ketoconazole level and resistance to antifungal treatment

rifampin and pyrazinamide

cyclosporine: Possibly decreased blood level and therapeutic effects of cyclosporine

rifampin

aminophylline, oxtriphylline, theophylline: Increased metabolism and clearance of these theophylline preparations

beta blockers, chloramphenicol, clofibrate, corticosteroids, cyclosporine, dapsone, digitalis glycosides, disopyramide, hexocbarbital, itraconazole, mexiletine, oral anticoagulants, oral antidiabetic drugs, phenytoin, propafenone, quinidine, tocainide, verapamil (oral): Increased metabolism, resulting in lower blood levels of these drugs

bone marrow depressants: Increased leukopenic or thrombocytopenic effects

clofazimine: Reduced absorption of rifampin

diazepam: Enhanced elimination of diazepam and decreased effectiveness

estramustine, estrogens, oral contraceptives: Decreased estrogenic effects

methadone: Possibly impaired methadone absorption, leading to withdrawal symptoms

probenecid: Increased blood level or prolonged duration of rifampin, increasing risk of toxicity

nonnucleoside reverse transcriptase inhibitors, protease inhibitors (indinavir, nelfinavir, ritonavir, saquinavir): Accelerated metabolism of these drugs in patients with HIV, resulting in subtherapeutic levels. Also delayed metabolism of rifampin, increasing the risk of toxicity

trimethoprim: Increased elimination and shortened elimination half-life of trimethoprim

isoniazid
acetaminophen: Increased risk of hepatotoxicity and possibly nephrotoxicity
alfentanil: Decreased alfentanil clearance and increased duration of alfentanil's effects
aluminum-containing antacids: Decreased isoniazid absorption
benzodiazepines: Decreased benzodiazepine clearance
carbamazepine: Increased blood carbamazepine level and toxicity, and increased risk of isoniazid toxicity
corticosteroids: Decreased isoniazid effects
cycloserine: Increased risk of adverse CNS effects and CNS toxicity
disulfiram: Changes in behavior and coordination
enflurane: Increased risk of high-output renal failure
meperidine: Risk of hypotensive episodes or CNS depression
nephrotoxic drugs: Increased risk of nephrotoxicity
oral anticoagulants: Increased anticoagulant effects
phenytoin: Increased blood phenytoin level and risk of phenytoin toxicity
theophylline: Increased blood theophylline level
pyrazinamide
allopurinol, colchicine, probenecid, sulfinpyrazone: Possibly increased blood uric acid level and decreased efficacy of antigout therapy
FOODS
isoniazid
tyramine-containing foods, such as cheese and fish: Increased responses to tyramine contained in foods, possibly resulting in chills, diaphoresis, headache, light-headedness, and red, itchy, clammy skin
ACTIVITIES
rifampin and pyrazinamide
alcohol use: Increased risk of hepatotoxicity

Adverse Reactions
CNS: Chills, clumsiness, confusion, dizziness, drowsiness, encephalopathy, fatigue, fever, hallucinations, headache, neurotoxicity, paresthesia, peripheral neuritis, psychosis, seizures, weakness
CV: Vasculitis
EENT: Discolored saliva, tears, and sputum; mouth or tongue soreness; optic neuritis; periorbital edema
ENDO: Gynecomastia, hyperglycemia
GI: Abdominal cramps, anorexia, diarrhea, discolored feces, elevated liver function test results, epigastric discomfort, flatulence, hearburn, hepatitis, hepatotoxicity, jaundice, nausea, pseudomembranous colitis, vomiting

GU: Discolored urine, dysuria, interstitial nephritis
HEME: Agranulocytosis, aplastic anemia, decreased hemoglobin, eosinophilia, hemolytic anemia, leukopenia, porphyria, sideroblastic anemia, thrombocytopenia
MS: Arthralgia, gout, joint stiffness, myalgia
SKIN: Acne, discolored skin and sweat, photosensitivity, pruritus, rash, urticaria
Other: Angioedema, flulike symptoms, hypocalcemia, hypophosphatemia

Nursing Considerations

- Review liver function test results before and every 2 to 4 weeks during rifampin, isoniazid, and pyrazinamide therapy because the drug can cause hepatotoxicity. Monitor patient for signs of hepatotoxicity, such as darkened urine, fever, jaundice, malaise, nausea and vomiting.
- Be aware that about 50% of patients metabolize isoniazid slowly, which may lead to increased toxic effects of the combination drug. Monitor patient for such adverse reactions as peripheral neuritis; if adverse reactions occur, notify prescriber and expect to decrease dosage.
- Be aware that patients with advanced HIV infection may experience more adverse reactions and in greater severity.
- Expect to also give pyridoxine (vitamin B_6) to patients who are malnourished or predisposed to developing neuropathy, such as diabetics.
- Be aware that the pyrazinamide component of the drug can affect the accuracy of certain urine ketone strip test results.

PATIENT TEACHING

- Instruct patient to take rifampin, isoniazid, and pyrazinamide exactly as prescribed and not to stop without consulting prescriber. Explain that interruptions can increase adverse reactions. Remind patient that treatment may take months or years.
- Direct patient to take this combination drug on an empty stomach 1 hour before or 2 hours after meals with a full glass of water. If GI distress occurs, instruct him to take the drug with food or an antacid that doesn't contain aluminum.
- Advise patient to report signs of hepatic dysfunction, including darkened urine, decreased appetite, fatigue, and jaundice.
- Warn that drug may turn urine, feces, saliva, sputum, sweat, tears, and skin reddish orange to reddish brown.
- Caution patient against wearing soft contact lenses during therapy because drug may permanently stain them.

- Advise female patients who take an oral conceptive to use an additional form of birth control during therapy with rifampin, isoniazid, and pyrazinamide.
- Caution patient not to drink alcohol while taking drug because alcohol increases the risk of hepatotoxicity.
- Give patient a list of tyramine-containing foods to avoid while taking combination drug, such as cheese, fish, salami, red wine, and yeast extracts. Explain that consuming these foods during drug therapy may cause unpleasant adverse reactions, such as chills, a pounding heartbeat, and sweating.
- Instruct patient to keep appointments for periodic laboratory tests and physical examinations.
- Urge patient to notify prescriber about fever, nausea, numbness and tingling in arms and legs, rash, visual changes, vomiting, and yellow skin.
- Advise diabetic patient to use alternative methods of ketone determination while taking drug.
- Urge patient to minimize exposure to sun and to wear protective clothing, hat, sunglasses, and sunscreen when outdoors.

sulfadoxine and pyrimethamine

Fansidar

Class and Category

Chemical: Folic acid antagonist (sulfadoxine, pyrimethamine)
Therapeutic: Antimalarial (sulfadoxine, pyrimethamine)
Pregnancy category: C

Indications and Dosages

▶ *To treat acute, uncomplicated* Plasmodium falciparum *malaria when chloroquine resistance is suspected*

TABLETS

Adults and adolescents age 18 and over. 1,000 mg sulfadoxine and 50 mg pyrimethamine (2 tablets) as a single dose. Alternatively, 1,500 mg sulfadoxine and 75 mg pyrimethamine (3 tablets) as a single dose.

Children over age 2 months weighing more than 45 kg (99 lb). 1,500 mg sulfadoxine and 75 mg pyrimethamine (3 tablets) as a single dose.

Children over age 2 months weighing 31 to 45 kg (68 to 99 lb). 1,000 mg sulfadoxine and 50 mg pyrimethamine (2 tablets) as a single dose.

Children over age 2 months weighing 21 to 30 kg (46 to 66 lb). 750 mg sulfadoxine and 37.5 mg pyrimethamine (1½ tablets) as a single dose.

Children over age 2 months weighing 11 to 20 kg (24 to 44 lb). 500 mg sulfadoxine and 25 mg pyrimethamine (1 tablet) as a single dose.

Children over age 2 months weighing 5 to 10 kg (11 to 22 lb). 250 mg sulfadoxine and 12.5 mg pyrimethamine (½ tablet) as a single dose.

▶ *To prevent P.* falciparum *malaria when patient is traveling to areas where chloroquine-resistant* P. falciparum *malaria is endemic and alternative drugs are not available or are contraindicated*

TABLETS

Adults and adolescents age 18 and over. 500 mg sulfadoxine and 25 mg pyrimethamine (1 tablet) 1 to 2 days before arrival in endemic area, followed by 500 mg sulfadoxine and 25 mg pyrimethamine (1 tablet) once weekly during stay and for 4 to 6 wk after departure from endemic area. Alternatively, 1,000 mg sulfadoxine and 50 mg pyrimethamine (2 tablets) 1 to 2 days before arrival in endemic area, followed by 1,000 mg sulfadoxine and 50 mg pyrimethamine (2 tablets) every 2 wk throughout stay and continued for 4 to 6 weeks after departure from endemic area. Therapy should last no longer than 2 years.

Children over age 2 months weighing more than 45 kg. 750 mg sulfadoxine and 37.5 mg pyrimethamine (1½ tablets) as a single dose 1 to 2 days before arrival in endemic area, followed by 750 mg sulfadoxine and 37.5 mg pyrimethamine (1½ tablets) every wk throughout stay and continued for 4 to 6 weeks after leaving endemic area. Therapy should last no longer than 2 years.

Children over age 2 months weighing 31 to 45 kg. 500 mg sulfadoxine and 25 mg pyrimethamine (1 tablet) as a single dose 1 to 2 days before arrival in endemic area, followed by 500 mg sulfadoxine and 25 mg pyrimethamine (1 tablet) every wk throughout stay and continued for 4 to 6 weeks after departure from endemic area. Therapy should last no longer than 2 years.

Children over age 2 months weighing 21 to 30 kg. 375 mg sulfadoxine and 18.75 mg pyrimethamine (¾ tablet) as a single dose 1 to 2 days before arrival in endemic area, followed by 375 mg sulfadoxine and 18.75 mg (¾ tablet) pyrimethamine every wk throughout stay and continued 4 to 6 weeks after departure from endemic area. Therapy should last no longer than 2 years.

Children over age 2 months weighing 11 to 20 kg. 250 mg sulfadoxine and 12.5 mg pyrimethamine (½ tablet) as a single dose 1 to 2 days before arrival in endemic area, followed by 250 mg sulfadoxine and 12.5 mg pyrimethamine (½ tablet) every wk throughout stay and continued for 4 to 6 weeks after departure from endemic area. Therapy should last no longer than 2 years.

Children over age 2 months weighing 5 to 10 kg. 125 mg sulfadoxine and 6.25 mg pyrimethamine (¼ tablet) as a single dose 1 to 2 days before arrival in endemic area, followed by 125 mg sulfadoxine and 6.25 mg pyrimethamine (¼ tablet) every wk throughout stay and continued for 4 to 6 weeks after departure from endemic area. Therapy should last no longer than 2 years.

Mechanism of Action

Sulfadoxine and pyrimethamine are both folic acid antagonists. Sulfadoxine inhibits the activity of dihydropteroate.

Pyrimethamine inhibits the activity of dihydrofolate reductase, a folic acid enzyme. These actions take place during the asexual erythrocytic stages of malaria caused by *Plasmodium falciparum,* thus preventing the *P. falciparum* organism from replicating.

Contraindications

Breast-feeding; hypersensitivity to pyrimethamine, sulfadoxine, sulfonamides or their components; megaloblastic anemia caused by folate deficiency; pregnancy at term (prophylaxis use); prolonged use in patients with blood dyscrasias or renal or hepatic failure

Interactions

DRUGS

sulfadoxine and pyrimethamine

antifolic drugs such as sulfonamides, trimethoprim, trimethoprim-sulfamethoxazole: Increased risk of adverse reactions

chloroquine: Increased incidence and severity of adverse reactions

pyrimethamine

antifolic drugs such as sulfonamides, trimethoprim, trimethoprim-sulfamethoxazole: Increased risk of bone marrow suppression

lorazepam: Increased risk of mild hepatotoxicity

p-aminobenzoic acid (PABA): Decreased effectiveness of pyrimethamine

Adverse Reactions

CNS: Apathy, ataxia, chills, depression, drug fever, fatigue, hallucinations, headache, insomnia, nervousness, peripheral neuritis, polyneuritis, seizures, vertigo
CV: Allergic myocarditis and pericarditis, periarteritis nodosa
EENT: Glossitis, periorbital edema, stomatitis, tinnitus
GI: Abdominal pain, bloating, diarrhea, hepatitis, hepatocellular necrosis, nausea, pancreatitis, transient liver enzyme elevation, vomiting
GU: Anuria, elevated BUN and serum creatinine levels, crystalluria, interstitial nephritis, oliguria, renal failure, toxic nephrosis
HEME: Agranulocytosis, aplastic anemia, eosinophilia, hemolytic anemia, hypoprothrombinemia, leukopenia, megaloblastic anemia, methemoglobinemia, purpura, thrombocytopenia
MS: Arthralgia, muscle weakness
RESP: Pulmonary infiltrates
SKIN: Alopecia, erythema multiforme, exfoliative dermatitis, generalized skin eruptions, photosensitivity, pruritus, Stevens-Johnson syndrome, toxic epidermal necrolysis, urticaria
Other: Anaphylaxis, lupus erythematosus phenomenon, Lyell's syndrome, serum sickness

Nursing Considerations

- Use cautiously in patients with impaired renal or hepatic function, possible folate deficiency, or severe allergy or bronchial asthma because of an increased risk of adverse effects.
- Monitor a patient who has glucose-6-phosphate dehydrogenase deficiency closely for pain, shortness of breath, and fatigue because hemolysis may occur when a sulfonamide drug such as sulfadoxine is administered.
- **WARNING** Stop therapy and notify prescriber immediately if the patient shows any sign of a rash, if routine monitoring shows a significant reduction in any blood element, or if the patient develops an active bacterial or fungal infection. Severe reactions such as Stevens-Johnson syndrome or toxic epidermal necrolysis may have occurred.
- Monitor patient's hematologic status, as ordered, and report abnormalities. When drug is used prophylactically for 2 months or longer, a mild but reversible leukopenia may occur. Although rare, severe reactions such as agranulocytosis, aplastic anemia, and other blood dyscrasias may occur.
- If the patient has impaired renal function or if therapy is expected to last longer than 3 months, routinely monitor the pa-

tient's BUN and serum creatinine levels and obtain urine samples for microscopic examination.

PATIENT TEACHING

• Instruct patient to avoid excessive sun exposure.
• Stress the importance of stopping drug and notifying prescriber immediately at the first sign of rash.
• Tell patient to drink at least 8 glasses of fluid daily to prevent crystalluria and stone formation.
• Instruct patient to notify prescriber immediately if he develops a sore throat, fever, achy joints, cough, shortness of breath, pallor, bruising, jaundice, or glossitis because the drug may need to be stopped and medical treatment given.
• Urge female patients of childbearing age to avoid pregnancy and not to breast-feed their infants during sulfadoxine and pyrimethamine therapy because sulfadoxine crosses the placenta and appears in breast milk, possibly causing kernicterus.

sulfamethoxazole and trimethoprim (co-trimoxazole)

Apo-Sulfatrim (CAN), Bactrim, Bactrim-DS, Bactrim Pediatric, Cofatrim Forte, Cotrim, Cotrim DS, Cotrim Pediatric, Novo-Trimel (CAN), Nu-Cotrimox (CAN), Roubac (CAN), Septra, Septra DS, Septra Pediatric, Sulfatrim, Sulfatrim DS, Sulfatrim S/S, Sulfatrim Suspension

Class and Category

Chemical: Sulfonamide derivative (sulfamethoxazole), dihydrofolic acid analogue (trimethoprim)
Therapeutic: Antibiotic
Pregnancy category: C

Indications and Dosages

▶ *To treat acute otitis media, shigellosis, UTI, and other infections caused by gram-negative organisms (including* Enterobacter *species,* Escherichia coli, Haemophilus ducreyi, Haemophilus influenzae, *indole-positive* Proteus *species,* Klebsiella pneumoniae, Neisseria gonorrhoeae, Proteus mirabilis, Providencia *species,* Salmonella *species,* Serratia *species, and* Shigella *species) and gram-positive organisms (including group A beta-hemolytic streptococci,* Nocardia *species,* Staphylococcus aureus, *and* Streptococcus pneumoniae)

ORAL SUSPENSION, TABLETS

Adults. 800 mg of sulfamethoxazole and 160 mg of trimetho-

prim every 12 hr for 10 to 14 days (5 days for shigellosis).
Children age 2 months and over. 40 mg/kg of sulfamethoxazole and 8 mg/kg of trimethoprim daily in two divided doses every 12 hr for 10 days (5 days for shigellosis).
DOSAGE ADJUSTMENT If creatinine clearance is 15 to 30 ml/min/1.73 m², dosage reduced by one-half. If creatinine clearance is less than 15 ml/min/1.73 m², drug should be avoided.
I.V. INFUSION
Adults and children over age 2 months. 40 to 50 mg/kg of sulfamethoxazole and 8 to 10 mg/kg of trimethoprim daily in divided doses every 6, 8, or 12 hr for up to 5 days for shigellosis, 14 days for UTI.
▶ *To treat acute exacerbation of chronic bronchitis*
ORAL SUSPENSION, TABLETS
Adults. 800 mg of sulfamethoxazole and 160 mg of trimethoprim every 12 hr for 14 days.
▶ *To treat traveler's diarrhea*
ORAL SUSPENSION, TABLETS
Adults. 800 mg of sulfamethoxazole and 160 mg of trimethoprim every 12 hr for 5 days.
▶ *To prevent* Pneumocystis jiroveci (carinii) *pneumonia*
ORAL SUSPENSION, TABLETS
Adults. 800 mg of sulfamethoxazole and 160 mg of trimethoprim every 24 hr.
Children. 750 mg/m² of sulfamethoxazole and 150 mg/m² of trimethoprim daily in two divided doses on 3 consecutive days weekly. *Maximum:* 1,600 mg of sulfamethoxazole and 320 mg of trimethoprim daily.
▶ *To treat* P. jiroveci (carinii) *pneumonia*
ORAL SUSPENSION, TABLETS
Adults. 100 mg/kg of sulfamethoxazole and 15 to 20 mg/kg of trimethoprim daily in divided doses every 6 hr for 14 to 21 days.
I.V. INFUSION
Adults and children over age 2 months. 75 to 100 mg/kg of sulfamethoxazole and 15 to 20 mg/kg of trimethoprim daily in three or four divided doses every 6 to 8 hr for up to 14 days.

Incompatibilities
Don't mix co-trimoxazole with other drugs or solutions.

Contraindications
Age under 2 months; hypersensitivity to sulfamethoxazole, sul-

fonamides, trimethoprim, or their components; megaloblastic anemia caused by folate deficiency

---

Mechanism of Action

Blocks two consecutive steps in the formation of essential nucleic acids and proteins in susceptible organisms. Sulfamethoxazole inhibits synthesis of dehydrofolic acid (a nucleic acid) by competing with para-aminobenzoic acid. Trimethoprim inhibits the action of the enzyme dihydrofolate reductase, thus blocking production of tetrahydrofolic acid.

Interactions

DRUGS

ACE inhibitors: Possibly increased risk of hyperkalemia in elderly patients

cyclosporine: Decreased blood level and effectiveness of cyclosporine; increased risk of nephrotoxicity

digoxin: Possibly increased blood digoxin level and increased risk of digoxin toxicity

diuretics: Increased risk of thrombocytopenic purpura in elderly patients

indomethacin: Possibly increased blood co-trimoxazole level

methotrexate: Increased blood methotrexate level and risk of methotrexate toxicity

phenytoin: Possibly decreased hepatic clearance and prolonged half-life of phenytoin

pyrimethamine (dosage greater than 25 mg/wk): Increased risk of megaloblastic anemia

sulfonylureas: Possibly increased hypoglycemic effects

tricyclic antidepressants: Decreased antidepressant effectiveness

warfarin: Increased anticoagulant effects

Adverse Reactions

CNS: Anxiety, aseptic meningitis, ataxia, chills, depression, fatigue, hallucinations, headache, insomnia, seizures, vertigo

EENT: Glossitis, stomatitis

GI: Abdominal pain, anorexia, diarrhea, hepatitis, nausea, pancreatitis, pseudomembranous enterocolitis, vomiting

GU: Crystalluria, renal failure, toxic nephrosis

HEME: Agranulocytosis, eosinophilia, hemolytic anemia, leukopenia, methemoglobinemia, neutropenia, thrombocytopenia

RESP: Cough, dyspnea
SKIN: Dermatitis, erythema, photosensitivity, rash, Stevens-Johnson syndrome, toxic epidermal necrolysis, urticaria
Other: Anaphylaxis, hyperkalemia, injection site inflammation and pain

Nursing Considerations

- Use cautiously in patients with impaired hepatic or renal function, severe allergy or bronchial asthma, or possible folate deficiency (the elderly, long-term alcoholics, patients taking anticonvulsants, patients who are malnourished or have malabsorption).
- Expect to obtain culture and sensitivity test results before starting co-trimoxazole.
- For I.V. infusion, dilute each 5 ml of co-trimoxazole with 75 to 125 ml of D₅W before administration.
- When giving drug to neonates, don't mix with solutions that contain benzyl alcohol because this preservative has been linked to a fatal toxic syndrome involving circulatory, CNS, renal, and respiratory impairment and metabolic acidosis.
- Infuse slowly over 60 to 90 minutes.
- Watch for evidence of blood dyscrasia, including bleeding, ecchymosis, and joint pain, especially in elderly patients who are also taking a thiazide diuretic.
- Monitor elderly patients closely because they have an increased risk of bone marrow suppression, hyperkalemia, and severe skin reactions.
- Monitor patient closely for diarrhea, which may indicate pseudomembranous colitis. If diarrhea occurs, notify prescriber and expect to withhold drug. Expect to treat pseudomembranous colitis with fluids, electrolytes, protein, and an antibiotic effective against *Clostridium difficile.*

PATIENT TEACHING

- To minimize photosensitivity, advise patient to avoid direct sunlight and to use sunscreen.
- Instruct patient to notify prescriber immediately if rash or other serious adverse reactions occur.
- Urge patient to tell prescriber about diarrhea that's severe or lasts longer than 3 days. Remind patient that watery or bloody stools can occur 2 months or more after sulfamethoxale and trimethoprim therapy and can be serious, requiring prompt treatment.

ticarcillin disodium and clavulanate potassium

Timentin

Class and Category

Chemical: Penicillin
Therapeutic: Antibiotic combination
Pregnancy category: B

Indications and Dosages

▶ *To treat moderate to severe infections, such as appendicitis, bacteremia, bone and joint infections (including osteomyelitis), diabetic foot ulcer, diverticulitis, gynecologic infections (including endometritis), infectious arthritis, intra-abdominal infection, lower respiratory tract infections (including pneumonia), peritonitis, septicemia, skin and soft-tissue infections (including cellulitis), and UTI caused by susceptible organisms; to manage febrile neutropenia*

I.V. INFUSION

Adults and children age 12 and over weighing 60 kg (132 lb) or more. 3.1 grams (3 grams ticarcillin and 100 mg clavulanic acid) infused over 30 min every 4 to 6 hr.

Adults and children age 12 and over weighing less than 60 kg. 200 to 300 mg/kg/day (based on ticarcillin content) in divided doses every 4 to 6 hr.

Children and infants over age 3 months. For mild to moderate infections, 200 mg/kg/day (based on ticarcillin content) in divided doses every 6 hr; for severe infections, 300 mg/kg/day (based on ticarcillin content) in divided doses every 4 to 6 hr.

▶ *To treat pulmonary infections caused by complications of cystic fibrosis, such as bronchiectasis or pneumonia*

I.V. INFUSION

Children. 350 to 450 mg/kg/day (based on ticarcillin content) in divided doses.

DOSAGE ADJUSTMENT For patients with renal impairment, loading dose of 3.1 g; then dosage adjusted based on creatinine clearance.

Incompatibilities

Don't give ticarcillin and clavulanate through the same I.V. line as amikacin, gentamicin, or tobramycin. Don't give within 1 hour of aminoglycosides.

Contraindications

Hypersensitivity to ticarcillin, clavulanic acid, or their components

Mechanism of Action

Ticarcillin inhibits bacterial cell wall synthesis by binding to specific penicillin-binding proteins located inside bacterial cell walls. In this way, the drug ultimately leads to cell wall lysis and death.

Clavulanic acid, which doesn't alter the action of ticarcillin, binds with bound and extracellular beta-lactamase, preventing beta-lactamase from inactivating ticarcillin.

Interactions

DRUGS

aminoglycosides: Additive or synergistic activity against some bacteria, possibly mutual inactivation
anticoagulants: Possibly interference with platelet aggregation
methotrexate: Prolonged blood methotrexate level, increased risk of methotrexate toxicity
oral estrogen and progesterone combination contraceptives: Decreased contraceptive effectiveness
probenecid: Prolonged blood ticarcillin level

Adverse Reactions

CV: Thrombophlebitis, vasculitis
GI: Elevated liver function test results, nausea, pseudomembranous colitis, vomiting
GU: Proteinuria
HEME: Anemia, eosinophilia, hemorrhage, leukopenia, neutropenia, prolonged bleeding time, thrombocytopenia
SKIN: Erythema nodosum, exfoliative dermatitis, pruritus, rash, toxic epidermal necrolysis, urticaria
Other: Anaphylaxis, hypernatremia, hypokalemia, infusion site pain

Nursing Considerations

- Keep in mind that 3.1 grams of combination drug ticarcillin and clavulanate corresponds to 3 grams ticarcillin and 100 mg clavulanic acid.
- Dilute reconstituted I.V. solution to 10 to 100 mg/ml with compatible I.V. solution. To minimize vein irritation, don't exceed 100 mg/ml. Concentrations of 50 mg/ml or greater are preferred. Infuse appropriate I.V. dose over 30 to 120 minutes.
- Know that ticarcillin and clavulanate may worsen symptoms in patients with a history of GI disease or colitis.

- For patients with renal impairment, implement seizure precautions according to facility policy because they're at increased risk for seizures.
- Watch for evidence of superinfection, such as oral candidiasis and rash, in a breast-feeding infant.
- Monitor patient closely for diarrhea, which may indicate pseudomembranous colitis. If diarrhea occurs, notify prescriber and expect to withhold drug. Expect to treat pseudomembranous colitis with fluids, electrolytes, protein, and an antibiotic effective against *Clostridium difficile.*
- Monitor serum electrolyte levels for hypernatremia because of this drug's high sodium content. Monitor patient for hypokalemia from increased urinary potassium loss.
- **WARNING** Monitor patient's platelet count, PT, and APTT because drug may increase bleeding time and, in rare cases, may induce thrombocytopenia.
- Be aware that patient receiving high doses of ticarcillin may develop pseudoproteinuria.

PATIENT TEACHING
- Instruct patient taking ticarcillin and clavulanate to report past allergies to penicillins and to notify prescriber immediately about adverse reactions, including fever.
- Advise patient to decrease sodium intake to reduce the risk of electrolyte imbalance.
- Urge patient to tell prescriber about diarrhea that's severe or lasts longer than 3 days. Remind patient that watery or bloody stools can occur 2 months or more after ticarcillin and clavulanate therapy and can be serious, requiring prompt treatment.

Cardiovascular Drugs

aliskiren and hydrochlorothiazide
Tekturna HCT

Class and Category
Chemical: Hemifumarate salt (aliskiren), benzothiadiazide (hydrochlorothiazide)
Therapeutic: Antihypertensive, direct renin inhibitor (aliskiren), thiazide diuretic (hydrochlorothiazide)
Pregnancy category: D

Indications and Dosages
▶ *To treat hypertension when either drug alone fails to control blood pressure, when dose-related adverse reactions occur, or when hypokalemia occurs with hydrochlorothiazide monotherapy therapy despite adequate blood pressure control*
TABLETS
Adults. *Initial:* 150 mg aliskiren and 12.5 mg hydrochlorothiazide (one tablet) once daily. May be increased as needed every 2 to 4 weeks. *Maximum:* 300 mg aliskiren and 25 mg hydrochlorothiazide (one 300/25-mg tablet or two 150/12.5-mg tablets) once daily.

Contraindications
Anuria, hypersensitivity to aliskiren, hydrochlorothiazide, or sulfonamide derived drugs, or their components; pregnancy; renal impairment, disease, or failure

Interactions
DRUGS
aliskiren
ACE inhibitors, potassium-sparing diuretics, angiotensin receptor blockers, potassium supplements: Increased risk of hyperkalemia
atorvastatin, cyclosporine, ketoconazole: Increased aliskiren blood level
furosemide: Decreased blood furosemide levels

irbesartan: Decreased aliskiren blood level

hydrochlorothiazide

adrenocorticotropic hormone, amphotericin B, corticosteroids: Increased electrolyte depletion, especially of potassium

amantadine: Possibly increased amantadine blood level and risk of toxicity

amiodarone: Increased risk of arrhythmias from hypokalemia

antihypertensives: Increased antihypertensive effects

barbiturates, opioids: Possibly orthostatic hypotension

calcium: Possibly increased serum calcium level

cholestyramine, colestipol: Reduced GI absorption of hydrochlorothiazide

diazoxide: Increased antihypertensive and hyperglycemic effects of hydrochlorothiazide

diflunisal: Possibly increased blood hydrochlorothiazide level

digoxin: Increased risk of digitalis toxicity from hypokalemia

dopamine: Possibly increased diuretic effects of both drugs

insulin, oral antidiabetic drugs: Possibly increased blood glucose level

lithium: Decreased lithium clearance; increased risk of lithium toxicity

neuromuscular blockers: Possibly increased neuromuscular blockade from hypokalemia

nondepolarizing skeletal muscle relaxants: Possibly increased response to muscle relaxants

NSAIDs: Decreased diuretic effect of hydrochlorothiazide; increased risk of renal failure

oral anticoagulants: Possibly decreased oral anticoagulant effect

sympathomimetics: Possibly decreased antihypertensive effect of hydrochlorothiazide

vitamin D: Increased risk of hypercalcemia

ACTIVITIES

alcohol use: Possibly orthostatic hypotension

Adverse Reactions

CNS: Asthenia, dizziness, fatigue, fever, headache, insomnia, paresthesia, restlessness, seizures, vertigo, weakness

CV: Hypotension, orthostatic hypotension, vasculitis

EENT: Blurred vision, dry mouth, nasopharyngitis

ENDO: Hyperglycemia

GI: Abdominal cramps or pain, anorexia, constipation, diarrhea, dyspepsia, elevated liver ezyme levels, gastroesophageal reflux, jaundice, nausea, pancreatitis, vomiting

GU: Decreased libido, elevated blood urea nitrogen or creatinine levels, impotence, interstitial nephritis, nocturia, polyuria, renal calculi or failure
HEME: Agranulocytosis, aplastic anemia, decreased hemoglobin and hematocrit, hemolytic anemia, leukopenia, neutropenia, thrombocytopenia
MS: Arthralgia, back pain, muscle spasms and weakness
RESP: Increased cough, upper respiratory tract infection
SKIN: Alopecia, cutaneous vasculitis, erythema multiforme, exfoliative dermatitis, photosensitivity, purpura, rash, Stevens-Johnson syndrome, toxic epidermal necrolysis, urticaria
Other: Anaphylaxis, angioedema, dehydration, elevated creatine kinase or uric acid level, flulike symptoms, gout, hypercalcemia, hyperkalemia, hyperuricemia, hypochloremia, hypokalemia, hyponatremia, hypovolemia, metabolic alkalosis, weight loss

---

Mechanism of Action

Aliskiren inhibits renin secreted by the kidneys in response to decreased blood volume and renal perfusion. Renin cleaves angiotensinogen to form angiotensin I, which is converted to angiotensin II by ACE and non-ACE pathways. Angiotension II is a powerful vasoconstrictor that induces release of catecholamines from the adrenal medulla and prejunctional nerve endings. It also promotes aldosterone secretion and sodium reabsorption. Together, these actions increase blood pressure. By inhibiting renin release, aliskiren impairs the renin-angiotensin-aldosterone system. Without the vasoconstrictive effect of angiotension II, blood pressure decreases.

Hydrochlorothiazide, a thiazide diuretic, promotes movement of sodium (Na+), chloride (Cl-), and water (H$_2$O) from blood in the peritubular capillaries into the nephron's distal convoluted tubule. Initially, hydrochlorothiazide may decrease extracellular fluid volume, plasma volume, and cardiac output, which helps explain blood pressure reduction. It also may reduce blood pressure by directly dilating arteries. After several weeks, extracellular fluid volume, plasma volume, and cardiac output return to normal, and peripheral vascular resistance remains decreased.

Nursing Considerations

- To prevent hypotension, take measures to correct volume or salt depletion from high-dose diuretic therapy before starting aliskiren and hydrochlorothiazide. If hypotension occurs during therapy, place patient in a supine position and give normal saline solution intravenously, as needed and prescribed.

- Use aliskiren and hydrochlorothiazide cautiously in patients with hepatic impairment because hydrochlorothiazide may cause hepatic coma with even minor alterations of fluid and electrolyte balance.
- Give drug in the morning to avoid nocturia.
- **WARNING** The risk of angioedema with aliskiren is unknown. Watch closely for angioedema, especially in high-risk populations, such as African-Americans. If angioedema occurs, discontinue aliskiren and hydrochlorothiazide, notify prescriber, and provide supportive therapy until swelling has ceased. If swelling involves tongue, glottis, or larynx, be prepared to give epinephrine solution 1:1,000 (0.3 ml to 0.5 ml), as prescribed, and ensure a patent airway.
- Monitor fluid intake and output, daily weight, blood pressure, and serum levels of electrolytes, especially potassium.
- Assess patient for evidence of hypokalemia, such as muscle spasms and weakness.
- Check BUN and serum creatinine levels regularly.
- Monitor blood glucose level often, as ordered, in diabetic patients, and expect to increase antidiabetic drug dosage, as needed.
- If patient has a history of gouty arthritis, expect an increased risk of gout attacks during therapy.
- Monitor patient with systemic lupus erythematosus because hydrochlorothiazide may worsen it.

PATIENT TEACHING

- Advise patient to take aliskiren and hydrochorothiazide in the morning to avoid needing to urinate during the night. Also advise against eating a high-fat meal within 2 hours of taking the drug because doing so decreases drug absorption substantially.
- Instruct patient to take the drug with low-fat milk or food if adverse GI reactions occur.
- Direct patient to weigh himself at the same time each day wearing the same amount of clothing and to notify prescriber if he gains more than 2 lb (0.9 kg) per day or 5 lb (2.3 kg) per week.
- Teach patient how to monitor blood pressure to determine effectiveness of aliskiren and hydrochlorothiazide therapy.
- Stress the need to stop aliskiren and hydrochlorothiazide and seek immediate medical attention for swelling of face, limbs, eyes, lips, or tongue or trouble swallowing or breathing.
- Instruct patient not to increase potassium intake through supplements or potassium-containing salt substitutes without con-

sulting prescriber.
• Advise patient to change position slowly to minimize effects of orthostatic hypotension.
• Urge patient to notify prescriber about decreased urination, muscle cramps and weakness, and unusual bleeding or bruising.
• Instruct female patient to notify prescriber immediately if she is or could be pregnant because drug will need to be discontinued and another antihypertensive chosen.

amiloride hydrochloride and hydrochlorothiazide
Moduretic

Class and Category
Chemical: Pyrazine-carbonyl-guanidine (amiloride), benzothiadiazide (hydrochlorothiazide)
Therapeutic: Antihypertensive (amiloride, hydrochlorothiazide), potassium-sparing diuretic (amiloride), diuretic (hydrochlorothiazide)
Pregnancy category: B

Indications and Dosages
▶ *To manage hypertension or heart failure while preventing diuretic-induced hypokalemia*
TABLETS
Adults. 5 mg amiloride and 50 mg hydrochlorothiazide (1 tablet) daily; increased, as needed, to 10 mg amiloride and 100 mg hydrochlorothiazide (2 tablets) daily or 5 mg amiloride and 50 mg hydrochlorothiazide (1 tablet) b.i.d.

Mechanism of Action
Amiloride inhibits sodium reabsorption in the distal convoluted tubules and cortical collecting ducts of the kidneys. This results in sodium and water loss, which reduces blood pressure and enhances potassium retention.

Hydrochlorothiazide promotes the movement of sodium, chloride, and water from blood in the peritubular capillaries into the nephron's distal convoluted tubule. Initially, it may decrease extracellular fluid volume, plasma volume, and cardiac output, which helps explain blood pressure reduction. It also may reduce blood pressure by causing direct dilation of arteries. After several weeks, extracellular fluid volume, plasma volume, and cardiac output return to normal, and peripheral vascular resistance remains decreased.

Contraindications

Hypersensitivity to amiloride, hydrochlorothiazide, other sulfonamides or thiazides, or their components; impaired renal function; serum potassium level above 5.5 mEq/L; therapy with another potassium-sparing diuretic, such as spironolactone or triamterene; or use of a potassium supplement

Interactions

DRUGS

amiloride and hydrochlorothiazide
antihypertensives: Increased antihypertensive effects
digoxin: Decreased effectiveness of digoxin
lithium: Reduced renal clearance of lithium and increased risk of lithium toxicity
NSAIDs: Reduced diuretic effect of amiloride and hydrochlorothiazide

amiloride
ACE inhibitors, angiotensin II receptor antagonists, cyclosporine, potassium products, spironolactone, tacrolimus: Increased risk of hyperkalemia

hydrochlorothiazide
amantadine: Possibly increased amantadine blood level and risk of toxicity
amiodarone: Increased risk of arrhythmias from hypokalemia
amphotericin B, corticosteroids: Intensified electrolyte depletion, especially hypokalemia
barbiturates, opioids: May potentiate orthostatic hypotension
calcium: Possibly increased serum calcium level
cholestyramine, colestipol resins: Reduced GI absorption of hydrochlorothiazide
diazoxide: Increased antihypertensive and hyperglycemic effects of hydrochlorothiazide
diflunisal: Possibly increased blood hydrochlorothiazide level
digoxin: Increased risk of digitalis toxicity from hypokalemia
dopamine: Possibly increased diuretic effects of both drugs
insulin, oral antidiabetics: Possibly increased blood glucose level
neuromuscular blockers: Possibly increased neuromuscular blockade from hypokalemia
nondepolarizing skeletal muscle relaxants (such as tubocurarine): Possibly increased responsiveness to the muscle relaxant
pressor amines (such as norepinephrine): Possibly decreased response to pressor amines
oral anticoagulants: Possibly decreased anticoagulant effects

sympathomimetics: Possibly decreased antihypertensive effect of hydrochlorothiazide

vitamin D: Increased risk of hypercalcemia

FOODS

amiloride

high-potassium foods: Increased risk of hyperkalemia

Adverse Reactions

CNS: Confusion, depression, dizziness, drowsiness, encephalopathy, fatigue, headache, insomnia, nervousness, paresthesia, somnolence, tremor, vertigo, weakness

CV: Angina, arrhythmia, hypotension, palpitations, orthostatic hypotension, vasculitis

EENT: Blurred vision, dry mouth, increased intraocular pressure, nasal congestion, tinnitus, visual disturbances

ENDO: Hyperglycemia

GI: Abdominal pain, anorexia, constipation, diarrhea, GI bleeding, heartburn, indigestion, jaundice, nausea, vomiting

GU: Bladder spasms, decreased libido, dysuria, impotence, interstitial nephritis, nocturia, polyuria, renal failure

HEME: Agranulocytosis, aplastic anemia, hemolytic anemia, leukopenia, neutropenia, thrombocytopenia

MS: Arthralgia, leg pain, muscle spasms and weakness

RESP: Cough, dyspnea

SKIN: Alopecia, exfoliative dermatitis, photosensitivity, pruritus, purpura, rash, urticaria

Other: Anaphylaxis, dehydration, hypercalcemia, hyperchloremia, hyperkalemia, hyperuricemia, hypochloremia, hypokalemia, hyponatremia, hypovolemia, metabolic alkalosis, weight loss

Nursing Considerations

• Monitor blood pressure often to assess effectiveness of amiloride and hydrochlorothiazide therapy.

• Monitor fluid intake and output, daily weight, blood pressure, and serum levels of electrolytes, especially potassium, to detect volume depletion or electrolyte imbalance.

• **WARNING** Don't give amiloride and hydrochlorothiazide with other potassium-sparing diuretics.

• Watch for increased BUN and serum creatinine levels, especially in patients with impaired renal function, because drug may cause acute renal failure. If increases are significant or persistent, notify prescriber immediately.

• Monitor blood glucose level often in diabetic patients, and expect to increase antidiabetic dosage, as needed and ordered.

- If patient has a history of gouty arthritis, monitor patient for gout attacks during therapy.

PATIENT TEACHING

- Advise patient to take amiloride and hydrochlorothiazide with food in the morning or early evening to avoid the need to urinate during the night.
- Teach patient to monitor her blood pressure and to report consistently elevated measurements to prescriber.
- Direct patient to weigh herself at the same time each day wearing the same amount of clothing and to notify prescriber if she gains more than 2 lb (0.9 kg) per day or 5 lb (2.3 kg) per week.
- Instruct patient to avoid eating a diet high in potassium-rich foods, including citrus fruits, bananas, tomatoes, dates, and salt substitutes that contain potassium.
- To reduce the risk of dehydration and hypotension, advise patient to avoid exercise in hot weather and alcohol use. Also instruct her to notify prescriber if she has prolonged diarrhea, nausea, or vomiting.
- Advise patient to change positions slowly to minimize effects of orthostatic hypotension.
- Caution patient to avoid hazardous activities until drug's CNS effects are known.
- Explain the importance of regular exercise, proper diet, and other lifestyle changes in controlling hypertension.
- Warn patient about possibility of reversible hair loss and for male patients the additional possibility of impotence.

amlodipine besylate and atorvastatin calcium

Caduet

Class and Category

Chemical: Dihydropyridine (amlodipine) and synthetically derived fermentation product (atorvastatin)

Therapeutic: Antianginal, antihypertensive (amlodipine); antihyperlipidemic, HMG-CoA reductase inhibitor (atorvastatin)

Pregnancy category: X

Indications and Dosages

▶ *To continue treatment of hyperlipidemia and either hypertension or angina previously treated individually; to continue treatment with one component and start treatment with a second component*

TABLETS

Adults. Highly individualized. Dosage may be equivalent to monotherapy with either drug, or both dosages may be higher than previously prescribed for additional effects, or dosage may be based on the component currently being prescribed plus the recommended starting dose for the added drug. (See monotherapy details below for usual adult dosages.)

Monotherapy with amlodipine

▶ *To control hypertension*

TABLETS

Adults. *Initial:* 5 mg daily, increased gradually over 10 to 14 days p.r.n. *Maximum:* 10 mg daily.

DOSAGE ADJUSTMENT Initial dosage of 2.5 mg daily for elderly patients or patients with impaired hepatic function. Increased gradually over 7 to 14 days based on response.

▶ *To treat chronic stable angina and Prinzmetal's (variant) angina*

TABLETS

Adults. 5 to 10 mg daily.

DOSAGE ADJUSTMENT 5 mg daily for elderly patients and patients with impaired hepatic function.

Monotherapy with atorvastatin

▶ *To control lipid levels as an adjunct to diet in primary (heterozygous familial and nonfamilial) hypercholesterolemia and mixed dyslipidemia*

TABLETS

Adults. *Initial:* 10 to 20 mg daily, increased according to lipid level. *Maintenance:* 10 to 80 mg daily.

DOSAGE ADJUSTMENT Initial dosage may be increased to 40 mg daily for patients who need significant reduction (more than 45%) of cholesterol levels.

▶ *To control lipid levels in homozygous familial hypercholesterolemia*

TABLETS

Adults. 10 to 80 mg daily.

▶ *To start treatment of hyperlipidemia and either hypertension or angina*

TABLETS

Adults. *Initial:* Dosage based on recommendations for monotherapies of amlodipine and atorvastatin. (See monotherapy details for usual adult dosages.) *Maximum:* 10 mg for amlodipine; 80 mg for atorvastatin.

Contraindications

Active liver disease; breast-feeding; hypersensitivity to atorvastatin, amlodipine, or their components; pregnancy; unexplained persistently elevated serum transaminase level

Mechanism of Action

Amlodipine binds to dihydropyridine and nondihydropyridine cell membrane receptor sites on myocardial and vascular smooth-muscle cells and inhibits the influx of extracellular calcium ions across slow calcium channels. This decrease in intracellular calcium level inhibits smooth-muscle cell contraction, relaxes coronary and vascular smooth muscles, and decreases peripheral vascular resistance and systolic and diastolic blood pressure. Decreased peripheral vascular resistance also reduces myocardial workload and oxygen demand, which may relieve angina. Also, by inhibiting coronary artery muscle cell contractions and restoring blood flow, amlodipine may relieve Prinzmetal's angina.

Atorvastatin reduces serum cholesterol and lipoprotein levels by inhibiting HMG-CoA reductase and cholesterol synthesis in the liver and by increasing the number of LDL receptors on liver cells, thus enhancing LDL uptake and breakdown.

Interactions

DRUGS

amlodipine

beta blockers: Possibly excessive hypotension
fentanyl: Increased risk of severe hypotension and increased fluid volume requirements during surgery

atorvastatin

antacids, colestipol: Possibly decreased blood atorvastatin level
azole antifungals, clarithromycin, cyclosporine, erythromycin, fibric acid derivatives, lopinavir and ritonavir, ritonavir and saquinavir: Increased risk of severe myopathy or rhabdomyolysis
digoxin: Possibly increased blood digoxin level, causing toxicity
erythromycin: Increased blood atorvastatin level
oral contraceptives (such as ethinyl estradiol and norethindrone): Increased hormone level

Adverse Reactions

CNS: Amnesia, anxiety, dizziness, emotional lability, facial paralysis, fatigue, fever, headache, hyperkinesia, lack of coordination, lethargy, light-headedness, malaise, paresthesia, peripheral neuropathy, somnolence, stroke, syncope, tremor, unusual dreams, weakness

CV: Arrhythmias, elevated serum CK level, hot flashes, hypotension, orthostatic hypotension, palpitations, peripheral edema, phlebitis, vasodilation

EENT: Amblyopia, altered refraction, cheilitis, dry eyes or mouth, epistaxis, eye hemorrhage, gingival hemorrhage, glaucoma, glossitis, hearing loss, pharyngitis, sinusitis, stomatitis, taste loss or perversion, tinnitus

ENDO: Hyperglycemia, hypoglycemia

GI: Abdominal cramps or pain, anorexia, bilary pain, colitis, constipation, diarrhea, duodenal or stomach ulcers, dysphagia, elevated liver enzymes, eructation, esophagitis, flatulence, gastroenteritis, hepatitis, increased appetite, indigestion, melena, nausea, pancreatitis, rectal hemorrhage, tenesmus, vomiting

GU: Abnormal ejaculation; albuminuria; cystitis; decreased libido; dysuria; epididymitis; hematuria; impotence; nephritis; nocturia; renal calculi; urinary frequency, incontinence, or urgency; urine retention; UTI; vaginal hemorrhage

HEME: Anemia, thrombocytopenia

MS: Arthralgia, back pain, bursitis, gout, leg cramps, myalgia, myasthenia gravis, myositis, neck rigidity, tendon contractures or rupture, tenosynovitis, torticollis

RESP: Dyspnea, pneumonia

SKIN: Acne, alopecia, contact dermatitis, diaphoresis, dry skin, ecchymosis, eczema, flushing, jaundice, petechiae, photosensitivity, pruritus, rash, seborrhea, ulceration, urticaria

Other: Allergic reaction, facial or generalized edema, flulike symptoms, infection, lymphadenopathy, weight gain or loss

Nursing Considerations

- Use amlodipine and atorvastatin cautiously in patients with heart block, heart failure, impaired renal function, or hepatic disorder.
- Monitor blood pressure when adjusting amlodipine, especially in patients with heart failure.
- If patient is receiving atorvastatin for the first time, expect to obtain liver function tests before therapy starts, after 6 and 12 weeks, every 6 months thereafter, and whenever the dosage increases.
- Expect to measure blood levels 2 to 4 weeks after first atorvastatin dose and to adjust dosage, as directed. Repeat this process periodically until levels are within desired range.
- Monitor elderly patients closely for changes in neurologic status because they may be at higher risk of hemorrhagic stroke while on amlopine and atorvastatin therapy.

PATIENT TEACHING

- Emphasize that amlodipine and atorvastatin is an adjunct to—

not a substitute for—a low-cholesterol diet and any other prescribed dietary restrictions.
- Tell patient to immediately notify prescriber about dizziness, arm or leg swelling, trouble breathing, hives, or rash. Also advise patient to notify prescriber immediately if he develops unexplained muscle pain, tenderness, or weakness, especially if accompanied by fatigue or fever.
- Suggest taking drug with food to reduce GI upset that may be caused by amlodipine.
- Advise patient to routinely have his blood pressure checked and his blood monitored to verify the effectiveness of therapy with amlodipine and atorvastatin.

amlodipine besylate and benazepril hydrochloride
Lotrel

Class and Category
Chemical: Dihydropyridine (amlodipine), ethylester of benazeprilat (benazepril)
Therapeutic: Antihypertensive (amlodipine, benazepril)
Pregnancy category: D

Indications and Dosages
▶ *To treat hypertension in patients not adequately controlled with amlodipine or benazepril therapy alone*
CAPSULES
Adults. *Initial:* Depending on patient's previous dosage of amlodipine or benazepril, 2.5 mg amlodipine and 10 mg benazepril (1 capsule) to 10 mg amlodipine and 20 mg benazepril (1 capsule) daily. If dosage is started at lower end, may be gradually increased, as needed, based on response. *Maximum:* 10 mg amlodipine and 20 mg benazepril daily.
DOSAGE ADJUSTMENT Initial dosage of 2.5 mg amlodipine and 10 mg benazepril daily for elderly patients or patients with impaired hepatic function. Dosage increased gradually based on response.

Contraindications
History of hereditary or idiopathic angioedema; hypersensitivity to amlodipine, benazepril, other ACE inhibitors or their components; pregnancy

Mechanism of Action
Amlodipine binds to dihydropyridine and nondihydropyridine cell membrane receptor sites on myocardial and vascular smooth-muscle cells and inhibits the influx of extracellular calcium ions across slow calcium channels. This decreases the intracellular calcium level, inhibiting smooth-muscle cell contractions, relaxing coronary and vascular smooth muscles, decreasing peripheral vascular resistance, and reducing systolic and diastolic blood pressure.

Benazepril may reduce blood pressure by affecting the renin-angiotensin-aldosterone system. By inhibiting ACE, benazepril:
- prevents conversion of angiotensin I to angiotensin II, a potent vasoconstrictor that also stimulates adrenal cortex to secrete aldosterone.
- may inhibit renal and vascular production of angiotensin II.
- decreases serum angiotensin II level and increases serum renin activity. This decreases aldosterone secretion, slightly increasing serum potassium level and fluid loss.
- decreases vascular tone and blood pressure.
- inhibits aldosterone release, which reduces sodium and water reabsorption and increases their excretion, further reducing blood pressure.

Interactions
DRUGS
amlodipine and benazepril
diuretics: Possibly excessive reduction of blood pressure when amlodipine and benazepril therapy starts.
lithium: Possibly increased serum lithium level and risk of toxicity
potassium supplements, potassium-sparing diuretics: Possibly increased serum potassium level
amlodipine
beta blockers: Possibly excessive hypotension
fentanyl: Increased risk of severe hypotension and increased fluid volume requirements during surgery
benazepril
antacids: Possibly decreased benazepril bioavailability
capsaicin: Possibly induced or exacerbated ACE inhibitor cough
digoxin: Increased serum digoxin level
phenothiazines: Possibly increased intended and adverse benazepril effects

Adverse Reactions
CNS: Anxiety, asthenia, dizziness, fatigue, headache, insomnia, nervousness, somnolence, tremor

CV: Edema, orthostatic hypotension, palpitations
EENT: Dry mouth, pharyngitis
ENDO: Hot flashes
GI: Abdominal pain, constipation, diarrhea, dyspepsia, esophagitis, nausea
GU: Decreased libido, elevated plasma BUN and serum creatinine levels, impotence, polyuria
MS: Back pain, musculoskeletal pain or cramps
RESP: Cough
SKIN: Dermatitis, flushing, rash, skin nodule
Other: Anaphylaxis, angioedema, hypokalemia

Nursing Considerations
- Use amlodipine and benazepril cautiously in patients with heart block, heart failure, impaired renal function, or heptatic disorder because amlodipine can cause fluid retention.
- Before starting amlodipine and benazepril, evaluate blood pressure with patient lying down, sitting, and standing. Then monitor it throughout therapy to evaluate drug effectiveness.
- Check urine output and BUN and serum creatinine levels, as appropriate, before therapy begins. Drug should not be used if serum creatinine level is less than 30 ml/min/1.73 m^2.
- **WARNING** Be alert for anaphylactoid reactions, including angioedema, especially after the first dose. If angioedema extends to larynx and patient has laryngeal stridor or signs of airway obstruction, stop drug and prepare to give epinephrine subcutaneously immediately, as prescribed.
- Monitor WBC count periodically, especially in patients with collagen-vascular disease, to detect neutropenia and agranulocytosis. Although they aren't known to occur with benazepril, they have occurred with captropril, another ACE inhibitor.
- Check liver enzymes and monitor patient for jaundice because hepatic failure, although rare, has occurred with other ACE inhibitors. If liver enzymes increase or patient develops jaundice, notify prescriber and expect to stop amlodipine and benazepril.

PATIENT TEACHING
- Teach patient how to monitor blood pressure, if appropriate, and how to recognize signs of hypertension and hypotension.
- **WARNING** Urge patient to contact prescriber before using potassium supplements or OTC salt substitutes, which may contain potassium. They increase the risk of hyperkalemia.
- Inform patient that a persistent dry cough may develop and may not subside unless amlodipine and benazepril therapy is

stopped. If cough becomes bothersome or interferes with sleep or activities, instruct patient to notify prescriber.

• **WARNING** Instruct patient to contact prescriber immediately if she develops evidence of hypersensitivity, especially angioedema, (swelling of the face, eyes, lips, or tongue), difficulty breathing, hives, or rash.

• Urge patient to change position slowly and to rise slowly from a sitting or lying position to minimize orthostatic hypotension.

• Tell patient to notify prescriber if she is, could be, or is planning to become pregnant because amlodopine and benazepril may adversely affect fetal development; therapy should be stopped.

amlodipine besylate and olmesartan medoxomil

Azor

Class and Category

Chemical: Dihydropyridine calcium channal blocker (amlodipine), angiotensin II receptor antagonist (olmesartan)
Therapeutic: Antihypertensive (amlodipine, olmesartan)
Pregnancy category: C (1st trimester); D (2nd and 3rd trimesters)

Indications and Dosages

▶ *To treat hypertension when initial therapy with amlodipine monotherapy, olmesartan monotherapy or other antihypertensive agents fails; as adjunct therapy to control hypertension*

TABLETS

Adults. *Initial:* 5 mg amlodipine and 20 mg olmesartan (1 tablet) once daily, increased as needed every 2 to 4 weeks. *Maximum:* 10 mg amlodipine and 40 mg olmesartan (1 tablet of 10/40 mg strength or 2 tablets of 5/20 mg strength) once daily.

Contraindications

Hypersensitivity to amlodipine, olmesartan, or their components

Interactions

DRUGS

amlodipine

aminoglutethimide, carbamazepine, nafcillin, nevirapine, phenobarbital, phenytoin, rifampin: Possibly decreased amlodipine level and effects
aminophylline, cyclosporine, fluvoxamine, mexiletine, mirtazapine, ropinirole, theophylline, trifluoperazine: Increased levels and effects of these drugs

azole antifungals, clarithromycin, diclofenac, doxycycline, erythromycin, imatinib, isoniazid, nefazodone, nicardipine, propofol, protease inhibitors, quinidine, telithromycin, verapamil: Increased amlodipine effects
beta blockers: Possibly excessive hypotension
calcium: Possibly decreased hypotensive effects of amlodipine
fentanyl: Increased risk of severe hypotension and increased fluid volume requirements during surgery
olmesartan
ACE inhibitors, potassium-sparing diuretics, angiotensin receptor blockers, potassium supplements: Increased risk of hyperkalemia
lithium: Possibly increased lithium toxicity
NSAIDs: Possibly decreased olmesartan effectiveness

Mechanism of Action

Amlodipine binds to dihydropyridine cell membrane receptor sites on myocardial and vascular smooth-muscle cells and inhibits influx of extracellular calcium ions across slow calcium channels. This decreases intracellular calcium level, inhibiting smooth-muscle cell contractions and relaxing coronary and vascular smooth muscles, decreasing peripheral vascular resistance and reducing systolic and diastolic blood pressure.

Olmesartan blocks the hormone angiotensin II from binding to receptor sites in vascular smooth muscle, adrenal glands, and other tissues. This action inhibits the vasoconstrictive and aldosterone-secreting of angiotensin II, thereby reducing blood pressure.

Adverse Reactions

CNS: Anxiety, asthenia, dizziness, fatigue, headache, insomnia, lethargy, light-headedness, paresthesia, somnolence, syncope, tremor, vertigo
CV: Arrhythmias, chest pain, hypercholesterolemia, hyperlipidemia, hypertriglyceridemia, hypotension, palpitations, peripheral edema, tachycardia
EENT: Dry mouth, pharyngitis, rhinitis, sinusitis
ENDO: Hot flashes, hyperglycemia, hyperuricemia
GI: Abdominal cramps or pain, constipation, diarrhea, elevated liver enzyme levels, esophagitis, gastroenteritis, indigestion, jaundice, nausea, vomiting
GU: Acute renal failure, decreased libido, elevated BUN and serum creatinine levels, hematuria, impotence, nocturia, urinary frequency, UTI
HEME: Decreased hemoglobin and hematocrit levels

MS: Arthralgia, arthritis, back pain, myalgia, rhabdomyolysis, skeletal pain
RESP: Bronchitis, cough, dyspnea, upper respiratory tract infection
SKIN: Alopecia, dermatitis, flushing, pruritus, rash, urticaria
Other: Angioedema, hyperkalemia, increased creatine kinase level, flulike symptoms, generalized pain, weight loss

Nursing Considerations

- Use cautiously in patients with heart block, heart failure, impaired renal function, hepatic disorder, or severe aortic stenosis because of amlodipine.
- Expect to provide treatment such as normal saline solution I.V., as prescribed, to correct known or suspected hypovolemia before starting amlodipine and olmesartan.
- Monitor blood pressure while adjusting dosage, especially in patients with heart failure or severe aortic stenosis.
- Expect to discontinue drug temporarily if patient has hypotension. Place patient in supine position immediately and prepare to administer normal saline solution I.V., as prescribed. Expect to resume drug therapy after blood pressure stabilizes.
- Watch for increased BUN and serum creatinine levels, especially in a patient with impaired renal function, because drug may cause acute renal failure. If increased levels are significant or persist, notify prescriber immediately.
- **WARNING** Monitor patient's blood pressure often if she receives a diuretic or other antihypertensive during therapy because of an increased risk of hypotension.
- If patient receives a diuretic, provide adequate hydration, as appropriate, to help prevent hypovolemia. Watch for evidence of hypovolemia, such as hypotension with dizziness and fainting.
- **WARNING** Monitor patient with severe obstructive coronary artery disease for increased frequency, duration, or severity of angina or development of acute MI, especially when amlodipine and olmesartan therapy starts or dosage is increased.

PATIENT TEACHING

- Tell patient to immediately notify prescriber of dizziness, arm or leg swelling, trouble breathing, hives, or rash.
- Advise patient to routinely have blood pressure checked to monitor drug effectiveness and detect hypotension.
- Advise patient to avoid exercise in hot weather and excessive consumption of alcohol to reduce the risk of dehydration and hypotension. Also instruct her to notify prescriber if she has prolonged diarrhea, nausea, or vomiting.

- Caution patient to avoid hazardous activities until drug's CNS effects are known.
- Explain the importance of regular exercise, proper diet, and other lifestyle changes in controlling hypertension.
- Advise female patient to notify prescriber immediately about known or suspected pregnancy. Explain that if she becomes pregnant, presriber may replace drug with another antihypertensive that is safe to use during pregnancy.

amlodipine and valsartan
Exforge

Class and Category
Chemical: Dihydropyridine (amlodipine), nonpeptide tetrazole derivative (valsartan)
Therapeutic: Antihypertensive, dihydropyridine calcium channel blocker (amlodipine), angiotension II receptor blocker (valsartan)
Pregnancy category: D

Indications and Dosages
▶ *To treat hypertension*
TABLETS
Adults. *Initial:* 5 mg amlodipine and 160 mg valsartan (1 tablet) daily, increased in 2 to 4 weeks as needed. *Maximum:* 10 mg amlodopine and 320 mg valsartan (1 tablet) daily.
DOSAGE ADJUSTMENT Initial dosage of 2.5 mg amlodopine and 160 mg valsartan (½ tablet of 5 mg/320 mg strength) daily for elderly patients. Dosage increased gradually for elderly patients and patients with hepatic or severe renal dysfunction.

Mechanism of Action
Amlodipine binds to dihydropyridine cell membrane receptor sites on myocardial and vascular smooth-muscle cells and inhibits influx of extracellular calcium ions across slow calcium channels. This decreases intracellular calcium level, inhibiting smooth-muscle cell contraction and relaxing coronary and vascular smooth muscles, decreasing peripheral vascular resistance, and reducing systolic and diastolic blood pressure.

Valsartan blocks the hormone angiotensin II from binding to receptor sites in vascular smooth muscle, adrenal glands, and other tissues. This action inhibits angiotensin II's vasoconstrictive and aldosterone-secreting effects, thereby reducing blood pressure.

Contraindications

Hypersensitivity to amlodipine, valsartan, or their components

Interactions

DRUGS

amlodipine and valsartan

other antihypertensives: Additive hypotensive effect

amlodipine

aminoglutethimide, carbamazepine, nafcillin, nevirapine, phenobarbital, phenytoin, rifampin: Possibly decreased amlodipine level and effects

aminophylline, cyclosporine, fluvoxamine, mexiletine, mirtazapine, ropinirole, theophylline, trifluoperazine: Increased levels and effects of these drugs

azole antifungals, clarithromycin, diclofenac, doxycycline, erythromycin, imatinib, isoniazid, nefazodone, nicardipine, propofol, protease inhibitors, quinidine, telithromycin, verapamil: Increased amlodipine level and effects

beta blockers: Possibly excessive hypotension

calcium: Possibly decreased hypotensive effects of amlodipine

fentanyl: Increased risk of severe hypotension and increased fluid volume requirements during surgery

valsartan

ACE inhibitors, potassium-sparing diuretics, angiotensin receptor blockers, potassium supplements: Increased risk of hyperkalemia

lithium: Possibly increased lithium toxicity

NSAIDs: Possibly decreased olmesartan effectiveness

diuretics: Additive hypotensive effects

FOODS

valsartan

potassium-containing salt substitutes: Possibly hyperkalemia

Adverse Reactions

CNS: Anxiety, dizziness, fatigue, headache, insomnia, lethargy, light-headedness, neuropathy, paresthesia, somnolence, syncope, tremor, vertigo

CV: Arrhythmias, cardiac failure, chest pain, hypotension, palpitations, peripheral edema or ischemia, vascultitis

EENT: Dry mouth, pharyngitis, rhinitis, sinusitis

ENDO: Hot flashes, hyperglycemia

GI: Abdominal cramps or pain, constipation, diarrhea, elevated liver enzyme levels, esophagitis, hepatitis, indigestion, nausea, pancreatitis, vomiting

GU: Decreased libido, impaired renal function, impotence, urinary frequency

HEME: Leukopenia, thrombocytopenia
MS: Arthralgia, myalgia
RESP: Cough, dyspnea, upper respiratory infection
SKIN: Dermatitis, flushing, pruritus, rash, urticaria
Other: Angioedema, hyperkalemia, hypersensitivity reaction, viral infection, weight loss

Nursing Considerations

- Amlodipne and valsartan shouldn't be given to patients who have hypovolemia or are taking a diuretic because of the increased risk of severe hypotension from volume depletion.
- Use drug cautiously in patients with heart block, heart failure, impaired renal function, hepatic disorder, severe aortic stenosis, recent myocardial infarction, dialysis, or surgery because it may induce hypotension under these conditions.
- Check blood pressure often during therapy to determine effectiveness and detect hypotension, which may be pronounced, especially in patients with heart failure or severe aortic stenosis.
- If hypotension occurs, place patient in a supine position and, if ordered, give an intravenous infusion of normal saline solution.
- **WARNING** Although uncommon, patients with severe obstructive coronary artery disease may develop increased frequency, duration, or severity of angina or acute myocardial infarction when therapy starts or dosage increases. Monitor patient closely.
- Be aware that maximal blood pressure reduction typically occurs after 4 weeks. If patient's blood pressure remains uncontrolled, notify prescriber and expect dosage to be increased or drug to be discontinued.
- Monitor serum potassium level because drug may elevate it by blocking aldosterone secretion.

PATIENT TEACHING
- Instruct patient to take amlodipine and valsartan exactly as prescribed at the same time every day to maintain its effects.
- Tell patient to immediately notify prescriber of dizziness, arm or leg swelling, trouble breathing, hives, or rash.
- Suggest taking amlodipine and valsartan with food if gastrointestinal upset occurs.
- Advise patient to routinely monitor blood pressure.
- Tell patient to avoid hazardous activities until drug's CNS effects are known.
- Instruct patient not to use potassium-containing salt substitutes without consulting prescriber.

- Advise female patient of childbearing age to use reliable birth control during therapy and to notify prescriber immediately if she is or could be pregnant; valsartan will need to be stopped.
- Urge patient to keep follow-up appointments with prescriber to monitor progress.

aspirin (buffered) and pravastatin sodium

Pravigard PAC

Class and Category

Chemical: Salicylate (aspirin), mevinic acid derivative (pravastatin)
Therapeutic: Antiplatelet (aspirin), antihyperlipidemic (pravastatin)
Pregnancy category: X

Indications and Dosages

▶ *To reduce the occurrence of cardiovascular events such as death, MI, and stroke in patients with cardiovascular or cerebrovascular disease*
TABLETS

Adults. *Initial:* 81 mg or 325 mg aspirin and 40 mg pravastatin daily. Pravastatin dosage may be increased every 4 wk, as needed. *Maintenance:* 81 mg or 325 mg aspirin and 40 to 80 mg pravastatin daily.

DOSAGE ADJUSTMENT For patients with significant renal or hepatic impairment, those taking immunosuppressants, and elderly patients, initial pravastatin dosage reduced to 10 mg daily. For elderly patients and those taking immunosuppressants, pravastatin maintenance dosage usually limited to 20 mg daily.

Mechanism of Action

Aspirin inhibits platelet aggregation by interfering with production of thromboxane A2, a substance that stimulates platelet aggregation. It also blocks the activity of cyclooxygenase, the enzyme needed for prostaglandin synthesis. Prostaglandins, important mediators in the inflammatory response, cause local vasodilation with swelling and pain. By blocking cyclooxygenase and inhibiting prostaglandins, aspirin causes inflammatory symptoms to subside.

Pravastatin inhibits cholesterol synthesis in the liver by blocking the enzyme needed to convert hydroxymethylglutaryl (HMG)-CoA to mevalonate, an early precursor of cholesterol. When cholesterol synthesis is blocked, the liver increases breakdown of LDL cholesterol.

Contraindications

Active hepatic disease or unexplained, persistent elevated liver function test results; allergy to tartrazine dye; asthma; bleeding problems such as hemophilia; breast-feeding; hypersensitivity to aspirin, pravastatin, or their components; peptic ulcer disease; pregnancy

Interactions

DRUGS

aspirin and pravastatin

anticoagulants: Increased bleeding or prolonged PT

pravastatin

cholestyramine, colestipol: Decreased pravastatin bioavailability

cyclosporine, erythromycin, gemfibrozil, immunosuppressants, niacin: Increased risk of rhabdomyolysis and acute renal failure

aspirin

ACE inhibitors: Decreased antihypertensive effect

activated charcoal: Decreased aspirin absorption

antacids, urine alkalinizers: Decreased aspirin effectiveness

ascorbic acid, furosemide, para-aminosalicylic acid: Increased risk of aspirin toxicity

carbonic anhydrase inhibitors: Salicylism

corticosteroids: Increased excretion and decreased blood level of aspirin

heparin: Increased risk of bleeding

methotrexate: Increased blood level and decreased excretion of methotrexate, causing toxicity

nizatidine: Increased blood aspirin level

NSAIDs: Possibly decreased blood NSAID level and increased risk of adverse GI effects

oral antidiabetics, insulin: Increased risk of hypoglycemia

penicillins, sulfonamides: Increased blood levels of penicillins and sulfonamides *probenecid, sulfinpyrazone:* Decreased effectiveness in treating gout

urine acidifiers (such as ammonium chloride and ascorbic acid): Decreased aspirin excretion

vancomycin: Increased risk of ototoxicity

ACTIVITIES

alcohol use: Increased risk of ulcers

Adverse Reactions

CNS: Anxiety, confusion, depression, dizziness, fatigue, headache, nervousness, sleep disturbance

CV: Angina pectoris, chest pain

EENT: Blurred vision, diplopia, hearing loss, rhinitis, tinnitus
GI: Abdominal pain, constipation, diarrhea, flatulence, GI bleeding, heartburn, hepatotoxicity, indigestion, nausea, pancreatitis, stomach pain, vomiting
GU: Dysuria, nocturia, urinary frequency
HEME: Decreased blood iron level, leukopenia, prolonged bleeding time, shortened RBC lifespan, thrombocytopenia
MS: Arthralgia, musculoskeletal cramps or pain, myalgia, myopathy, rhabdomyolysis
RESP: Cough, dyspnea, upper respiratory tract infection
SKIN: Ecchymosis, rash, urticaria
Other: Angioedema, Reye's syndrome

Nursing Considerations

• Use aspirin and pravastatin cautiously in patients with renal or hepatic impairment and in elderly patients.
• Give aspirin and pravastatin 1 hour before or 4 hours after giving cholestyramine or colestipol.
• Monitor BUN and serum creatinine levels and liver function test results periodically for abnormal elevations.
• Monitor lipoprotein level, as indicated, to evaluate drug effects.

PATIENT TEACHING

• Instruct patient to take aspirin with food or after meals because it may cause GI upset if taken on an empty stomach.
• Advise patient to consult prescriber before taking aspirin and pravastatin with any other prescription drug for blood disorder, diabetes, gout, or arthritis.
• Tell patient not to take aspirin that has a strong vinegar odor but to replace it with tablets that don't smell like vinegar.
• Instruct patient to notify prescriber immediately about development of muscle pain, tenderness, weakness, and other symptoms of myopathy.
• Urge female patient of childbearing age to use a reliable method of contraception during therapy and to notify prescriber at once if she becomes or suspects she might be pregnant.

atenolol and chlorthalidone
Tenoretic

Class and Category

Chemical: Cardioselective beta blocker (atenolol), phthalimidine derivative of benzenesulfonadmide (thiazide-like diuretic) (chlorthalidone)

Therapeutic: Antihypertensive (atenolol, chlorthalidone), diuretic (chlorthalidone)
Pregnancy category: D

Indications and Dosages

▶ *To treat hypertension*

TABLETS

Adults. 50 mg atenolol and 25 mg chlorthalidone (1 tablet) daily, increased, as needed, to 100 mg atenolol and 25 mg chlorthalidone (1 tablet) daily.

DOSAGE ADJUSTMENT For patients with creatinine clearance of 15 to 35 ml/min/1.73 m^2, atenolol dosage shouldn't exceed 50 mg daily. For patients with creatinine clearance below 15 ml/min/1.73 m^2, atenolol dosage shouldn't exceed 50 mg every other day.

Mechanism of Action

Atenolol inhibits stimulation of beta$_1$-receptor sites, which are located mainly in the heart, causing a decrease in cardiac excitability, cardiac output and myocardial oxygen demand. Atenolol also decreases release of renin from the kidneys, aiding in reducing blood pressure. At high doses, it inhibits stimulation of beta$_2$ receptors in the lungs, which may cause bronchoconstriction.

Chlorthalidone may promote sodium, chloride, and water excretion by inhibiting sodium reabsorption in the kidneys' distal tubules. Initially, it may decrease extracellular fluid volume, plasma volume, and cardiac output, which helps explain how it reduces blood pressure. It also may dilate arteries directly, helping reduce peripheral vascular resistance and blood pressure. After several weeks, extracelllar fluid and plasma volume and cardiac output return to normal, but peripheral vascular resistance remains decreased.

Contraindications

Anuria; breast-feeding; cardiogenic shock; heart block greater than first degree; hypersensitivity to atenolol, chlorthalidone, other sulfonamide-derived drugs, or their components; overt cardiac failure: sinus bradycardia

Interactions

DRUGS

atenolol and chlorthalidone

antihypertensives, catecholamine-depleting drugs (such as reserpine): Increased antihypertensive effect leading to hypotension, marked bradycardia, or both

clonidine: Increased risk of rebound hypertension
atenolol
calcium channel blockers (such as verapamil and diltiazem): Possibly symptomatic bradycardia and conduction abnormalities
chlorthalidone
allopurinol: Increased risk of allopurinol hypersensitivity
amphotericin B, glucocorticoids: Intensified electrolyte depletion
anesthetics: Potentiated effects of anesthetics
anticholinergics: Increased chlorthalidone absorption
antidiabetics, methenamines, oral anticoagulants, sulfonylureas: Decreased effects of these drugs
antineoplastics: Prolonged antineoplastic-induced leukopenia
cholestyramine, colestipol: Decreased chlorthalidone absorption
diazoxide: Increased risk of hyperglycemia and hypotension
digitalis glycosides: Increased risk of digitalis-induced arrhythmias
lithium: Decreased renal lithium clearance and increased risk of lithium toxicity
loop diuretics: Increased synergistic effects, resulting in profound diuresis and serious electrolyte imbalances
methyldopa: Potential development of hemolytic anemia
neuromuscular blockers: Increased neuromuscular blockade
NSAIDs: Possibly reduced diuretic effect of chlorthalidone
vitamin D: Enhanced vitamin D action

Adverse Reactions

CNS: Depression, dizziness, dreaming, drowsiness, fatigue, hallucinations, headache, lethargy, light-headedness, paresthesia, psychosis, restlessness, tiredness, weakness, vertigo
CV: Bradycardia, orthostatic hypotension, Raynaud's phenomenon, sick sinus syndrome, vasculitis
EENT: Dry eyes or mouth, visual disturbance
ENDO: Hyperglycemia
GI: Abdominal cramping, anorexia, constipation, diarrhea, elevated bilirubin and liver enzymes, gastric irritation, jaundice, nausea, pancreatitis, vomiting
GU: Impotence
HEME: Agranulocytosis, aplastic anemia, leukopenia, thrombocytopenia
MS: Cold extremities, leg pain, muscle spasm
RESP: Dyspnea, wheezing
SKIN: Alopecia (reversible), cutaneous vasculitis, exacerbation of psoriasis, photosensitivity, psoriasis type rash, purpura, toxic epidermal necrolysis, urticaria

Other: Antinuclear antibody formation, hyperuricemia, hypochloremic alkalosis, hypokalemia, hyponatremia, lupus syndrome, Peyronie's disease

Nursing Considerations

- Use atenolol and chlorthalidone cautiously in patients with impaired hepatic function or progressive hepatic disease because minor changes in fluid and electrolyte balance may cause hepatic coma.
- Use atenolol and chlorthalidone cautiously in patients with heart failure controlled by cardiac glycosides, conduction abnormalities, or left ventricular dysfunction who take verapamil or diltiazem and in patients with arterial circulatory disorders, bronchospastic disease, or impaired renal function.
- Assess patient's blood pressure regularly to determine effectiveness of therapy.
- Monitor patient for evidence of heart failure. At first sign of heart failure, expect patient to receive a cardiac glycoside, a diuretic, or both and to be monitored closely. If failure continues, expect atenolol and chlorthalidone to be stopped.
- Assess BUN, serum electrolytes, uric acid, and blood glucose level before and periodically during therapy. Monitor patient for signs of fluid and electrolyte imbalance.
- Monitor diabetic patients closely because atenolol may mask tachycardia caused by hypoglycemia. Unlike other beta blockers, atenolol doesn't mask other signs of hypoglycemia, cause hypoglycemia, or delay return of blood glucose to normal.
- Closely monitor patient with hyperthyroidism because atenolol may mask some signs of thyrotoxicosis. Avoid abrupt withdrawal of atenolol and chlorthalidone because it may prompt thyrotoxicosis or ischemic heart disease.
- Expect to stop drug several days before gradually withdrawing clonidine therapy, if prescribed. Then expect to restart atenolol and chlorthalidone several days after clonidine has been stopped because clonidine can cause rebound hypertension.
- Notify prescriber immediately if patient develops bradycardia, hypotension, or other serious adverse reactions.
- Stop atenolol and chlorthalidone, as ordered, before parathyroid function studies are performed because the chlorthalidone portion of the drug decreases calcium excretion.

PATIENT TEACHING

- Stress the importance of taking atenolol and chlorthalidone even when feeling well.

- Tell patient to take drug in the morning with food or milk to avoid gastric irritation.
- Caution patient not to stop taking atenolol and chlorthalidone abruptly because serious adverse effects may occur. Also tell patient that while being weaned from the drug, he should perform minimal physical activity to prevent chest pain.
- Inform diabetic patient that atenolol may alter his blood glucose level and mask a rapid heartbeat during a hypoglycemic reaction. Urge the patient to test his blood glucose level regularly.
- Instruct patient to rise slowly from a seated or lying position to minimize the effects of orthostatic hypotension.
- Teach patient to monitor his blood pressure and to report consistently elevated measurements to prescriber.
- Tell patient to protect his skin from the sun to avoid sunburn while taking atenolol and chlorthalidone.
- Urge patient to report sudden joint pain to prescriber immediately because drug can cause sudden gout attacks.
- Encourage patient to eat high-potassium foods, such as bananas, apricots, grapefruits, tomato juice, and orange juice.
- Advise patient to notify prescriber about symptoms of low potassium level (such as irregular heartbeat, muscle weakness, fatigue) or low sodium level (such as confusion, fatigue, irritability, muscle cramps).
- Advise female patient of childbearing age to notify prescriber if she is, could be, or plans to become pregnant or if she's breastfeeding because drug may cause serious adverse reactions in the fetus or newborn.

benazepril hydrochloride and hydrochlorothiazide
Lotensin HCT

Class and Category
Chemical: Ethylester of benazeprilat (benazepril), benothiadiazide (hydrochlorothiazide)
Therapeutic: Antihypertensive (benazepril, hydrochlorothiazide), diuretic (hydrochlorothiazide)
Pregnancy category: D

Indications and Dosages
▶ *To treat hypertension uncontrolled by benazepril or hydrochlorothiazide alone*

TABLETS

Adults. *Initial:* 10 or 20 mg benazepril and 12.5 mg (10-mg/ 12.5-mg tablet or 20-mg/12.5-mg tablet) hydrochlorothiazide daily, increased as needed based on response (hydrochlorothiazide increased only every 2 to 3 wk). *Maximum:* 20 mg benazepril and 50 mg hydrochlorothiazide daily

▶ *To treat hypertension for patients adequately controlled by hydrochloro-thiazide but who develop significant potassium loss with monotherapy*

TABLETS

Adults. 5 mg benazepril and 6.25 mg hydrochlorothiazide (1 tablet) daily.

Mechanism of Action

Benazepril may reduce blood pressure by affecting the renin-angiotensin-aldosterone system. By inhibiting ACE, benazepril:

- prevents conversion of angiotensin I to angiotensin II, a potent vasocon-strictor that also stimulates adrenal cortex to secrete aldosterone.
- may inhibit renal and vascular production of angiotensin II.
- decreases serum angiotensin II level and increases serum renin activity. This decreases aldosterone secretion, slightly increasing serum potassium level and fluid loss.
- decreases vascular tone and blood pressure.
- inhibits aldosterone release, which reduces sodium and water reabsorption and increases their excretion, further reducing blood pressure.

Hydrochlorothiazide promotes movement of sodium, chloride, and water from blood in the peritubular capillaries into the nephron's distal convoluted tubule. Initially, it may decrease extracellular fluid volume, plasma volume, and cardiac output, which helps explain blood pressure reduction. It also may reduce blood pressure by dilating arteries. After several weeks, extracellular fluid volume, plasma volume, and cardiac output return to normal, and pe-ripheral vascular resistance remains decreased.

Contraindications

Anuria; hypersensitivity to benazepril, other ACE inhibitors, hy-drochlorothiazide, other sulfonamide-derived drugs or their com-ponents

Interactions

DRUGS

benazepril and hydrochlorothiazide

antihypertensives, diuretics: Increased antihypertensive effects

digoxin: Increased serum digoxin level and risk of toxicity *lithium:* Increased serum lithium level and risk of toxicity

benazepril

antacids: Possibly decreased bioavailability of benazepril

capsaicin: Possibly induced or worsened ACE inhibitor cough

indomethacin: Reduced hypotensive effects of benazepril

insulin, oral antidiabetics: Increased risk of hypoglycemia

phenothiazines: Possibly increased therapeutic and adverse effects of benazepril

potassium-sparing diuretics (such as amiloride, spironolactone, triamterene), potassium supplements: Increased risk of hyperkalemia

hydrochlorothiazide

amantadine: Possibly increased amantadine level and toxicity

amiodarone: Increased risk of arrhythmias from hypokalemia

amphotericin B, corticosteroids: Intensified electrolyte depletion, especially hypokalemia

barbiturates, opioids: Possibly potentiated orthostatic hypotension

calcium: Possibly increased serum calcium level

carbamazepine: Increased risk of hyponatremia

cholestyramine, colestipol resins: Reduced GI absorption of hydrochlorothiazide

diazoxide: Increased antihypertensive and hyperglycemic effects of hydrochlorothiazide

diflunisal: Possibly increased blood hydrochlorothiazide level

dopamine: Possibly increased diuretic effects of both drugs

insulin, oral antidiabetics: Possibly increased blood glucose level

neuromuscular blockers: Possibly enhanced neuromuscular blockade from hypokalemia

nondepolarizing skeletal muscle relaxants (such as tubocurarine): Possibly increased responsiveness to the muscle relaxant

NSAIDs: Decreased diuretic effect of hydrochlorothiazide, increased risk of renal failure

pressor amines (such as norepinephrine): Possibly decreased response to pressor amines

oral anticoagulants: Possibly decreased anticoagulant effects

sympathomimetics: Possibly decreased antihypertensive effect of hydrochlorothiazide

vitamin D: Increased risk of hypercalcemia

Adverse Reactions

CNS: Anxiety, asthenia, dizziness, fatigue, fever, headache, hypertonia, insomnia, nervousness, parethesia, somnolence, syncope, vertigo, weakness

CV: Angina, chest pain, ECG changes, hypotension, orthostatic hypotension, palpitations, peripheral edema, vasculitis

EENT: Blurred vision, dry mouth, epistaxis, taste perversion, sinusitis, tinnitus, voice alteration

ENDO: Hyperglycemia

GI: Abdominal pain, anorexia, constipation, diarrhea, dyspepsia, elevated liver function test results, gastritis, jaundice, melena, nausea, pancreatitis, vomiting

GU: Decreased libido, elevated BUN and serum creatinine levels, impotence, interstitial nephritis, nephritic syndrome, nocturia, polyuria, proteinuria, renal insufficiency, urinary frequency, UTI

HEME: Agranulocytosis, aplastic anemia, decreased hemoglobin level, hemolytic anemia, leukopenia, neutropenia, thrombocytopenia

MS: Arthralgia, arthritis, muscle spasms and weakness, myalgia

RESP: ACE inhibitor cough, asthma, bronchitis, bronchospasm, dyspnea

SKIN: Alopeica, exfoliative dermatitis, diaphoresis, flushing, photosensitivity, purpura, rash, urticaria

Other: Anaphylaxis, angioedema, dehydration, flu syndrome, gout, hypercalemia, hyperkalemia, hyperuricemia, hypochloremia, hypokalemia, hyponatremia, metabolic alkalosis, weight loss

Nursing Considerations

- Use benazepril and hydrochlorothiazide cautiously in patients with impaired renal function because this drug can alter renal function.
- Use cautiously in patients with impaired hepatic function because hydrochlorothiazide may alter fluid and electrolyte balance and precipitate hepatic coma.
- Use cautiously in patients with systemic lupus erythematosus because hydrochlorothiazide may activate or worsen it.
- Monitor blood pressure often to assess effectiveness of therapy.
- Watch for excessive hypotension, especially in patients with heart failure. If present, notify prescriber, place patient in supine position, and give normal saline intravenously if needed and ordered, until blood pressure is restored.
- **WARNING** Monitor patient closely for signs and symptoms of angioedema or allergic reactions such as rash, urticaria, or difficulty breathing. If present, withhold drug, notify prescriber immediately, and expect to treat symptomatically. If airway obstruction threatens, promptly give 0.3 to 0.5 ml of epinephrine solution 1:1,000 subcutaneously, as prescribed.

- Provide adequate hydration, as appropriate, to help prevent hypovolemia.
- Monitor fluid intake and output, daily weight, and serum electrolyte levels (especially potassium) to detect volume depletion or electrolyte imbalance.
- Monitor patient for increased BUN and serum creatinine levels, especially in patients with impaired renal function, because drug may cause acute renal failure. If increases are significant or persistent, notify prescriber immediately.
- Monitor blood glucose level often in diabetic patients, and expect to increase antidiabetic dosage, as needed and ordered.
- Check WBC count periodically, especially in patients with collagen-vascular disease, to detect neutropenia and agranulocytosis. Although they aren't known to occur with benazepril, they have occurred with captropril, another ACE inhibitor.
- Assess liver enzymes periodically and monitor patient for jaundice because hepatic failure, although rare, has occurred with other ACE inhibitors. If liver enzymes develop marked elevation or patient develops jaundice, notify prescriber and expect to stop benazepril and hydrochlorothiazide.

PATIENT TEACHING

- Advise patient to take benazepril and hydrochlorothiazide in the morning or early evening to avoid the need to urinate during the night.
- Teach patient to monitor her blood pressure and pulse rate and to report consistently elevated measurements to prescriber.
- Instruct patient to weigh herself at the same time each day wearing the same amount of clothing and to notify prescriber if she gains more than 2 lb (0.9 kg) per day or 5 lb (2.3 kg) per week.
- To reduce the risk of dehydration and hypotension, advise patient to avoid exercise in hot weather and to avoid alcohol. Also instruct her to notify prescriber if she has prolonged diarrhea, nausea, or vomiting.
- Caution patient to avoid hazardous activities until drug's CNS effects are known.
- WARNING Strongly urge patient to contact prescriber before using any OTC salt substitutes, which may contain potassium or potassium supplements. These substances increase the risk of hyperkalemia.
- Advise female patient to notify prescriber immediately if she is or could be pregnant because benazepril and hydrochloroth-

iazide will need to be replaced with another antihypertensive.
- Warn patient with gout that drug may precipitate an acute gout attack.
- Inform patient that a persistent dry cough may develop and may not subside unless therapy is stopped. If cough becomes bothersome or interferes with her sleep or activities, instruct her to notify prescriber.
- **WARNING** Instruct patient to contact prescriber immediately if she has signs of hypersensitivity, especially angioedema, (swelling of the face, eyes, lips, or tongue), difficulty breathing, hives, or rash.
- Caution patient to avoid sudden position changes and to rise slowly from a seated or reclining position to minimize orthostatic hypotension.

bisoprolol fumarate and hydrochlorothiazide

Ziac

Class and Category

Chemical: Selective beta₁-adrenergic blocker (bisoprolol), benothiadiazide (hydrochlorothiazide)
Therapeutic: Antihypertensive (bisoprolol, hydrochlorothiazide), diuretic (hydrochlorothiazide)
Pregnancy category: C

Indications and Dosages

▶ *To treat hypertension uncontrolled by bisoprolol or hydrochlorothiazide alone; to treat hypertension in patients adequately controlled by hydrochlorothiazide alone but who develop significant potassium loss as a result*

TABLETS

Adults. *Initial:* 2.5 mg bisoprolol and 6.25 mg hydrochlorothiazide (1 tablet) daily, increased as needed every 14 days based on response. *Maximum:* 20 mg bisoprolol and 12.5 mg hydrochlorothiazide daily.

Contraindications

Anuria; cardiogenic shock; heart failure unless caused by tachyarrhythmia; hypersensitivity to bisoprolol, hydrochlorothiazide, or their components; marked sinus bradycardia; overt heart failure unless compensated; second- or third-degree heart block

Mechanism of Action

Bisoprolol inhibits stimulation of beta$_1$-receptors mainly in the heart, which decreases cardiac excitability, cardiac output, and myocardial oxygen demand. Bisoprolol also decreases renin release from the kidneys, which helps reduce blood pressure.

Hydrochlorothiazide promotes movement of sodium, chloride, and water from blood in the peritubular capillaries into the nephron's distal convoluted tubule. Initially, it may decrease extracellular fluid volume, plasma volume, and cardiac output, which helps explain blood pressure reduction. It also may reduce blood pressure by dilating arteries. After several weeks, extracellular fluid volume, plasma volume, and cardiac output return to normal, and peripheral vascular resistance remains decreased.

Interactions

DRUGS

beta blockers, digitalis glycosides: Decreased heart rate and slowed atrioventricular conduction

bisoprolol and hydrochlorothiazide

antihypertensives: Increased additive antihypertensive effect

clonidine: Rebound hypertension

bisoprolol

aluminum salts, barbiturates, calcium salts, cholestyramine, colestipol, NSAIDs, penicillins, rifampin, salicylates, sulfinpyrazone: Possibly decreased therapeutic and adverse effects of bisoprolol

antiarrhythmics, calcium channel blockers (such as verapamil and diltiazem): Possibly symptomatic bradycardia and conduction abnormalities

calcium channel blockers: Possibly increased therapeutic and adverse effects of bisoprolol

catecholamine-depleting drugs (such as reserpine and guanethidine): Possibly enhanced reduction of sympathetic activity

ciprofloxacin, quinolones: Possibly increased bioavailability of bisoprolol

epinephrine: Possibly hypertension followed by bradycardia

ergot alkaloids: Possibly peripheral ischemia and gangrene

flecainide: Possibly increased therapeutic and adverse effects of either drug

lidocaine: Possibly increased risk of lidocaine toxicity

oral contraceptives: Possibly increased bioavailability and plasma level of bisoprolol

prazosin: Possibly increased orthostatic hypotension
quinidine: Possibly increased effects of bisoprolol
sulfonylureas: Possibly masked hypoglycemic symptoms

hydrochlorothiazide

amantadine: Possibly increased blood amantadine level and risk of toxicity
amiodarone: Increased risk of arrhythmias from hypokalemia
amphotericin B, corticosteroids: Intensified electrolyte depletion, especially hypokalemia
barbiturates, opioids: May potentiate orthostatic hypotension
calcium: Possibly increased serum calcium level
cholestyramine, colestipol resins: Reduced GI absorption of hydrochlorothiazide
diazoxide: Increased antihypertensive and hyperglycemic effects of hydrochlorothiazide
diflunisal: Possibly increased blood hydrochlorothiazide level
digoxin: Increased risk of digitalis toxicity from hypokalemia
dopamine: Possibly increased diuretic effects of both drugs
insulin, oral antidiabetics: Possible increased blood glucose level
lithium: Decreased lithium clearance and increased risk of toxicity
neuromuscular blockers: Possibly enhanced neuromuscular blockade from hypokalemia
nondepolarizing skeletal muscle relaxants (such as tubocurarine): Possibly increased responsiveness to the muscle relaxant
NSAIDs: Decreased diuretic effect of hydrochlorothiazide and increased risk of renal failure
pressor amines (such as norepinephrine): Possibly decreased response to pressor amines
oral anticoagulants: Possibly decreased anticoagulant effects
sympathomimetics: Possibly decreased antihypertensive effect of hydrochlorothiazide
vitamin D: Increased risk of hypercalcemia

Adverse Reactions

CNS: Anxiety, asthenia, confusion, depression, dizziness, emotional lability, fatigue, fever, hallucinations, headache, insomnia, malaise, nightmares, paresthesia, tremor, somnolence, vertigo, weakness

CV: Arrhythmia, bradycardia, chest pain, claudication, edema, heart block, heart failure, hypercholesterolemia, hyperlipidemia, hypotension, MI, orthostatic hypotension, palpitations, peripheral vascular insufficiency, renal and mesenteric artery thrombosis, vasculitis

EENT: Altered taste, blurred vision, dry mouth, eye pain or pressure, increased salivation, larynospasm, pharyngitis, rhinitis, sinusitis, tinnitus

ENDO: Hyperglycemia

GI: Abdominal cramps, constipation, diarrhea, dyspepsia, diarrhea, epigastric pain, gastritis, indigestion, jaundice, ischemic colitis, nausea, vomiting

GU: Cystitis, impotence, interstitial nephritis, loss of libido, nocturia, Peyronie's disease, polyuria, renal colic

HEME: Agranulocytosis, aplastic anemia, eosinophilia, hemolytic anemia, leukopenia, neutropenia, thrombocytopenia, thrombocytopenic purpura

MS: Arthralgia; muscle cramps, twitching, and weakness; myalgia; neck pain

RESP: Asthma, bronchitis, bronchospasm, cough, dyspnea, respiratory distress, upper respiratory infection

SKIN: Alopecia, diaphoresis, eczema, exfoliative dermatitis, flushing, photosensitivity, pruritus, purpura, rash, urticaria

Other: Anaphylaxis, angioedema, dehydration, gout, hypercalcemia, hyperkalemia, hyperuricemia, hypochloremia, hypokalemia, hyponatremia, hypovolemia, metabolic alkalosis, weight gain or loss

Nursing Considerations

- Use bisoprolol and hydrochlorothiazide cautiously in patients with heart failure, arterial circulatory disorders, bronchospastic disease, or impaired renal function.
- Use cautiously in patients with impaired hepatic function because hydrochlorothiazide may alter fluid and electrolyte balance, which may precipitate hepatic coma.
- Use cautiously in patients with systemic lupus erythematosus because hydrochlorothiazide may activate or worsen it.
- Monitor blood pressure often to assess effectiveness of bisoprolol and hydrochlorothiazide therapy.
- Provide adequate hydration, as appropriate, to help prevent hypovolemia.
- Monitor fluid intake and output, daily weight, blood pressure, and serum electrolyte levels (especially potassium) to detect volume depletion or electrolyte imbalance.
- Watch for increased BUN and serum creatinine levels, especially in patients with impaired renal function, because drug may cause acute renal failure. If increases are significant or persistent, notify prescriber immediately.

- Monitor blood glucose level often in diabetic patients, and expect to increase antidiabetic dosage, as needed and ordered.
- Monitor patient for evidence of heart failure. At first sign of heart failure, expect patient to receive a cardiac glycoside, a diuretic, or both and to be monitored closely. If failure continues, expect bisoprolol and hydrochlorothiazide to be stopped.
- Monitor diabetic patient closely because bisoprolol may mask signs of hypoglycemia, cause hypoglycemia, or delay the return of blood glucose to a normal level.
- Monitor patient with hyperthyroidism closely because bisoprolol may mask some signs of thyrotoxicosis. Avoid abrupt withdrawal of bisoprolol and hydrochlorothiazide because it may precipitate thyrotoxicosis or ischemic heart disease.
- Expect to stop bisoprolol and hydrochlorothiazide several days before gradually withdrawing clonidine therapy, if prescribed. Then expect to restart bisoprolol and hydrochlorothiazide several days after clonidine has been stopped because clonidine can cause rebound hypertension.
- Notify prescriber immediately if patient develops bradycardia, hypotension, or other serious adverse reactions.

PATIENT TEACHING
- Advise patient to take bisoprolol and hydrochlorothiazide in the morning or early evening to avoid the need to urinate during the night.
- Warn patient to take bisoprolol and hydrochlorothiazide exactly as prescribed and not to abruptly stop therapy because serious adverse effects could occur, such as an MI or arrhythmia.
- Teach patient to monitor her blood pressure and to report consistently elevated measurements to prescriber.
- Direct patient to weigh herself at the same time each day wearing the same amount of clothing and to notify prescriber if she gains more than 2 lb (0.9 kg) per day or 5 lb (2.3 kg) per week.
- Instruct patient to eat a diet high in potassium-rich food, such as citrus fruits, bananas, tomatoes, and dates.
- To reduce the risk of dehydration and hypotension, advise patient to avoid exercise in hot weather and to avoid alcohol. Also instruct her to notify prescriber if she has prolonged diarrhea, nausea, or vomiting.
- Caution patient to avoid hazardous activities until drug's CNS effects are known.
- Caution diabetic patient that the drug may mask some signs of hypoglycemia; tell her to test her blood glucose level regularly.

candesartan cilexetil and hydrochlorothiazide
Atacand HCT

Class and Category
Chemical: Angiotensin II receptor antagonist (candesartan), benothiadiazide (hydrochlorothiazide)
Therapeutic: Antihypertensive (candesartan, hydrochlorothiazide), diuretic (hydrochlorothiazide)
Pregnancy category: C (first trimester), D (second and third trimesters)

Indications and Dosages
▶ *To treat hypertension when candesartan or hydrochlorothiazide alone has failed to control blood pressure*
TABLETS
Adults whose blood pressure hasn't been controlled with 32 mg of candesartan. 32 mg candesartan and 12.5 mg hydrochlorothiazide (1 tablet) daily. Increased, as needed, to 32 mg candesartan and 25 mg hydrochlorothiazide (2 tablets) daily.
Adults whose blood pressure hasn't been controlled with 25 mg of hydrochlorothiazide or whose blood pressure has been controlled with 25 mg of hydrochlorothiazide but who develop hypokalemia as a result. 16 mg candesartan and 12.5 mg hydrochlorothiazide (1 tablet) daily.

Contraindications
Anuria; hypersensitivity to candesartan, hydrochlorothiazide, other sulfonamide-derived drugs or their components

---

Mechanism of Action
Candesartan selectively blocks binding of the potent vasoconstrictor angiotensin II to angiotensin 1 (a subtype of angiotensin II) receptor sites in many tissues, including vascular smooth muscle and adrenal glands. This inhibits vasoconstrictive and aldosterone-secreting effects of angiotensin II, which reduces blood pressure.

Hydrochlorothiazide promotes movement of sodium, chloride, and water from blood in the peritubular capillaries into the nephron's distal convoluted tubule. Initially, it may decrease extracellular fluid volume, plasma volume, and cardiac output, which helps explain blood pressure reduction. It also may reduce blood pressure by dilating arteries. After several weeks, extracellular fluid volume, plasma volume, and cardiac output return to normal, and peripheral vascular resistance remains decreased.

Interactions

DRUGS

candesartan and hydrochlorothiazide

antihypertensives, diuretics: Additive antihypertensive effects, possibly increasing risk of hypotension

lithium: Increased serum lithium level and risk of toxicity

candesartan

cyclosporine, potassium-sparing diuretics, potassium supplements: Increased risk of hyperkalemia

hydrochlorothiazide

amantadine: Possibly increased blood amantadine level and risk of toxicity

amiodarone: Increased risk of arrhythmias from hypokalemia

amphotericin B, corticosteroids: Intensified electrolyte depletion, especially hypokalemia

barbiturates, opioids: May potentiate development of orthostatic hypotension

calcium: Possibly increased serum calcium level

cholestyramine, colestipol resins: Reduced GI absorption of hydrochlorothiazide

diazoxide: Increased antihypertensive and hyperglycemic effects of hydrochlorothiazide

diflunisal: Possibly increased blood hydrochlorothiazide level

digoxin: Increased risk of digitalis toxicity from hypokalemia

dopamine: Possibly increased diuretic effects of both drugs

insulin, oral antidiabetics: Possibly increased blood glucose level

neuromuscular blockers: Possibly enhanced neuromuscular blockade from hypokalemia

nondepolarizing skeletal muscle relaxants, such as tubocurarine: Possibly increased responsiveness to the muscle relaxant

NSAIDs: Decreased diuretic effect of hydrochlorothiazide, increased risk of renal failure

pressor amines, such as norepinephrine: Possibly decreased response to pressor amines

oral anticoagulants: Possibly decreased anticoagulant effects

sympathomimetics: Possibly decreased antihypertensive effect of hydrochlorothiazide

vitamin D: Increased risk of hypercalcemia

FOODS

candesartan

high-potassium diet, potassium-containing salt substitutes: Increased risk of hyperkalemia

Adverse Reactions

CNS: Anxiety, asthenia, dizziness, fatigue, headache, hypesthesia, insomnia, paresthesia, vertigo, weakness

CV: Abnormal ECG, angina, bradycardia, chest pain, depression, extrasystoles, hypotension, MI, orthostatic hypotension, palpitations, peripheral edema, tachycardia, vasculitis

EENT: Blurred vision, conjunctivitis, dry mouth, epistaxis, pharyngitis, rhinitis, sinusitis, tinnitus

ENDO: Hyperglycemia

GI: Abdominal pain or cramps, anorexia, constipation, diarrhea, dyspepsia, gastritis, gastroenteritis, hepatitis, increased liver enzymes, indigestion, jaundice, nausea, vomiting

GU: Acute renal failure, cystitis, decreased libido, hematuria, impotence, increased BUN and serum creatinine levels, interstitial nephritis, nocturia, polyuria, renal failure, UTI

HEME: Agranulocytosis, aplastic or hemolytic anemia, leukopenia, neutropenia

MS: Arthralgia, arthrosis, arthritis, back pain, muscle spasms or weakness, myalgia, leg cramps, sciatica

RESP: Bronchitis, cough, dyspnea, upper respiratory infection

SKIN: Alopecia, dermatitis, diaphoresis, eczema, exfoliative dermatitis, photosensitivity, pruritus, purpura, rash, urticaria

Other: Anaphylaxis, angioedema, dehydration, flulike symptoms, hypercalcemia, hyperuricemia, hypochloremia, hypokalemia, hyponatremia, hypovolemia, increased CK level, infection, metabolic alkalosis, viral infection, weight loss

Nursing Considerations

- Use cautiously in patients with impaired hepatic or renal function because candesartan and hydrochlorothiazide may cause acute renal failure or alter fluid and electrolyte balance, which may precipitate hepatic coma.
- Also use cautiously in patients with systemic lupus erythematosus because hydrochlorothiazide may activate or worsen it.
- If patient has known or suspected hypovolemia, expect to correct it with I.V. normal saline solution, as prescribed, before starting candesartan and hydrochlorothiazide.
- Provide hydration, as appropriate, during therapy to help prevent hypovolemia.
- Monitor blood pressure often to assess effectiveness of candesartan and hydrochlorothiazide therapy.
- Watch for hypotension, especially in patients undergoing major surgery and anesthesia because angiotensin II receptor antago-

nists like candesartan can cause blockade of the renin-angiotensin system. If patient develops hypotension, expect to stop drug temporarily. Immediately place patient in supine position, and prepare to give I.V. normal saline solution, as prescribed. Expect to resume therapy after blood pressure stabilizes.

- Monitor fluid intake and output, daily weight, and serum electrolyte levels (especially potassium) to detect volume depletion or electrolyte imbalance.
- Check for increased BUN and serum creatinine levels, especially in patients with impaired renal function, because drug may cause acute renal failure. If increases are significant or persistent, notify prescriber immediately.
- Monitor blood glucose level often in diabetic patients, and expect to increase antidiabetic dosage, as needed and ordered.
- Check patient's CBC routinely, as ordered, for abnormalities. If they're significant or persistent, notify prescriber immediately.

PATIENT TEACHING

- Advise patient to take candesartan and hydrochlorothiazide in the morning or early evening to avoid nighttime urination.
- Teach patient to monitor her blood pressure and to report consistently elevated measurements to prescriber.
- Alert patient that full effects of therapy may take up to 4 weeks.
- Caution patient that light-headedness may occur, especially early in therapy, and should be reported to the prescriber.
- Direct patient to weigh herself at the same time each day wearing the same amount of clothing and to notify prescriber if she gains more than 2 lb (0.9 kg) per day or 5 lb (2.3 kg) per week.
- **WARNING** Strongly urge patient to contact prescriber before using potassium supplements or OTC salt substitutes, which may contain potassium and increase the risk of hyperkalemia.
- To reduce the risk of dehydration and hypotension, advise patient to avoid exercise in hot weather and to avoid alcohol. Also tell her to notify prescriber if she has prolonged diarrhea, nausea, or vomiting.
- Caution patient to avoid hazardous activities until drug's CNS effects are known.
- Explain the importance of regular exercise, proper diet, and other lifestyle changes in controlling hypertension.
- Advise female patient to notify prescriber immediately if she is or could be pregnant. Candesartan and hydrochlorothiazide will need to be replaced with another antihypertensive.

captopril and hydrochlorothiazide
Capozide

Class and Category

Chemical: ACE inhibitor (captopril), benothiadiazide (hydrochlorothiazide)

Therapeutic: Antihypertensive (captopril, hydrochlorothiazide), diuretic (hydrochlorothiazide)

Pregnancy category: C (first trimester), D (second and third trimesters)

Indications and Dosages

▶ *To treat hypertension uncontrolled with captopril or hydrochlorothiazide alone*

TABLETS

Adults. *Initial:* 25 mg captopril and 15 mg hydrochlorothiazide (1 tablet) daily, increased as needed. *Maximum:* 150 mg captropril and 50 hydrochlorothiazide daily.

Mechanism of Action

Captopril may reduce blood pressure by affecting the renin-angiotensin-aldosterone system. By inhibiting ACE, captopril:

- prevents conversion of angiotensin I to angiotensin II, a potent vasoconstrictor that also stimulates adrenal cortex to secrete aldosterone.
- may inhibit renal and vascular production of angiotensin II.
- decreases serum angiotensin II level and increases serum renin activity. This decreases aldosterone secretion, slightly increasing serum potassium level and fluid loss.
- decreases vascular tone and blood pressure.
- inhibits aldosterone release, which reduces sodium and water reabsorption and increases their excretion, further reducing blood pressure.

Hydrochlorothiazide promotes movement of sodium, chloride, and water from blood in peritubular capillaries into the nephron's distal convoluted tubule. Initially, it may decrease extracellular fluid volume, plasma volume, and cardiac output, which helps explain blood pressure reduction. It also may reduce blood pressure by dilating arteries. After several weeks, extracellular fluid volume, plasma volume, and cardiac output return to normal, and peripheral vascular resistance remains decreased.

Contraindications

Anuria; hypersensitivity to captopril, hydrochlorothiazide, other ACE inhibitors or sulfonamide-derived drugs, or their components

Interactions

DRUGS

captopril and hydrochlorothiazide

antihypertensives, diuretics: Increased antihypertensive effects

digoxin: Increased blood digoxin level and risk of toxicity

lithium: Increased blood lithium level and toxicity

NSAIDs, sympathomimetics: Possibly reduced antihypertensive effects of captopril and hydrochlorothiazide and increased risk of renal toxicity

captopril

allopurinol: Increased risk of hypersensitivity reactions, including Stevens-Johnson syndrome, skin eruptions, fever, and arthralgia; possibly increased risk of fatal neutropenia or agranulocytosis

antacids: Possibly impaired captopril absorption

bone marrow depressants (such as amphotericin B and methotrexate), procainamide, systemic corticosteroids: Possibly increased risk of fatal neutropenia or agranulocytosis

capsaicin: Possibly induced or worsened ACE inhibitor cough

cyclosporine, potassium-sparing diuretics, potassium supplements: Increased risk of hyperkalemia

probenecid: Increased blood level and decreased total clearance of captopril

hydrochlorothiazide

amantadine: Possibly increased blood amantadine level and risk of toxicity

amiodarone: Increased risk of arrhythmias from hypokalemia

amphotericin B, corticosteroids: Intensified electrolyte depletion, especially hypokalemia

barbiturates, opioids: May potentiate orthostatic hypotension

calcium: Possibly increased serum calcium level

cholestyramine, colestipol resins: Reduced GI absorption of hydrochlorothiazide

diazoxide: Increased antihypertensive and hyperglycemic effects of hydrochlorothiazide

diflunisal: Possibly increased blood hydrochlorothiazide level

dopamine: Possibly increased diuretic effects of both drugs

insulin, oral antidiabetics: Possibly increased blood glucose level

neuromuscular blockers: Possibly enhanced neuromuscular blockade from hypokalemia

nondepolarizing skeletal muscle relaxants (such as tubocurarine): Possibly increased responsiveness to the muscle relaxant

pressor amines (such as norepinephrine): Possibly decreased response to pressor amines

oral anticoagulants: Possibly decreased anticoagulant effects
vitamin D: Increased risk of hypercalcemia
FOODS
captopril
potassium-containing salt substitutes: Increased risk of hyperkalemia
ACTIVITIES
captopril
alcohol use: Additive hypotensive effects

Adverse Reactions

CNS: Dizziness, fever, headache, insomnia, paresthesia, vertigo, weakness
CV: Chest pain, hypotension, orthostatic hypotension, palpitations, tachycardia, vasculitis
EENT: Blurred vision, dry mouth, loss of taste
ENDO: Hyperglycemia
GI: Abdominal cramps, anorexia, constipation, diarrhea, indigestion, jaundice, nausea, vomiting
GU: Decreased libido, dysuria, impotence, interstitial nephritis, nephritic syndrome, nocturia, oliguria, polyuria, proteinuria, renal failure, urinary frequency
HEME: Agranulocytosis, aplastic and hemolytic anemia, eosinophilia, leukopenia, neutropenia, thrombocytopenia
MS: Arthraliga, muscle spasms and weakness
RESP: Cough
SKIN: Alopecia, exfoliative dermatitis, photosensitivity, purpura, pruritus, rash, urticaria
Other: Anaphylaxis, angioedema, dehydration, hypercalcemia, hyperkalemia, hyperuricemia, hypochloremia, hypokalemia, hyponatremia, hypovolemia, metabolic alkalosis, positive ANA titer, weight loss

Nursing Considerations

- Use cautiously in patients with impaired hepatic function because hydrochlorothiazide may alter fluid and electrolyte balance, which may precipitate hepatic coma.
- Also use cautiously in patients with systemic lupus erythematosus because hydrochlorothiazide may activate or worsen the diesease.
- Monitor blood pressure often to assess effectiveness of captropril and hydrochlorothiazide therapy. If hypotension occurs, keep patient supine until resolved.
- Provide adequate hydration, as appropriate, to help prevent hypovolemia.

- Monitor fluid intake and output, daily weight, and serum electrolyte levels (especially potassium) to detect volume depletion or electrolyte imbalance.
- Watch for increased BUN and serum creatinine levels, especially in patients with impaired renal function, because drug may cause renal dysfunction. If increases are significant or persistent or patient has renal symptoms such as oliguria, polyuria, or urinary frequency, notify prescriber immediately.
- Monitor blood glucose level often in diabetic patients, and expect to increase antidiabetic dosage, as needed and ordered.
- Monitor patient's WBC counts regularly, as ordered, especially in patients with collagen vascular disease or renal disease.
- **WARNING** Monitor patient closely for angioedema of the face, lips, tongue, glottis, larynx, or limbs. For angioedema of the face and lips, stop drug and give an antihistamine, as prescribed. If tongue, glottis, or larynx is involved, assess patient for airway obstruction, prepare to give epinephrine 1:1,000 (0.3 to 0.5 ml) subcutaneously, and maintain a patent airway.

PATIENT TEACHING
- Advise patient to take captropril and hydrochlorothiazide in the morning or early evening to avoid the need to urinate during the night. Also tell patient to take drug 1 hour before a meal.
- Teach patient to monitor her blood pressure and to report consistently elevated measurements to prescriber.
- Direct patient to weigh herself at the same time each day wearing the same amount of clothing and to notify prescriber if she gains more than 2 lb (0.9 kg) per day or 5 lb (2.3 kg) per week.
- To reduce the risk of dehydration and hypotension, advise patient to avoid exercise in hot weather and to avoid alcohol. Also instruct her to notify prescriber if she has prolonged diarrhea, nausea, or vomiting.
- Caution patient to avoid hazardous activities until drug's CNS effects are known.
- Explain the importance of regular exercise, proper diet, and other lifestyle changes in controlling hypertension.
- Tell patient to avoid sunlight or to wear sunscreen in direct sunlight because photosensitivity may occur.
- Advise patient not to use salt substitutes that contain potassium and to consult prescriber before increasing dietary potassium intake to avoid increasing the risk of hyperkalemia.
- Stress importance of notifying prescriber about possible indicators of, such as a sore throat or fever occurs.
- Warn patient not to stop taking drug abruptly.

clonidine and chlorthalidone
Clorpres, Combipres

Class and Category
Chemical: Imidazoline derivative (clonidine), phthalimidine derivative of benzenesulfonamide (thiazide-like diuretic) (chlorthalidone)
Therapeutic: Antihypertensive, diuretic
Pregnancy category: C

Indications and Dosages
▶ *To treat hypertension uncontrolled with clonidine or chlorthalidone monotherapy*
TABLETS
Adults. *Initial:* 0.1 mg clonidine and 15 mg chlorthalidone (1 tablet) daily or b.i.d., increased as needed. *Maximum:* 0.6 mg clonidine and 30 mg chlorthalidone

---

Mechanism of Action
Clonidine stimulates alpha-adrenergic receptors in the brain stem to reduce sympathetic outflow from the CNS and a decrease in peripheral vascular resistance, heart rate, and systolic and diastolic blood pressure.

Chlorthalidone may promote sodium, chloride, and water excretion by inhibiting sodium reabsorption in the kidneys' distal tubules. Initially, chlorthalidone may decrease extracellular fluid volume, plasma volume, and cardiac output, which helps explain how it reduces blood pressure. It also may dilate arteries directly, which helps reduce peripheral vascular resistance and blood pressure. After several weeks, extracellular fluid and plasma volume and cardiac output return to normal, but peripheral vascular resistance remains decreased to lower blood pressure.

Contraindications
Anuria; hypersensitivity to clonidine, chlorthalidone, other sulfonamide-derived drugs, or their components

Interactions
DRUGS
clonidine and chlorthalidone
antihypertensives, diuretics: Increased antihypertensive effects
digoxin: Increased risk of digitalis toxicity from hypokalemia
clonidine
barbituratres, other CNS depressants: Increased depressant effects of these drugs

beta blockers, calcium channel blockers: Additive effects, such as bradycardia and AV block; increased risk of exacerbated hypertensive response when clonidine is withdrawn (beta blockers only)

levodopa: Decreased levodopa effectiveness

prazosin, tricyclic antidepressants: Decreased antihypertensive effect of clonidine

chlorthalidone

allopurinol: Increased risk of allopurinol hypersensitivity

amphotericin B, corticosteroids: Intensified electrolyte depletion, especially hypokalemia

anesthetics: Potentiated effects of anesthetics

anticholinergics: Increased chlorthalidone absorption

antineoplastics: Prolonged antineoplastic-induced leukopenia

cholestyramine, colestipol resins: Reduced GI absorption of chlorthalidone

diazoxide: Increased antihypertensive and hyperglycemic effects of chlorthalidone

insulin, oral antidiabetics: Possibly increased blood glucose level

lithium: Decreased lithium clearance and increased risk of toxicity

loop diuretics: Increased synergistic effects, resulting in profound diuresis and serious electrolyte imbalances

methenamines: Decreased effects of methenamines

metyldopa: Potential development of hemolytic anemia

neuromuscular blockers: Possibly enhanced neuromuscular blockade

NSAIDs: Decreased diuretic effect of chlorthalidone

oral anticoagulants: Possibly decreased anticoagulant effects

sympathomimetics: Possibly decreased antihypertensive effect of clorthalidone

vitamin D: Enhanced vitamin D action

ACTIVITIES

clonidine

alcohol use: Enhanced depressive effectives of clonidine

Adverse Reactions

CNS: Agitation, depression, dizziness, drowsiness, fatigue, headache, insomnia, light-headedness, malaise, nervousness, paresthesia, restlessness, sedation, vertigo, weakness

CV: Chest pain, orthostastic hypotension, vasculitis

EENT: Blurred or yellow vision, burning eyes, dry eyes and mouth

ENDO: Hyperglycemia

GI: Abdominal cramps or pain, anorexia, bloating, constipation, diarrhea, gastric irritation, mildly elevated liver function test results, nausea, pancreatitis, vomiting

GU: Decreased libido, impotence, nocturia
HEME: Agranulocytosis, aplastic anemia, hypoplastic anemia, leukopenia, thromboyctopenia
MS: Muscle spasms
SKIN: Cutaneous vasculitis, exfoliative dermatitis, jaundice, necrotizing vasculitis, photosensitivity, purpura, rash, urticaria
Other: Gout, hyperuricemia, hypochloremic alkalosis, hypokalemia, hyponatremia, weight gain, withdrawal symptoms

Nursing Considerations

- Use clonidine and chlorthalidone cautiously in patients with impaired hepatic function because minor changes in fluid and electrolyte balance may cause hepatic coma.
- Also use clonidine and chlorthalidone cautiously in elderly patients, who may be more sensitive to its hypotensive effect, and in patients with severe coronary insufficiency, recent MI, cerebrovascular disease, or chronic renal faiulre.
- Monitor blood pressure and heart rate often during clonidine and chlorthalidone therapy to assess effectiveness.
- Assess BUN, serum electrolyte, uric acid, and blood glucose levels before and periodically during therapy. Monitor patient for signs of fluid and electrolyte imbalance.
- **WARNING** Monitor renal function periodically to detect cumulative drug effects, which may cause azotemia in patients with impaired renal function.
- **WARNING** Be aware that stopping drug abruptly can elevate serum catecholamine level and cause such withdrawal symptoms as nervousness, agitation, headache, confusion, tremor, and rebound hypertension.
- If patient has had an allergic reaction to transdermal clonidine, be aware that he also may have an allergic reaction to oral clonidine. Monitor him closely.

PATIENT TEACHING
- Advise patient to take drug exactly as prescribed and not to stop taking it abruptly because withdrawal symptoms and severe hypertension may occur.
- Tell patient to take drug with food or milk and to take it earlier in the day to avoid the need to urinate during the night.
- Urge patient to eat high-potassium foods (such as bananas, apricots, grapefruits, tomato juice, and orange juice) and to report signs of a low potassium level (such as an irregular heartbeat, muscle weakness, and fatigue) or a low sodium level (such as confusion, irritability, and muscle cramps).

- Teach patient to monitor blood pressure and to report consistently elevated measurements to prescriber.
- Caution patient to avoid hazardous activities until drug's CNS effects are known.
- Advise male patients about possibly decreased libido.
- Tell patient to notify prescriber about urine retention, vision changes, excessive drowsiness, rash, chest pain, and dizziness with position changes. Urge tell patient to rise slowly to avoid hypotensive effects.
- Instruct patient to protect his skin from the sun.
- Urge patient to immediately report sudden joint pain to prescriber because drug can cause sudden gout attacks.
- To reduce the risk of dehydration and hypotension, advise patient to avoid exercise in hot weather and to avoid alcohol. Tell her to report about prolonged diarrhea, nausea, or vomiting.
- Advise diabetic patient to monitor blood glucose level closely because drug may cause hyperglycemia, which may warrant a change in treatment plan.

dipyridamole and aspirin
Aggrenox

Class and Category
Chemical: Salicylate (aspirin), pyrimidine (dipyridamole)
Therapeutic: Platelet aggregation inhibitor
Pregnancy category: NR (aspirin D, dipyridamole B)

Indications and Dosages
▶ *To prevent recurrence of thromboembolic stroke*
CAPSULES
Adults. *Initial:* 25 mg aspirin and 200 mg extended-release dipyridamole (1 capsule) b.i.d.

Mechanism of Action
Dipyridamole inhibits platelet uptake of adenosine, thus increasing the amount of adenosine in surrounding blood. The increased adenosine acts on platelet A_2 receptors, stimulating the activity of intraplatelet adenylate cyclase. This action in turn increases the level of cyclic adenosine monophosphate in platelets, which decreases platelet activation and aggregation.

Aspirin inhibits platelet aggregation by interfering with production of thromboxane A_2, a substance that stimulates platelet aggregation.

Contraindications

Allergy to NSAIDs or tartrazine dye; hypersensitivity to aspirin, dipyridamole, or their components

Interactions

DRUGS

aspirin

ACE inhibitors, beta blockers: Decreased antihypertensive effect

acetazolamide: Increased blood acetazolamide level and risk of toxicity

activated charcoal: Decreased aspirin absorption

antacids, urine alkalinizers: Decreased aspirin effectiveness

carbonic anhydrase inhibitors: Salicylism

corticosteroids: Increased excretion and decreased blood level of aspirin

heparin: Increased risk of bleeding

methotrexate: Increased blood level and decreased excretion rate of methotrexate, causing toxicity

nizatidine: Increased blood aspirin level

NSAIDs: Possibly decreased blood NSAID level and increased risk of bleeding

oral anticoagulants: Increased risk of bleeding; prolonged bleeding time

phenytoin: Decreased blood phenytoin level

sulfonylureas: Possibly enhanced effect of sulfonylureas with large doses of aspirin

urine acidifiers (such as ammonium chloride and ascorbic acid): Decreased aspirin excretion

valproic acid: Increased blood valproic acid level

vancomycin: Increased risk of ototoxicity

dipyridamole

adenosine: Increased blood adenosine level; potentiated effects of adenosine

cefamandole, cefoperazone, cefotetan, plicamyin, valproic acid: Possibly hypoprothrombinemia and increased risk of bleeding

cholinesterase inhibitors: Possibly counteracted effects of these drugs and aggravation of myasthenia gravis

heparin, NSAIDs, thrombolytics: Possibly increased risk of bleeding

ACTIVITIES

aspirin

alcohol use: Increased risk of GI bleeding

Adverse Reactions

CNS: Amnesia, asthenia, headache, seizures, somnolence, syncope

EENT: Epistaxis
GI: Abdominal pain, anorexia, diarrhea, dyspepsia, esophageal irritation, GI bleeding, hemorrhoids, hepatic impairment, nausea, vomiting
HEME: Anemia
MS: Arthralgia, arthritis, back pain
SKIN: Purpura

Nursing Considerations

- Be aware that combination aspirin and dipyridamole isn't interchangeable with individual aspirin or dipyridamole tablets.
- **WARNING** Monitor patients with severe hepatic impairment for evidence of bleeding, such as easy bruising, tarry stools, and epistaxis. Monitor coagulation test results as appropriate, and notify prescriber immediately about significant changes. These patients already have an increased risk of bleeding, and platelet inhibition increases the risk further.
- Monitor liver function test results as appropriate if patient has hepatic impairment because dipyridamole may increase hepatic enzyme levels and cause hepatic failure.
- Monitor renal function test results, such as glomerular filtration rate (GFR), if patient has renal impairment. Because aspirin is excreted by the kidneys, it should be avoided in patients with a GFR below 10 ml/min. Otherwise, patient may develop aspirin toxicity.
- If patient consumes three or more alcoholic beverages daily or has hypoprothrombinemia, peptic ulcer disease, or vitamin K deficiency, monitor him closely for signs and symptoms of bleeding.
- If patient has coronary artery disease, assess for chest pain and hypotension because of dipyridamole's vasodilatory effect.

PATIENT TEACHING
- Advise patient to swallow capsule whole and not to break, chew, or crush it.
- Instruct patient to take drug with a full glass of water and to avoid lying down for 15 to 30 minutes afterward to prevent esophageal irritation.
- Warn patient to consult prescriber before taking any drug to treat pain, fever, or arthritis.
- Urge patient not to stop taking drug for any reason without first consulting prescriber.
- Advise patient to notify other health care providers that he takes aspirin and dipyridamole.

enalapril maleate and felodipine ER
Lexxel

Class and Category
Chemical: Dicarbocyl-containing ACE inhibitor (enalapril), dihy-dropyridine derivative (felodipine)
Therapeutic: Antihypertensive (enalapril, felodipine)
Pregnancy category: C (first trimester), D (second and third trimesters)

Indications and Dosages
▶ *To treat hypertension when enalapril or felodipine alone has failed to control blood pressure*
TABLETS
Adults. 5 mg enalapril and 5 mg felodipine (1 tablet) daily; in-creased as needed in 7 to 14 days to 10 mg enalapril and 10 mg felodipine (2 tablets) daily; increased again, as needed, in 7 to 14 days to 20 mg enalapril and 10 mg felodipine (4 tablets, each containing 5 mg enalipril and 2.5 mg felodipine) daily.

Mechanism of Action
Enalapril may reduce blood pressure by affecting the renin-angiotensin-aldosterone system. By inhibiting ACE, enalapril:
- prevents conversion of angiotensin I to angiotensin II, a potent vasocon-strictor that also stimulates adrenal cortex to secrete aldosterone.
- may inhibit renal and vascular production of angiotensin II.
- decreases serum angiotensin II level and increases serum renin activity. This decreases aldosterone secretion, slightly increasing serum potassium level and fluid loss.
- decreases vascular tone and blood pressure.
- inhibits aldosterone release, which reduces sodium and water reabsorption and increases their excretion, further reducing blood pressure.

Felodipine may slow movement of extracellular calcium into myocardial and vascular smooth-muscle cells by deforming calcium channels in cell membranes, inhibiting ion-controlled gating mechanisms, and interfering with calcium release from the sacroplasmic reticulum. The effect of these actions is a decrease in intracellular calcium ions, which inhibits contraction of smooth-muscle cells and dilates coronary and systemic arteries. As with other calcium channel blockers, felodipine increases oxygen to the myocardium and reduces peripheral resistance, blood pressure, and afterload.

Contraindications
Hereditary or idiopathic angioedema; history of angioedema from

previous ACE inhibitor; hypersensitivity to enalapril, felodipine, or their components

Interactions

DRUGS

enalapril and felodipine

antihypertensives, diuretics: Additive hypotensive effects
lithium: Increased blood lithium level and toxicity
NSAIDs, sympathomimetics: Possibly reduced antihypertensive effects of enalapril and felodipine

enalapril

allopurinol, bone marrow depressants (such as amphotericin B and methotrexate), procainamide, systemic corticosteroids: Possibly increased risk of fatal neutropenia or agranulocytosis
cyclosporine, potassium-sparing diuretics, potassium supplements: Increased risk of hyperkalemia

felodopine

anesthetics (hydrocarbon inhalation): Possibly hypotension
anticonvulsants: Decreased plasma felodipine level and effectiveness
beta blockers: Increased adverse effects of beta blockers
cimetidine, erythromycin, itraconazole, ketoconazole: Increased felodipine bioavailability
digoxin: Transient increase in blood digoxin level and risk of toxicity
estrogens: Possibly increased fluid retention and decreased therapeutic effect of felodopine
procainamide, quinidine: Increased risk of prolonged QT interval
tacrolimus: Possibly increased serum tacrolimus level

FOODS

enalapril

potassium-containing salt substitutes: Increased risk of hyperkalemia

felodopine

grapefruit juice: Doubled felodipine bioavailability

ACTIVITIES

enalapril

alcohol use: Possibly additive hypotensive effect

Adverse Reactions

CNS: Asthenia, ataxia, confusion, depression, dizziness, dream disturbances, fatigue, headache, insomnia, nervousness, paresthesia, peripheral neuropathy, somnolence, stroke, syncope, vertigo, weakness
CV: Angina, arrhythmias, cardiac arrest, chest pain, edema, hypotension, MI, orthostatic hypotension, palpitations, Raynaud's

phenomenon, tachycardia

EENT: Blurred vision, conjunctivitis, dry eyes and mouth, gingival hyperplasia, glossitis, hoarseness, lacrimation, loss of smell, pharyngitis, rhinorrhea, rhinitis, stomatitis, taste perversion, tinnitus

ENDO: Gynecomastia

GI: Abdominal cramps or pain, anorexia, constipation, diarrhea, hepatic failure, hepatitis, ileus, indigestion, melena, nausea, pancreatitis, vomiting

GU: Flank pain, impotence, oliguria, renal failure, UTI

HEME: Agranulocytosis

MS: Back pain, muscle spasms

RESP: Asthma; bronchitis; bronchospasm; cough; dyspnea; pneumonia; pulmonary edema, embolism, infarction, and infiltrates; upper respiratory tract infection

SKIN: Alopecia, diaphoresis, erythema multiforme, exfoliative dermatitis, flushing, pemphigus, photosensitivity, pruritus, rash, Stevens-Johnson syndrome, toxic epidermal necrolysis, urticaria

Other: Anaphylaxis, angioedema, herpes zoster, hyperkalemia

Nursing Considerations

- Use enalapril and felodipine cautiously in patients with heart failure, reduced ventricular function, or impaired hepatic or renal function.
- Monitor blood pressure during therapy and when dosage changes, especially in elderly patients, to assess effectiveness.
- Monitor laboratory test results to check hepatic and renal function, leukocyte count, and serum potassium level.
- Expect felodipine bioavailability to increase by up to twofold when taken with grapefruit juice.
- WARNING Be aware that felodipine may cause severe hypotension with syncope, which may lead to reflex tachycardia and angina in patients with coronary artery disease or a history of angina.
- WARNING Monitor patient closely for angioedema of the face, lips, tongue, glottis, larynx, or limbs. For angioedema of the face and lips, stop drug and give an antihistamine, as prescribed. If tongue, glottis, or larynx is involved, assess patient for airway obstruction, prepare to give epinephrine 1:1,000 (0.3 to 0.5 ml) subcutaneously, and maintain a patent airway.
- Monitor patient for signs of felodopine overdose, such as excessive peripheral vasodilation, marked hypotension, and possibly bradycardia. If you detect such signs, place patient in supine

position with legs elevated and give I.V. fluids, as prescribed. Expect to give I.V. atropine for bradycardia.

PATIENT TEACHING

- Instruct patient to swallow tablets whole and not to crush or chew them.
- Caution patient not to fluctuate her intake of grapefruit juice during therapy.
- Instruct patient to monitor her pulse rate and blood pressure and to report consistent changes to prescriber.
- Teach patient how to minimize gingival hyperplasia by following good dental hygiene practices.
- Advise patient to notify prescriber immediately if she has palpitations; pronounced dizziness; swelling of face, hands, or feet; or a persistent, dry cough.
- Advise female patient to notify prescriber immediately if she is or could be pregnant. Enalapril and felodipine will need to be replaced with another antihypertensive immediately.
- Advise patient to change positions slowly and avoid hazardous activities until the drug's effects are known.
- Tell patient to consult prescriber before using salt substitutes, potassium supplements, or other drugs (including OTC drugs) during therapy.
- Alert patient to notify prescriber about any signs of infection, such as a sore throat or fever.

enalapril maleate and hydrochlorothiazide

Vaseretic

Class and Category

Chemical: Dicarbocyl-containing ACE inhibitor (enalapril), benothiadiazine (hydrochlorothiazide)

Therapeutic: Antihypertensive (enalapril, hydrochlorothiazide), diuretic (hydrochlorothiazide)

Pregnancy category: C (first trimester), D (second and third trimesters)

Indications and Dosages

▶ *To treat hypertension not adequately controlled by enalapril or hydrochlorothiazide alone*

TABLETS

Adults. *Initial:* 5 mg enalapril and 12.5 mg hydrochlorothiazide (1 tablet) daily. Alternatively, 10 mg enalapril and 25 mg hydrochlorothiazide (1 tablet) daily. Dosoage increased, as needed, every 2 to 3 wk. *Maximum:* 20 mg enalapril and 50 mg hydrochlorothiazide.

Mechanism of Action

Enalapril may reduce blood pressure by affecting the renin-angiotensin-aldosterone system. By inhibiting inhibiting ACE, enalapril:

- prevents conversion of angiotensin I to angiotensin II, a potent vasoconstrictor that also stimulates adrenal cortex to secrete aldosterone.
- may inhibit renal and vascular production of angiotensin II.
- decreases serum angiotensin II level and increases serum renin activity. This decreases aldosterone secretion, slightly increasing serum potassium level and fluid loss.
- decreases vascular tone and blood pressure.
- inhibits aldosterone release, which reduces sodium and water reabsorption and increases their excretion, further reducing blood pressure.

Hydrochlorothiazide promotes movement of sodium, chloride, and water from blood in the peritubular capillaries into the nephron's distal convoluted tubule. Initially, it may decrease extracellular fluid volume, plasma volume, and cardiac output, which helps explain blood pressure reduction. It also may reduce blood pressure by dilating arteries. After several weeks, extracellular fluid volume, plasma volume, and cardiac output return to normal, and peripheral vascular resistance remains decreased.

Contraindications

Anuria; hereditary or idiopathic angioedema; history of angioedema from previous ACE inhibitor; hypersensitivity to enalapril, hydrochlorothiazide, other sulfonamide-derived drugs or their components

Interactions

DRUGS

enalapril and hydrochlorothiazide

antihypertensives, diuretics: Additive hypotensive effects
lithium: Increased blood lithium level and toxicity
NSAIDs, sympathomimetics: Possibly reduced antihypertensive effects and increased risk of renal toxicity

enalapril

allopurinol, bone marrow depressants (such as amphotericin B and methotrexate), procainamide, systemic corticosteroids: Possibly increased risk of fatal neutropenia or agranulocytosis *cyclosporine, potassium-sparing diuretics, potassium supplements:* Increased risk of hyperkalemia

sodium aurothiomalate: Increased risk of nitritoid reactions, such as facial flushing, hypotension, nausea, vomiting

hydrochlorothiazide

amantadine: Possibly increased blood level and risk of toxicity of amantadine

amiodarone: Increased risk of arrhythmias from hypokalemia

amphotericin B, corticosteroids: Intensified electrolyte depletion, especially hypokalemia

antihypertensives: Increased antihypertensive effects

barbiturates, opioids: May potentiate orthostatic hypotension

calcium: Possibly increased serum calcium level

cholestyramine, colestipol resins: Reduced GI absorption of hydrochlorothiazide

diazoxide: Increased antihypertensive and hyperglycemic effects of hydrochlorothiazide

diflunisal: Possibly increased blood hydrochlorothiazide level

digoxin: Increased risk of digitalis toxicity from hypokalemia

dopamine: Possibly increased diuretic effects of both drugs

insulin, oral antidiabetics: Possibly increased blood glucose level

neuromuscular blockers: Possibly enhanced neuromuscular blockade from hypokalemia

nondepolarizing skeletal muscle relaxants (such as tubocurarine): Possibly increased responsiveness to the muscle relaxant

pressor amines (such as norepinephrine): Possibly decreased response to pressor amines

oral anticoagulants: Possibly decreased anticoagulant effects

vitamin D: Increased risk of hypercalcemia

FOODS

enalapril

potassium-containing salt substitutes: Increased risk of hyperkalemia

ACTIVITIES

enalapril

alcohol use: Possibly additive hypotensive effect

Adverse Reactions

CNS: Asthenia, ataxia, confusion, depression, dizziness, dream disturbances, fatigue, headache, insomnia, nervousness, paresthesia, peripheral neuropathy, somnolence, stroke, syncope, vertigo, weakness

CV: Angina, arrhythmias, cardiac arrest, chest pain, hypotension, MI, orthostatic hypotension, palpitations, Raynaud's phenome-

non, tachycardia, vasculitis
EENT: Blurred vision, conjunctivitis, dry eyes and mouth, glossitis, hoaseness, lacrimation, loss of smell, pharyngitis, rhinorrhea, stomatitis, taste perversion, tinnitus
ENDO: Gynecomastia, hyperglycemia
GI: Abdominal pain, anorexia, constipation, diarrhea, dyspepsia, flatulence, hepatic failure, hepatitis, ileus, indigestion, jaundice, melena, nausea, pancreatitis, vomiting
GU: Decreased libido, flank pain, impotence, interstitial nephritis, nocturia, polyuria, oliguria, renal failure, UTI
HEME: Agranulocytosis, aplastic anemia, hemolytic anemia, leukopenia, neutropenia, thrombocytopenia
MS: Arthralgia; muscle cramps, spasms, and weakness
RESP: Asthma; back pain; bronchitis; bronchospasm; cough; dyspnea; pneumonia; pulmonary edema, embolism, infarction and infiltrates; upper respiratory tract infection
SKIN: Alopecia, diaphoresis, erythema multiforme, exfoliative dermatitis, flushing, pemphigus, photosensitivity, pruritus, rash, Stevens-Johnson syndrome, toxic epidermal necrolysis, urticaria
Other: Anaphylaxis, angioedema, dehydration, gout, herpes zoster, hypercalcemia, hyperkalemia, hyperuricemia, hypochloremia, hypokalemia, hyponatremia, hypovolemia, metabolic alkalosis, weight loss

Nursing Considerations
- Use cautiously in patients with impaired renal or hepatic function because enalapril and hydrochlorothiazide may alter fluid and electrolyte balance and cause renal failure or hepatic coma.
- Also use cautiously in patients with systemic lupus erythematosus because hydrochlorothiazide may activate or worsen it.
- Monitor blood pressure frequently to assess effectiveness of enalapril and hydrochlorothiazide therapy.
- WARNING Be aware that enalapril and hydrochlorothiazide may cause severe hypotension with syncope, leading to reflex tachycardia and angina in patients with coronary artery disease or a history of angina.
- WARNING Monitor patient closely for angioedema of the face, lips, tongue, glottis, larynx, or limbs. For angioedema of the face and lips, stop drug and give an antihistamine, as prescribed. If tongue, glottis, or larynx is involved, assess patient for airway obstruction, prepare to give epinephrine 1:1,000 (0.3 to 0.5 ml) subcutaneously, and maintain a patent airway.
- Provide hydration, as appropriate, to help prevent hypovolemia.

- Monitor fluid intake and output, daily weight, and serum electrolyte levels (especially potassium) to detect volume depletion or electrolyte imbalance.
- Watch for increased BUN and serum creatinine levels, especially in patients with impaired renal function, because drug may cause acute renal failure. If increases are significant or persistent, notify prescriber immediately.
- Monitor blood glucose level often in diabetic patients, and expect to increase antidiabetic dosage, as needed and ordered.
- Monitor WBC count periodically, especially in patients with collagen-vascular disease, to detect neutropenia and agranulocytosis. Although they aren't known to occur with enalapril, they have occurred with captropril, another ACE inhibitor.
- Assess liver enzymes periodically and monitor patient for jaundice because hepatic failure, although rare, has occurred with other ACE inhibitors. If liver enzymes develop marked elevation or patient develops jaundice, notify prescriber and expect to stop benazepril and hydrochlorothiazide.

PATIENT TEACHING

- Advise patient to take enalapril and hydrochlorothiazide in the morning or early evening to avoid needing to urinate during the night.
- Teach patient to monitor her blood pressure and to report consistently elevated measurements to prescriber.
- Direct patient to weigh herself at the same time each day wearing the same amount of clothing and to notify prescriber if she gains more than 2 lb (0.9 kg) per day or 5 lb (2.3 kg) per week.
- To reduce the risk of dehydration and hypotension, advise patient to avoid exercise in hot weather and to avoid alcohol. Also instruct her to notify prescriber if she has prolonged diarrhea, nausea, or vomiting.
- Caution patient to avoid hazardous activities until drug's CNS effects are known.
- Explain the importance of regular exercise, proper diet, and other lifestyle changes in controlling hypertension.
- WARNING Strongly urge patient to contact prescriber before using potassium supplements or OTC salt substitutes, which may contain potassium, increasing the risk of hyperkalemia.
- Advise female patient to notify prescriber right away if she is or could be pregnant. Enalapril and hydrochlorothiazide will need to be replaced with another antihypertensive immediately.
- Warn patient with gout that drug may cause acute gout attack.

eprosartan mesylate and hydrochlorothiazide
Teveten

Class and Category
Chemical: Nonbiphenyl nontetrazole angiotensin II receptor antagonist (eprosartan), benothiadiazide (hydrochlorothiazide)
Therapeutic: Antihypertensive (eprosartan, hydrochlorothiazide), diuretic (hydrochlorothiazide)
Pregnancy category: C (first trimester), D (second and third trimesters)

Indications and Dosages
▶ *To treat hypertension uncontrolled by eprosartan or hydrochlorothiazide alone*
TABLETS
Adults. *Initial:* 600 mg eprosartan and 12.5 mg hydrochlorothiazide (1 tablet) daily; increased as needed to 600 mg eprosartan and 25 mg hydrochlorothiazide (1 tablet) daily.

Mechanism of Action
Eprosartan blocks the effects of angiotensin II (a potent vasoconstrictor that's part of the renin-angiotensin-aldosterone system) by blocking it from binding to angiotensin I receptors in vascular smooth muscles, adrenal glands, and other tissues. This action halts angiotensin II's negative feedback on renin secretion. Thus, circulating renin and angiotensin II levels rise and vascular resistance declines, reducing blood pressure.

Hydrochlorothiazide promotes movement of sodium, chloride, and water from blood in the peritubular capillaries into the nephron's distal convoluted tubule. Initially, the drug may decrease extracellular fluid volume, plasma volume, and cardiac output, which helps explain blood pressure reduction. It also may reduce blood pressure by dilating arteries. After several weeks, extracellular fluid volume, plasma volume, and cardiac output return to normal, and peripheral vascular resistance remains decreased.

Contraindications
Anuria; hypersensitivity to eprosartan, hydrochlorothiazide, other sulfonamide-derived drugs, or their components

Interactions
DRUGS

eprosartan and hydrochlorothiazide

diuretics, other antihypertensives: Increased antihypertensive effects

eprosartan

cyclosporine, potassium-sparing diuretics, potassium supplements: Increased risk of hyperkalemia

hydrochlorothiazide

amantadine: Possibly increased blood level and risk of toxicity of amantadine

amiodarone: Increased risk of arrhythmias from hypokalemia

amphotericin B, corticosteroids: Intensified electrolyte depletion, especially hypokalemia

antihypertensives: Increased antihypertensive effects

barbiturates, opioids: May potentiate orthostatic hypotension

calcium: Possibly increased serum calcium level

cholestyramine, colestipol resins: Reduced GI absorption of hydrochlorothiazide

diazoxide: Increased antihypertensive and hyperglycemic effects of hydrochlorothiazide

diflunisal: Possibly increased blood hydrochlorothiazide level

digoxin: Increased risk of digitalis toxicity from hypokalemia

dopamine: Possibly increased diuretic effects of both drugs

insulin, oral antidiabetics: Possibly increased blood glucose level

lithium: Decreased lithium clearance and increased risk of lithium toxicity

neuromuscular blockers: Possibly enhanced neuromuscular blockade from hypokalemia

nondepolarizing skeletal muscle relaxants (such as tubocurarine): Possible increased responsiveness to the muscle relaxant

NSAIDs: Decreased diuretic effect of hydrochlorothiazide and increased risk of renal failure

pressor amines (such as norepinephrine): Possibly decreased response to pressor amines

oral anticoagulants: Possibly decreased anticoagulant effects

sympathomimetics: Possibly decreased antihypertensive effect of hydrochlorothiazide

vitamin D: Increased risk of hypercalcemia

FOODS

eprosartan

high-potassium diet, potassium-containing salt substitutes: Increased risk of hyperkalemia

Adverse Reactions

CNS: Depression, dizziness, drowsiness, fatigue, headache, insomnia, paresthesia, vertigo, weakness

CV: Angina pectoris, atrial fibrillation, bradycardia, extrasystole, hypertriglyceridemia, hypotension, orthostatic hypotension, palpitations, tachycardia, vasculitis
EENT: Blurred vision, dry mouth, pharyngitis, rhinitis
ENDO: Hyperglycemia
GI: Abdominal cramps or pain, anorexia, constipation, diarrhea, indigestion, jaundice, nausea, vomiting
GU: Decreased libido, impotence, interstitial nephritis, nocturia, polyuria, oliguria, renal failure, UTI
HEME: Agranulocytosis, aplastic and hemolytic anemia, leukopenia, neutropenia, thrombocytopenia
MS: Muscle spasms and weakness, myalgia, rhabdomyolysis
RESP: Cough, upper respirator tract infection
SKIN: Alopecia, exfoliative dermatitis, photosensitivity, purpura, rash, urticaria
Other: Anaphylaxis, angioedema, dehydration, hypercalcemia, hyperuricemia, hypochloremia, hypokalemia, hyponatremia, hypovolemia, metabolic alkalosis, weight loss

Nursing Considerations

- Use cautiously in patients with impaired hepatic function because hydrochlorothiazide may alter fluid and electrolyte balance and lead to hepatic coma.
- Also use cautiously in patients with systemic lupus erythematosus because hydrochlorothiazide may activate or worsen it.
- If patient has known or suspected hypovolemia, expect to correct it with I.V. normal saline solution, as prescribed, before starting eprosartan and hydrochlorothiazide.
- Monitor blood pressure often to assess effectiveness of eprosartan and hydrochlorothiazide therapy.
- If patient develops hypotension, expect to stop drug temporarily. Immediately place patient in supine position, and prepare to give I.V. normal saline solution, as prescribed. Expect to resume therapy after blood pressure stabilizes.
- Provide hydration, as appropriate, to help prevent hypovolemia.
- Monitor fluid intake and output, daily weight, and serum electrolyte levels (especially potassium) to detect volume depletion or electrolyte imbalance.
- **WARNING** Monitor patient closely for angioedema of the face, lips, tongue, glottis, larynx, or limbs. For angioedema of the face and lips, stop drug and give an antihistamine, as prescribed. If tongue, glottis, or larynx is involved, assess patient for airway obstruction, prepare to give epinephrine 1:1,000

(0.3 to 0.5 ml) subcutaneously, and maintain a patent airway.

- Watch for increased BUN and serum creatinine levels, especially in patients with impaired renal function, because drug may cause acute renal failure. If increases are significant or persistent, notify prescriber immediately.
- Monitor blood glucose level often in diabetic patients, and expect to increase antidiabetic dosage, as needed and ordered.

PATIENT TEACHING

- Advise patient to take drug in the morning or early evening to avoid the need to urinate during the night.
- Teach patient to monitor her blood pressure and to report consistently elevated measurements to prescriber.
- **WARNING** Strongly urge patient to contact prescriber before using potassium supplements or OTC salt substitutes, which may contain potassium and increase the risk of hyperkalemia.
- Direct patient to weigh herself at the same time each day wearing the same amount of clothing and to notify prescriber if she gains more than 2 lb (0.9 kg) per day or 5 lb (2.3 kg) per week.
- To reduce the risk of dehydration and hypotension, advise patient to avoid exercise in hot weather and to avoid alcohol. Tell her to report prolonged diarrhea, nausea, or vomiting.
- Caution patient to avoid hazardous activities until drug's CNS effects are known.
- Explain the importance of regular exercise, proper diet, and other lifestyle changes in controlling hypertension.
- Advise female patient to notify prescriber immediately if she is or could be pregnant because eprosartan and hydrochlorothiazide will need to be replaced with another antihypertensive that's safe during the second and third trimesters of pregnancy.

ezetimibe and simvastatin

Vytorin

Class and Category

Chemical: Azetidinone (ezetimibe), synthetically derived fermentation product of *Aspergillus terreus* (simvastatin)
Therapeutic: Antihyperlipidemic
Pregnancy category: X

Indications and Dosages

▶ *To treat primary hypercholesterolemia*

TABLETS

Adults. *Initial:* 10 mg ezetimibe and 10 mg simvastatin daily for mild LDL cholesterol level reduction, 10 mg ezetimibe and 20 mg simvastatin daily for moderate LDL cholesterol level reduction, or 10 mg ezetimibe and 40 mg simvastatin daily for aggressive (more than 55%) LDL cholesterol level reduction. Dosage adjusted, as needed, after 2 or more weeks. *Maximum:* 10 mg ezetimibe and 80 mg simvastatin daily.

▶ *To treat homozygous familial hypercholesterolemia*

TABLETS

Adults. 10 mg ezetimibe and 40 mg simvastatin daily or 10 mg ezetimibe and 80 mg simvastatin daily at bedtime.

DOSAGE ADJUSTMENT For patients with severe renal insufficiency, ezetimibe and simvastatin are given only if patient has already taken simvastatin at a dose of 5 mg or higher. For patients taking cyclosporine, ezetimibe and simvastatin are given only if patient has already taken simvastatin at a dose of 5 mg or higher, and the dosage shouldn't exceed 10 mg ezetimibe and 10 mg simvastatin daily. For patients taking danazol, dosage shouldn't exceed 10 mg ezetimibe and 10 mg simvastatin daily. For patients taking amiodarone or verapamil, dosage shouldn't exceed 10 mg ezetimibe and 20 mg simvastatin daily.

Mechanism of Action

Ezetimibe and simvastatin work together to decrease the serum cholesterol level. Normally, lipids in the intestinal lumen break down into cholesterol and other substances that create smaller droplets called micelles. Micelles enter intestinal epithelial cells (called enterocytes), where they combine with triglycerides, cholesterol, and other substances to form chylomicrons. Chylomicrons enter the lymphatic system and are carried to the bloodstream.

Ezetimibe blocks cholesterol absorption into enterocytes. This decreased movement of cholesterol through the intestinal wall decreases chylomicron and LDL cholesterol levels in the bloodstream.

Simvastatin interferes with the hepatic enzyme hydroxymethylglutaryl-coenzyme A reductase. This action reduces formation of mevalonic acid, a cholesterol precursor, thus interrupting cholesterol synthesis. When the cholesterol level declines in hepatic cells, LDLs are consumed, which in turn reduces the levels of circulating total cholesterol and serum triglycerides.

Contraindications

Active liver disease; breast-feeding; concurrent therapy with clarithromycin, erythromycin, fibrates, HIV protease inhibitors, itraconazole, ketoconazole, nefazodone, or telithromycin; hypersensitivity to ezetimibe, simvastatin, or their components; ingestion of more than 1 quart of grapefruit juice daily; pregnancy

Interactions

DRUGS

ezetimibe

cholestyramine: Reduced ezetimibe effectiveness
cyclosporine: Increased blood ezetimibe and cyclosporine levels
fenofibrate, gemfibrozil: Increased blood ezetimibe level

simvastatin

amiodarone, clarithromycin, cyclosporine, danazol, erythromycin, gemfibrozil and other fibrates, itraconazole, ketoconazole, nefazodone, niacin at 1 gram or more daily, protease inhibitors (amprenavir, indinavir, nelfinavir, ritonavir, saquinavir), telithromycin, verapamil: Increased risk of myopathy or rhabdomyolysis

azole antifungals, cyclosporine, gemfibrozil, immunosuppressants, macrolide antibiotics (including erythromycin), niacin, verapamil: Increased risk of acute renal failure

bile acid sequestrants, cholestyramine, colestipol: Decreased bioavailability of simvastatin

digoxin: Possibly slight elevation in blood digoxin level
diltiazem, verapamil: Possibly increased blood simvastatin level and increased risk of myopathy
oral anticoagulants: Increased risk of bleeding or prolonged PT

FOODS

simvastatin

grapefruit juice (1 or more quarts/day): Possibly increased blood simvastatin level; increased risk of myopathy or rhabdomyolysis

Adverse Reactions

CNS: Asthenia, depression, dizziness, fatigue, headache, memory impairment, paresthesia, peripheral neuropathy
CV: Chest pain
EENT: Pharyngitis, rhinitis, sinusitis, taste alteration
GI: Abdominal cramps or pain, cholelithiasis, cholecystitis, constipation, diarrhea, elevated liver function test results, flatulence, heartburn, hepatic failure, hepatitis, nausea, pancreatitis, vomiting
HEME: Anemia, thrombocytopenia
MS: Arthralgia, back pain, myalgia, myopathy, rhabdomyolysis
RESP: Cough, upper respiratory tract infection
SKIN: Alopecia, eczema, pruritus, rash, urticaria
Other: Anaphylaxis, angioedema, viral infection

Nursing Considerations

- Use ezetimibe and simvastatin cautiously in elderly patients and those with hepatic or renal impairment.
- Monitor patient's liver function test results before and every 3 to 6 months during therapy, as ordered.
- Give ezetimibe and simvastatin 2 hours before or 4 hours after giving a bile acid sequestrant such as cholestyramine or colestipol).
- Monitor serum lipoprotein level, as ordered, to evaluate patient's response to therapy.
- Monitor patient closely for evidence of myopathy, such as unexplained muscle pain, tenderness, or weakness, especially when therapy starts or dosage increases. If present, notify prescriber and stop drug immediately, as ordered.
- Expect to temporarily stop ezetimibe and simvastatin before elective major surgery or if patient develops any major medical-surgical condition because of the increased risk of myopathy.

PATIENT TEACHING
- Advise patient to take ezetimibe and simvastatin in the evening.
- Encourage patient to follow a low-fat and low-cholesterol diet.
- Instruct patient who's taking a bile acid sequestrant (cholestyramine, colestipol) to take ezetimibe and simvastatin 2 hours before or 4 hours after taking the bile acid sequestrant.
- Urge patient to notify prescriber immediately about symptoms of myopathy, such as muscle pain, tenderness, and weakness.
- Instruct female patient of childbearing age to use reliable contraception while taking drug. Instruct her to notify prescriber at once if she suspects pregnancy.
- Urge patient to avoid grapefruit juice to decrease risk of toxicity.

fosinopril sodium and hydrochlorothiazide
Monopril HCT

Class and Category
Chemical: Phosphinic acid derivative (fosinopril), benothiadiazide (hydrochlorothiazide)
Therapeutic: Antihypertensive (fosinopril, hydrochlorothiazide), diuretic (hydrochlorothiazide)
Pregnancy category: C (first trimester), D (second and third trimesters)

Indications and Dosages

▶ *To treat hypertension uncontrolled by fosinopril or hydrochlorothiazide alone*

TABLETS

Adults. *Initial:* 10 mg fosinopril and 12.5 mg hydrochlorothiazide (1 tablet) daily. Increased, as needed, to 20 mg fosinopril and 12.5 mg hydrochlorothiazide (1 tablet) daily.

Mechanism of Action

Fosinopril may reduce blood pressure by affecting the renin-angiotensin-aldosterone system. By inhibiting ACE, fosinopril:

- prevents conversion of angiotensin I to angiotensin II, a potent vasoconstrictor that also stimulates adrenal cortex to secrete aldosterone.
- may inhibit renal and vascular production of angiotensin II.
- decreases serum angiotensin II level and increases serum renin activity. This decreases aldosterone secretion, slightly increasing serum potassium level and fluid loss.
- decreases vascular tone and blood pressure.
- inhibits aldosterone release, which reduces sodium and water reabsorption and increases their excretion, further reducing blood pressure.

Hydrochlorothiazide promotes movement of sodium, chloride, and water from blood in the peritubular capillaries into the nephron's distal convoluted tubule. Initially, it may decrease extracellular fluid volume, plasma volume, and cardiac output, which helps explain blood pressure reduction. It also may reduce blood pressure by dilating arteries. After several weeks, extracellular fluid volume, plasma volume, and cardiac output return to normal, and peripheral vascular resistance remains decreased.

Contraindications

Anuria; hypersensitivity to fosinopril, hydrochlorothiazide, other ACE inhibitors or sulfonamide-derived drugs, or their components

Interactions

DRUGS

fosinopril and hydrochlorothiazide

antihypertensives, diuretics: Increased antihypertensive effects
digoxin: Increased serum digoxin level and risk of digitalis toxicity
lithium: Increased serum lithium levels and toxicity

fosinopril

allopurinol, bone marrow depressants, procainaminde, systemic corticoste-

roids: Increased risk of potentially fatal neutropenia or agranulocytosis

antacids: Possibly decreased bioavailability of fosinopril from impaired absorption

cyclosporine, potassium-sparing diuretics (amiloride, spironolactone, triamterene), potassium supplements: Increased risk of hyperkalemia

hydrochlorothiazide

amantadine: Possibly increased blood amantadine level and risk of toxicity

amiodarone: Increased risk of arrhythmias from hypokalemia

amphotericin B, corticosteroids: Intensified electrolyte depletion, especially hypokalemia

antihypertensives: Increased antihypertensive effects

barbiturates, opioids: May potentiate orthostatic hypotension

calcium: Possibly increased serum calcium level

cholestyramine, colestipol resins: Reduced GI absorption of hydrochlorothiazide

diazoxide: Increased antihypertensive and hyperglycemic effects of hydrochlorothiazide

diflunisal: Possibly increased blood hydrochlorothiazide level

digoxin: Increased risk of digitalis toxicity from hypokalemia

dopamine: Possibly increased diuretic effects of both drugs

insulin, oral antidiabetics: Possibly increased blood glucose level

lithium: Decreased lithium clearance and increased risk of toxicity

neuromuscular blockers: Possibly enhanced neuromuscular blockade from hypokalemia

nondepolarizing skeletal muscle relaxants (such as tubocurarine): Possibly increased responsiveness to the muscle relaxant

NSAIDs: Decreased diuretic effect of hydrochlorothiazide, increased risk of renal failure

pressor amines (such as norepinephrine): Possibly decreased response to pressor amines

oral anticoagulants: Possibly decreased anticoagulant effects

sympathomimetics: Possibly decreased antihypertensive effect of hydrochlorothiazide

vitamin D: Increased risk of hypercalcemia

FOODS

fosinopril

salt substitutes that contain potassium: Increased risk of hyperkalemia

ACTIVITIES

fosinopril

alcohol use: Possibly additive hypotension

Adverse Reactions

CNS: Confusion, depression, dizziness, drowsiness, fatigue, fever, headache, insomnia, mood swings, paresthesia, sleep disturbance, syncope, tremor, vertigo, weakness

CV: Angina, arrhythmias (including AV conduction disorders, bradycardia, and tachycardia), claudication, hypotension, MI, orthostatic hypotension, palpitations, vasculitis

EENT: Blurred vision, dry mouth, epistaxis, eye irritation, hoarseness, rhinitis, sinus problems, taste perversion, tinnitus, vision changes

ENDO: Hyperglycemia

GI: Abdominal cramps, distention, or pain; anorexia; constipation; diarrhea; flatulence; hepatic failure; hepatitis; hepatomegaly; indigestion; jaundice; nausea; pancreatitis; vomiting

GU: Decreased libido, flank pain, impotence, interstitial nephritis, nocturia, polyuria, renal insufficiency or failure, urinary frequency

HEME: Agranulocytosis, aplastic and hemolytic anemia, leukopenia, neutropenia, thrombocytopenia

MS: Arthralgia, muscle spasms and weakness, myalgia

RESP: Asthma; bronchitis; bronchospasm; dry, persistent, tickling cough; dyspnea; tracheobronchitis; upper respiratory tract infection

SKIN: Alopecia, diaphoresis, exfoliative dermatitis, photosensitivity, pruritus, purpura, rash, urticaria

Other: Anaphylaxis, angioedema, dehydration, gout, hypercalcemia, hyperkalemia, hyperuricemia, hypochloremia, hypokalemia, hyponatremia, hypovolemia, metabolic alkalosis, weight gain or loss

Nursing Considerations

- Use cautiously in patients with impaired hepatic function because hydrochlorothiazide may alter fluid and electrolyte balance and cause hepatic coma.
- Also use cautiously in patients with systemic lupus erythematosus because hydrochlorothiazide may activate or worsen it.
- Monitor blood pressure often to assess effectiveness of fosinopril and hydrochlorothiazide therapy.
- Assess patient for hypotension for at least 2 hours after giving fosinopril and hydrochlorothiazide. If present, notify precriber and monitor patient until blood pressure stabilizes. Provide supportive measures, as indicated and ordered.
- If patient receives an antacid, separate administration times by at least 2 hours.

- **WARNING** Monitor patient closely for signs and symptoms of angioedema or allergic reactions such as rash, urticaria, or difficulty breathing. If present, withhold drug, notify prescriber immediately, and expect to treat symptomatically. If airway obstruction threatens, promptly give 0.3 to 0.5 ml of epinephrine solution 1:1,000 subcutaneously, as prescribed.
- Provide adequate hydration, as appropriate, to help prevent hypovolemia.
- Monitor fluid intake and output, daily weight, and serum electrolyte levels (especially potassium) to detect volume depletion or electrolyte imbalance.
- Watch for increased BUN and serum creatinine levels, especially in patients with impaired renal function, because drug may cause acute renal failure. If increases are significant or persistent, notify prescriber immediately.
- Monitor blood glucose level often in diabetic patients, and expect to increase antidiabetic dosage, as needed and ordered.
- Check WBC count periodically, especially in patients with collagen-vascular disease, to detect neutropenia and agranulocytosis. Although they aren't known to occur with fosinopril, they have occurred with captropril, another ACE inhibitor.
- Assess liver enzymes periodically, and monitor patient for jaundice because hepatic failure, although rare, has occurred with other ACE inhibitors. If liver enzymes develop marked elevation or patient develops jaundice, notify prescriber and expect to stop fosinopril and hydrochlorothiazide.

PATIENT TEACHING
- Advise patient to take drug in the morning or early evening to avoid the need to urinate during the night.
- Teach patient to monitor her blood pressure and pulse rate and to report consistently elevated measurements to prescriber.
- **WARNING** Instruct patient to contact prescriber immediately if she has evidence of hypersensitivity, especially angioedema (swelling of the face, eyes, lips or tongue), difficulty breathing, hives, or rash.
- Direct patient to weigh herself at the same time each day wearing the same amount of clothing and to notify prescriber if she gains more than 2 lb (0.9 kg) per day or 5 lb (2.3 kg) per week.
- To reduce the risk of dehydration and hypotension, advise patient to avoid exercise in hot weather and to avoid alcohol. Also tell her to notify prescriber if she has prolonged diarrhea, nausea, or vomiting.

- Caution patient to avoid hazardous activities until drug's CNS effects are known.
- Explain the importance of regular exercise, proper diet, and other lifestyle changes in controlling hypertension.
- **WARNING** Strongly urge patient to contact prescriber before using potassium supplements or OTC salt substitutes, which may contain potassium. These products increase the risk of hyperkalemia.
- Advise female patient to notify prescriber immediately if she is or could be pregnant because fosinopril and hydrochlorothiazide will need to be replaced with another antihypertensive that's safe to use during the second and third trimesters of pregnancy.
- Warn patient with gout that drug may precipitate an acute gout attack.
- Inform patient that a persistent dry cough may develop and may not subside unless fosinopril and hydrochlorothiazide therapy is stopped. If cough becomes bothersome or interferes with her sleep or activities, instruct her to notify prescriber.
- Tell patient to avoid sudden position changes and to rise slowly from a seated or reclining position to minimize orthostatic hypotension.

hydralazine and hydrochlorothiazide
Apresazide, Hydra-Zide

Class and Category
Chemical: Phthalazine derivative (hydralazine), benzothiadiazide (hydrochlorothiazide)
Therapeutic: Antihyperthenisve (hydralazine, hydrochlorothiazide), diuretic (hydrochlorothiazide)
Pregnancy category: C

Indications and Dosages
▶ *To treat hypertension*
CAPSULES
Adults. 25 to 100 mg hydralazine and 25 to 50 mg hydrochlorothiazide (1 to 2 capsules depending on product) b.i.d.

Contraindications
Anuria; coronary artery or rheumatic heart disease; hypersensitivity to hydralazine, hydrochlorothiazide, other sulfonamide-derived drugs or their components; mitral valve disease

Mechanism of Action

Hydralazine exerts a direct vasodilating effect on smooth muscle in arterioles, interferes with calcium movement in arteriole smooth muscle by altering cellular calcium metabolism, and dilates arteries to lower blood pressure.

Hydrochlorothiazide promotes movement of sodium, chloride, and water from blood in the peritubular capillaries into the nephron's distal convoluted tubule. Initially, it may decrease extracellular fluid volume, plasma volume, and cardiac output, which helps explain blood pressure reduction. It also may reduce blood pressure by dilating arteries. After several weeks, extracellular fluid volume, plasma volume, and cardiac output return to normal, and peripheral vascular resistance remains decreased.

Interactions

DRUGS

hydralazine and hydrochlorothiazide
antihypertensives, diazoxide: Risk of severe hypotension
NSAIDs, sympathomimetics: Decreased antihypertensive effect
hydralazine
beta blockers: Increased effects of both drugs
epinephrine: Possibly decreased vasopressor effect of epinephrine
hydrochlorothiazide
amantadine: Possibly increased blood amantadine level and risk of toxicity
amiodarone: Increased risk of arrhythmias from hypokalemia
amphotericin B, corticosteroids: Intensified electrolyte depletion, especially hypokalemia
antihypertensives: Increased antihypertensive effects
barbiturates, opioids: May potentiate orthostatic hypotension
calcium: Possibly increased serum calcium level
cholestyramine, colestipol resins: Reduced GI absorption of hydrochlorothiazide
diazoxide: Increased hyperglycemic effects of hydrochlorothiazide
diflunisal: Possibly increased blood hydrochlorothiazide level
digoxin: Increased risk of digitalis toxicity from hypokalemia
dopamine: Possibly increased diuretic effects of both drugs
insulin, oral antidiabetics: Possibly increased blood glucose level
lithium: Decreased lithium clearance and increased risk of toxicity
MAO inhibitors: Risk of severe hypotension
neuromuscular blockers: Possibly enhanced neuromuscular blockade from hypokalemia

nondepolarizing skeletal muscle relaxants (such as tubocurarine): Possibly increased responsiveness to the muscle relaxant

NSAIDs: Increased risk of renal failure

pressor amines (such as norepinephrine): Possibly decreased response to pressor amines

oral anticoagulants: Possibly decreased anticoagulant effects

vitamin D: Increased risk of hypercalcemia

FOODS

hydralazine

all foods: Possibly increased bioavailability of hydralazine

ACTIVITIES

hydralazine and hydrochlorothiazide

alcohol use: Potentiated hypotensive effect

Adverse Reactions

CNS: Chills, dizziness, fever, headache, insomnia, paresthesia, peripheral neuritis, vertigo, weakness

CV: Angina, edema, hypotension, orthostatic hypotension, palpitations, tachycardia, vasculitis

EENT: Blurred vision, dry mouth, lacrimation, nasal congestion

ENDO: Hyperglycemia

GI: Abdominal cramps, anorexia, constipation, diarrhea, indigestion, jaundice, nausea, vomiting

GU: Decreased libido, impotence, interstitial nephritis, nocturia, polyuria, proteinurea, renal failure

HEME: Agranulocytosis, aplastic and hemolytic anemia, leukopenia, neutropenia, thrombocytopenia

MS: Muscle spasms and weakness

RESP: Dyspnea

SKIN: Alopecia, blisters, exfoliative dermatitis, flushing, photosensitivity, pruritus, purpura, rash, urticaria

Other: Anaphylaxis, dehydration, gout, hypercalcemia, hyperuricemia, hypochloremia, hypokalemia, hyponatremia, hypovolemia, lupus-like symptoms, lymphadenopathy, metabolic alkalosis, weight loss

Nursing Considerations

- Use cautiously in patients with impaired hepatic function because hydrochlorothiazide may alter fluid and electrolyte balance, which may lead to hepatic coma.
- Also use cautiously in patients with systemic lupus erythematosus because hydrochlorothiazide may activate or worsen the disorder and hydralazine may cause lupus-like symptoms.
- Give drug with food to increase bioavailability.

- Monitor CBC, lupus erythematosus cell preparation, and ANA titer before and periodically during long-term treatment.
- **WARNING** Expect to stop drug immediately if patient develops lupus-like symptoms, such as arthralgia, fever, myalgia, pharyngitis, and splenomegaly.
- Check blood pressure often to assess effectiveness of hydralazine and hydrochlorothiazide therapy.
- Provide hydration, as appropriate, to help prevent hypovolemia.
- Monitor fluid intake and output, daily weight, and serum electrolyte levels (especially potassium) to detect volume depletion or electrolyte imbalance.
- Monitor for increased BUN and serum creatinine levels, especially in patients with impaired renal function, because drug may cause acute renal failure. If increases are significant or persistent, notify prescriber immediately.
- Monitor blood glucose level often in diabetic patients, and expect to increase antidiabetic dosage, as needed and ordered.
- Expect prescriber to withdraw drug gradually to avoid a rapid increase in blood pressure.
- Expect to treat peripheral neuritis with pyridoxine if it occurs.

PATIENT TEACHING

- Advise patient to take hydralazine and hydrochlorothiazide with food to increase absorption and in the morning or early evening to avoid the need to urinate during the night.
- Direct patient to weigh herself at the same time each day wearing the same amount of clothing and to notify prescriber if she gains more than 2 lb (0.9 kg) per day or 5 lb (2.3 kg) per week.
- Instruct patient to eat a diet high in potassium-rich foods, such as citrus fruits, bananas, tomatoes, and dates.
- To reduce the risk of dehydration and hypotension, advise patient to avoid exercise in hot weather and top avoid alcohol. Also instruct her to notify prescriber if she has prolonged diarrhea, nausea, or vomiting.
- Urge patient to change position slowly, especially in the morning. Caution her that hot showers may increase hypotension.
- Instruct patient to immediately notify prescriber about fever, muscle and joint aches, and sore throat.
- Urge patient to report numbness and tingling in her limbs, which may require treatment with another drug.
- Caution patient to avoid hazardous activities until drug's CNS effects are known.
- Caution patient against stopping drug abruptly because doing so may cause severe rise in her blood pressure.

- Advise patient to avoid direct sunlight including ultraviolet light as much as possible and to wear protective clothing including a hat and use a sunscreen when exposure can not be avoided.

hydrochlorothiazide and triamterene
Dyazide, Maxzide

Class and Category
Chemical: benothiadiazide (hydrochlorothiazide), pterdine derivative (triamterene)
Therapeutic: Antihypertensive (hydrochlorothiazide, triamterene), diuretic (hydrochlorothiazide)
Pregnancy category: C

Indications and Dosages
▶ *To treat hypertension or edema in patients adequately controlled by hydrochlorothiazide alone but who develop significant potassium loss; to treat hypertension in patients uncontrolled with triamterene monotherapy*
CAPSULES
Adults. 25 mg hydrochlorothiazide and 37.5 mg triamterene (1 capsule) daily. Increased, as needed, to 50 mg hydrochlorothiazide and 75 mg triamterene (2 capsules) daily.

Mechanism of Action
Hydrochlorothiazide promotes movement of sodium, chloride, and water from blood in the peritubular capillaries into the nephron's distal convoluted tubule. Initially, it may decrease extracellular fluid volume, plasma volume, and cardiac output, which helps explain blood pressure reduction. It also may reduce blood pressure by dilating arteries. After several weeks, extracellular fluid volume, plasma volume, and cardiac output return to normal, and peripheral vascular resistance remains decreased.

Triamterene inhibits sodium reabsorption in distal convoluted tubules and cortical collecting ducts, causing sodium and water loss, which reduces blood pressure. It also enhances potassium retention.

Contraindications
Anuria; diabetic nephropathy or renal disease linked to renal insufficiency; hyperkalemia (potassium level of 5.5 mEq/L or more); hypersensitivity to hydrochlorothiazide, triamterene, other sulfonamide-derived drugs, or their components; severe hepatic dysfunction

Interactions
DRUGS
hydrochlorothiazide and triamterene
amantadine: Possibly increased blood level and risk of toxicity of amantadine

antihypertensives, diuretics: Increased antihypertensive effects

chlorpropamide: Increased risk of severe hyponatremia

exchange resins (such as sodium polystyrene sulfonate): Decreased serum potassium levels; increased fluid retention

insulin, oral antidiabetics: Possibly increased blood glucose level

lithium: Decreased lithium clearance and increased risk of toxicity

NSAIDs: Decreased diuretic effect of hydrochlorothiazide and triamterene, increased risk of renal failure

hydrochlorothiazide
amiodarone: Increased risk of arrhythmias from hypokalemia

amphotericin B, corticosteroids: Intensified electrolyte depletion, especially hypokalemia

barbiturates, opioids: May potentiate orthostatic hypotension

calcium: Possibly increased serum calcium level

cholestyramine, colestipol resins: Reduced GI absorption of hydrochlorothiazide

diazoxide: Increased antihypertensive and hyperglycemic effects of hydrochlorothiazide

diflunisal: Possibly increased blood hydrochlorothiazide level

digoxin: Increased risk of digitalis toxicity from hypokalemia

dopamine: Possibly increased diuretic effects of both drugs

methenamine: Possibly decreased effectiveness of methenamine

neuromuscular blockers: Possibly enhanced neuromuscular blockade from hypokalemia

nondepolarizing skeletal muscle relaxants (such as tubocurarine): Possibly increased responsiveness to the muscle relaxant

pressor amines (such as norepinephrine): Possibly decreased response to pressor amines

oral anticoagulants: Possibly decreased anticoagulant effects

sympathomimetics: Possibly decreased antihypertensive effect of hydrochlorothiazide

vitamin D: Increased risk of hypercalcemia

triamterene
ACE inhibitors, amiloride, angiotensin-II receptor antagonists, cyclosporine, heparin, potassium-containing drugs, potassium salts, potassium supplements, spironolactone: Increased risk of hyperkalemia

folic acid: Possibly antagonized action of folic acid

laxatives: Possibly reduced potassium-retaining effects of triamterene

Adverse Reactions

CNS: Dizziness, fatigue, headache, insomnia, paresthesia, vertigo, weakness

CV: Hypotension, orthostatic hypotension, vasculitis

EENT: Blurred vision, dry mouth

ENDO: Hyperglycemia, hypoglycemia

GI: Abdominal cramps, anorexia, constipation, diarrhea, indigestion, jaundice, nausea, vomiting

GU: Azotemia, decreased libido, impotence, elevated BUN and serum creatinine levels, interstitial nephritis, nocturia, polyuria, renal calculi, renal failure

HEME: Agranulocytosis, aplastic and hemolytic anemia, leukopenia, neutropenia, thrombocytopenia

MS: Muscle spasms and weakness

SKIN: Alopecia, exfoliative dermatitis, photosensitivity, purpura, rash, subacute cutaneous lupus erythematosus–like reactions, urticaria

Other: Anaphylaxis, dehydration, hypercalcemia, hyperkalemia, hyperuricemia, hypochloremia, hypokalemia, hyponatremia, hypovolemia, metabolic alkalosis, weight loss

Nursing Considerations

• Use cautiously in patients with impaired hepatic function because hydrochlorothiazide may alter fluid and electrolyte balance and lead to hepatic coma.

• Also use cautiously in patients with systemic lupus erythematosus because hydrochlorothiazide may activate or worsen it.

• Be aware that hydrochlorothiazide and triamterene shouldn't be given to patients with creatinine clearance below 10 ml/min/1.73 m^2 because they have an increased risk of drug-induced hyperkalemia.

• Check blood pressure often to assess effectiveness of hydrochlorothiazide and triamterene therapy.

• Provide hydration, as appropriate, to help prevent hypovolemia.

• Monitor fluid intake and output, daily weight, and serum electrolyte levels (especially potassium) to detect volume depletion or electrolyte imbalance.

• Monitor patient for evidence of hyperkalemia, such as irregular heartbeat (usually the first sign), paresthesia, muscle weakness, fatigue, flaccid paralysis of the limbs, bradycardia, and shock. In suspected hyperkalemia, obtain an ECG tracing, as ordered. A widened QRS complex or an arrhythmia warrants prompt treatment. If hyperkalemia is confirmed, hydrochlorothiazide and triamterene must be stopped.

- Watch for increased BUN and serum creatinine levels, especially in patients with impaired renal function, because drug may cause acute renal failure. If increases are significant or persistent, notify prescriber immediately.
- Monitor blood glucose level frequently in diabetic patients, and expect to increase the antidiabetic dosage, as needed and ordered.
- Assess patient for evidence of metabolic or respiratory acidosis, which may occur suddenly in patients with cardiac disease or uncontrolled diabetes mellitus.
- Monitor patient's serum uric acid level, as ordered, because drug may reduce uric acid clearance and increase the risk of gout and hyperuricemia. It also may worsen hyponatremia.
- Monitor CBC with differential because hydrochlorothiazide may increase the risk of serious hematologic adverse effects and triamterene may increase the risk of megaloblastic anemia in a patient with folic acid deficiency.

PATIENT TEACHING

- Teach patient to monitor her blood pressure and pulse rate and to report consistent changes to prescriber.
- Advise patient to take hydrochlorothiazide and triamterene in the morning or early evening to avoid the need to urinate during the night.
- Instruct patient to take drug with milk or food to minimize stomach upset.
- Instruct patient to weigh herself at the same time each day wearing the same amount of clothing and to notify prescriber if she gains more than 2 lb (0.9 kg) per day or 5 lb (2.3 kg) per week.
- To reduce the risk of dehydration and hypotension, advise patient to avoid exercise in hot weather and to avoid alcohol. Also instruct her to notify prescriber if she has prolonged diarrhea, nausea, or vomiting.
- Caution patient to avoid hazardous activities until drug's CNS effects are known.
- Explain the importance of regular exercise, proper diet, and other lifestyle changes in controlling hypertension.
- Instruct patient to minimize exposure to sunlight.
- Explain to patient with a history of gout that drug may increase the risk of an attack.

irbesartan and hydrochlorothiazide
Avalide

Class and Category
Chemical: Nonpeptide angiotensin II antagonist (irbesartan), benothiadiazide (hydrochlorothiazide)
Therapeutic: Antihypertensive (irbesartan, hydrochlorothiazide), diuretic (hydrochlorothiazide)
Pregnancy category: D

Indications and Dosages
▶ *To provide initial hypertension treatment for patients who will likely need multiple drugs to achieve adequate blood pressure control; to treat hypertension in patients uncontrolled by irbesartan or hydrochlorothiazide alone*
TABLETS
Adults. *Initial:* 150 mg irbesartan and 12.5 mg hydrochlorothiazide (1 tablet) daily. May be increased to 300 mg irbesartan and 12.5 mg hydrcholorothiazide (1 tablet) daily, as needed, in 2 to 4 wk. *Maximum:* 300 mg irbesartan and 25 mg hydrochlorothiazide daily.

Mechanism of Action
Irbesartan selectively blocks binding of the potent vasoconstrictor angiotension (AT) II to AT1 receptor sites in many tissues, including vascular smooth muscle and adrenal glands. This inhibits the vasoconstrictive and aldosterone-secreting effects of AT II, which reduces blood pressure.

Hydrochlorothiazide promotes movement of sodium, chloride, and water from blood in peritubular capillaries into the nephron's distal convoluted tubule. Initially, it may decrease extracellular fluid volume, plasma volume, and cardiac output, which helps explain blood pressure reduction. It also may reduce blood pressure by dilating arteries. After several weeks, extracellular fluid volume, plasma volume, and cardiac output return to normal, and peripheral vascular resistance remains decreased.

Contraindications
Anuria; hypersensitivity to irbesartan, hydrochlorothiazide, other sulfonamide-derived drugs, or their components

Interactions
DRUGS
irbesartan and hydrochlorothiazide
diuretics, other antihypertensives: Increased antihypertensive effects

hydrochlorothiazide

amantadine: Possibly increased blood amantadine level and risk of toxicity

amiodarone: Increased risk of arrhythmias from hypokalemia

amphotericin B, corticosteroids: Intensified electrolyte depletion, especially hypokalemia

barbiturates, opioids: May potentiate orthostatic hypotension

calcium: Possibly increased serum calcium level

cholestyramine, colestipol resins: Reduced GI absorption of hydrochlorothiazide

diazoxide: Increased antihypertensive and hyperglycemic effects of hydrochlorothiazide

diflunisal: Possibly increased blood hydrochlorothiazide level

digoxin: Increased risk of digitalis toxicity from hypokalemia

dopamine: Possibly increased diuretic effects of both drugs

insulin, oral antidiabetics: Possibly increased blood glucose level

lithium: Decreased lithium clearance and increased risk of toxicity

neuromuscular blockers: Possibly enhanced neuromuscular blockade from hypokalemia

nondepolarizing skeletal muscle relaxants (such as tubocurarine): Possibly increased responsiveness to the muscle relaxant

NSAIDs: Decreased diuretic effect of hydrochlorothiazide, increased risk of renal failure

pressor amines (such as norepinephrine): Possible decreased response to pressor amines

oral anticoagulants: Possibly decreased anticoagulant effects

sympathomimetics: Possibly decreased antihypertensive effect of hydrochlorothiazide

vitamin D: Increased risk of hypercalcemia

Adverse Reactions

CNS: Anxiety, dizziness, fatigue, headache, insomnia, nervousness, paresthesia, vertigo, weakness

CV: Chest pain, hypotension, orthostatic hypotension, peripheral edema, tachycardia, vasculitis

EENT: Blurred vision, dry mouth, pharyngitis, rhinitis

ENDO: Hyperglycemia

GI: Abdominal cramps or pain, anorexia, constipation, diarrhea, heartburn, hepatitis, indigestion, jaundice, nausea, vomiting

GU: Decreased libido, impotence, interstitial nephritis, nocturia, polyuria, renal failure, UTI

HEME: Agranulocytosis, aplastic and hemolytic anemia, leukopenia, neutropenia, thrombocytopenia

MS: Muscle spasms and weakness, musculoskeletal pain, myopathy, rhabdomyolysis
RESP: Upper respiratory tract infection
SKIN: Alopecia, exfoliative dermatitis, photosensitivity, purpura, rash, urticaria
Other: Anaphylaxis, angioedema, dehydration, hypercalcemia, hyperkalemia, hyperuricemia, hypochloremia, hypokalemia, hyponatremia, hypovolemia, metabolic alkalosis, weight loss

Nursing Considerations
• Use cautiously in patients with impaired hepatic function because hydrochlorothiazide may alter fluid and electrolyte balance and lead to hepatic coma.
• Also use cautiously in patients with systemic lupus erythematosus because hydrochlorothiazide may activate or worsen it.
• If patient has known or suspected hypovolemia, expect to correct it with I.V. normal saline solution, as prescribed, before starting irbesartan and hydrochlorothiazide. Provide hydration as needed during therapy to help prevent hypovolemia.
• Monitor blood pressure often to assess effectiveness of therapy with irbesartan and hydrochlorothiazide.
• If patient develops hypotension, expect to stop drug temporarily. Immediately place patient in supine position, and prepare to give I.V. normal saline solution, as prescribed. Expect to resume therapy after blood pressure stabilizes.
• **WARNING** Monitor patient closely for angioedema of the face, lips, tongue, glottis, larynx, or limbs. For angioedema of the face and lips, stop drug and give an antihistamine, as prescribed. If tongue, glottis, or larynx is involved, assess patient for airway obstruction, prepare to give epinephrine 1:1,000 (0.3 to 0.5 ml) subcutaneously, and maintain a patent airway.
• Monitor fluid intake and output, daily weight, and serum electrolyte levels (especially potassium) to detect volume depletion or electrolyte imbalance.
• Watch for increased BUN and serum creatinine levels, especially in patients with impaired renal function, because drug may cause acute renal failure. If increases are significant or persistent, notify prescriber immediately.
• Monitor blood glucose level often in diabetic patients, and expect to increase antidiabetic dosage, as needed and ordered.
PATIENT TEACHING
• Advise patient to take drug in the morning or early evening to avoid the need to urinate during the night.

- Teach patient to monitor her blood pressure and to report consistently elevated measurements to prescriber.
- Direct patient to weigh herself at the same time each day wearing the same amount of clothing and to notify the prescriber if she gains more than 2 lb (0.9 kg) per day or 5 lb (2.3 kg) per week.
- To reduce the risk of dehydration and hypotension, advise patient to avoid exercise in hot weather and to avoid alcohol. Also instruct her to notify prescriber if she has prolonged diarrhea, nausea, or vomiting.
- Caution patient to avoid hazardous activities until drug's CNS effects are known.
- Explain the importance of regular exercise, proper diet, and other lifestyle changes in controlling hypertension.
- Advise female patient to notify prescriber immediately if she is or could be pregnant; irbesartan and hydrochlorothiazide will need to be replaced with another antihypertensive that's safe to use during pregnancy.

isosorbide dinitrate and hydralazine hydrochloride
BiDil

Class and Category
Chemical: Organic nitrate (isosorbide dinitrate), phthalazine (hydralazine)
Therapeutic: Vasodilator (isosorbide dinitrate, hydralazine)
Pregnancy category: C

Indications and Dosages
▶ *As adjunct to improve survival, prolong time between hospitalizations and improve functional status in black patients with heart failure*
TABLETS
Adults. *Initial:* 20 mg isosorbide dinitrate and 37.5 mg hydralazine (1 tablet) three times daily, increased as needed in 3 to 5 days. *Maximum:* 40 mg isosorbide and 75 mg hydralazine (2 tablets) three times daily.
DOSAGE ADJUSTMENT Initial dosage reduced to 10 mg isosorbide dinitrate and 18.75 mg hydralazine (½ tablet) three times daily, as needed, if patient has intolerable adverse reactions

Mechanism of Action

Isosorbide may interact with nitrate receptors in vascular smooth-muscle cell membranes. By interacting with nitrate receptors' sulfhydryl groups, the drug is reduceed to nitric oxide, which activates the enzyme guanylate cyclase, increasing intracellular formation of cyclic guanosine monophosphate (cGMP). An increased cGMP leavel may relax vascular smooth muscle by forcing calcium out of muscle cells, causing vasodilation. This improves cardiac output by reducing mainly preload and also afterload.

Hydralazine may act in a manner that resembles organic nitrates and sodium nitroprusside, except that hydralazine is selective for arteries. It:

- exerts a direct vasodilating effect on vascular smooth muscle
- interferes with calcium movement in vascular smooth muscle by altering cellular calcium metabolism
- dilates arteries rather than veins, which minimizes orthostatic hypotension and increases cardiac output and cerebral blood flow
- causes a reflex autonomic response that increases heart rate, cardiac output, and left ventricular ejection fraction
- has a positive inotropic effect on the heart.

Although the exact mechanism of action for both isosorbide and hydralazine in the improvement of heart failure in black patients is not known, it is thought that these combined actions play a role.

Contraindications

Angle-closure glaucoma; cerebral hemorrhage; concurrent use of phosphodiesterase-5 (PDE-5) inhibitors (sildenafil, tadalafil, vardenafil); head trauma; hypersensitivity to isosorbide, other nitrates, hydralazine, and their components; mitral valve rheumatic heart disease

Interactions

DRUGS

isosorbide dinitrate and hydralazine

antihypertensives: Increased risk of orthostatic or severe hypotension

isosorbide dinitrate

acetylcholine, norepinephrine: Possibly decreased effectiveness of these drugs

aminoglutethimide, carbamazepine, nafcillin, nevirapine, phenobarbital, phenytoin, rifampin: Decreased isosorbide level and effects

aspirin: Increased blood level and action of isosorbide

azole antifungals, clarithromycin, diclofenac, doxycycline, erythromycin, imatinib, isoniazid, nefazodone, nicardipine, propofol, protease inhibitors, quinidine, telithromycin, verapamil: Increased isosorbide dinitrate level and effects

calcium channel blockers, opioid analgesics, other vasodilators: Increased risk of orthostatic hypotension

sildenafil, tadalafil, vardenafil: Increased risk of hypotension and death

sympathomimetics: Increased risk of hypotension and possibly decreased therapeutic effects of isosorbide

hydralazine

diazoxide, MAO inhibitors: Risk of severe hypotension

epinephrine: Possibly decreased vasopressor effect of epinephrine

metoprolol, propranolol: Increased effects of both drugs

NSAIDs: Decreased hydralazine effects

sympathomimetics: Possibly decreased antihypertensive effect of hydralazine

ACTIVITIES

isosorbide dinitrate and hydralazine

alcohol use: Additive vasodilation effects; Increased risk of orthostatic hypotension

FOODS

hydralazine

all foods: Possibly increased bioavailability of hydralazine

Adverse Reactions

CNS: Agitation, asthenia, chills, confusion, dizziness, fever, headache, insomnia, malaise, paresthesia, peripheral neuritis, restlessness, somnolence, syncope, vertigo, weakness

CV: Angina, arrhythmias, edema, hypercholesteremia, hyperlipidemia, orthostatic hypotension, palpitations, peripheral edema, tachycardia, ventricular tachycardia

EENT: Amblyopia, blurred vision, diplopia, lacrimation, nasal congestion, rhinitis, sinusitis

ENDO: Hyperglycemia

GI: Abdominal pain, anorexia, cholecystitis, constipation, diarrhea, indigestion, nausea, vomiting

GU: Dysuria, impotence, urinary frequency

HEME: Hemolytic anemia

MS: Arthralgia, muscle twitching, myalgia, tendon disorder

RESP: Bronchitis, dyspnea, pneumonia, upper respiratory tract infection

SKIN: Alopecia, blisters, diaphoresis, flushing, pruritus, rash, urticaria

Other: Allergic reaction; angioedema; lupus-like symptoms, especially with high doses; lymphadenopathy

Nursing Considerations

- Use isosorbide and hydralazine cautiously in patients with hypovolemia or even mild hypotension because drug may decrease blood pressure even more.
- Monitor CBC, lupus erythematosus cell preparation, and ANA titer before therapy and periodically during long-term treatment, as indicated.
- Weigh patient daily during therapy.
- Check patient's blood pressure in lying, sitting, and standing positions, and watch for signs of orthostatic hypotension. Expect orthostatic hypotension to be most common in the morning, during hot weather, and with exercise.
- Monitor patient's heart rate because drug may cause tachycardia and possible myocardial ischemia and angina.
- Be aware that isosorbide may aggravate angina in patients with hypertrophic cardiomyopathy.
- **WARNING** Expect to stop drug if patient has lupus-like symptoms, such as arthralgia, fever, myalgia, pharyngitis, and splenomegaly.
- Expect prescriber to withdraw drug gradually to avoid a rapid increase in blood pressure.
- Monitor patient for evidence of peripheral neuritis, such as paresthesia, numbness, and tingling. Notify prescriber if peripheral neuritis develops, and expect pyridoxine to be prescribed.
- Patient may have daily headaches at start of therapy from drug's vasodilating effects. Give acetaminophen, as prescribed, to relieve pain.
- **WARNING** Stopping drug abruptly may cause angina and increase the risk of MI.

PATIENT TEACHING

- Teach patient and family to recognize signs and symptoms of angina, including chest pain, fullness, or pressure, commonly with sweating and nausea. Pain may radiate down the left arm or into the neck or jaw. Inform female patients and those with diabetes mellitus or hypertension that they may have only fatigue and shortness of breath.
- Advise patient to change positions slowly, especially in the morning. Explain that hot showers may increase hypotension.
- Instruct patient to immediately notify prescriber about fever, muscle and joint aches, and sore throat.

- Urge patient to report numbness and tingling in her limbs, which may require treatment with another drug.
- Caution patient against stopping drug abruptly because doing so may cause severe changes in blood pressure, chest pain, or heart attack.
- Instruct patient to report blurred vision, fainting, increased anginal attacks, rash, and severe or persistent headaches. Reassure patient that headaches usually subside with continued therapy. Instruct her to notify prescriber if they don't.
- Caution patient to avoid hazardous activities until drug's CNS effects are known.
- Urge patient to avoid alcohol consumption.
- Tell patient to drink adequate fluids and to avoid excessive fluid loss from sweating. Tell patient to notify prescriber about diarrhea or vomiting because fluid loss may cause a severe decrease in blood pressure, light-headedness, or even fainting.
- Caution men to avoid erectile dysfunction drugs while taking isosorbide and hydralazine because they may interact to cause a severe drop in blood pressure, chest pain, or a heart attack.

lisinopril and hydrochlorothiazide
Prinzide, Zestoretic

Class and Category
Chemical: Lysine ester of enalaprilat (lisinopril), benothiadiazide (hydrochlorothiazide)
Therapeutic: Antihypertensive (lisinopril, hydrochlorothiazide), diuretic (hydrochlorothiazide)
Pregnancy category: C (first trimester), D (second and third trimesters)

Indications and Dosages
▶ *To treat hypertension uncontrolled by lisinopril or hydrochlorothiazide*
TABLETS
Adults. *Initial:* Depending on current lisinopril or hydrochlorothiazide dose, 10 mg lisinopril and 12.5 mg hydrochlorothiazide (1 tablet) or 20 mg lisinopril and 12.5 mg hydrochlorothiazide (1 tablet) daily. May be increased, as needed, every 2 to 3 wk. *Maximum:* 20 mg lisinopril and 25 mg hydrochlorothiazide daily.

Contraindications
Anuria; hereditary or idiopathic angioedema; history of angioedema from previous ACE inhibitor use; hypersensitivity to lisinopril, hydrochlorothiazide, other ACE inhibitors, other

sulfonamide-derived drugs, or their components; severe renal dysfunction

---

Mechanism of Action

Lisinopril may reduce blood pressure by affecting the renin-angiotensin-aldosterone system. By inhibiting ACE, lisinopril:

- prevents conversion of angiotensin I to angiotensin II, a potent vasoconstrictor that also stimulates adrenal cortex to secrete aldosterone.
- may inhibit renal and vascular production of angiotensin II.
- decreases serum angiotensin II level and increases serum renin activity. This decreases aldosterone secretion, slightly increasing serum potassium level and fluid loss.
- decreases vascular tone and blood pressure.
- inhibits aldosterone release, which reduces sodium and water reabsorption and increases their excretion, further reducing blood pressure.

Hydrochlorothiazide promotes movement of sodium, chloride, and water from blood in peritubular capillaries into the nephron's distal convoluted tubule. Initially, it may decrease extracellular fluid volume, plasma volume, and cardiac output, which helps explain blood pressure reduction. It also may reduce blood pressure by dilating arteries. After several weeks, extracellular fluid volume, plasma volume, and cardiac output return to normal, and peripheral vascular resistance remains decreased.

Interactions

DRUGS

lisinopril and hydrochlorothiazide

antihypertensives, diuretics: Increased antihypertensive effects

lithium: Increased blood lithium level and toxicity

NSAIDs, sympathomimetics: Possibly reduced antihypertensive effects of lisinopril and hydrochlorothiazide and increased risk of renal toxicity

lisinopril

allopurinol, bone marrow depressants (such as amphotericin B and methotrexate), procainamide, systemic corticosteroids: Possibly increased risk of fatal neutropenia or agranulocytosis

cyclosporine, potassium-sparing diuretics, potassium supplements: Increased risk of hyperkalemia

sodium aurothiomalate: Increased risk of nitritoid reactions, such as facial flushing, nausea, vomiting, and hypotension

hydrochlorothiazide

amantadine: Possibly increased amantadine level and risk of toxicity
amiodarone: Increased risk of arrhythmias from hypokalemia
amphotericin B, corticosteroids: Intensified electrolyte depletion, especially hypokalemia
antihypertensives: Increased antihypertensive effects
barbiturates, opioids: May potentiate orthostatic hypotension
calcium: Possibly increased serum calcium level
cholestyramine, colestipol resins: Reduced GI absorption of hydrochlorothiazide
diazoxide: Increased antihypertensive and hyperglycemic effects of hydrochlorothiazide
diflunisal: Possibly increased blood hydrochlorothiazide level
digoxin: Increased risk of digitalis toxicity from hypokalemia
dopamine: Possibly increased diuretic effects of both drugs
insulin, oral antidiabetics: Possibly increased blood glucose level
neuromuscular blockers: Possibly enhanced neuromuscular blockade from hypokalemia
nondepolarizing skeletal muscle relaxants (such as tubocurarine): Possibly increased responsiveness to muscle relaxant
pressor amines (such as norepinephrine): Possibly decreased response to pressor amines
oral anticoagulants: Possibly decreased anticoagulant effects
sympathomimetics: Possibly decreased antihypertensive effect of hydrochlorothiazide
vitamin D: Increased risk of hypercalcemia
FOODS
lisinopril
potassium-containing salt substitutes: Increased risk of hyperkalemia
ACTIVITIES
lisinopril
alcohol use: Possibly additive hypotensive effect

Adverse Reactions

CNS: Asthenia, ataxia, confusion, depression, dizziness, dream disturbances, fatigue, headache, insomnia, nervousness, paresthesia, peripheral neuropathy, somnolence, stroke, syncope, vertigo, weakness
CV: Angina, arrhythmias, cardiac arrest, chest pain, hypotension, MI, orthostatic hypotension, palpitations, Raynaud's phenomenon, tachycardia, vasculitis
EENT: Blurred vision, conjunctivitis, dry eyes and mouth, glossitis, hoarseness, lacrimation, loss of smell, pharyngitis, rhinorhea, stomatitis, taste perversion, tinnitus

ENDO: Hyperglycemia

GI: Abdominal pain, anorexia, constipation, diarrhea, dyspepsia, flatulence, hepatic failure, hepatitis, ileus, indigestion, jaundice, melena, nausea, pancreatitis, vomiting

GU: Decreased libido, flank pain, impotence, interstitial nephritis, nocturia, polyuria, oliguria, renal failure, UTI

HEME: Agranulocytosis, aplastic anemia, hemolytic anemia, leukopenia, neutropenia, thrombocytopenia

MS: Arthralgia; muscle cramps, spasms, and weakness

RESP: Asthma; back pain; bronchitis; bronchospasm; cough; dyspnea; pneumonia; pulmonary edema, embolism, infarction and infiltrates; upper respiratory tract infection

SKIN: Alopecia, cutaneous pseudolymphoma, diaphoresis, erythema multiforme, exfoliative dermatitis, flushing, pemphigus, photosensitivity, pruritus, rash, Stevens-Johnson syndrome, toxic epidermal necrolysis, urticaria

Other: Anaphylaxis, angioedema, dehydration, gout, herpes zoster, hypercalcemia, hyperkalemia, hyperuricemia, hypochloremia, hypokalemia, hyponatremia, hypovolemia, metabolic alkalosis, weight loss

Nursing Considerations

- Use cautiously in patients with impaired hepatic function because hydrochlorothiazide may alter fluid and electrolyte balance and lead to hepatic coma.
- Also use cautiously in patients with systemic lupus erythematosus because hydrochlorothiazide may activate or worsen it.
- Don't give drug to patients with severe renal dysfunction because, although rare, anaphylaxis has occurred in some patients dialyzed with high-flux membranes while being treated with an ACE inhibitor such as lisinopril.
- Monitor blood pressure often to assess effectiveness of lisinopril and hydrochlorothiazide therapy.
- WARNING Be aware that the drug may cause severe hypotension with syncope, which may lead to MI or stroke.
- If patient develops hypotension, expect to stop drug temporarily. Immediately place patient in supine position, and prepare to give I.V. normal saline solution, as prescribed. Expect to resume therapy after blood pressure stabilizes.
- WARNING Monitor patient—especially a black patient—closely for angioedema of the face, lips, tongue, glottis, larynx, or limbs. For angioedema of the face and lips, stop drug and give an antihistamine, as prescribed. If tongue, glottis, or

larynx is involved, assess patient for airway obstruction, prepare to give epinephrine 1:1,000 (0.3 to 0.5 ml) subcutaneously, and maintain a patent airway.

- Provide hydration, as appropriate, to help prevent hypovolemia.
- Monitor fluid intake and output, daily weight, and serum electrolyte levels (especially potassium) to detect volume depletion or electrolyte imbalance.
- Watch for increased BUN and serum creatinine levels, especially in patients with impaired renal function, because drug may cause acute renal failure. If increases are significant or persistent, notify prescriber immediately.
- Monitor blood glucose level often in diabetic patients, and expect to increase antidiabetic dosage, as needed and ordered.
- Check WBC count periodically, especially in patients with collagen-vascular disease, to detect neutropenia and agranulocytosis. Although they aren't known to occur with lisinopril, they have occurred with captropril, another ACE inhibitor.
- Assess liver enzymes periodically, and monitor patient for jaundice because hepatic failure, although rare, has occurred with other ACE inhibitors. If liver enzymes develop marked elevation or patient develops jaundice, notify prescriber and expect to stop lisinopril and hydrochlorothiazide.

PATIENT TEACHING

- Advise patient to take drug in the morning or early evening to avoid the need to urinate during the night.
- Teach patient to monitor her blood pressure and to report consistently elevated measurements to prescriber.
- Direct patient to weigh herself at the same time each day wearing the same amount of clothing and to notify prescriber if she gains more than 2 lb (0.9 kg) per day or 5 lb (2.3 kg) per week.
- To reduce the risk of dehydration and hypotension, advise patient to avoid exercise in hot weather and alcohol use. Also instruct her to notify prescriber if she experiences prolonged diarrhea, nausea, or vomiting.
- Caution patient to avoid hazardous activities until drug's CNS effects are known.
- Explain the importance of regular exercise, proper diet, and other lifestyle changes in controlling hypertension.
- **WARNING** Strongly urge patient to contact prescriber before using potassium supplements or OTC salt substitutes, which may contain potassium. These products increase the risk of hyperkalemia.

- Advise female patient to notify prescriber immediately if she is or could be pregnant. Lisinopril and hydrochlorothiazide will need to be replaced with another antihypertensive that's safe to use during pregnancy.
- Warn patient with gout that drug may precipitate an acute gout attack.

losartan potassium and hydrochlorothiazide

Hyzaar

Class and Category

Chemical: Angiotensin II receptor antagonist (losartan), benothiadiazide (hydrochlorothiazide)

Therapeutic: Antihypertensive (losartan, hydrochlorothiazide), diuretic (hydrochlorothiazide)

Pregnancy category: C (first trimester), D (second and third trimesters)

Indications and Dosages

▶ *To treat hypertension uncontrolled by losartan or hydrochlorothiazide alone; to treat hypertension in a patient whose blood pressure was controlled with 25 mg hydrochlorothiazide but who developed hypokalemia as a result; to provide initial treatment of severe hypertension*

TABLETS

Adults. *Initial:* 50 mg losartan and 12.5 mg hydrochlorothiazide (1 tablet) daily. After 3 wk, increased as needed to 100 mg losartan and 25 mg hydrochlorothiazide (1 tablet) daily.

DOSAGE ADJUSTMENT For patients who are volume-depleted, start with 25 mg losartan and 12.5 mg hydrochlorothiazide (1 tablet) daily.

▶ *To reduce the risk of stroke in patients with hypertension and left ventricular hypertrophy*

TABLETS

Adults. *Initial:* 50 mg losartan and 12.5 mg hydrochlorothiazide (1 tablet) daily; increased, as needed, to 100 mg losartan and 12.5 mg hydrochlorothiazide (1 tablet) daily and then to 100 mg losartan and 25 mg hydrochlorothiazide (1 tablet) daily, if needed.

Contraindications

Anuria; hypersensitivity to losartan, hydrochlorothiazide, other sulfonamide-derived drugs, or their components

Mechanism of Action

Losartan blocks the effects of angiotensin II (a potent vasoconstrictor that's part of the renin-angiotensin-aldosterone system) by blocking its binding to angiotensin I receptors in vascular smooth muscles, adrenal glands, and other tissues. This action halts angiotensin II's negative feedback on renin secretion. Thus, circulating renin and angiotensin II levels rise and vascular resistance declines, reducing blood pressure.

Hydrochlorothiazide promotes movement of sodium, chloride, and water from blood in peritubular capillaries into the nephron's distal convoluted tubule. Initially, it may decrease extracellular fluid volume, plasma volume, and cardiac output, which helps explain blood pressure reduction. It also may reduce blood pressure by dilating arteries. After several weeks, extracellular fluid volume, plasma volume, and cardiac output return to normal, and peripheral vascular resistance remains decreased.

Interactions

DRUGS

losartan and hydrochlorothiazide

antihypertensives, diuretics: Increased antihypertensive effects
indomethacin, NSAIDs, smpathomimetics: Possibly decreased antihypertensive effects, increased risk of renal failure
lithium: Decreased lithium clearance, increased risk of lithium toxicity

losartan

cyclosporine, potassium-sparing diuretics, potassium supplements: Increased risk of hyperkalemia

hydrochlorothiazide

amantadine: Possibly increased blood amantadine level and risk of toxicity
amiodarone: Increased risk of arrhythmias from hypokalemia
amphotericin B, corticosteroids: Intensified electrolyte depletion, especially hypokalemia
antihypertensives: Increased antihypertensive effects
barbiturates, opioids: May potentiate orthostatic hypotension
calcium: Possibly increased serum calcium level
cholestyramine, colestipol resins: Reduced GI absorption of hydrochlorothiazide
diazoxide: Increased antihypertensive and hyperglycemic effects of hydrochlorothiazide
diflunisal: Possibly increased blood hydrochlorothiazide level

digoxin: Increased risk of digitalis toxicity from hypokalemia
dopamine: Possibly increased diuretic effects of both drugs
insulin, oral antidiabetics: Possibly increased blood glucose level
neuromuscular blockers: Possibly enhanced neuromuscular blockade from hypokalemia
nondepolarizing skeletal muscle relaxants (such as tubocurarine): Possibly increased responsiveness to the muscle relaxant
pressor amines (such as norepinephrine): Possibly decreased response to pressor amines
oral anticoagulants: Possibly decreased anticoagulant effects
vitamin D: Increased risk of hypercalcemia

FOODS

losartan
high-potassium diet, potassium-containing salt substitutes: Increased risk of hyperkalemia

Adverse Reactions

CNS: Asthenia, depression, dizziness, drowsiness, fatigue, headache, insomnia, paresthesia, vertigo, weakness
CV: Angina pectoris, atrial fibrillation, bradycardia, edema, extrasystole, hypertriglyceridemia, hypotension, orthostatic hypotension, palpitations, tachycardia, vasculitis
EENT: Blurred vision, dry mouth, pharyngitis, rhinitis, sinusitis
ENDO: Hyperglycemia
GI: Abdominal cramps or pain, anorexia, constipation, diarrhea, hepatitis, indigestion, jaundice, nausea, vomiting
GU: Decreased libido, impotence, interstitial nephritis, nocturia, polyuria, renal failure, UTI
HEME: Agranulocytosis, aplastic and hemolytic anemia, leukopenia, neutropenia, thrombocytopenia
MS: Back or leg pain, muscle spasms and weakness, rhabdomyolysis
RESP: Bronchitis, dry cough, upper respiratory tract infection
SKIN: Alopecia, erythroderma, exfoliative dermatitis, photosensitivity, purpura, rash, urticaria
Other: Anaphylaxis, angioedema, dehydration, hypercalcemia, hyperkalemia, hyperuricemia, hypochloremia, hypokalemia, hyponatremia, hypovolemia, metabolic alkalosis, weight loss

Nursing Considerations

• Use cautiously in patients with impaired hepatic function because hydrochlorothiazide may alter fluid and electrolyte balance and lead to hepatic coma.

- Also use cautiously in patients with systemic lupus erythematosus because hydrochlorothiazide may activate or worsen it.
- If patient has known or suspected hypovolemia, expect to correct it with I.V. normal saline solution, as prescribed, before starting losartan and hydrochlorothiazide therapy.
- Monitor blood pressure often to assess effectiveness of losartan and hydrochlorothiazide therapy.
- If patient develops hypotension, expect to stop drug temporarily. Immediately place patient in supine position, and prepare to give I.V. normal saline solution, as prescribed. Expect to resume therapy after blood pressure stabilizes.
- Provide hydration, as appropriate, to help prevent hypovolemia.
- Monitor fluid intake and output, daily weight, and serum electrolyte levels (especially potassium) to detect volume depletion or electrolyte imbalance.
- Watch for increased BUN and serum creatinine levels, especially in patients with impaired renal function, because drug may cause acute renal failure. If increases are significant or persistent, notify prescriber immediately.
- Monitor blood glucose level often in diabetic patients, and expect to increase antidiabetic dosage, as needed and ordered.

PATIENT TEACHING
- Advise patient to take drug in the morning or early evening to avoid the need to urinate during the night.
- Teach patient to monitor her blood pressure and to report consistently elevated measurements to prescriber.
- **WARNING** Strongly urge patient to contact prescriber before using potassium supplements or OTC salt substitutes, which may contain potassium, which increases risk of hyperkalemia.
- Direct patient to weigh herself at the same time each day wearing the same amount of clothing and to notify prescriber if she gains more than 2 lb (0.9 kg) per day or 5 lb (2.3 kg) per week.
- **WARNING** Monitor patient closely for angioedema of the face, lips, tongue, glottis, larynx, or limbs. For angioedema of the face and lips, stop drug and give an antihistamine, as prescribed. If tongue, glottis, or larynx is involved, assess patient for airway obstruction, prepare to give epinephrine 1:1,000 (0.3 to 0.5 ml) subcutaneously, and maintain a patent airway.
- To reduce the risk of dehydration and hypotension, advise patient to avoid exercise in hot weather and to avoid alcohol. Also instruct her to notify prescriber if she has prolonged diarrhea, nausea, or vomiting.

- Caution patient to avoid hazardous activities until drug's CNS effects are known.
- Explain the importance of regular exercise, proper diet, and other lifestyle changes in controlling hypertension.
- Advise female patient to notify prescriber immediately if she is or could be pregnant; drug will need to be replaced with another antihypertensive that's safe to use during pregnancy.

methyldopa and hydrochlorothiazide
Aldoril 15, Aldoril 25, Aldoril D30, Aldoril D50

Class and Category
Chemical: 3,4-dihdroxyphenylalainine (DOPA) analogue (methyldopa), benothiadiazide (hydrochlorothiazide)
Therapeutic: Antihypertensive (methyldopa, hydrochlorothiazide), diuretic (hydrochlorothiazide)
Pregnancy category: C

Indications and Dosages
▶ *To treat hypertension uncontrolled by methyldopa or hydrochlorothiazide alone*
TABLETS
Adults. 250 mg methyldopa and 15 mg hydrochlorothiazide (1 Aldoril 15 tablet) b.i.d. or t.i.d. Or, 250 mg methyldopa and 25 mg hydrochlorothiazide (1 Aldoril 25 tablet) b.i.d. Increased, as needed, to 500 mg methyldopa and 30 mg hydrochlorothiazide (1 Aldoril D30 tablet) daily or 500 mg methyldopa and 50 mg hydrochlorothiazide (1 Aldoril D50 tablet) daily.

Mechanism of Action
Methyldopa is decarboxylated in the body to produce alpha-methylnorepinephrine, a metabolite that stimulates central inhibitory alpha-adrenergic receptors. This action may reduce blood pressure by decreasing sympathetic stimulation of the heart and peripheral vascular system.

Hydrochlorothiazide promotes movement of sodium, chloride, and water from blood in peritubular capillaries into the nephron's distal convoluted tubule. Initially, it may decrease extracellular fluid volume, plasma volume, and cardiac output, which helps explain blood pressure reduction. It also may reduce blood pressure by dilating arteries. After several weeks, extracellular fluid volume, plasma volume, and cardiac output return to normal, and peripheral vascular resistance remains decreased.

Contraindications

Active hepatic disease; anuria; hypersensitivity to methyldopa, hydrochlorothiazide, other sulfonamide-derived drugs, or their components; impaired hepatic function from previous methyldopa therapy; use within 14 days of MAO inhibitor therapy

Interactions

DRUGS

methyldopa and hydrochlorothiazide

diuretics, other antihypertensives: Increased antihypertensive effects
lithium: Decreased lithium clearance and increased risk of toxicity
NSAIDs, sympathomimetics: Decreased antihypertensive effects, increased risk of renal failure

methyldopa

appetite suppressants, tricyclic antidepressants: Possibly decreased therapeutic effects of methyldopa
central anesthetics: Possibly need for reduced anesthetic dosage
CNS depressants: Possibly increased CNS depression
haloperidol: Increased risk of adverse CNS effects
levodopa: Possibly decreased therapeutic effects of levodopa and increased risk of adverse CNS effects
MAO inhibitors: Possibly hallucinations, headaches, hyperexcitability, and severe hypertension
oral anticoagulants: Possibly decreased effects of anticoagulants

hydrochlorothiazide

amantadine: Possibly increased blood level and risk of toxicity of amantadine
amiodarone: Increased risk of arrhythmias from hypokalemia
amphotericin B, corticosteroids: Intensified electrolyte depletion, especially hypokalemia
barbiturates, opioids: May potentiate orthostatic hypotension
calcium: Possibly increased serum calcium level
cholestyramine, colestipol resins: Reduced GI absorption of hydrochlorothiazide
diazoxide: Increased antihypertensive and hyperglycemic effects of hydrochlorothiazide
diflunisal: Possibly increased blood hydrochlorothiazide level
digoxin: Increased risk of digitalis toxicity from hypokalemia
dopamine: Possibly increased diuretic effects of both drugs
insulin, oral antidiabetics: Possibly increased blood glucose level
neuromuscular blockers: Possibly enhanced neuromuscular blockade from hypokalemia
nondepolarizing skeletal muscle relaxants (such as tubocurarine): Possi-

bly increased responsiveness to the muscle relaxant
pressor amines (such as norepinephrine): Possibly decreased response
to pressor amines
oral anticoagulants: Possibly decreased anticoagulant effects
vitamin D: Increased risk of hypercalcemia
ACTIVITIES
methyldopa
alcohol use: Possibly increased CNS depression

Adverse Reactions

CNS: Decreased concentration, depression, dizziness, drowsiness,
fever, headache, insomnia, involuntary motor activity, memory
loss (transient), nightmares, paresthesia, parkinsonism, sedation,
vertigo, weakness
CV: Angina, bradycardia, edema, heart failure, hypotension, myocarditis, orthostatic hypotension, vasculitis
EENT: Black or sore tongue, blurred vision, dry mouth, nasal
congestion
ENDO: Gynecomastia, hyperglycemia
GI: Abdominal cramps, anorexia, constipation, diarrhea, flatulence, hepatic necrosis, hepatitis, indigestion, jaundice, nausea,
pancreatitis, vomiting
GU: Decreased libido, impotence, interstitial nephritis, nocturia,
polyuria, renal failure
HEME: Agranulocytosis, aplastic and hemolytic anemia, leukopenia, neutropenia, positive Coombs' test, positive tests for ANA
and rheumatoid factor, thrombocytopenia
MS: Muscle spasms and weakness
SKIN: Alopecia, eczema, exfoliative dermatitis, photosensitivity,
purpura, rash, urticaria
Other: Anaphylaxis, dehydration, hypercalcemia, hyperuricemia,
hypochloremia, hypokalemia, hyponatremia, hypovolemia, metabolic alkalosis, weight gain or loss

Nursing Considerations

- Use cautiously in patients with impaired hepatic function because drug may alter fluid and electrolyte balance and lead to
  hepatic coma.
- Use cautiously in patients with systemic lupus erythematosus
  because hydrochlorothiazide may activate or worsen it.
- Check patient's CBC results before therapy, as ordered, to estab-
  lish a baseline and check for asnemia. Monitor CBC periodically
  during therapy, as ordered, to detect adverse hematologic reactions to the drug.

- Monitor blood pressure often to assess effectiveness of methyldopa and hydrochlorothiazide.
- Provide hydration, as appropriate, to help prevent hypovolemia.
- Monitor fluid intake and output, daily weight, and serum electrolyte levels (especially potassium) to detect volume depletion or electrolyte imbalance.
- Monitor for increased BUN and serum creatinine levels, especially in patients with impaired renal function, because drug may cause acute renal failure. If increases are significant or persistent, notify prescriber immediately.
- Monitor blood glucose level often in diabetic patients, and expect to increase antidiabetic dosage, as needed and prescribed.
- Monitor results of Coombs' test; a positive result after several months of treatment indicates that patient has hemolytic anemia. Expect prescriber to discontinue drug.
- Notify prescriber if patient experiences signs of heart failure (dyspnea, edema, hypertension) or involuntary, rapid, jerky movements.

PATIENT TEACHING
- Advise patient to take methyldopa and hydrochlorothiazide in the morning or early evening to avoid awakening during the night to urinate.
- Teach patient how to monitor her blood pressure and to report consistently elevated measurements to prescriber.
- Tell patient to take drug exactly as prescribed and not to abruptly stop it. Explain that hypertension can return within 48 hours after stopping drug.
- Direct patient to weigh herself at the same time each day wearing the same amount of clothing and to notify prescriber if she gains more than 2 lb (0.9 kg) per day or 5 lb (2.3 kg) per week.
- Instruct patient to eat a diet high in potassium-rich food, including citrus fruits, bananas, tomatoes, and dates.
- To reduce the risk of dehydration and hypotension, advise patient to avoid exercise in hot weather and alcohol use. Also instruct her to notify prescriber if she experiences prolonged diarrhea, nausea, or vomiting.
- Caution patient to avoid hazardous activities until drug's CNS effects are known.
- Explain the importance of regular exercise, proper diet, and other lifestyle changes in controlling hypertension.
- Direct patient to notify prescriber about bruising, chest pain, fever, involuntary jerky movements, prolonged dizziness, rash, and yellow eyes or skin.

metoprolol tartrate and hydrochlorothiazide
Lopressor HCT

Class and Category
Chemical: Beta$_1$-adrengeric antagonist (metoprolol), benothiadiazide (hydrochlorothiazide)
Therapeutic: Antihypertensive, diuretic
Pregnancy category: C

Indications and Dosages
▶ *To manage hypertension*
TABLETS
Adults. Based on previous dosage of metoprolol or hydrochlorthiazide monotherapy, 100 mg to 200 mg metoprolol and 25 mg to 50 mg hydrochlorothiazide once daily or in divided doses.

Mechanism of Action
Metoprolol helps reduce blood pressure by decreasing release of renin from the kidneys and by antagonizing the effects of neurotransmitters that compete for the beta receptor sites. Also, metoprolol decreases cardiac output and adrenergic activity.

Hydrochlorothiazide promotes movement of sodium, chloride, and water from blood in peritubular capillaries into the nephron's distal convoluted tubule. Initially, it may decrease extracellular fluid volume, plasma volume, and cardiac output, which helps explain blood pressure reduction. It also may reduce blood pressure by dilating arteries. After several weeks, extracellular fluid volume, plasma volume, and cardiac output return to normal, and peripheral vascular resistance remains decreased.

Contraindications
Acute heart failure; anuria; bradycardia (heart rate less than 45 beats/minute); cardiogenic shock; hypersensitivity to metoprolol, other beta blockers, hydrochlorothiazide, other sulfonamide-derived drugs, or their components; second- or third-degree AV block.

Interactions
DRUGS
metoprolol and hydrochlorothiazide
antihypertensives, diuretics: Increased antihypertensive effect

insulin, oral antidiabetics: Decreased blood glucose control; possibly masking of signs and symptoms of hypoglcemia by metoprolol
neuromuscular blockers: Possibly enhanced and prolonged neuromuscular blockade
NSAIDs, sympathomimetics: Possibly decreased antihypertensive effect of hydrochlorothiazide and metoprolol

metoprolol

aluminum salts, barbiturates, calcium salts, cholestyramine, colestipol, rifampin, salicylates, sulfinpyrazone: Decreased therapeutic effects of metoprolol
amiodarone, digoxin, diltiazem, verapamil: Increased risk of complete AV block
beta blockers, digioxin: Increased risk of bradycardia and slowed atrioventricular conduction
bupropion, cimetidine, diphenhydramine, fluoxetine, hydroxychloroquine, paroxetine, quinidine, thioridazine, terbinafine: Possibly increased blood metoprolol level
calcium channel blockers: Increased risk of heart failure and increased therapeutic effects of both drugs
cimetidine: Increased blood metoprolol level
clonidine: Increased risk of rebound hypertension when clonidine is discontinued
clonidine, diazoxide, guanabenz: Increased risk of hypotension
estrogens: Possibly decreased antihypertensive effect of metoprolol
general anesthetics: Increased risk of hypotension and heart failure
lidocaine: Increased risk of lidocaine toxicity
MAO inhibitors: Increased risk of hypertension
phenothiazines: Possibly increased blood levels of both drugs
propafenone: Increased blood level and half-life of metoprolol
xanthines: Possibly decreased effects of these drugs or metoprolol

hydrochlorothiazide

amantadine: Possibly increased amantadine level and risk of toxicity
amiodarone: Increased risk of arrhythmias from hypokalemia
amphotericin B, corticosteroids: Intensified electrolyte depletion, especially hypokalemia
antihypertensives: Increased antihypertensive effects
barbiturates, opioids: May potentiate orthostatic hypotension
calcium: Possibly increased serum calcium level
cholestyramine, colestipol resins: Reduced GI absorption of hydrochlorothiazide
diazoxide: Increased antihypertensive and hyperglycemic effects of hydrochlorothiazide

diflunisal: Possibly increased blood hydrochlorothiazide level
digoxin: Increased risk of digitalis toxicity from hypokalemia
dopamine: Possibly increased diuretic effects of both drugs
lithium: Decreased lithium clearance and increased risk of toxicity
nondepolarizing skeletal muscle relaxants (such as tubocurarine): Possibly increased responsiveness to the muscle relaxant
pressor amines (such as norepinephrine): Possibly decreased response to pressor amines
oral anticoagulants: Possibly decreased anticoagulant effects
vitamin D: Increased risk of hypercalcemia
FOODS
metoprolol
all foods: Increased bioavailability of metoprolol

Adverse Reactions

CNS: Anxiety, confusion, depression, dizziness, drowsiness, fatigue, hallucinations, headache, insomnia, lethargy, nightmares, paresthesia, restlessness, somnolence, vertigo, weakness
CV: Arrhythmias (including AV block and bradycardia), arterial insuffiency, chest pain, edema, gangrene of extremity (with preexisting severe peripheral circulatory disorder), heart failure, hypotension, orthostatic hypotension, palpitations, vasculitis
EENT: Blurred vision, dry mouth, ear ache, nasal congestion, rhinitis, tinnitus
ENDO: Hyperglycemia
GI: Abdominal cramps, anorexia, constipation, diarrhea, indigestion, jaundice, nausea, pancreatitis, vomiting
GU: Decreased libido, impotence, interstitial nephritis, nocturia, polyuria, renal failure
HEME: Agranulocytosis, aplastic and hemolytic anemia, leukopenia, neutropenia, thrombocytopenia
MS: Back pain; muscle pain, spasms and weakness; myalgia
RESP: Bronchospasms, dsypnea, respiratory distress
SKIN: Alopecia, diaphoresis, exfoliative dermatitis, necrotizing angiitis, photosensitivity, purpura, rash, Stevens-Johnson syndrome, urticaria, worsening of psoriasis
Other: Anaphylaxis, dehydration, flulike syndrome, gout, hypercalcemia, hyperuricemia, hypochloremia, hypokalemia, hyponatremia, hypovolemia, metabolic alkalosis, weight loss

Nursing Considerations

- Use cautiously in patients with heart failure controlled by digitalis and diuretics because both digitalis and metoprolol slow AV conduction.

- Use cautiously in patients with impaired hepatic function because hydrochlorothiazide may alter fluid and electrolyte balance and lead to hepatic coma.
- Also use cautiously in patients with systemic lupus erythematosus because hydrochlorothiazide may activate or worsen it.
- Patients with bronchospastic disease are less likely to develop adverse respiratory effects if drug is given in smaller doses three times daily instead of larger doses twice daily.
- Check blood pressure often to assess effectiveness of therapy.
- Provide hydration, as appropriate, to help prevent hypovolemia.
- Patients who take metoprolol and hydrochlorothiazide may be at risk for AV block. If AV block results from depressed AV node conduction, prepare to give appropriate drug, as prescribed, or assist with insertion of a temporary pacemaker.
- Monitor fluid intake and output, daily weight, and serum electrolyte levels (especially potassium) to detect heart failure, volume depletion, or electrolyte imbalance.
- Watch for increased BUN and serum creatinine levels, especially in patients with impaired renal function, because drug may cause acute renal failure. If increases are significant or persistent, notify prescriber immediately.
- Monitor blood glucose level often in diabetic patients, and expect to increase antidiabetic dosage, as needed and ordered. Metoprolol may mask the tachycardia usually present in hypoglycemia but not the other signs of hypoglycemia, such as dizziness and sweating.
- **WARNING** Stopping this drug abruptly can cause myocardial ischemia, MI, ventricular arrhythmias, or severe hypertension, especially in patients with cardiac disease, and can cause thyroid storm in patients with hyperthyroidism or thyrotoxicosis. Expect to taper the drug when therapy ends.

PATIENT TEACHING

- Advise patient to take metoprolol and hydrochlorothiazide with food in the morning or early evening to avoid the need to urinate during the night.
- Advise patient to notify prescriber if pulse rate is less than 60 beats/minute or is significantly lower than usual.
- Teach patient to monitor her blood pressure and to report consistently elevated measurements to prescriber.
- Direct patient to weigh herself at the same time each day wearing the same amount of clothing and to notify prescriber if she gains more than 2 lb (0.9 kg) per day or 5 lb (2.3 kg) per week.

- Instruct patient to eat a diet high in potassium-rich foods, such as citrus fruits, bananas, tomatoes, and dates.
- To reduce the risk of dehydration and hypotension, advise patient to avoid alcohol and exercising in hot weather. Urge her to notify prescriber about prolonged diarrhea, nausea, or vomiting.
- Caution patient to avoid hazardous activities until drug's CNS effects are known.
- Explain the importance of regular exercise, proper diet, and other lifestyle changes in controlling hypertension.
- Caution patient not tot stop taking metoprolol and hydrochlorothiazide abruptly.
- Alert patient with diabetes that drug may mask a rapid heart beat caused by hypoglycemia and that the only symptom of hypoglycemia may be sweating. Advise her to check her blood glucose level regularly.

moexipril hydrochloride and hydrochlorothiazide
Uniretic

Class and Category
Chemical: Prodrug of moexiprilat (moexipril), benothiadiazide (hydrochlorothiazide)
Therapeutic: Antihypertensive (moexipril, hydrochlorothiazide), diuretic (hydrochlorothiazide)
Pregnancy category: C (first trimester), D (second and third trimesters)

Indications and Dosages
▶ *To treat hypertension uncontrolled by moexipril or hydrochlorothiazide alone*
TABLETS
Adults. *Initial:* Depending on previous dosage of moexipril or hydrochlorothiazide monotherapy, 7.5 mg or 15 mg moexipril and 12.5 mg or 25 mg hydrochlorothiazide (1 or 2 tablets depending on strength) daily, 1 hr before meal. Dosage increased as needed every 2 to 3 wk. *Maximum:* 30 mg moexipril and 50 mg hydrochlorothiazide daily 1 hr before meal.
▶ *To treat patients with hypertension controlled by hydrochlorothiazide but who develop hypokalemia*
TABLETS
Adults. 3.75 mg moexipril and 6.25 mg hydrochlorothiazide

(½ tablet of the 7.5-mg moexipril and 12.5-mg hydrochlorothiazide strength) daily 1 hr before meal

DOSAGE ADJUSTMENT For patients who have an excessive drop in blood pressure while taking 7.5 mg moexipril and 12.5 mg hydrochlorothiazide, dosage reduced to 3.75 mg moexipril and 6.25 mg hydrochlorothiazide daily 1 hr before meal.

Mechanism of Action

Moexipril may reduce blood pressure by affecting the renin-angiotensin-aldosterone system. By inhibiting ACE, moexipril:

- prevents conversion of angiotensin I to angiotensin II, a potent vasoconstrictor that also stimulates adrenal cortex to secrete aldosterone.
- may inhibit renal and vascular production of angiotensin II.
- decreases serum angiotensin II level and increases serum renin activity. This decreases aldosterone secretion, slightly increasing serum potassium level and fluid loss.
- decreases vascular tone and blood pressure
- inhibits aldosterone release, which reduces sodium and water reabsorption and increases their excretion, further reducing blood pressure.

Hydrochlorothiazide promotes movement of sodium, chloride, and water from blood in peritubular capillaries into the nephron's distal convoluted tubule. Initially, it may decrease extracellular fluid volume, plasma volume, and cardiac output, which helps explain blood pressure reduction. It also may reduce blood pressure by dilating arteries. After several weeks, extracellular fluid volume, plasma volume, and cardiac output return to normal, and peripheral vascular resistance remains decreased.

Contraindications

Anuria; history of angioedema with previous ACE inhibitor use; hypersensitivity to moexipril, hydrochlorothiazide, other sulfonamide-derived drugs, or their components

Interactions

DRUGS

moexipril and hydrochlorothiazide

antihypertensives, diuretics: Increased antihypertensive effect

digoxin: Possibly increased blood digoxin level and toxicity

lithium: Increased blood lithium level and risk of toxicity

NSAIDs, sympathomimetics: Possibly reduced antihypertensive effects of and increased risk of renal toxicity

moexipril

allopurinol, bone marrow depressants (such as amphotericin B and methotrexate), procainamide, systemic corticosteroids: Possibly increased risk of fatal neutropenia or agranulocytosis

antacids: Possibly decreased moexipril bioavailability

cyclosporine, potassium-sparing diuretics, potassium supplements: Increased risk of hyperkalemia

phenothiazines: Increased pharmacologic effects of moexipril

hydrochlorothiazide

amantadine: Possibly increased blood amantadine level and risk of toxicity

amiodarone: Increased risk of arrhythmias from hypokalemia

amphotericin B, corticosteroids: Intensified electrolyte depletion, especially hypokalemia

barbiturates, opioids: May potentiate orthostatic hypotension

calcium: Possibly increased serum calcium level

cholestyramine, colestipol resins: Reduced GI absorption of hydrochlorothiazide

diazoxide: Increased antihypertensive and hyperglycemic effects of hydrochlorothiazide

diflunisal: Possibly increased blood hydrochlorothiazide level

dopamine: Possibly increased diuretic effects of both drugs

insulin, oral antidiabetics: Possibly increased blood glucose level

neuromuscular blockers: Possibly enhanced neuromuscular blockade from hypokalemia

nondepolarizing skeletal muscle relaxants (such as tubocurarine): Possibly increased responsiveness to the muscle relaxant

pressor amines (such as norepinephrine): Possibly decreased response to pressor amines

oral anticoagulants: Possibly decreased anticoagulant effects

vitamin D: Increased risk of hypercalcemia

FOODS

moexipril

all foods: Decreased moexipril absorption

potassium-containing salt substitutes: Increased risk of hyperkalemia

ACTIVITIES

moexipril

alcohol use: Possibly additive hypotensive effect

Adverse Reactions

CNS: Anxiety, chills, confusion, dizziness, drowsiness, fatigue, fever, headache, hypertonia, insomnia, malaise, mood changes, nervousness, paresthesia, sleep disturbance, stroke, syncope, vertigo, weakness

CV: Abnormal ECG, angina, arrhythmias, chest pain, hypotension, MI, orthostatic hypotension, palpitations, periperal edema, vasculitis

EENT: Blurred vision, dry mouth, hoarseness, laryngeal edema, mouth or tongue swelling, pharnygitis, rhinitis, sinusitis, taste perversion, tinnitus

ENDO: Hyperglycemia

GI: Abdominal cramps, distention or pain; anorexia; constipation; diarrhea; dyspepsia; dysphagia; elevated liver function test results; hepatitis; increased appetite; indigestion; jaundice; nausea; vomiting

GU: Azotemia; decreased libido; elevated BUN, serum creatinine and uric acid levels; impotence; interstitial nephritis; nocturia; oliguria; proteinuria; polyuria; pyuria; renal failure or insufficiency; urinary frequency; UTI

HEME: Agranulocytosis, aplastic and hemolytic anemia, bone marrow depression, elevated erythrocyte sedimentation rate, leukocytosis, leukopenia, neutropenia, thrombocytopenia

MS: Arthralgia, back pain, leg heaviness or weakness, muscle spasms and weakness, myalgia, myositis

RESP: Bronchitis, bronchospasm, cough, dyspnea, upper respiratory infection

SKIN: Alopecia, diaphoresis, exfoliative dermatitis, flushing, pallor, pemphigus, photosensitivity, pruritus, purpura, rash, Stevens-Johnson syndrome, urticaria

Other: Anaphylaxis, angioedema, dehydration, flulike syndrome, hypercalcemia, hyperkalemia, hyperuricemia, hypochloremia, hypokalemia, hyponatremia, hypovolemia, increased SGPT, metabolic alkalosis, positive ANA titer, weight loss

Nursing Considerations

- Use moexipril and hydrochlorothiazide cautiously in patients with impaired hepatic function because hydrochlorothiazide may alter fluid and electrolyte balance and lead to hepatic coma.
- Also use cautiously in patients with systemic lupus erythematosus because hydrochlorothiazide may activate or worsen it.
- **WARNING** Contact prescriber if patient is or may be pregnant. Moexipril may cause fetal or neonatal harm or death if taken during the second or third trimester.
- Check blood pressure often to assess effectiveness of moexipril and hydrochlorothiazide therapy.
- Provide hydration, as appropriate, to help prevent hypovolemia.
- Monitor fluid intake and output, daily weight, and serum elec-

trolyte levels (especially potassium) to detect volume depletion or electrolyte imbalance.

- Watch for increased BUN and serum creatinine levels, especially in patients with impaired renal function, because drug may cause acute renal failure. If increases are significant or persistent, notify prescriber immediately.
- **WARNING** Monitor patient closely for angioedema of the face, lips, tongue, glottis, larynx, or limbs. For angioedema of the face and lips, stop drug and give an antihistamine, as prescribed. If tongue, glottis, or larynx is involved, assess patient for airway obstruction, prepare to give epinephrine 1:1,000 (0.3 to 0.5 ml) subcutaneously, and maintain a patent airway.
- Monitor blood glucose level often in diabetic patients, and expect to increase antidiabetic dosage, as needed and ordered.

PATIENT TEACHING
- Advise patient to take moexipril and hydrochlorothiazide in the morning or early evening 1 hour before a meal to avoid the need to urinate during the night.
- Teach patient to monitor her blood pressure and to report consistently elevated measurements to prescriber.
- Urge female patient to notify prescriber immediately if she is or could be pregnant.
- **WARNING** Instruct patient to stop drug and seek immediate medical care for hoarseness; swelling of tongue, glottis, larynx, face, or feet; or sudden difficulty swallowing or breathing.
- Caution patient not to stop drug without consulting prescriber, even if she feels better.
- Direct patient to weigh herself at the same time each day wearing the same amount of clothing and to notify prescriber if she gains more than 2 lb (0.9 kg) per day or 5 lb (2.3 kg) per week.
- Urge patient to avoid potassium supplements and potassium-containing salt substitutes unless prescriber allows them.
- To reduce the risk of dehydration and hypotension, advise patient to avoid alcohol and exercising in hot weather. Urge her to report prolonged diarrhea, nausea, or vomiting.
- Caution patient to avoid hazardous activities until drug's CNS effects are known.
- Tell patient to report evidence of infection (such as chills, fever, and sore throat) as well as diarrhea, nausea, or vomiting, which may lead to dehydration-induced hypotension.
- Explain the importance of regular exercise, proper diet, and other lifestyle changes in controlling hypertension.

nadolol and bendroflumethiazide
Corzide

Class and Category
Chemical: Nonselective beta blocker (nadolol), thiazide (bendroflumethiazide)
Therapeutic: Antihypertensive (nadolol, bendroflumethiazide), diuretic (bendroflumethiazide)
Pregnancy category: C

Indications and Dosages
▶ *To treat hypertension*
TABLETS
Adults. *Initial:* 40 mg nadolol and 5 mg bendroflumethiazide (1 tablet) daily. Increased, as needed, to 80 mg nadolol and 5 mg bendroflumethiazide (1 tablet) daily.
DOSAGE ADJUSTMENT For patients with a creatinine clearance of 31 to 50 ml/min/1.73 m^2, dosage interval increased to q 36 hours. For patients with a creatinine clearance of 30 ml/min/1.73 m^2 or less, combination therapy with a thiazide diuretic such as bendroflumethiazide isn't recommended.

Contraindications
Anuria; asthma; bronchospasm; cardiogenic shock; heart failure; hypersensitivity to nadolol, bendroflumethiazide, other beta blockers or sulfonamide-derived drugs, or their components; second- or third-degree AV block; severe COPD; sinus bradycardia

---

Mechanism of Action
Nadolol causes competitive antagonism of catecholamines at peripheral adrenergic neuron sites, leading to decreased cardiac output. It has a central effect leading to reduced tonic-sympathetic nerve outflow to the periphery, and it suppresses renin secretion by blocking beta-adrenergic receptors responsible for renin release from the kidneys. Combined, these effects work together to lower blood pressure.

Bendroflumethiazide promotes movement of sodium, chloride, and water from blood in peritubular capillaries into the nephron's distal convoluted tubule. Initially, it may decrease extracellular fluid volume, plasma volume, and cardiac output, which helps explain blood pressure reduction. It also may reduce blood pressure by dilating arteries. After several weeks, extracellular fluid volume and plasma volume return to near normal, cardiac output returns to normal, and peripheral vascular resistance remains decreased.

Interactions

DRUGS

nadolol and bendroflumethiazide

amiodarone: Additive depressant effects on conduction, negative inotropic effects, and increased risk of arrhythmias from hypokalemia

antihypertensives, diuretics: Increased antihypertensive effects

insulin, oral antidiabetics: Possible increased blood glucose level

neuromuscular blockers: Possibly enhanced neuromuscular blockade from hypokalemia

NSAIDs: Decreased hypotensive effects

sympathomimetics: Possibly mutual inhibition of therapeutic effects

nadolol

allergen immunotherapy, allergenic extracts for skin testing: Increased risk of serious systemic adverse reactions or anaphylaxis

anesthetics (general): Increased risk of hypotension and myocardial depression

beta blockers: Additive beta blockade effects

calcium channel blockers: Increased risk of bradycardia

catecholamine-depleting drugs (such as reserpine): Increased catecholamine-blocking action which may result in hypotension, marked bradycardia, vertigo, syncopal attacks, or orthostatic hypotension

cimetidine: Possibly interference with nadolol clearance, resulting in elevated plasma levels

clonidine, guanabenz: Impaired blood pressure control

diazoxide, nitroglycerin: Increased risk of hypotension

digoxin: Decreased heart rate and slowed AV conduction

estrogens: Decreased antihypertensive effect of nadolol

fentanyl, fentanyl derivatives: Possibly increased risk of initial bradycardia after induction of fentanyl or a derivative (with long-term nadolol use)

insulin, oral antidiabetics: Possibly impaired recovery from hypoglycemia, masking of signs of hypoglycemia

lidocaine: Decreased lidocaine clearance; increased risk of toxicity

phenothiazines: Increased blood levels of both drugs

xanthines: Possibly mutual inhibition of therapeutic effects

bendroflumethiazide

amantadine: Possibly increased blood amantadine level and risk of toxicity

amiodarone: Increased risk of arrhythmias from hypokalemia

amphotericin B, corticosteroids: Intensified electrolyte depletion, especially hypokalemia

antihypertensives: Increased antihypertensive effects

barbiturates, opioids: May potentiate orthostatic hypotension

calcium: Possibly increased serum calcium level

cholestyramine, colestipol resins: Reduced GI absorption of bendroflumethiazide

diazoxide: Increased antihypertensive and hyperglycemic effects of bendroflumethiazide

diflunisal: Possibly increased blood bendroflumethiazide level

digoxin: Increased risk of digitalis toxicity from hypokalemia

dopamine: Possibly increased diuretic effects of both drugs

insulin, oral antidiabetics: Possibly increased blood glucose level

lithium: Decreased lithium clearance and increased risk of toxicity

MAO inhibitors: Enhanced antihypertensive effect

methenamine: Possibly decreased effectiveness of methenamine

neuromuscular blockers: Possibly enhanced neuromuscular blockade from hypokalemia

nondepolarizing skeletal muscle relaxants (such as tubocurarine): Possibly increased responsiveness to the muscle relaxant

pressor amines (such as norepinephrine): Possibly decreased response to pressor amines

oral anticoagulants: Possibly decreased anticoagulant effects

vitamin D: Increased risk of hypercalcemia

ACTIVITIES

bendroflumethiazide

alcohol use: Possibly potentiated orthostatic hypotension

Adverse Reactions

CNS: Anxiety, depression, dizziness, drowsiness, fatigue, headache, insomnia, paresthesia, syncope, vertigo, weakness, yawning

CV: Bradycardia, chest pain, edema, heart block, heart failure, hypotension, orthostatic hypotension, vasculitis, ventricular arrhythmias

EENT: Blurred vision, dry mouth, nasal congestion, taste perversion

ENDO: Hyperglycemia

GI: Abdominal cramps, anorexia, constipation, diarrhea, dyspepsia, elevated liver function test results, hepatic necrosis, hepatitis, indigestion, jaundice, nausea, vomiting

GU: Decreased libido, ejaculation failure, impotence, interstitial nephritis, nocturia, polyuria, renal failure

HEME: Agranulocytosis, aplastic and hemolytic anemia, leukopenia, neutropenia, thrombocytopenia

MS: Muscle spasms and weakness
RESP: Cough, dyspnea, wheezing
SKIN: Alopecia, exfoliative dermatitis, photosensitivity, pruritus, purpura, rash, scalp tingling, urticaria
Other: Anaphylaxis, dehydration, hypercalcemia, hyperuricemia, hypochloremia, hypokalemia, hyponatremia, hypovolemia, metabolic alkalosis, weight loss

Nursing Considerations
- Use nadolol and bendroflumethiazide cautiously in patients with impaired hepatic function because bendroflumethiazide may alter fluid and electrolyte balance and lead to hepatic coma.
- Also use cautiously in patients with systemic lupus erythematosus because bendroflumethiazide may activate or worsen it.
- Monitor blood pressure often to assess effectiveness of nadolol and bendroflumethiazide therapy.
- Anticipate that nadolol may worsen psoriasis. In patients with myasthenia gravis, it may worsen muscle weakness and diplopia.
- Provide hydration, as appropriate, to help prevent hypovolemia.
- Monitor fluid intake and output, daily weight, and serum electrolyte levels (especially potassium) to detect volume depletion or electrolyte imbalance.
- Watch for increased BUN and serum creatinine levels, especially in patients with impaired renal function, because drug may cause acute renal failure. If increases are significant or persistent, notify prescriber immediately.
- Check blood glucose level often in diabetic patients, and expect to increase antidiabetic dosage, as needed and ordered.
- **WARNING** Withdraw drug gradually over 2 weeks, or as ordered, to avoid MI caused by unopposed beta stimulation or thyroid storm caused by underlying hyperthyroidism. Expect drug to mask tachycardia caused by hyperthyroidism.

PATIENT TEACHING
- Advise patient to take nadolol and bendroflumethiazide in the morning or early evening to avoid the need to urinate during the night.
- Teach patient how to monitor her blood pressure and how to take her pulse. Tell her to report consistent abnormalities to prescriber.
- Caution patient not to stop drug abruptly or change dosage without consulting prescriber.

- Direct patient to weigh herself at the same time each day wearing the same amount of clothing and to notify prescriber if she gains more than 2 lb (0.9 kg) per day or 5 lb (2.3 kg) per week.
- Instruct patient to eat a diet high in potassium-rich foods, such as citrus fruits, bananas, tomatoes, and dates.
- To reduce the risk of dehydration and hypotension, advise patient to avoid exercise in hot weather and to avoid alcohol. Also instruct her to notify prescriber if she has prolonged diarrhea, nausea, or vomiting.
- Caution patient to avoid hazardous activities until drug's CNS effects are known.
- Explain the importance of regular exercise, proper diet, and other lifestyle changes in controlling hypertension.
- Advise diabetic patient to monitor blood glucose level closely; drug may alter control and mask some signs of hypoglycemia.
- Instruct patient to notify prescriber about shortness of breath.

niacin extended-release and lovastatin
Advicor

Class and Category
Chemical: Vitamin B_3 (niacin), mevinic acid derivative (lovastatin)
Therapeutic: Antiyperlipidemic (niacin, lovastatin)
Pregnancy category: X

Indications and Dosages
▶ *To treat primary hypercholesterolemia (heterozygous familial and nonfamilial) and mixed dyslipidemia when monotherapy with niacin or lovastatin has failed*
TABLETS
Adults. *Initial:* 500 mg niacin and 20 mg lovastatin (1 tablet) daily at bedtime. Dosage increased as needed, every 4 wk, first to 1,000 mg niacin and 20 mg lovastatin (1 tablet) daily at bedtime, and then to 1,500 mg niacin and 40 mg lovastatin (1 tablet containing 500 mg niacin and 20 mg lovastatin and 1 tablet containing 1,000 mg niacin and 20 mg lovastatin) daily at bedtime, and finally to 2,000 mg niacin and 40 mg lovastatin (2 tablets) daily at bedtime. *Maximum:* 2,000 mg niacin and 40 mg lovastatin.

Contraindications
Active peptic ulcer disease; arterial bleeding; breast-feeding; hepatic impairment (significant or unexplained); hypersensitivity to lovastatin, niacin, niacinamide, or their components; pregnancy

Mechanism of Action

Niacin lowers serum cholesterol and triglyceride levels by inhibiting synthesis of very-low-density lipoproteins, which are needed to form low-density lipoproteins, the primary carrier of blood cholesterol.

Lovastatin interferes with the hepatic enzyme hydroxymethylglutaryl-coenzyme A reductase. By doing so, lovastatin reduces formation of mevalonic acid (a cholesterol precursor), thus interrupting the pathway by which cholesterol is synthesized. When the cholesterol level declines in hepatic cells, LDLs are consumed, which also reduces the amount of circulating total cholesterol. The decrease in LDLs may result in a decreased level of apolipoprotein B, which is found in each LDL particle.

Interactions

DRUGS

niacin and lovastatin

bile acid sequestrants (cholestyramine, colestipol): Decreased niacin and lovastatin bioavailability and effectiveness

amiodarone, clarithromycin, cyclosporine, danazol, erythromycin, fibric acid derivatives, gemfibrozil and other fibrates, immunosuppressants, itraconazole, ketoconazole, nefazodone, protease inhibitors, telithromycin, verapamil: Increased risk of severe myopathy or rhabdomyolysis

niacin

chenodiol, ursodiol: Decreased antihyperlipidemic effects of niacin

ganglionic blocking and vasoactive antihypertensives: Potentiated antihypertensive effects and possible postural hypotension

nutritional supplements containing large doses of niacin or related compounds, such as nicotinamide; vitamins: Possibly potentiated adverse effects of niacin

lovastatin

antifungal azoles such as ketoconazole and itraconazole, clarithromycin, cyclosporine, erythromycin, HIV protease inhibitors, nefazodone, telithromycin: Increased blood lovastatin level

isradipine: Increased hepatic clearance of lovastatin

oral anticoagulants: Possibly increased anticoagulant effect and risk of bleeding

FOODS

niacin

hot drinks: Increased risk of flushing and pruritus

lovastatin

all foods: Increased lovastatin absorption

grapefruit juice (more than 1 quart daily): Increased risk of develop-

ing myopathy or rhabdomyolysis
ACTIVITIES
niacin
alcohol use: Increased risk of flushing and pruritus
lovastatin
alcohol use: Increased blood lovastatin level

Adverse Reactions

CNS: Asthenia, chills, dizziness, fatigue, headache, insomnia, syncope
CV: Arrhythmias, edema, palpitations, peripheral vasodilation, tachycardia
EENT: Blurred vision, cataracts, dry eyes, pharyngitis, rhinitis, sinusitis
ENDO: Hyperglycemia
GI: Abdominal cramps and pain, cholestasis, constipation, diarrhea, dyspepsia, elevated liver function test results, epigastric pain, flatulence, hepatotoxicity, indigestion, nausea, vomiting
MS: Arthritis, back pain, myalgia, myopathy, myositis, rhabdomyolysis
RESP: Cough, shortness of breath, upper respiratory tract infection
SKIN: Dermatomyositis, diaphoresis, dry skin, erythema multiforme, flushing, pruritus, rash, sensation of warmth, Stevens-Johnson syndrome, toxic epidermal necrolysis
Other: Anaphylaxis, angioedema, flulike syndrome, hyperuricemia

Nursing Considerations

- Use cautiously in patients who consume substantial quantities of alcohol or have a history of liver disease because active liver disease and unexplained transaminase elevations contraindicate use of the niacin and lovastatin combination.
- Also use cautiously in patients with unstable angina or who are in the acute phase of MI, particularly if they take vasoactive drugs such as nitrates, calcium channel blockers, or adrenergic blockers because of increased risk of vasodilation.
- Give niacin and lovastatin at bedtime after a low-fat snack to minimize stomach upset and 1 hour before or 4 hours after giving a bile acid sequestrant, cholestyramine, or colestipol.
- WARNING Expect to monitor liver function tests every 6 months during therapy or as indicated. Monitor patient for evidence of hepatotoxicity or cholestasis, including darkening of urine, gray stools, loss of appetite, severe stomach pain, and yellow eyes or skin. If present, notify prescriber. Expect drug to be discontinued if serum transaminase level rises to

three times the upper limit of normal or if patient has evidence of hepatic dysfunction.

- Monitor patient for flushing, a reaction to niacin caused by dilation of peripheral cutaneous blood vessels, which increases blood flow and causes redness, mainly in the face, neck, and chest. Expect patient to develop tolerance to this effect after 2 weeks of therapy. Notify prescriber about persistent flushing; effects may be controlled with aspirin, as prescribed, taken before each niacin and lovastatin dose.

- Assess patients with peptic ulcer disease for possible worsening of symptoms because nicotinic acid can stimulate histamine release, leading to increased gastric acid production.

- Watch patients with or predisposed to gout for worsening of symptoms because drug can cause hyperuricemia when given in high doses.

- **WARNING** Monitor patient for myopathy and rhabdomyolysis, characterized by unexplained muscle pain, tenderness, or weakness, especially early in therapy or during periods of dosage increases. Be aware that a CK level more than 10 times the upper limit of normal in a patient with unexplained muscle symptoms indicates myopathy. Notifiy prescriber immediately, and be prepared to discontinue therapy if myopathy or rhabdomyolysis is suspected or present.

- Monitor patients with diabetes mellitus for altered glucose control because high doses of niacin may cause hyperglycemia.

- Monitor CBC, especially in patients with thrombocytopenia or coagulopathy and in those who are on anticoagulant therapy, because niacin may promote slight decreases in platelet counts or increased prothrombin times.

- Be prepared to temporarily stop niacin and lovastatin therapy, as ordered, for a few days before elective major surgery or when any major acute medical or surgical condition occurs.

PATIENT TEACHING

- Advise patient not to break, crush, or chew tablets but to swallow them whole.

- Tell patient to take drug at bedtime after a low-fat snack to minimize stomach upset and flushing.

- To minimize flushing, urge patient to avoid hot drinks around the time she takes a dose. Explain that she may experience skin flushing, mainly in the face, neck, and chest, but that she may develop tolerance to this effect after 2 weeks of therapy. Advise her to notify prescriber about persistent or intolerable flushing because prescriber may adjust dosage or recommend that patient take aspirin or another NSAID 30 minutes before each dose to control flushing. If patient awakens because of flushing, warn her to rise slowly to minimize the risk of dizziness and syncope.

- Instruct patient to avoid activities requiring mental alertness, such as driving or operating machinery, until full effects of drug are known because vasodilatory response to niacin may be dramatic at start of therapy.
- Emphasize importance of following a standard low-cholesterol diet during therapy.
- Tell patient to report muscle aches, pains, tenderness, or weakness; severe GI distress; and vision changes promptly.
- Urge patient to avoid consuming alcohol or more than 1 quart of grapefruit juice daily while taking drug.
- Stress the importance of periodic eye examinations during therapy because lovastatin has caused optic nerve degeneration in animals, and similar effects have occurred in patients taking other statin drugs.
- Teach female patient of childbearing age appropriate contraceptive methods. Tell her to report suspected pregnancy immediately because drug may harm fetus and will need to be stopped.
- Tell patient to consult prescriber before taking vitamins or nutritional supplements containing niacin or nicotinamide.
- Advise patient with diabetes to monitor her blood glucose level closely and to notify prescriber of any significant and persistent changes.

niacin extended-release and simvastatin
Simcor

Class and Category
Chemical: Vitamin B_3 (niacin), synthetically derived fermentation product of *Aspergillus terreus* (simvastatin)
Therapeutic: Antihyperlipidemic, vitamin B_3 (niacin), HMG-CoA reductase inhibitor, statin (simvastatin)
Pregnancy category: X

Indications and Dosages
▶ *To treat hyperlipidemia in patients with primary hypercholesterolemia and mixed dyslipidemia (Fredrickson type IIa and IIb) when monotherapy with simvastatin or niacin is inadequate; to treat hypertriglyceridemia in patients with Fredrickson type IV hyperlipidemia when monotherapy with simvastatin or niacin is inadaquate*

TABLETS

Adults. *Initial:* 500 mg niacin extended-release and 20 mg simvastatin (1 tablet) at bedtime with a low-fat snack. Dosage increased, as needed, in 4 weeks, to 1,000 mg niacin extended-release and 20 mg simvastatin (1 tablet) at bedtime with a low-fat snack. Further increases in niacin extended-release dosage should not exceed 500 mg every 4 weeks. *Maximum:* 2,000 mg niacin extended-release and 40 mg simvastatin (2 tablets) at bedtime with low-fat snack.

Mechanism of Action

Niacin lowers serum cholesterol and triglyceride levels by inhibiting synthesis of very-low-density lipoproteins, which are needed to form low-density lipoproteins, the primary carrier of blood cholesterol.

Simvastatin interferes with the hepatic enzyme hydroxymethylglutaryl-coenzyme A reductase, which reduces formation of mevalonic acid, a cholesterol precursor, and interrupts cholesterol synthesis. When the cholesterol level declines in hepatic cells, low-density lipoproteins are consumed, which reduces the level of circulating total cholesterol and serum triglycerides. Simvastatin also may increase removal of chylomicron triglyceride from plasma.

Contraindications

Active hepatic disease; active peptic ulcer disease; arterial bleeding; breast-feeding; concurrent use of clarithromycin, erythromycin, HIV protease inhibitors, itraconazole, ketoconazole, nefazodone, telithromycin, or more than 1 quart of grapefruit juice daily; hypersensitivity to niacin, simvastatin, or their components; pregnancy

Interactions

DRUGS

niacin and simvastatin

bile acid sequestrant (cholestyramine, colestipol): Decreased niacin and simvastatin bioavailability

niacin

chenodiol, ursodiol: Decreased antihyperlipidemic effects of niacin
ganglionic-blocking and vasoactive antihypertensives: Potentiated antihypertensive effects and possible orthostatic hypotension
nutritional supplements containing large doses of niacin or related compounds, such as nicotinamide; vitamins: Possibly potentiated adverse effects of niacin

simvastatin

amiodarone, azole antifungals, clarithromycin, cyclosporine, danazol, diclofenac, diltiazem, doxycycline, gemfibrozil and other fibrates, erythromycin, imatinib, isoniazid, nefazodone, niacin (1 gram daily or more), nicardipine, propofol, protease inhibitors (amprenavir, indinavir, lopinavir, nelfinavir, ritonavir, saquinavir), proton pump inhibitors, ranolazine, sildenafil, telithromycin, verapamil: Increased risk of myopathy or rhabdomyolysis

azole antifungals, cyclosporine, gemfibrozil, immunosuppressants, macrolide antibiotics (including erythromycin), niacin, verapamil: Increased risk of acute renal failure

bosentan, phenutoin, rifampin: Possibly decreased simvastatin level and effects

digoxin: Possibly slight elevation in blood digoxin level

oral anticoagulants (warfarin): Increased bleeding or prolonged PT

ACTIVITIES

niacin

alcohol use: Risk of flushing and pruritus

FOODS

niacin

hot drinks: Increased risk of flushing and pruritus

simvastatin

grapefruit juice (1 or more quarts daily): Possibly increased blood simvastatin level

Adverse Reactions

CNS: Asthenia, chills, dizziness, fatigue, fever, global amnesia, headache, insomnia, memory impairment, peripheral neuropathy, syncope

CV: Chest pain, orthostatic hypotension, palpitations, peripheral edema, tachycardia, vasculitis

EENT: Amblyopia; cataracts; facial, laryngeal, or tongue edema; rhinitis

ENDO: Abnormal thyroid function studies, hyperglycemia

GI: Abdominal pain, constipation, diarrhea, dyspepsia, elevated liver enzyme levels, flatulence, heartburn, hepatitis, hepatic failure, indigestion, nausea, pancreatitis, vomiting

HEME: Decreased platelet count, eosinophilia, hemolytic anemia, leukopenia, prolonged prothrombin time, thrombocytopenia

MS: Arthralgia, arthritis, back pain, elevated creatine kinase levels, myalgia, myopathy, rhabdomyolysis, tendon rupture

RESP: Dyspnea, shortness of breath, upper respiratory tract infection

SKIN: Diaphoresis, eczema, erythema multiforme, flushing, photosensitivity, pruritus, rash, skin discoloration, Stevens-Johnson syndrome, toxic epidermal necrolysis, urticaria

Other: Anaphylaxis, angioedema, gout, lupus erythematous–like syndrome

Nursing Considerations

- Use niacin extended-release and simvastatin cautiously in elderly patients, those with renal or hepatic impairment, and those with a history of gout.
- Give drug at bedtime with a low-fat snack.
- Expect to check patient's liver function test results before therapy starts, when dosage changes, and every 3 to 6 months, as clinically indicated.
- Monitor serum lipid panel, as ordered, to evaluate response to therapy.
- If patient is receiving amiodarone or verapamil, expect to limit simvastatin dose to 20 mg daily. If patient is receiving cyclosporine, danazol, or gemfibrozil, expect to limit simvastatin dose to 10 mg daily.
- Report any suspicion of myopathy—such as muscle pain, tenderness, or weakness—immediately to prescriber. Expect patient's CK level to be measured and drug to be discontinued.
- Briefly stop niacin extended-release and simvastatin therapy, as ordered, for a few days before elective major surgery or if patient develops an acute medical disorder, such as sepsis, hypotension, dehydration, trauma, a severe metabolic or endocrine problem, electrolyte imbalance, or uncontrolled seizures.
- Monitor blood glucose level in diabetic patients and, if it changes, expect adjustment to the diabetes treatment regimen. If glucose level shows pronounced changes, expect niacin extended-release and simvastatin to be discontinued.

PATIENT TEACHING

- Instruct patient to take niacin extended-release and simvastatin at bedtime with a low-fat snack.
- Advise patient not to break, crush, or chew tablets but to swallow them whole.
- Instruct patient to notify prescriber if therapy is interrupted because it may need to be tapered upward.
- Encourage patient to follow a low-fat, cholesterol-lowering diet.
- Urge patient to notify prescriber immediately about symptoms of myopathy, such as muscle pain, tenderness, or weakness.
- Inform female patient of childbearing age of need to use reli-

able contraceptive methods while taking drug. Instruct her to notify prescriber at once if she suspects pregnancy.

- Advise patient to avoid large quantities of grapefruit juice to decrease risk of drug toxicity.
- Alert patient that drug may cause flushing but reassure her that it usually subsides after several weeks. If patient is awakened at night with flushing, instruct her to get up slowly, especially if feeling dizzy or faint. If flushing is problematic, have patient check with the prescriber about possibility of taking aspirin or a non-steroidal anti-inflammatory agent 30 minutes before taking the drug and to avoid ingestion of alcohol, hot beverages and spicy foods around bedtime.
- Instruct diabetic patients to monitor her blood glucose level closely.

olmesartan medoxomil and hydrochlorothiazide
Benicar HCT

Class and Category
Chemical: AT1 subtype angiotensin II receptor antagonist (olmesartan, benothiadiazine (hydrochlorothiazide)
Therapeutic: Antihypertensive (olmesartan, hydrochlorothiazide), diuretic (hydrochlorothiazide)
Pregnancy category: C (first trimester), D (second and third trimesters)

Indications and Dosages
▶ *To manage hypertension when olmesartan or hydrochlorothiazide alone has failed*
TABLETS
Adults who aren't taking hydrochlorothiazide. *Initial:* 40 mg olmesartan and 12.5 mg hydrochlorothiazide (1 tablet) daily, increased in 2 to 4 wk to 40 mg olmesartan and 25 mg hydrochlorothiazide (1 tablet) daily, if needed.
Adults who aren't taking olmesartan. *Initial:* 20 mg olmesartan and 12.5 mg hydrochlorothiazide (1 tablet) daily, increased every 2 to 4 wk to 40 mg olmesartan and 25 mg hydrochlorothiazide (1 tablet) daily, if needed.

Contraindications
Anuria; hypersensitivity to olmesartan, hydrochlorothiazide, other sulfonamide-derived drugs, or their components; pregnancy; renal failure

Mechanism of Action

Olmesartan blocks binding of angiotensin II to receptor sites in many tissues, including vascular smooth muscle and adrenal glands. Angiotensin II is a potent vasoconstrictor that also stimulates the adrenal cortex to secrete aldosterone. The inhibiting effects of angiotensin II reduce blood pressure.

Hydrochlorothiazide promotes movement of sodium, chloride, and water from blood in peritubular capillaries into the nephron's distal convoluted tubule. Initially, it may decrease extracellular fluid volume, plasma volume, and cardiac output, which helps explain blood pressure reduction. It also may reduce blood pressure by dilating arteries. After several weeks, extracellular fluid volume, plasma volume, and cardiac output return to normal, and peripheral vascular resistance remains decreased.

Interactions

DRUGS

olmesartan

potassium-sparing diuretics: Increased risk of hyperkalemia

hydrochlorothiazide

amantadine: Possibly increased blood amantadine level and risk of toxicity

amiodarone: Increased risk of arrhythmias from hypokalemia

amphotericin B, corticosteroids: Intensified electrolyte depletion, especially hypokalemia

antihypertensives: Increased antihypertensive effects

barbiturates, opioids: May potentiate orthostatic hypotension

calcium: Possibly increased serum calcium level

cholestyramine, colestipol resins: Reduced GI absorption of hydrochlorothiazide

diazoxide: Increased antihypertensive and hyperglycemic effects of hydrochlorothiazide

diflunisal: Possibly increased blood hydrochlorothiazide level

digoxin: Increased risk of digitalis toxicity from hypokalemia

dopamine: Possibly increased diuretic effects of both drugs

insulin, oral antidiabetics: Possibly increased blood glucose level

lithium: Decreased lithium clearance and increased risk of toxicity

neuromuscular blockers: Possibly increased neuromuscular blockade from hypokalemia

nondepolarizing skeletal muscle relaxants (such as tubocurarine): Possibly increased responsiveness to the muscle relaxant

NSAIDs: Decreased diuretic effect of hydrochlorothiazide and increased risk of renal failure

pressor amines (such as norepinephrine): Possibly decreased response to pressor amines

oral anticoagulants: Possibly decreased anticoagulant effects

sympathomimetics: Possibly decreased antihypertensive effect of hydrochlorothiazide

vitamin D: Increased risk of hypercalcemia

Adverse Reactions

CNS: Asthenia, dizziness, headache, vertigo

CV: Chest pain, hypercholesterolemia, hyperlipemia, increased liver enzymes, orthostatic hypotension, peripheral edema, tachycardia

ENDO: Hyperglycemia

GI: Abdominal pain, diarrhea, dyspepsia, gastroenteritis, nausea, vomiting

GU: Acute renal failure, elevated BUN and serum creatinine levels, hematuria, interstitial nephritis, renal failure, urinary tract infection

MS: Arthralgia, arthritis, back pain, muscle spasm, myalgia

RESP: Cough, upper respiratory tract infection

SKIN: Alopecia, pruritus, rash,urticaria

Other: Angioedema, hypercalcemia, hyperkalemia, hyperuricemia, hypokalemia, hypomagnesemia

Nursing Considerations

- Use cautiously in patients with impaired hepatic function because hydrochlorothiazide may alter fluid and electrolyte balance and lead to hepatic coma.
- Also use cautiously in patients with systemic lupus erythematosus because hydrochlorothiazide may activate or worsen it.
- Monitor blood pressure often to assess effectiveness of olmesartan and hydrochlorothiazide therapy.
- Provide hydration, as appropriate, to help prevent hypovolemia.
- Monitor fluid intake and output, daily weight, blood pressure, and serum electrolyte levels (especially potassium) to detect volume depletion or electrolyte imbalance.
- **WARNING** Monitor patients who are volume- or sodium-depleted closely because symptomatic hypotension may occur when therapy starts. If hypotension occurs, place patient in supine position and, if needed, give an intravenous infusion of normal saline, as prescribed. Expect to resume drug therapy after blood pressure stabilizes.
- Watch for increased BUN and serum creatinine levels, especially in patients with impaired renal function, because drug may cause acute renal failure. If increases are significant or persist-

ent, notify prescriber immediately.

• Be aware that loop diuretics are preferred to thiazide diuretics in patients with a creatinine clearance greater than 30 ml/min/1.73 m^2; expect olmesartan and hydrochlorothiazide to be stopped in patients who develop significant renal impairment during therapy.

• Monitor blood glucose level frequently in diabetic patients, and expect to increase the antidiabetic dosage, as needed and ordered.

PATIENT TEACHING

• Advise patient to take drug in the morning or early evening to avoid the need to urinate during the night.

• Instruct patient to take drug with food or milk if adverse GI reactions occur.

• Teach patient to monitor her blood pressure and to report consistently elevated measurements to prescriber.

• Direct patient to weigh herself at the same time each day wearing the same amount of clothing and to notify the prescriber if she gains more than 2 lb (0.9 kg) per day or 5 lb (2.3 kg) per week.

• Instruct patient to eat a diet high in potassium-rich foods, such as citrus fruits, bananas, tomatoes, and dates.

• To reduce the risk of dehydration and hypotension, advise patient to avoid exercise in hot weather and to avoid alcohol. Also instruct her to notify prescriber if she has prolonged diarrhea, nausea, or vomiting.

• Caution patient to avoid hazardous activities until drug's CNS effects are known.

• Explain the importance of regular exercise, proper diet, and other lifestyle changes in controlling hypertension.

• Advise female patient to notify prescriber immediately about known or suspected pregnancy because olmesartan and hydrochlorothiazide will need to be replaced with another antihypertensive that's safe to use during the second and third trimesters of pregnancy.

prazosin hydrochloride and polythiazide
Minizide

Class and Category

Chemical: Quinazoline derivative (prazosin), benothiadiazide (polythiazide)

Therapeutic: Antihypertensive (prazosin, polythiazide), diuretic (polythiazide)
Pregnancy category: C

Indications and Dosages

▶ *To treat hypertension*

CAPSULES

Adults. *Initial:* 1 mg prazosin and 0.5 mg polythiazide (1 tablet) b.i.d. or t.i.d., increased as needed. *Maximum:* 5 mg prazosin and 0.5 mg polythiazide b.i.d. or t.i.d.

Mechanism of Action

Prazosin selectively and competitively inhibits $alpha_1$-adrenergic receptors. This action promotes peripheral arterial and venous dilation and reduces peripheral vascular resistance, thereby lowering blood pressure.

Polythiazide promotes movement of sodium, chloride, and water from blood in peritubular capillaries into the nephron's distal convoluted tubule. Initially, it may decrease extracellular fluid volume, plasma volume, and cardiac output, which helps explain blood pressure reduction. It also may reduce blood pressure by dilating arteries. After several weeks, extracellular fluid volume, plasma volume, and cardiac output return to normal, and peripheral vascular resistance remains decreased to account for lowering of blood pressure.

Contraindications

Angina; anuria; hypersensitivity to prazosin, polythiazide, other quinazolines or sulfonamide-derived drugs, or their components

Interactions

DRUGS

prazosin and polythiazide

antihypertensives, diuretics: Increased antihypertensive effects
NSAIDs, sympathomimetics: Decreased effectiveness of prazosin

prazosin

beta blockers: Increased risk of hypotension and syncope
dopamine: Antagonized peripheral vasoconstrictive effect of dopamine (with high doses)
ephedrine: Decreased vasopressor response to ephedrine
epinephrine: Possibly severe hypotension and tachycardia
metaraminol: Decreased vasopressor effect of metaraminol
methoxamine, phenylephrine: Possibly decreased vasopressor effect and shortened duration of action of these drugs

sildenafil, tadalafil, vardenafil: Increased risk of hypotension
polythiazide
amantadine: Possibly increased blood level and risk of toxicity of amantadine
amiodarone: Increased risk of arrhythmias from hypokalemia
amphotericin B, corticosteroids: Intensified electrolyte depletion, especially hypokalemia
barbiturates, opioids: May potentiate orthostatic hypotension
calcium: Possibly increased serum calcium level
cholestyramine, colestipol resins: Reduced GI absorption of polythiazide
diazoxide: Increased antihypertensive and hyperglycemic effects of polythiazide
diflunisal: Possibly increased blood polythiazide level
digoxin: Increased risk of digitalis toxicity from hypokalemia
dopamine: Possibly increased diuretic effects of both drugs
insulin, oral antidiabetics: Possibly increased blood glucose level
lithium: Decreased lithium clearance and increased risk of toxicity
neuromuscular blockers: Possibly increased neuromuscular blockade from hypokalemia
nondepolarizing skeletal muscle relaxants (such as tubocurarine): Possibly increased responsiveness to the muscle relaxant
pressor amines (such as norepinephrine): Possibly decreased response to pressor amines
oral anticoagulants: Possibly decreased anticoagulant effects
vitamin D: Increased risk of hypercalcemia

Adverse Reactions

CNS: Dizziness, drowsiness, fatigue, headache, insomnia, malaise, nervousness, paresthesia, syncope, vertigo, weakness
CV: Angina, edema, hypotension, orthostatic hypotension, palpitations, vasculitis
EENT: Blurred vision, dry mouth
ENDO: Hyperglycemia
GI: Abdominal cramps, anorexia, constipation, diarrhea, indigestion, jaundice, nausea, vomiting
GU: Decreased libido, impotence, interstitial nephritis, nocturia, polyuria, renal failure, urinary frequency or incontinence
HEME: Agranulocytosis, aplastic and hemolytic anemia, leukopenia, neutropenia, thrombocytopenia
MS: Muscle spasms and weakness
SKIN: Alopecia, exfoliative dermatitis, photosensitivity, priapism, purpura, rash, urticaria

Other: Anaphylaxis, dehydration, gout, hypercalcemia, hyperuricemia, hypochloremia, hypokalemia, hyponatremia, hypovolemia, metabolic alkalosis, weight loss

Nursing Considerations

- Use cautiously in patients with impaired hepatic function because polythiazide may alter fluid and electrolyte balance and cause hepatic coma.
- Also use cautiously in patients with systemic lupus erythematosus because polythiazide may activate or worsen it.
- Use cautiously in patients with renal impairment because of increased sensitivity to prazocin, in those with angina pectoris because drug may induce or aggravate angina, in those with narcolepsy because prazosin may worsen cataplexy, and in elderly patients because of their increased risk of hypotension.
- Monitor patient closely for the first 90 minutes of first dose because syncope may occur. If so, place patient in recumbent position and treat supportively until blood pressure normalizes.
- Check blood pressure often to assess effectiveness of prazosin and polythiazide therapy.
- Provide hydration, as appropriate, to help prevent hypovolemia.
- Monitor fluid intake and output, daily weight, and serum electrolyte levels (especially potassium) to detect volume depletion or electrolyte imbalance.
- Watch for increased BUN and serum creatinine levels, especially in patients with impaired renal function, because drug may cause acute renal failure. If increases are significant or persistent, notify prescriber immediately.
- Monitor blood glucose level often in diabetic patients, and expect to increase antidiabetic dosage, as needed and ordered.

PATIENT TEACHING

- Teach patient to monitor her blood pressure and to report consistently elevated measurements to prescriber.
- Direct patient to weigh herself at the same time each day wearing the same amount of clothing and to notify the prescriber if she gains more than 2 lb (0.9 kg) per day or 5 lb (2.3 kg) per week.
- Instruct patient to eat a diet high in potassium-rich foods, such as citrus fruits, bananas, tomatoes, and dates.
- To reduce the risk of dehydration and hypotension, advise patient to avoid exercise in hot weather and to avoid alcohol. Also instruct her to notify prescriber if she has prolonged diarrhea, nausea, or vomiting.

- Caution patient to avoid hazardous activities until drug's CNS effects are known.
- Suggest rising slowly from a lying or sitting position to minimize the effects of orthostatic hypotension.
- Advise patient to notify prescriber immediately about adverse reactions, especially dizziness and fainting.
- Instruct patient not to take any drugs, including OTC drugs,, without first consulting prescriber to avoid serious interactions.
- Warn patient that drug may precipitate gout and to report toe pain to prescriber.
- Explain the importance of regular exercise, proper diet, and other lifestyle changes in controlling hypertension.

propranolol hydrochloride and hydrochlorothiazide

Inderide, Inderide LA

Class and Category

Chemical: Beta-adrenergic blocker (propranolol), benothiadiazide (hydrochlorothiazide)
Therapeutic: Antihypertensisve (propranolol, hydrochlorothiazide), diuretic (hydrochlorothiazide)
Pregnancy category: C

Indications and Dosages

▶ *To treat hypertension*
TABLETS
Adults. *Initial:* 40 mg propranolol and 25 mg hydrochlorothiazide (1 tablet) b.i.d., increased as needed to 80 mg propranolol and 25 mg hydrochlorothiazide (1 tablet) b.i.d., as needed.
E.R. CAPSULES
Adults. 80 to 160 mg propranolol and 50 mg hydrochlorothiazide (1 capsule containing 50 mg hydrochlorothiazide and 80, 120, or 160 mg propranolol) daily.

Contraindications

Anuria; asthma including acute bronchospasm; cardiogenic shock; greater than first-degree AV block; heart failure (unless secondary to tachyarrhythmia that's responsive to propranolol); hypersensitivity to propranolol, hydrochlorothiazide, other sulfonamide-derived drugs, or their components; pulmonary edema; sinus bradycardia

Mechanism of Action

Propranolol competes with adrenergic neurotransmitters for binding at sympathetic receptor sites. Beta$_1$-receptor blockade decreases resting and exercise heart rate and cardiac output and decreases systolic and diastolic blood pressure.

Hydrochlorothiazide promotes movement of sodium, chloride, and water from blood in peritubular capillaries into the nephron's distal convoluted tubule. Initially, it may decrease extracellular fluid volume, plasma volume, and cardiac output, which helps explain blood pressure reduction. It also may reduce blood pressure by dilating arteries. After several weeks, extracellular fluid volume, plasma volume, and cardiac output return to normal, and peripheral vascular resistance remains decreased.

Interactions

DRUGS

propranolol and hydrochlorothiazide

amiodarone: Additive depressant effects on conduction, negative inotropic effects, and increased risk of arrhythmias from hypokalemia

antihypertensives, diuretics: Increased antihypertensive effects

insulin, oral antidiabetics: Possibly increased blood glucose level

neuromuscular blockers: Possibly enhanced neuromuscular blockade from hypokalemia

NSAIDs: Decreased hypotensive effects

sympathomimetics: Possibly mutual inhibition of therapeutic effects

propranolol

allergen immunotherapy, allergenic extracts for skin testing: Increased risk of serious systemic adverse reactions or anaphylaxis

aluminum hydroxide: Decreased intestinal absorption of propranolol

anesthetics (hydrocarbon inhalation): Increased risk of myocardial depression and hypotension

beta blockers: Additive beta-blockade effects

calcium channel blockers: Possibly depressed myocardial contractility or atrioventricular conduction

catecholamine-depleting drugs (such as reserpine): Increased catecholamine-blocking action which may result in hypotension, marked bradycardia, vertigo, syncopal attacks, or orthostatic hypotension

chlorpromazine: Increased plasma levels of both drugs

cimetidine: Possibly interference with propranolol clearance, resulting in elevated plasma levels *digoxin:* Decreased heart rate, slowed AV conduction

estrogens: Decreased antihypertensive effect of propranolol

fentanyl, fentanyl derivatives: Possibly increased risk of initial brady-cardia after induction of fentanyl or a derivative (with long-term propranolol use)

glucagon: Possibly blunted hyperglycemic response

haloperidol: Increased risk of hypotension and cardiac arrest

lidocaine: Decreased lidocaine clearance, increased risk of lidocaine toxicity

MAO inhibitors: Increased risk of significant hypertension

phenothiazines: Increased blood levels of both drugs

phenytoin, phenobarbitone, rifampin: Additive cardiac depressant effects (with parenteral phenytoin), accelerated propranolol clearance

propafenone: Increased blood level and half-life of propranolol

thyroxine: Lowered T_3 level

xanthines: Possibly mutual inhibition of therapeutic effects

hydrochlorothiazide

amantadine: Possibly increased blood amantadine level and risk of toxicity

amphotericin B, corticosteroids: Intensified electrolyte depletion, especially hypokalemia

barbiturates, opioids: May potentiate orthostatic hypotension

calcium: Possibly increased serum calcium level

cholestyramine, colestipol resins: Reduced GI absorption of hydrochlorothiazide

diazoxide: Increased antihypertensive and hyperglycemic effects of hydrochlorothiazide

diflunisal: Possibly increased blood hydrochlorothiazide level

digoxin: Increased risk of digitalis toxicity from hypokalemia

dopamine: Possibly increased diuretic effects of both drugs

lithium: Decreased lithium clearance and increased risk of toxicity

nondepolarizing skeletal muscle relaxants (such as tubocurarine): Possibly increased responsiveness to the muscle relaxant

pressor amines (such as norepinephrine): Possibly decreased response to pressor amines

oral anticoagulants: Possibly decreased anticoagulant effects

vitamin D: Increased risk of hypercalcemia

ACTIVITIES

propranolol

alcohol use: Slowed rate of propranolol absorption, possibly increased plasma propranolol level

nicotine chewing gum, smoking cessation, smoking deterrents: Increased therapeutic effects of propranolol

Adverse Reactions

CNS: Anxiety, depression, dizziness, drowsiness, fatigue, headache, insomnia, lethargy, nervousness, paresthesia, vertigo, weakness

CV: AV conduction disorders, cold extremities, heart failure, hypotension, orthostatic hypotension, sinus bradycardia, vasculitis

EENT: Blurred vision, dry mouth, nasal congestion

ENDO: Hyperglycemia

GI: Abdominal cramps or pain, anorexia, constipation, diarrhea, indigestion, jaundice, nausea, vomiting

GU: Decreased libido, impotence, interstitial nephritis, nocturia, polyuria, renal failure

HEME: Agranulocytosis, aplastic and hemolytic anemia, leukopenia, neutropenia, thrombocytopenia

MS: Muscle spasms and weakness

RESP: Bronchospasm, dyspnea, wheezing

SKIN: Alopecia, erythema multiforme, exfoliative dermatitis, photosensitivity, purpura, rash, Stevens-Johnson syndrome, toxic epidermal necrolysis, urticaria

Other: Anaphylaxis, dehydration, hypercalcemia, hyperuricemia, hypochloremia, hypokalemia, hyponatremia, hypovolemia, metabolic alkalosis, weight loss

Nursing Considerations

- Use cautiously in patients with impaired hepatic function because hydrochlorothiazide may alter fluid and electrolyte balance and lead to hepatic coma.
- Also use cautiously in patients with systemic lupus erythematosus because hydrochlorothiazide may activate or worsen it.
- Monitor blood pressure, apical and radial pulses, respiration, and circulation in limbs before and during therapy to assess effectiveness and detect adverse reactions of therapy.
- Monitor patient closely for hypersensitivity reactions. If patient develops a rash, urticaria, or has trouble breathing, notify prescriber and withhold drug, as ordered. Be aware that patient may be unresponsive to doses of epinephrine usually given to treat allergic reaction.
- Provide adequate hydration, as appropriate, to help prevent hypovolemia.
- Monitor fluid intake and output, daily weight, and serum electrolyte levels (especially potassium) to detect volume depletion or electrolyte imbalance.

- Because propranolol's negative inotropic effect can depress cardiac output, monitor cardiac output in patients with heart failure, particularly those with severely compromised left ventricular dysfunction.
- Be aware that propranolol can mask tachycardia that occurs in hyperthyroidism. Abrupt withdrawal in patients with hyperthyroidism or thyrotoxicosis can precipitate thyroid storm.
- Watch for increased BUN and serum creatinine levels, especially in patients with impaired renal function, because drug may cause acute renal failure. If increases are significant or persistent, notify prescriber immediately.
- Monitor blood glucose level often in diabetic patients. Propranolol may prolong and mask signs of hypoglycemia (especially tachycardia, palpitations, and tremor), but it doesn't suppress diaphoresis or hypertensive response to hypoglycemia. Propranolol and hydrochlorothiazide also may increase blood glucose level. Notify prescriber if hyperglycemia occurs, and expect to increase antidiabetic dosage, as needed and ordered.
- **WARNING** Be aware that stopping propranolol and hydrochlorothiazide abruptly may cause myocardial ischemia, MI, ventricular arrhythmias, or severe hypertension, particularly in patients with cardiac disease.

PATIENT TEACHING
- Teach patient to monitor her blood pressure and take her pulse. Tell her to report consistent abnormalities to prescriber.
- Direct patient to weigh herself at the same time each day wearing the same amount of clothing and to notify prescriber if she gains more than 2 lb (0.9 kg) per day or 5 lb (2.3 kg) per week.
- Instruct patient to eat a diet high in potassium-rich foods, such as citrus fruits, bananas, tomatoes, and dates.
- To reduce the risk of dehydration and hypotension, advise patient to avoid exercise in hot weather and alcohol use. Also instruct her to notify prescriber if she experiences prolonged diarrhea, nausea, or vomiting.
- Caution patient to avoid hazardous activities until drug's CNS effects are known.
- Explain the importance of regular exercise, proper diet, and other lifestyle changes in controlling hypertension.
- Caution patient not to change dosage without consulting prescriber and not to stop taking drug abruptly.
- Advise patient to notify prescriber immediately if she experiences shortness of breath.

- Advise patient to consult prescriber before taking OTC drugs, especially cold remedies.
- Tell smoker to notify prescriber immediately if she stops smoking because smoking cessation may decrease propranolol metabolism, calling for dosage adjustments.
- Urge diabetic patient to monitor blood glucose level closely because drug may alter control and mask signs of hypoglycemia.
- Advise female patient of childbearing age to notify prescriber if she is or could be pregnant.

quinapril and hydrochlorothiazide
Accuretic

Class and Category
Chemical: Ethylester of quinaprilat (quinapril), benothiadiazine (hydrochlorothiazide)
Therapeutic: Antihypertensive, diuretic
Pregnancy category: C (first trimester), D (second and third trimesters)

Indications and Dosages
▶ *To treat hypertension uncontrolled with quinapril alone; to treat hypertension in patients adequately controlled with hydrochlorothiazide alone but who develop significant potassium loss*
TABLETS
Adults. *Initial:* 10 mg quinapril and 12.5 mg hydrochlorothiazide (1 tablet) or 20 mg quinapril and 12.5 mg hydrochlorothiaizide (1 tablet) daily. Increased as needed every 2 to 3 wk. *Maximum:* 20 mg quinapril and 25 mg hydrochlorothiaizide daily.

Contraindications
Anuria; hereditary or idiopathic angioedema; history of angioedema from previous ACE inhibitor; hypersensitivity to quinapril, hydrochlorothiazide, other sulfonamide-derived drugs, or their components

Interactions
DRUGS
quinapril and hydrochlorothiaizide
antihypertensives, diuretics: Additive hypotensive effects
lithium: Increased blood lithium level and lithium toxicity
NSAIDs, sympathomimetics: Possibly reduced antihypertensive effects of quinapril and hydrochlorizide and increased risk of renal toxicity

quinapril

allopurinol, bone marrow depressants (such as amphotericin B and methotrexate), procainamide, systemic corticosteroids: Possibly increased risk of fatal neutropenia or agranulocytosis

CNS depressants: Additive hypotensive effects

cyclosporine, potassium-sparing diuretics, potassium supplements: Increased risk of hyperkalemia

tetracyclines: Reduced tetracycline absorption

hydrochlorothiazide

amantadine: Possibly increased blood amantadine level and risk of toxicity

amiodarone: Increased risk of arrhythmias from hypokalemia

amphotericin B, corticosteroids: Intensified electrolyte depletion, especially hypokalemia

antihypertensives: Increased antihypertensive effects

barbiturates, opioids: May potentiate orthostatic hypotension

calcium: Possibly increased serum calcium level

cholestyramine, colestipol resins: Reduced GI absorption of hydrochlorothiazide

diazoxide: Increased antihypertensive and hyperglycemic effects of hydrochlorothiazide

diflunisal: Possibly increased blood hydrochlorothiazide level

digoxin: Increased risk of digitalis toxicity from hypokalemia

dopamine: Possibly increased diuretic effects of both drugs

insulin, oral antidiabetics: Possibly increased blood glucose level

lithium: Decreased lithium clearance and increased risk of toxicity

neuromuscular blockers: Possibly enhanced neuromuscular blockade from hypokalemia

nondepolarizing skeletal muscle relaxants (such as tubocurarine): Possibly increased responsiveness to the muscle relaxant

NSAIDs: Increased risk of renal failure

pressor amines (such as norepinephrine): Possibly decreased response to pressor amines

oral anticoagulants: Possibly decreased anticoagulant effects

sympathomimetics: Possibly decreased antihypertensive effect of hydrochlorothiazide

vitamin D: Increased risk of hypercalcemia

FOODS

quinapril

potassium-containing salt substitutes: Increased risk of hyperkalemia

ACTIVITIES

quinapril

alcohol use: Possibly additive hypotensive effect

Mechanism of Action

Quinapril may reduce blood pressure by affecting the renin-angiotensin-aldosterone system. By inhibiting ACE, quinapril:

- prevents conversion of angiotensin I to angiotensin II, a potent vasoconstrictor that also stimulates adrenal cortex to secrete aldosterone.
- may inhibit renal and vascular production of angiotensin II.
- decreases serum angiotensin II level and increases serum renin activity. This decreases aldosterone secretion, slightly increasing serum potassium level.
- decreases vascular tone and blood pressure.
- inhibits aldosterone release, which reduces sodium and water reabsorption and increases their excretion, further reducing blood pressure.

Hydrochlorothiazide promotes movement of sodium, chloride, and water from blood in peritubular capillaries into the nephron's distal convoluted tubule. Initially, it may decrease extracellular fluid volume, plasma volume, and cardiac output, which helps explain blood pressure reduction. It also may reduce blood pressure by dilating arteries. After several weeks, extracellular fluid volume, plasma volume, and cardiac output return to normal, and peripheral vascular resistance remains decreased.

Adverse Reactions

CNS: Depression, dizziness, drowsiness, fatigue, headache, insomnia, light-headedness, malaise, paresthesia, sleep disturbance, syncope, vertigo, weakness

CV: Chest pain, hypotension, orthostatic hypotension, palpitations, tachycardia, vasculitis

EENT: Amblyopia, blurred vision, dry mouth, loss of taste, pharyngitis

ENDO: Hyperglycemia

GI: Abdominal cramps or pain, anorexia, constipation, diarrhea, indigestion, jaundice, nausea, vomiting

GU: Decreased libido, impotence, interstitial nephritis, nocturia, polyuria, renal failure

HEME: Agranulocytosis, aplastic and hemolytic anemia, leukopenia, neutropenia, thrombocytopenia

MS: Arthralgia, back pain, muscle spasms and weakness, myalgia

RESP: Cough, dyspnea

SKIN: Alopecia, diaphoresis, exfoliative dermatitis, flushing, photosensitivity, pruritus, purpura, rash, urticaria

Other: Anaphylaxis, angioedema, dehydration, hypercalcemia, hyperkalemia, hyperuricemia, hypochloremia, hypokalemia, hypomagnesemia, hyponatremia, hypovolemia, metabolic alkalosis, weight loss

Nursing Considerations

- Use quinapril and hydrochlorothiazide cautiously in patients with impaired hepatic function because hydrochlorothiazide may alter fluid and electrolyte balance and lead to hepatic coma. Quinapril, an ACE inhibitor, may induce a syndrome that starts with cholestatic jaundice and progresses to fulminant hepatic necrosis that may be fatal.
- Also use drug cautiously in patients who have systemic lupus erythematosus because hydrochlorothiazide may activate or worsen it.
- **WARNING** Be aware that patients with heart failure, hyponatremia, or severe volume or sodium depletion; those who've recently received intensive diuresis or an increase in diuretic dosage; and those undergoing dialysis may be at risk of excessive hypotension. Monitor blood pressure often during first 2 weeks of therapy and whenever dosage increases. If excessive hypotension occurs, notify prescriber immediately, place patient in a supine position and, if prescribed, infuse normal saline solution.
- Monitor blood pressure often to assess effectiveness of of quinapril and hydrochlorothiazide therapy.
- **WARNING** Because of the risk of angioedema, be prepared to stop drug and administer emergency measures, including subcutaneous epinephrine 1:1,000 (0.3 to 0.5 ml) if swelling of tongue, glottis, or larynx causes airway obstruction.
- Provide adequate hydration, as appropriate, to help prevent hypovolemia.
- If pregnancy is suspected, notify prescriber immediately; drug will need to be stopped.
- Monitor fluid intake and output, daily weight, and serum electrolyte levels (especially potassium) to detect volume depletion or electrolyte imbalance.
- Watch for increased BUN and serum creatinine levels, especially in patients with impaired renal function, because drug may cause acute renal failure. If increases are significant or persistent, notify prescriber immediately.
- Monitor blood glucose level often in diabetic patients, and expect to increase antidiabetic dosage, as needed and ordered.
- Monitor patient's WBC counts regularly, as ordered, especially in patients with collagen vascular disease or renal disease.

PATIENT TEACHING

• Advise patient to take drug in the morning or early evening to avoid the need to urinate during the night.

• Teach patient to monitor her blood pressure and to report consistently elevated measurements to prescriber.

• Instruct patient to stop drug and tell prescriber immediately if she has swelling of face, eyes, lips, or tongue or trouble breathing.

• Direct patient to weigh herself at the same time each day wearing the same amount of clothing and to notify prescriber if she gains more than 2 lb (0.9 kg) per day or 5 lb (2.3 kg) per week.

• Instruct patient to consult prescriber before using potassium supplements or salt substitutes that contain potassium.

• To reduce the risk of dehydration and hypotension, advise patient to avoid exercise in hot weather and to avoid alcohol. Urge her to report prolonged diarrhea, nausea, or vomiting.

• Explain that drug may cause dizziness and light-headedness, especially during the first few days. Caution patient to avoid hazardous activities until drug's CNS effects are known and to notify prescriber immediately if he faints.

• Inform female patient of childbearing age about risks of taking quinapril and hydrochlorothiazide during pregnancy. Caution her to use effective contraception and to notify prescriber immediately about known or suspected pregnancy.

• Advise patient planning to undergo surgery or anesthesia to inform specialist that she takes quinapril and hydrochlorothiazide.

• Tell patient to notify prescriber about yellowing of the skin or whites of her eyes because drug may need to be stopped.

• Stress importance of notifying prescriber if any indications of infection, such as a sore throat or fever occurs.

• Explain the importance of regular exercise, proper diet, and other lifestyle changes in controlling hypertension.

spironolactone and hydrochlorothiazide
Aldactazide

Class and Category

Chemical: Aldosterone antagonist (spironolactone), benothiadiazine (hydrochlorothiazide)

Therapeutic: Antihypertensive (spironolactone, hydrochlorothiazide), potassium-sparing diuretic (spironolactone, hydrochlorothiazide)

Pregnancy category: C

Indications and Dosages

▶ *To treat hypertension*

TABLETS

Adults. *Initial:* 25 mg spironolactone and 25 mg hydrochlorothiazide (1 tablet) daily, increased as needed to 50 to 100 mg spironolactone and 50 to 100 mg hydrochlorothiazide (number of tablets variable depending on strength used) daily or b.i.d.

▶ *To relieve edema in patients with heart failure, hepatic cirrhosis, or nephrotic syndrome*

TABLETS

Adults. 25 to 200 mg spironolactone and 25 to 200 mg hydrochlorothiazide (number of tablets variable depending on strength used) once daily or in divided doses.

Mechanism of Action

Spironolactone competes with aldosterone for receptors on the walls of distal convoluted tubule cells, thereby preventing sodium and water reabsorption and causing their excretion through the distal convoluted tubules while limiting excretion of potassium and magnesium. Increased urinary excretion of sodium and water reduces blood volume and blood pressure.

Hydrochlorothiazide promotes movement of sodium, chloride, and water from blood in peritubular capillaries into the nephron's distal convoluted tubule. Initially, it may decrease extracellular fluid volume, plasma volume, and cardiac output, which helps explain blood pressure reduction. It also may reduce blood pressure by dilating arteries. After several weeks, extracellular fluid volume, plasma volume, and cardiac output return to normal, and peripheral vascular resistance remains decreased.

Contraindications

Acute renal insufficiency, anuria, hyperkalemia, hypersensitivity to spironolactone, hydrochlorothiazide, other sulfonamide-derived drugs, or their components

Interactions

DRUGS

spironolactone and hydrochlorothiazide

antihypertensives: Possibly potentiated antihypertensive or diuretic effects of spironolactone and hydrochlorothizide

digoxin: Possibly increased half-life of digoxin and increased risk of digitalis toxicity *heparin, oral anticoagulants:* Decreased anticoagulant effect of these drugs

lithium: Decreased lithium clearance and increased risk of toxicity

NSAIDs, sympathomimetics: Possibly decreased antihypertensive effect of spironolactone and hydrochlorothiazide

spironolactone

ACE inhibitors, cyclosporine, potassium-containing drugs, potassium-sparing diuretics, potassium supplements: Increased risk of hyperkalemia

exchange resins (sodium cycle), such as sodium polystyrene sulfonate: Increased risk of hypokalemia and fluid retention

hydrochlorothiazide

amantadine: Possibly increased blood amantadine level and risk of toxicity

amiodarone: Increased risk of arrhythmias from hypokalemia

amphotericin B, corticosteroids: Intensified electrolyte depletion, especially hypokalemia

barbiturates, opioids: May potentiate orthostatic hypotension

calcium: Possibly increased serum calcium level

cholestyramine, colestipol resins: Reduced GI absorption of hydrochlorothiazide

diazoxide: Increased antihypertensive and hyperglycemic effects of hydrochlorothiazide

diflunisal: Possibly increased blood hydrochlorothiazide level

dopamine: Possibly increased diuretic effects of both drugs

insulin, oral antidiabetics: Possibly increased blood glucose level

neuromuscular blockers: Possibly enhanced neuromuscular blockade from hypokalemia

nondepolarizing skeletal muscle relaxants (such as tubocurarine): Possibly increased responsiveness to the muscle relaxant

pressor amines (such as norepinephrine): Possibly decreased response to pressor amines

vitamin D: Increased risk of hypercalcemia

FOODS

spironolactone

low-salt milk, salt substitutes: Increased risk of hyperkalemia

Adverse Reactions

CNS: Dizziness, encephalopathy, fatigue, headache, insomnia, paresthesia, vertigo, weakness

CV: Hypotension, orthostatic hypotension, vasculitis

EENT: Blurred vision, dry mouth, increased intraocular pressure, nasal congestion, tinnitus, vision changes

ENDO: Gyncomastia, hyperglycemia

GI: Abdominal cramps or pain, anorexia, constipation, diarrhea, flatulence, indigestion, jaundice, nausea, vomiting

GU: Decreased libido, impotence, interstitial nephritis, nocturia, polyuria, renal failure

HEME: Agranulocytosis, aplastic and hemolytic anemia, leukopenia, neutropenia, thrombocytopenia

MS: Arthralgia, back and leg pain, muscle spasms and weakness, myalgia

RESP: Cough, dyspnea

SKIN: Alopecia, exfoliative dermatitis, photosensitivity, purpura, rash, Stevens-Johnson syndrome, urticaria

Other: Anaphylaxis, dehydration, hypercalcemia, hyperkalemia, hyperuricemia, hypochloremia, hypokalemia, hypomagnesemia, hyponatremia, hypovolemia, metabolic alkalosis, weight loss

Nursing Considerations

- Use spironolactone and hydrochlorothiazide cautiously in patients with impaired hepatic function because hydrochlorothiazide may alter fluid and electrolyte balance and lead to hepatic coma.
- Also use drug cautiously in patients who have systemic lupus erythematosus because hydrochlorothiazide may activate or worsen it.
- Monitor blood pressure often to assess effectiveness of spironolactone and hydrochlorothiazide.
- Provide hydration, as appropriate, to help prevent hypovolemia.
- Monitor fluid intake and output, daily weight, and serum electrolyte levels (especially potassium) to detect volume depletion or electrolyte imbalance.
- Watch for increased BUN and serum creatinine levels, especially in patients with impaired renal function, because drug may cause acute renal failure. If increases are significant or persistent, notify prescriber immediately.
- Monitor blood glucose level often in diabetic patients, and expect to increase antidiabetic dosage, as needed and ordered.

PATIENT TEACHING

- Advise patient to take spironolactone and hydrochlorothiazide in the morning or early evening to avoid the need to urinate during the night. Tell patient to take drug with meals or milk to minimize stomach upset.
- Teach patient to monitor her blood pressure and to report consistently elevated measurements to prescriber.

- Direct patient to weigh herself at the same time each day wearing the same amount of clothing and to notify prescriber if she gains more than 2 lb (0.9 kg) per day or 5 lb (2.3 kg) per week.
- Instruct patient to eat a diet high in potassium-rich foods, such as citrus fruits, bananas, tomatoes, and dates.
- To reduce the risk of dehydration and hypotension, advise patient to avoid alcohol and exercising in hot weather. Also instruct her to report prolonged diarrhea, nausea, or vomiting.
- Caution patient to avoid hazardous activities until drug's CNS effects are known.
- Explain the importance of regular exercise, proper diet, and other lifestyle changes in controlling hypertension.

telmisartan and hydrochlorothiazide
Micardis HCT

Class and Category
Chemical: AT1 angiotensin II receptor antagonist (telmisartan), benothiadiazide (hydrochlorothiazide)
Therapeutic: Antihypertensive (telmisartan, hydrochlorothiazide), diuretic (hydrochlorothiazide)
Pregnancy category: C (first trimester), D (second and third trimesters)

Indications and Dosages
▶ *To treat hypertension uncontrolled by 80 mg telmisartan daily*
TABLETS
Adults. *Initial:* 80 mg telmisartan and 12.5 mg hydrochlorothiazide (1 tablet) daily. Dosage gradually increased every 2 to 4 wk, as needed. *Maximum:* 160 mg telmisartan and 25 mg hydrochlorothiazide.
▶ *To treat hypertension uncontrolled by 25 mg hydrochlorothiazide daily*
TABLETS
Adults. *Initial:* 80 mg telmisartan and 12.5 mg hydrochlorothiazide (1 tablet) daily or 80 mg telmisartan and 25 mg hydrochlorothiazide (1 tablet) daily. Dosage gradually increased every 2 to 4 wk, as needed. *Maximum:* 160 mg telmisartan and 25 mg hydrochlorothiazide.
▶ *To treat hypertension for patients adequately controlled by hydrochlorothiazide alone but who develop significant potassium loss*
TABLETS
Adults. 80 mg telmisartan and 12.5 mg hydrochlorothiazide (1 tablet) daily.

Mechanism of Action

Telmisartan blocks angiotensin II from binding to AT1 receptor sites in many tissues, including vascular smooth muscle and adrenal glands. This inhibits the vasoconstrictive and aldosterone-secreting effects of angiotensin II, which reduces blood pressure.

Hydrochlorothiazide promotes movement of sodium, chloride, and water from blood in peritubular capillaries into the nephron's distal convoluted tubule. Initially, it may decrease extracellular fluid volume, plasma volume, and cardiac output, which helps explain blood pressure reduction. It also may reduce blood pressure by dilating arteries. After several weeks, extracellular fluid volume, plasma volume, and cardiac output return to normal, and peripheral vascular resistance remains decreased.

Contraindications

Anuria; hypersensitivity to telmisartan, hydrochlorothiazide, other sulfonamide-derived drugs, or their components; pregnancy; renal failure

Interactions

DRUGS

telmisartan and hydrochlorothiazide

antihypertensives, diuretics: Increased antihypertensive effects

digoxin: Increased risk of digitalis toxicity

telmisartan

potassium-sparing diuretics: Increased risk of hyperkalemia

warfarin: Possibly slight decrease in mean warfarin trough level

hydrochlorothiazide

amantadine: Possibly increased blood amantadine level and risk of toxicity

amiodarone: Increased risk of arrhythmias from hypokalemia

amphotericin B, corticosteroids: Intensified electrolyte depletion, especially hypokalemia

barbiturates, opioids: May potentiate orthostatic hypotension

calcium: Possibly increased serum calcium level

cholestyramine, colestipol resins: Reduced GI absorption of hydrochlorothiazide

diazoxide: Increased antihypertensive and hyperglycemic effects of hydrochlorothiazide

diflunisal: Possibly increased blood hydrochlorothiazide level

dopamine: Possibly increased diuretic effects of both drugs

insulin, oral antidiabetics: Possibly increased blood glucose level *lithium:* Decreased lithium clearance and increased risk of lithium toxicity

neuromuscular blockers: Possibly increased neuromuscular blockade from hypokalemia

nondepolarizing skeletal muscle relaxants (such as tubocurarine): Possibly increased responsiveness to the muscle relaxant

NSAIDs: Decreased diuretic effect of hydrochlorothiazide, increased risk of renal failure

pressor amines (such as norepinephrine): Possibly decreased response to pressor amines

oral anticoagulants: Possibly decreased anticoagulant effects

sympathomimetics: Possibly decreased antihypertensive effect of hydrochlorothiazide

vitamin D: Increased risk of hypercalcemia

Adverse Reactions

CNS: Asthenia, dizziness, fatigue, headache, insomnia, paresthesia, syncope, vertigo, weakness

CV: Atrial fibrillation, bradtcardia, chest pain, congestive heart failure, hyperkalemia, hypertension, hypotension, MI, orthostatic hypotension, peripheral edema, vasculitis

EENT: Blurred vision, dry mouth

ENDO: Hyperglycemia

GI: Abdominal cramps or pain, anorexia, constipation, diarrhea, elevated liver enzymes, hepatic dysfunction, indigestion, jaundice, nausea, vomiting

GU: Decreased libido, impotence, interstitial nephritis, nocturia, polyuria, renal failure, UTI

HEME: Agranulocytosis, aplastic and hemolytic anemia, eosinophilia, leukopenia, neutropenia, thrombocytopenia

MS: Back pain; muscle cramps, spasms, and weakness; myalgia; rhabdomyolysis

RESP: Coughing

SKIN: Alopecia, diaphoresis, erythema, exfoliative dermatitis, photosensitivity, purpura, rash, Stevens-Johnson syndrome, urticaria

Other: Anaphylaxis, angioedema, dehydration, hypercalcemia, hyperuricemia, hypochloremia, hypokalemia, hypomagnesemia, hyponatremia, hypovolemia, metabolic alkalosis, weight loss

Nursing Considerations

• Use telmisartan and hydrochlorothiazide cautiously in patients with impaired hepatic function.

- Also use this drug cautiously in patients with systemic lupus erythematosus because hydrochlorothiazide may activate or worsen it.
- Monitor liver function test results, as ordered. Assess for signs of drug toxicity and fluid and electrolyte imbalance in patients with severe hepatic disease because altered fluid and electrolyte balance may lead to hepatic coma.
- Monitor blood pressure often to assess effectiveness of telmisartan and hydrochlorothiazide therapy.
- Provide adequate hydration, as appropriate, to help prevent hypovolemia.
- Monitor fluid intake and output, daily weight, and serum electrolyte levels (especially potassium) to detect volume depletion or electrolyte imbalance.
- Watch for increased BUN and serum creatinine levels, especially in patients with impaired renal function, because drug may cause acute renal failure. If increases are significant or persistent, notify prescriber immediately.
- Check blood glucose level often in diabetic patients, and expect to increase antidiabetic dosage, as needed and ordered.

PATIENT TEACHING

- Advise patient to take telmisartan and hydrochlorothiazide in the morning or early evening to avoid the need to urinate during the night.
- Teach patient to monitor her blood pressure and report consistent elevations to prescriber.
- Instruct patient to weigh herself at the same time each day wearing the same amount of clothing and to notify prescriber if she gains more than 2 lb (0.9 kg) per day or 5 lb (2.3 kg) per week.
- Instruct patient to eat a diet high in potassium-rich foods, such as citrus fruits, bananas, tomatoes, and dates.
- To reduce the risk of dehydration and hypotension, advise patient to avoid exercise in hot weather and to avoid alcohol. Also instruct her to notify prescriber if she has prolonged diarrhea, nausea, or vomiting.
- Caution patient to avoid hazardous activities until drug's CNS effects are known.
- Explain the importance of regular exercise, proper diet, and other lifestyle changes in controlling hypertension.
- Advise female patients of childbearing age to notify prescriber immediately about known or suspected pregnancy.

timolol maleate and hydrochlorothiazide
Timolide

Class and Category
Chemical: Beta blocker (timolol), benothiadiazide (hydrochlorothiazide)
Therapeutic: Antihypertensive (timolol, hydrochlorothiazide), diuretic (hydrochlorothiazide)
Pregnancy category: C

Indications and Dosages
▶ *To treat hypertension*
TABLETS
Adults. 10 mg timolol and 25 mg hydrochlorothiazide (1 tablet) b.i.d. or 20 mg timiolol and 50 mg hydrochlorothiazide (2 tablets) daily.

Mechanism of Action
Timolol blocks beta$_1$ and beta$_2$ receptors in vascular smooth muscle and beta1 receptors in the heart. This reduces peripheral vascular resistance and blood pressure.

Hydrochlorothiazide promotes movement of sodium, chloride, and water from blood in peritubular capillaries into the nephron's distal convoluted tubule. Initially, it may decrease extracellular fluid volume, plasma volume, and cardiac output, which helps explain blood pressure reduction. It also may reduce blood pressure by dilating arteries. After several weeks, extracellular fluid volume, plasma volume, and cardiac output return to normal, and peripheral vascular resistance remains decreased.

Contraindications
Acute bronchospasm; anuria; asthma; cardiogenic shock; children; COPD (severe); heart failure; hypersensitivity to timolol, hydrochlorothiazide, other beta blockers or sulfonamide-derived drugs, or any of their components; pulmonary edema; second- or third-degree AV block; severe sinus bradycardia

Interactions
DRUGS
timolol and hydrochlorothiazide
amiodarone: Additive depressant effects on conduction, negative inotropic effects, increased risk of arrhythmias from hypokalemia,

antihypertensives, diuretics: Increased antihypertensive effects

insulin, oral antidiabetics: Possibly increased blood glucose level

neuromuscular blockers: Possibly increased neuromuscular blockade from hypokalemia

NSAIDs: Decreased hypotensive effects

sympathomimetics: Possibly mutual inhibition of therapeutic effects

timolol

allergen immunotherapy, allergenic extracts for skin testing: Increased risk of serious systemic adverse reactions or anaphylaxis

anesthetics (hydrocarbon inhalation): Increased risk of myocardial depression and hypotension

beta blockers: Additive beta-blockade effects

calcium channel blockers: Possibly depressed myocardial contractility or atrioventricular conduction.

catecholamine-depleting drugs (such as reserpine): Increased catecholamine-blocking action which may result in hypotension, marked bradycardia, vertigo, syncopal attacks or orthostatic hypotension

cimetidine: Possibly interference with timolol clearance, causing increased plasma levels

estrogens: Decreased antihypertensive effect of timolol

fentanyl, fentanyl derivatives: Possibly increased risk of initial bradycardia after induction of fentanyl or a derivative (with long-term timolol use)

glucagon: Possibly blunted hyperglycemic response

insulin, oral antidiabetics: Possibly masking of tachycardia in response to hypoglycemia

lidocaine: Decreased lidocaine clearance, increased risk of lidocaine toxicity

MAO inhibitors: Increased risk of significant hypertension

phenothiazines: Increased blood levels of both drugs

phenytoin (parenteral): Additive cardiac depressant effects, accelerated timolol clearance

xanthines: Possibly mutual inhibition of therapeutic effects

hydrochlorothiazide

amantadine: Possibly increased blood level and risk of toxicity of amantadine

amphotericin B, corticosteroids: Intensified electrolyte depletion, especially hypokalemia

barbiturates, opioids: May potentiate orthostatic hypotension

calcium: Possibly increased serum calcium level

cholestyramine, colestipol resins: Reduced GI absorption of hydrochlorothiazide

diazoxide: Increased antihypertensive and hyperglycemic effects of hydrochlorothiazide
diflunisal: Possibly increased blood hydrochlorothiazide level
digoxin: Increased risk of digitalis toxicity from hypokalemia
dopamine: Possibly increased diuretic effects of both drugs
lithium: Decreased lithium clearance and increased risk of toxicity
nondepolarizing skeletal muscle relaxants (such as tubocurarine): Possibly increased responsiveness to the muscle relaxant
pressor amines (such as norepinephrine): Possibly decreased response to pressor amines
oral anticoagulants: Possibly decreased anticoagulant effects
vitamin D: Increased risk of hypercalcemia

Adverse Reactions

CNS: Asthenia, decreased concentration, depression, dizziness, fatigue, hallucinations, headache, insomnia, nervousness, nightmares, paresthesia, stroke, syncope, vertigo, weakness
CV: Angina, arrhythmias, bradycardia, cardiac arrest, chest pain, edema, hypotension, orthostatic hypotension, palpitations, Raynaud's phenomenon, vasodilation, vasculitis
EENT: Blurred vision, diplopia, dry eyes or mouth, eye irritation, ptosis, tinnitus, vision changes
ENDO: Hyperglycemia, hypoglycemia
GI: Abdominal cramps or pain, anorexia, constipation, diarrhea, hepatomegaly, indigestion, jaundice, nausea, vomiting
GU: Decreased libido, impotence, interstitial nephritis, nocturia, polyuria, renal failure
HEME: Agranulocytosis, aplastic and hemolytic anemia, leukopenia, neutropenia, thrombocytopenia
MS: Arthralgia, muscle spasms and weakness
RESP: Bronchospasm, cough, crackles, dyspnea
SKIN: Alopecia, diaphoresis, exfoliative dermatitis, hyperpigmentation, photosensitivity, pruritus, psoriasis flare up, purpura, rash, urticaria
Other: Anaphylaxis, dehydration, hypercalcemia, hyperuricemia, hypochloremia, hypokalemia, hyponatremia, hypovolemia, metabolic alkalosis, weight loss

Nursing Considerations

- Use cautiously in patients with impaired hepatic function because hydrochlorothiazide may alter fluid and electrolyte balance and lead to hepatic coma.
- Also use cautiously in patients with systemic lupus erythematosus because hydrochlorothiazide may activate or worsen it.

- Monitor blood pressure often to assess effectiveness of therapy. Expect varied effectiveness in elderly patients; they may be less sensitive to drug's antihypertensive effect or more sensitive because of reduced drug clearance.
- **WARNING** Be aware that timolol and hydrochlorothiazide shouldn't be stopped abruptly because this may produce MI, myocardial ischemia, severe hypertension, or ventricular arrhythmias, particularly in patient with cardiovascular disease.
- Provide adequate hydration, as appropriate, to help prevent hypovolemia.
- Monitor fluid intake and output, daily weight, and serum electrolyte levels (especially potassium) to detect volume depletion or electrolyte imbalance.
- Watch for increased BUN and serum creatinine levels, especially in patients with impaired renal function, because drug may cause acute renal failure. If increases are significant or persistent, notify prescriber immediately.
- Be aware that timolol may mask signs and symptoms of acute hypoglycemia or prolong hypoglycemia. Monitor blood glucose level often in diabetic patients, and expect to increase antidiabetic dosage, as needed and ordered.
- Know that timolol may mask certain signs of hyperthyroidism, such as tachycardia. Monitor patient closely.
- Watch for impaired circulation in elderly patients with age-related peripheral vascular disease or patients with Raynaud's phenomenon. Alpha stimulation may worsen symptoms in such patients. Elderly patients also are at increased risk for beta-blocker-induced hypothermia.
- If patient develops a serious skin reaction, notify prescriber.

PATIENT TEACHING
- Advise patient to take timolol and hydrochlorothiazide in the morning or early evening to avoid the need to urinate during the night.
- Teach patient to monitor her blood pressure and pulse. Tell her to report consistent abnormalities to prescriber.
- Direct patient to weigh herself at the same time each day wearing the same amount of clothing and to notify prescriber if she gains more than 2 lb (0.9 kg) per day or 5 lb (2.3 kg) per week.
- Instruct patient to eat a diet high in potassium-rich foods, such as citrus fruits, bananas, tomatoes, and dates.
- To reduce the risk of dehydration and hypotension, advise patient to avoid exercise in hot weather and to avoid alcohol.

Also instruct her to notify prescriber if she has prolonged diarrhea, nausea, or vomiting.
* Caution patient to avoid hazardous activities until drug's CNS
effects are known.
* Explain the importance of regular exercise, proper diet, and
other lifestyle changes in controlling hypertension.
* Caution patient not to change dosage without consulting prescriber and not to stop taking drug abruptly.
* Advise patient to notify prescriber immediately if she experiences chest pain, fainting, light-headedness, or shortness of
breath, which may indicate a need for dosage adjustment.
* Advise patient to consult prescriber before taking OTC drugs,
especially cold remedies.
* Advise diabetic patient to monitor blood glucose level closely
because drug may alter control and mask some signs of hypoglycemia.
* Warn patient with psoriasis about possible flare-ups.

trandolapril and verapamil hydrochloride
Tarka

Class and Category
Chemical: Non–sulfhydryl-containing ACE inhibitor (trandolapril),
phenylalkylamine derivative (verapamil)
Therapeutic: Antihypertensive
Pregnancy: C (first trimester), D (later trimesters)

Indications and Dosages
▶ *To treat hypertension*
E.R. TABLETS
Adults. *Initial:* 1 mg trandolapril and 240 mg verapamil, 2 mg
trandolapril and 180 mg verapamil, 2 mg trandolapril and
240 mg verapamil, or 4 mg trandolapril and 240 mg verapamil
daily. *Maximum:* 4 mg trandolapril and 240 mg verapamil.
DOSAGE ADJUSTMENT Patients with hepatic impairment
given 30% of normal dosage. Dosage may be reduced in patients with cirrhosis and those with creatinine clearance less
than 30 ml/min/1.73 m^2.

Contraindications
Cardiogenic shock; history of angioedema from previous ACE inhibitor use; hypersensitivity to trandolapril, other ACE inhibitors,

verapamil, or their components; hypotension; severe heart failure; severe left ventricular dysfunction; sick sinus syndrome or second- or third-degree AV block (unless artificial pacemaker is in place)

Mechanism of Action

Trandolapril is the prodrug for trandolaprilat, which reduces blood pressure by inhibiting conversion of angiotensin I to angiotensin II. Angiotensin II is a potent vasoconstrictor that stimulates the renal cortex to secrete aldosterone. Decreased aldosterone release reduces sodium and water retention and increases their excretion, thereby reducing blood pressure. Trandolapril may also inhibit renal and vascular production of angiotensin II.

Verapamil inhibits calcium entry into coronary and vascular smooth-muscle cells by blocking slow calcium channels in cell membranes. The resulting decrease in intracellular calcium level inhibits smooth-muscle cell contractions and decreases myocardial oxygen demand by relaxing coronary and vascular smooth muscle, reducing peripheral vascular resistance, and decreasing systolic and diastolic blood pressures.

Interactions

DRUGS

trandolapril and verapamil

beta blockers: Increased risk of heart failure, hypotension, and severe bradycardia

carbamazepine, cyclosporine, theophylline: Possibly increased blood levels of these drugs and increased risk of toxicity

digoxin: Increased blood digoxin level and risk of digitalis toxicity

disopyramide, flecainide: Possibly additive negative inotropic effects

diuretics: Increased risk of hypotension

lithium: Increased risk of lithium-induced neurotoxicity

neuromuscular blockers: Prolonged recovery from neuromuscular blockade

potassium-sparing diuretics, potassium supplements: Increased risk of hyperkalemia

quinidine: Increased risk of quinidine toxicity, increased QT interval, additive negative inotropic effects

verapamil

anesthetics (inhaled): Enhanced cardiodepressive effects of verapamil

cimetidine: Decreased metabolism and increased blood verapamil level

phenobarbital: Increased verapamil clearance
rifampin: Decreased bioavailability of oral verapamil
FOODS
trandolapril and verapamil
high-potassium diet, potassium-containing salt substitutes: Increased risk of hyperkalemia
verapamil
all foods: Decreased verapamil bioavailability

Adverse Reactions

CNS: Dizziness, fatigue
CV: AV block, bradycardia, junctional rhythm, orthostatic hypotension
EENT: Dry mouth
GI: Constipation
RESP: Cough
Other: Angioedema

Nursing Considerations

- Be aware that disopyramide and flecainide should not be given within 48 hours before or 24 hours after trandolapril and verapamil because additive negative inotropic effects can result.
- **WARNING** Closely monitor blood pressure during first 2 weeks of therapy and whenever dosage or accompanying diuretic dosage is adjusted, especially in patients with heart failure, hyponatremia, or severe volume or sodium loss. If excessive hypotension occurs, notify prescriber immediately, place patient in supine position, and prepare to infuse I.V. normal saline solution, as prescribed.
- **WARNING** Be alert for signs and symptoms of angioedema. If swelling of tongue, glottis, or larynx causes airway obstruction, notify prescriber and be prepared to stop drug and administer emergency measures, including subcutaneous epinephrine 1:1,000 (0.3 to 0.5 ml).
- Assess patient for bradycardia and hypotension, which may indicate AV block, and notify prescriber if heart rate or blood pressure declines significantly.
- Continue to monitor blood pressure to assess drug's long-term effectiveness.

PATIENT TEACHING
- Instruct patient not to crush or chew E.R. trandolapril and verapamil tablet, but inform her that she may break tablet in half to aid in swallowing.
- Advise patient to take drug with food.

- Direct patient to monitor pulse rate before taking drug and to notify prescriber if pulse rate falls below 50 beats/min or as instructed by prescriber.
- Instruct patient to stop drug and notify prescriber immediately if she has swelling of face, eyes, lips, or tongue or has trouble breathing.
- Explain that drug may cause dizziness and light-headedness, especially during first few days of therapy. Urge patient to avoid hazardous activities until drug's adverse CNS effects are known and to notify prescriber immediately if she faints.
- Inform female patient of childbearing age about risks of taking trandolapril and verapamil during pregnancy, especially during second and third trimesters. Urge her to use effective contraception and to notify prescriber immediately if she is or could be pregnant.
- Advise patient planning to undergo surgery or anesthesia to inform specialist that she takes trandolapril and verapamil.
- Instruct patient to consult prescriber before using potassium supplements or salt substitutes containing potassium.
- Encourage patient to increase dietary fiber intake to prevent constipation. Advise her to notify prescriber if constipation persists.

valsartan and hydrochlorothiazide
Diovan HCT

Class and Category
Chemical: Nonpeptide tetrazole derivative (valsartan), benothiadiazide (hydrochlorothiazide)
Therapeutic: Antihypertensive (valsartan, hydrochlorothiazide), diuretic (hydrochlorothiazide)
Pregnancy category: D

Indications and Dosages
▶ *To treat hypertension in patients uncontrolled by valsartan or hydrochlorothiazide alone; to treat patients adequately controlled by 25 mg hydrochlorothiazide but who developed hypokalemia as a result; as initial treatment of hypertension in patients expected to need mutli-drug therapy*
TABLETS
Adults. *Initial:* 80 to 160 mg valsartan and 12.5 mg hydrochlorothiazide (1 tablet containing 12.5 mg hydrochlorothiazide

and either 80 or 160 mg valsartan) daily. Dosage may be increased, as needed, after 1 to 2 wk. *Maximum:* 320 mg valsartan and 25 mg hydrochlorothiazide daily.

Mechanism of Action

Valsartan blocks the hormone angiotensin II from binding to the receptor sites in vascular smooth muscle, adrenal glands, and other tissues. This action inhibits angiotensin II's vasoconstrictive and aldosterone-secreting effects, thereby reducing blood pressure.

Hydrochlorothiazide promotes movement of sodium, chloride, and water from blood in peritubular capillaries into the nephron's distal convoluted tubule. Initially, it may decrease extracellular fluid volume, plasma volume, and cardiac output, which helps explain blood pressure reduction. It also may reduce blood pressure by dilating arteries. After several weeks, extracellular fluid volume, plasma volume, and cardiac output return to normal, and peripheral vascular resistance remains decreased.

Contraindications

Anuria; hypersensitivity to valsartan, hydrochlorothiazide, other sulfonamide-derived drugs, or their components; pregnancy; renal failure

Interactions

DRUGS

valsartan and hydrochlorothiazide

antihypertensives, diuretics: Increased antihypertensive effects

valsartan

potassium salts, potassium-sparing diuretics: Possibly hyperkalemia

hydrochlorothiazide

amantadine: Possibly increased blood amantadine level and risk of toxicity

amiodarone: Increased risk of arrhythmias from hypokalemia

amphotericin B, corticosteroids: Intensified electrolyte depletion, especially hypokalemia

barbiturates, opioids: May potentiate orthostatic hypotension

calcium: Possibly increased serum calcium level

cholestyramine, colestipol resins: Reduced GI absorption of hydrochlorothiazide

diazoxide: Increased antihypertensive and hyperglycemic effects of hydrochlorothiazide

diflunisal: Possibly increased blood hydrochlorothiazide level

digoxin: Increased risk of digitalis toxicity from hypokalemia
dopamine: Possibly increased diuretic effects of both drugs
insulin, oral antidiabetics: Possibly increased blood glucose level
lithium: Decreased lithium clearance and increased risk of toxicity
neuromuscular blockers: Possibly increased neuromuscular blockade from hypokalemia
nondepolarizing skeletal muscle relaxants (such as tubocurarine): Possibly increased responsiveness to the muscle relaxant
NSAIDs: Decreased diuretic effect of hydrochlorothiazide and increased risk of renal failure
pressor amines (such as norepinephrine): Possibly decreased response to pressor amines
oral anticoagulants: Possibly decreased anticoagulant effects
sympathomimetics: Possibly decreased antihypertensive effect of hydrochlorothiazide
vitamin D: Increased risk of hypercalcemia
FOODS
valsartan
potassium-containing salt substitutes: Possibly hyperkalemia

Adverse Reactions
CNS: Anxiety, depression, dizziness, fatigue, fever, headache, insomnia, paresthesia, restlessness, somnolence, syncope, vertigo, weakness
CV: Chest pain, edema, hypotension, necrotizing angiitis, orthostatic hypotension, palpitations, tachycardia, vasculitis
EENT: Blurred vision, dry mouth, nasopharyngitis, pharyngitis, rhinitis, sinusitis, tinnitus
ENDO: Hyperglycemia
GI: Abdominal cramps or pain, anorexia, constipation, diarrhea, elevated liver enzymes, flatulence, hepatitis, indigestion, jaundice, nausea, pancreatitis, vomiting
GU: Decreased libido, impotence, interstitial nephritis, nocturia, polyuria, renal failure, UTI
HEME: Agranulocytosis, aplastic and hemolytic anemia, leukopenia, neutropenia, thrombocytopenia
MS: Arthralgia, muscle spasms and weakness
RESP: Bronchospasm, cough, dyspnea, respiratory distress, upper respiratory tract infection
SKIN: Alopecia, erythema multiforme, exfoliative dermatitis, photosensitivity, purpura, rash, Stevens Johnson syndrome, urticaria
Other: Anaphylaxis, angioedema, dehydration, hypercalcemia,

hyperkalemia, hyperuricemia, hypochloremia, hypokalemia, hypomagnesemia, hyponatremia, hypovolemia, metabolic alkalosis, viral infection, weight loss

Nursing Considerations

• Use valsartan and hydrochlorothiazide cautiously in patients with impaired hepatic function because hydrochlorothiazide may alter fluid and electrolyte balance and lead to hepatic coma.

• Also use drug cautiously in patients who have systemic lupus erythematosus because hydrochlorothiazide may activate or worsen it.

• Monitor blood pressure often to assess drug effectiveness.

• Provide hydration, as appropriate, to help prevent hypovolemia.

• Monitor fluid intake and output, daily weight, and serum electrolyte levels (especially potassium) to detect volume depletion or electrolyte imbalance.

• Watch for increased BUN and serum creatinine levels, especially in patients with impaired renal function, because drug may cause acute renal failure. If increases are significant or persistent, notify prescriber immediately.

• Monitor blood glucose level often in diabetic patients, and expect to increase antidiabetic dosage, as needed and ordered.

• Check patient's CBC routinely, as ordered, for abnormalities. If they are significant or persistent, notify prescriber immediately.

PATIENT TEACHING

• Advise patient to take drug in the morning or early evening to avoid the need to urinate during the night.

• Teach patient to monitor her blood pressure and to report consistently elevated measurements to prescriber.

• Alert patient that full effects of drug may take up to 4 weeks to occur.

• Direct patient to weigh herself at the same time each day wearing the same amount of clothing and to notify the prescriber if she gains more than 2 lb (0.9 kg) per day or 5 lb (2.3 kg) per week.

• **WARNING** Strongly urge patient to contact prescriber before using potassium supplements or OTC salt substitutes, which may contain potassium and will increase the risk of hyperkalemia.

• Instruct female patient of childbearing age to use reliable birth control during therapy and to notify prescriber immediately about known or suspected pregnancy.

- To reduce the risk of dehydration and hypotension, advise patient to avoid exercise in hot weather and to avoid alcohol. Also instruct her to notify prescriber if she has prolonged diarrhea, nausea, or vomiting.
- Caution patient to avoid hazardous activities until drug's CNS effects are known.
- Explain the importance of regular exercise, proper diet, and other lifestyle changes in controlling hypertension.

Central Nervous System Drugs

acetaminophen, caffeine, and butalbital

Americet, Esgic, Esgic Plus, Fioricet, Margesic, Medigesic, Repan

Class and Category

Chemical: Acetamide (acetaminophen), xanthine derivative (caffeine), barbiturate (butalbital)

Therapeutic: Analgesic (acetaminophen), CNS stimulant (caffeine), muscle relaxant (butalbital)

Pregnancy category: C

Indications and Dosages

▶ *To relieve tension or muscle contraction headache*

CAPSULES, TABLETS

Adults. 325 mg acetaminophen, 40 mg caffeine, and 50 mg butalbital (1 tablet or capsule) to 650 mg acetaminophen, 80 mg caffeine, and 100 mg butalbital (2 tablets or capsules) every 4 hr, as needed, not to exceed 4,000 mg acetaminophen daily. Or, 500 mg acetaminophen, 40 mg caffeine, and 50 mg butalbital (1 tablet or capsule) or 1,000 mg acetaminophen, 80 mg caffeine, and 100 mg butalbital (2 tablets or capsules) every 4 hr, as needed, not to exceed 4,000 mg acetaminophen daily.

Mechanism of Action

Acetaminophen inhibits the enzyme cyclooxygenase, blocking prostaglandin production and disrupting peripheral pain impulse generation.

Caffeine is a potent, competitive inhibitor of phosphodiesterase, an enzyme that degrades c3'5' AMP. Increased cAMP mediates most of its actions, including CNS stimulation to counteract the sedative properties of butalbital and cerebral vasoconstriction to relieve headache caused by increased blood volume from vasodilation.

Butalbital inhibits upward conduction of nerve impulses to the reticular formation of the brain, thereby disrupting impulse transmission to the cortex. This action depresses the CNS, producing drowsiness, hypnosis, and sedation.

Contraindications

History of barbiturate addiction; hypersensitivity to butalbital, acetaminophen, caffeine, other barbitrates or their components; porphyria; severe hepatic impairment; significant respiratory depression

Interactions

DRUGS

acetaminophen, caffeine, and butalbital

CNS depressants, general anesthetics, opioids, tranquilizers: Additive CNS effects

acetaminophen

barbiturates (except butalbital or primidone), carbamazepine, hydantoins, isoniazid, rifampin, sulfinpyrazone: Decreased therapeutic effects and increased hepatotoxic effects of acetaminophen

lamotrigine, loop diuretics: Possibly decreased therapeutic effects of these drugs

oral contraceptives: Decreased effectiveness of acetaminophen

probenecid: Possibly increased therapeutic effects of acetaminophen

propranolol: Possibly increased action of acetaminophen

zidovudine: Possibly decreased effects of zidovudine

caffeine

aspirin: Increased GI absorption of aspirin

beta-adrenergic agonists: Possibly enhanced cardiac inotropic effects of beta-adrenergic agonists

cimetidine, contraceptives (oral), disulfiram, fluoroquinolones: Decreased hepatic metabolism of caffeine and increased caffeine effect

clozapine: Possibly increased clozapine level and adverse reactions

lithium: Increased renal clearance of lithium

mexiletine: Decreased caffeine elimination resulting in increased caffeine effect

phenytoin: Increased caffeine clearance, resulting in decreased caffeine effect

theophylline: Reduced theophylline clearance with ingestion of more than 120 mg caffeine daily

butalbital

adrenocorticoids, anticoagulants (oral), tricyclic antidepressants: Decreased effectiveness of these drugs

disulfiram: Possibly increased risk of barbiturate (butalbital) toxicity

ketamine anesthesia: Increased risk of profound respiratory depression

MAO inhibitors: Increased CNS effects of butalbital

ACTIVITIES

acetaminophen, caffeine, and butalbital

alcohol use: Additive CNS effect; increased risk of hepatotoxicity

caffeine

smoking: Increased caffeine clearance resulting in decreased caffeine effect

Adverse Reactions

CNS: Anxiety, confusion, depression, dizziness, drowsiness, excitement, headache, insomnia, intoxicated feeling, irritability, lethargy light-headedness, nervousness, restlessness, tremor, twitching, vertigo

CV: Extrasystoles, orthostatic hypotension, palpitations, tachycardia

EENT: Epistaxis, laryngospasm, rhinitis, salivation, tinnitus

ENDO: Alterations in blood glucose level

GI: Abdominal pain, anorexia, constipation, diarrhea, flatulence, jaundice, hepatotoxicity, nausea, vomiting

HEME: Agranulocytosis, hemolytic anemia, leukopenia, neutropenia, pancytopenia, thrombocytopenia

RESP: Apnea, bronchospasm, respiratory depression, shortness of breath

SKIN: Erythema multiforme, exfoliative dermatitis, rash, toxic epidermal necrolysis, urticaria

Other: Angioedema, anaphylaxis, physical and psychological dependence

Nursing Considerations

- Before and during long-term therapy, monitor patient's liver function test results, including AST, ALT, and bilirubin levels, as ordered.
- Evaluate patient for therapeutic response, including reports of decreased pain and body movements that would indicate pain relief has occurred.
- Monitor renal function in patient on long-term therapy.
- Take safety precautions, as needed.
- Monitor patient for CNS depression.
- Monitor patient's respiratory depth, effort, and rate. Notify prescriber immediately if respiratory rate drops below 10 breaths/ minute.
- **WARNING** Assess patient for evidence of physical and psychological dependence.

PATIENT TEACHING
- Instruct patient to take drug with food or after meals to minimize stomach upset.
- Instruct patient to take acetaminophen, caffeine, and butalbital exactly as prescribed and not to adjust dose or frequency without consulting prescriber.
- Instruct patient to notify prescriber about worsening or breakthrough pain.
- Advise patient to notify prescriber if he becomes short of breath or has difficulty breathing.
- Caution patient to avoid hazardous activities until drug's CNS effects are known.
- Caution patient to avoid alcohol or other CNS depressants while taking drug. Also tell patient to contact prescriber before taking other prescription or OTC drugs because they may contain acetaminophen and lead to toxicity.
- Encourage patient to get up slowly from a sitting or lying position.
- To prevent constipation, encourage patient to consume plenty of fluids and high-fiber foods, if not contraindicated by another condition.
- Teach patient to recognize signs of hepatotoxicity, such as bleeding, easy bruising, and chronic overdose.

acetaminophen, caffeine, and dihydrocodeine bitartrate

Class and Category

Chemical: Acetamide (acetaminophen), xanthine derivative (caffeine), opioid agonist (dihydrocodeine)
Therapeutic: Analgesic (acetaminophen, dihydrocodeine), CNS stimulant (caffeine)
Pregnancy category: C

Indications and Dosages

▶ *To relieve moderate to moderately severe pain*
TABLETS
Adults. 712.8 mg acetaminophen, 60 mg caffeine, and 32 mg dihydrocodeine (1 tablet) every 4 hours, as needed. *Maximum:* 5 tablets in a 24-hour period.

Contraindications

Acute or severe bronchial asthma; hypercapnia; hypersensitivity to acetaminophen, caffeine, codeine, dihydrocodeine, or their components; paralytic ileus; significant respiratory depression

---

Mechanism of Action

Acetaminophen inhibits the enzyme cyclooxygenase, thereby blocking prostaglandin production and interfering with pain impulse generation in the peripheral nervous system.

Caffeine is a potent, competitive inhibitor of phosphodiesterase, an enzyme that degrades cAMP. Increased cAMP mediates most of its action, including CNS stimulation to counteract the sedative properties of dihydrocodeine and cerebral vasoconstriction to relieve headache caused by increased blood volume from vasodilation.

Dihydrocodeine may produce analgesia through partial metabolism to the opioid, morphine. Opioids bind and interact with opiate receptors in the CNS, altering the perception of and emotional response to pain and causing generalized CNS depression.

Interactions

DRUGS

acetaminophen, caffeine, and dihydrocodeine
CNS depressants, general anesthetics, opioids, tranquilizers: Additive CNS effects

acetaminophen
barbiturates (except butalbital or primidone), carbamazepine, hydantoins, isoniazid, rifampin, sulfinpyrazone: Decreased therapeutic effects and increased hepatotoxic effects of acetaminophen
cholestyramine: Decreased acetaminophen absorption
lamotrigine, loop diuretics: Possibly decreased therapeutic effects of these drugs
oral contraceptives: Decreased effectiveness of acetaminophen
phenothiazines: Increased risk of severe hypothermia
probenecid: Possibly increased therapeutic effects of acetaminophen
propranolol: Possibly increased action of acetaminophen
warfarin: Possibly slight increased action of warfarin
zidovudine: Possibly decreased effects of zidovudine

caffeine
aspirin: Increased GI absorption of aspirin; increased metabolism of aspirin
beta-adrenergic agonists: Possibly enhanced cardiac inotropic effects of beta-adrenergic agonists

cimetidine, contraceptives (oral), disulfiram, fluoroquinolones: Decreased hepatic caffeine metabolism and increased caffeine effect

clozapine: Possibly increased clozapine level resulting in increased risk of clozapine-induced adverse reactions

lithium: Increased renal clearance of lithium

mexiletine: Decreased caffeine elimination resulting in increased caffeine effect

phenobarbital: Increased phenobarbital metabolism

phenytoin: Increased caffeine clearance resulting in decreased caffeine effect

theophylline: Reduced theophylline clearance with ingestion of more than 120 mg caffeine daily

dihydrocodeine

anticholinergics, paregoric: Increased risk of severe constipation

antihypertensives, diuretics: Potentiated hypotensive effects

buprenorphine: Decreased effectiveness of dihydrocodeine

hydroxyzine: Increased codeine analgesic effect; increased CNS-depressant and hypotensive effects

MAO inhibitors: Increased risk of unpredictable, severe, and sometimes fatal reactions

metoclopramide: Antagonized effect of metoclopramide on GI motility

mixed agonist and antagonist opioid analgesics such as buprenorphine, butorphanol, nalbuphine, pentazocine: Possibly reduced analgesic effectiveness of dihydrocodeine

naloxone: Antagonized dihydrocodeine analgesic effect

naltrexone: Precipitated withdrawal symptoms in dihydrocodeine-dependent patients

neuromuscular blockers: Additive respiratory depressant effects

ACTIVITIES

acetaminophen, caffeine, and dihydrocodeine

alcohol use: Additive CNS effect; increased risk of hepatotoxicity

caffeine

smoking: Increased caffeine clearance resulting in decreased caffeine effect

Adverse Reactions

CNS: Anxiety, anxiety neurosis, confusion, dizziness, drowsiness, excitement, fatigue, hallucinations, headache, insomnia, irritability, lethargy, light-headedness, nervousness, restlessness, sedation, tenseness, tremor, vivid dreams

CV: Extrasystoles, orthostatic hypotension, palpitations, tachycardia

EENT: Dry mouth, laryngeal edema, laryngospasm, miosis, tinnitus

GI: Abdominal pain, anorexia, bilary tract spasm, constipation, diarrhea, flatulence, indigestion, jaundice, hepatotoxicity, nausea, vomiting

GU: Acute renal failure, diuresis, granulomatous interstitial nephritis, urine retention

HEME: Agranulocytosis, leukopenia, neutropenia, pancytopenia, thrombocytopenia

RESP: Apnea, bronchospasm, cough suppression, respiratory depression

SKIN: Diaphoresis, erythema multiforme, pruritus, rash, urticaria

Other: Anaphylaxis, angioedema, physical and psychological dependence

Nursing Considerations

- Use acetaminophen, caffeine, and dihydrocodeine cautiously in elderly or debilitated patients and patients with significant underlying medical conditions, especially renal or hepatic disorders and malnutrition.
- Use cautiously in patients with head injury or increased intracranial pressure because dihydrocodeine may obscure neurologic signs of increased intracranial pressure, especially in patients with head injuries.
- If therapy is prolonged, monitor liver function test results, including AST, ALT, and bilirubin levels, as ordered.
- Evaluate therapeutic response, including reports of decreased pain and presence of body movements that suggest pain relief.
- Monitor renal function during long-term therapy.
- Take safety precautions, as needed.
- Monitor patient for CNS depression.
- Monitor respiratory depth, effort, and rate. Notify prescriber immediately if respiratory rate drops below 10 breaths/minute. Respiratory depression may increase with head injury, intracranial lesions, or other causes of increased intracranial pressure.
- **WARNING** Assess patient for evidence of physical and psychological dependence.

PATIENT TEACHING

- Instruct patient to take drug with food or after meals to minimize stomach upset.
- Instruct patient to take acetaminophen, caffeine, and dihydrocodeine exactly as prescribed and not to adjust dose or frequency without consulting prescriber.

- Instruct patient to notify prescriber about worsening or break-through pain.
- Advise patient to notify prescriber if he has trouble breathing.
- Caution patient to avoid hazardous activities until drug's CNS effects are known.
- Caution patient to avoid alcohol and other CNS depressants during therapy. Also urge patient to contact prescriber before taking other prescription or OTC drugs because they may contain acetaminophen and lead to toxicity.
- Advise patient to get up slowly from a sitting or lying position.
- To prevent constipation, encourage patient to consume plenty of fluids and high-fiber foods, if not contraindicated by another condition.
- Teach patient to recognize signs of hepatotoxicity, such as bleeding, easy bruising, and chronic overdose.

acetaminophen and codeine phosphate

Aceta with Codeine, Capital with Codeine, Tylenol with Codeine Elixir, Tylenol with Codeine No. 2, Tylenol with Codeine No. 3, Tylenol with Codeine No. 4

Class, Category, and Schedule

Chemical: Acetamide (acetaminophen), phenanthrene derivative (codeine)
Therapeutic: Analgesic (acetaminophen, codeine)
Pregnancy category: C
Controlled substance schedule: III (tablets), V (oral solution and elixir)

Indications and Dosages

▶ *To relieve mild to moderately severe pain*
ORAL SOLUTION, ORAL SUSPENSION, TABLETS
Adults. 15 to 60 mg codeine and 300 to 1,000 mg acetaminophen (number of tablets or ml dependent on strength) every 4 hr, as needed. *Maximum:* 360 mg codeine and 4,000 mg acetaminophen in 24 hr.

Contraindications

Hypersensitivity to acetaminophen, codeine, other opioids, or their components; significant respiratory depression; upper airway obstruction

Mechanism of Action

Acetaminophen inhibits the enzyme cyclooxygenase, thereby blocking prostaglandin production and interfering with pain impulse generation in the peripheral nervous system.

Codeine may produce analgesia through partial metabolism to the opioid,
morphine. Opioids bind and interact with opiate receptors in the CNS, altering the perception of and emotional response to pain and causing generalized CNS depression.

Interactions

DRUGS

acetaminophen

*barbiturates, carbamazepine, hydantoins, isoniazid, rifampin, sulfinpyra-
zone:* Decreased therapeutic effects and increased hepatotoxic effects of acetaminophen

lamotrigine, loop diuretics: Possibly decreased therapeutic effects of
these drugs

oral contraceptives: Decreased effectiveness of acetaminophen

probenecid: Possibly increased therapeutic effects of acetaminophen

propranolol: Possibly increased action of acetaminophen

zidovudine: Possibly decreased effects of zidovudine

codeine

anticholinergics: Increased risk of paralytic ileus

antihypertensives, diuretics: Potentiated hypotensive effects

buprenorphine: Decreased effectiveness of codeine

CNS depressants: Additive CNS effects

hydroxyzine: Increased codeine analgesic effect; increased CNS depressant and hypotensive effects

MAO inhibitors: Increased risk of unpredictable, severe, and sometimes fatal reactions

metoclopramide: Antagonized effect of metoclopramide on GI motility

naloxone: Antagonized codeine analgesic effect

naltrexone: Precipitated withdrawal symptoms in codeine-
dependent patients

neuromuscular blockers: Additive respiratory depressant effects

opioids: Additive CNS and respiratory depressant effects and hypotensive effects

paregoric: Increased risk of severe constipation

ACTIVITIES

acetaminophen and codeine

alcohol use: Additive CNS effects of codeine, increased risk of hepatotoxicity with acetaminophen

Adverse Reactions

CNS: Coma, delirium, depression, disorientation, dizziness, drowsiness, euphoria, hallucinations, headache, lack of coordination, lethargy light-headedness, mental and physical impairment, mood changes, restlessness, sedation, seizures, tremor

CV: Bradycardia, heart block, orthostatic hypotension, palpitations, tachycardia

EENT: Altered taste, blurred vision, diplopia, dry mouth, laryngeal edema, laryngospasm, miosis

ENDO: Alterations in serum blood glucose level

GI: Abdominal cramps and pain, anorexia, constipation, flatulence, gastroesophageal reflux, jaundice, hepatotoxicity, ileus, indigestion, nausea, vomiting

GU: Decreased libido, difficult ejaculation, dysuria, impotence, oliguria, ureteral spasm, urinary incontinence, urine retention

HEME: Hemolytic anemia, leukopenia, neutropenia, pancytopenia, thrombocytopenia

RESP: Apnea, bronchoconstriction, bronchospasm, depressed cough reflex, respiratory depression

SKIN: Diaphoresis, flushing, pallor, pruritus, rash, urticaria

Other: Angioedema, anaphylaxis, physical and psychological dependence

Nursing Considerations

- Use cautiously in patients with head trauma intracranial lesions because codeine can cause exaggerated respiratory depression.
- Use cautiously in elderly and debilitated patients as well as patients with severe renal or hepatic dysfunction, gallbladder disease, respiratory impairment, cardiac arrhythmias, inflammatory disorders of the GI tract, hypothyroidism, Addison's disease, prostatic hypertrophy or urethral stricture, coagulation disorders, or acute abdominal conditions.
- **WARNING** Monitor patient closely for signs of overdose, even at normal dosage, because some patients metabolize codeine quickly, leading to a sudden rise in blood codeine level. This metabolic defect occurs in about 0.5 to 1% of patients who are Chinese, Japanese, or Hispanic; 1 to 10% of Caucasians; 3% of African Americans; and 16 to 28% of

North Africans, Ethiopians, and Arabs. Watch for extreme sleepiness, confusion, and shallow breathing after giving drug. If present, notify prescriber and be prepared to provide supportive care and discontinue drug, as ordered.

• Before and during long-term therapy, monitor patient's liver function test results, including AST, ALT, and bilirubin levels, as ordered.

• Evaluate patient for therapeutic response, including reports of decreased pain and body movements that would indicate pain relief has occurred.

• Monitor renal function in a patient on long-term therapy. Keep in mind that blood or albumin in urine may indicate nephritis or renal failure. Also monitor urine output; decreasing output may signal urine retention or decreased renal function.

• Take safety precautions, as needed.

• Assess patient's respiratory depth, effort and rate. Notify prescriber immediately if respiratory rate drops below 10 breaths/minute.

• **WARNING** Assess patient for evidence of physical and psychological dependence.

PATIENT TEACHING

• Instruct patient to take acetaminophen and codeine with food or after meals to minimize stomach upset.

• Instruct patient to take acetaminophen and codeine exactly as prescribed and not to adjust dose or frequency without consulting prescriber.

• Advise patient to only use manufacturer's dosage cup for liquid acetaminophen and codeine.

• Instruct patient to notify prescriber about worsening or breakthrough pain.

• Advise patient to notify prescriber if he becomes short of breath, has trouble breathing, or has extreme sleepiness or confusion.

• Caution patient to avoid hazardous activities until drug's CNS effects are known.

• Caution patient to avoid alcohol or other CNS depressants while taking acetaminophen and codeine; also to contact prescriber before taking other prescription or OTC drugs as they may contain acetaminophen and lead to toxicity.

• Advise patient to get up slowly from a sitting or lying position.

• To prevent constipation, encourage patient to consume plenty of fluids and high-fiber foods, if not contraindicated.

• Teach patient to recognize signs of hepatotoxicity, such as bleeding, easy bruising, and chronic overdose.

acetaminophen and hydrocodone bitartrate

Allay, Anexsia, Anolor DH 5, Bancap-HC, Co-Gesic, Dolacet, Dolagesic, Duocet, Hycomed, Hyco-Pap, Hydrocet, Hydrogesic, Lorcet-HD, Lorcet Plus, Lortab, Margesic-H, Oncet, Panacet, Panlor, Polygesic, Stagesic, T-Gesic, Ugesic, Vanacet, Vendone, Vicodin, Vicodin ES, Zydone

Class, Category, and Schedule

Chemical: Opioid and phenanthrene derivative (hydrocodone), para-aminophenol derivative (acetaminophen)
Therapeutic: Analgesic
Pregnancy category: C
Controlled substance schedule: III

Indications and Dosages

▶ *To treat moderate to severe back pain and pain from arthralgia, cancer, dental procedures, headache, and myalgia*

CAPSULES

Adults. 1 capsule (500 mg acetaminophen and 5 mg hydrocodone) every 4 to 6 hr, p.r.n. Or, 2 capsules (1,000 mg acetaminophen and 10 mg hydrocodone) every 6 hr, p.r.n. *Maximum:* 8 capsules (4,000 mg acetaminophen and 40 mg hydrocodone)/24 hr.

ORAL SOLUTION

Adults. 5 to 15 ml (167 mg acetaminophen and 2.5 mg hydrocodone/5 ml) every 4 to 6 hr, p.r.n., for up to 6 days.

TABLETS

Adults. 1 or 2 tablets (500 mg acetaminophen and 2.5 mg hydrocodone/tablet) every 4 to 6 hr, p.r.n. Or, 1 tablet (500 mg acetaminophen and 5 mg hydrocodone) every 4 to 6 hr, p.r.n., up to 2 tablets every 6 hr, p.r.n. Or, 1 tablet (650 mg acetaminophen and 7.5 mg hydrocodone) every 4 to 6 hr, p.r.n., up to 2 tablets every 6 hr, p.r.n. Or, 1 tablet (750 mg acetaminophen and 7.5 mg hydrocodone) every 4 to 6 hr, p.r.n. Or, 1 tablet (650 mg acetaminophen and 10 mg hydrocodone) every 4 to 6 hr, p.r.n. *Maximum:* 4,000 mg acetaminophen and 40 mg hydrocodone daily.

Mechanism of Action

Acetaminophen increases the pain threshold at the CNS level by inhibiting cyclooxygenase, an enzyme involved in prostaglandin synthesis. Prostaglandins, important mediators in the inflammatory response, cause local vasodilation with swelling and pain. They also play a role in pain transmission from the periphery to the spinal cord. With the inhibition of cyclooxygenase and prostaglandin synthesis, inflammatory symptoms subside.

Hydrocodone exerts a synergistic analgesic effect through two mechanisms of action. Hydrocodone, a mu opiate-receptor agonist, alters the perception of pain at the spinal cord and higher CNS levels by blocking the release of inhibitory neurotransmitters, such as gamma-aminobutyric acid and acetylcholine. It also alters the emotional response to pain.

Contraindications

Acute asthma; hypersensitivity to acetaminophen, aspirin, hydrocodone, opioids, NSAIDs, or their components; respiratory depression; upper airway obstruction

Interactions

DRUGS

anticholinergics: Increased risk of ileus, severe constipation, and urine retention

antidiarrheals (antiperistaltic): Increased risk of CNS depression and severe constipation

barbiturate anesthetics: Possibly increased respiratory and CNS depression

chlorpromazine, thioridazine: Increased risk of adverse and toxic effects of hydrocodone

CNS depressants: Increased risk of CNS and respiratory depression and hypotension

diuretics, other antihypertensives: Increased risk of hypotension

MAO inhibitors (such as furazolidone, phenelzine, procarbazine, selegiline, tranylcypromine) within 14 days of taking acetaminophen and hydrocodone: Increased risk of adverse CNS effects

metoclopramide: Possibly antagonized effect of metoclopramide on GI motility

naloxone: Possibly withdrawal symptoms in physically dependent patients

naltrexone: Possibly prolonged respiratory depression or cardiac arrest *opioid analgesics:* Risk of increased CNS and respiratory depression and hypotension

ACTIVITIES

alcohol use: Increased risk of CNS depression

Adverse Reactions

CNS: Confusion, dizziness, drowsiness, euphoria, headache, lethargy, restlessness, sedation, syncope

CV: Hypotension, orthostatic hypotension, tachycardia

EENT: Dry mouth, laryngeal edema, laryngospasm, vision changes

GI: Anorexia, constipation, nausea, vomiting

GU: Dysuria, urine retention

RESP: Atelectasis, bronchospasm, respiratory depression, wheezing

SKIN: Diaphoresis, flushing, pruritus, rash, urticaria

Other: Physical and psychological dependence

Nursing Considerations

- Expect prolonged use of acetaminophen and hydrocodone to produce physical and psychological dependence. Also, expect physical dependence may cause withdrawal symptoms when therapy stops.
- Assess elderly patients for adverse reactions because they're especially sensitive to drug and are at increased risk for constipation.
- **WARNING** Monitor patient for signs of overdose, such as blurred vision; cold, clammy skin; confusion; dizziness; dyspnea; headache; hearing loss; malaise; mental or mood changes; nausea; respiratory depression; sinus bradycardia; tinnitus; and vomiting. Notify prescriber immediately if they develop.

PATIENT TEACHING

- Inform patient that hydrocodone and acetaminophen may cause dizziness and drowsiness.
- Caution patient to avoid hazardous activities until drug's CNS effects are known.
- Caution patient not to take more than prescribed dosage because of risk of dependence.
- Urge patient to avoid using alcohol during drug therapy.
- Advise patient to change position slowly to minimize effects of orthostatic hypotension.
- If patient reports dry mouth, suggest that she use sugarless candy or gum or ice chips.

amphetamine and dextroamphetamine
Adderall, Adderall XR

Class, Category, and Schedule
Chemical: Phenylisopropylamine
Therapeutic: CNS stimulant
Pregnancy category: C
Controlled substance schedule: II

Indications and Dosages
▶ *To treat attention deficit hyperactivity disorder (ADHD)*
E.R. CAPSULES
Adults. 20 mg daily.
Adolescents ages 13 to 18. *Initial:* 10 mg daily. Dosage increased to 20 mg/day after 1 wk if needed.
Children age 6 and over. *Initial:* 5 or 10 mg daily. Dosage increased by 5 or 10 mg/day every wk until desired response occurs. *Maximum:* 30 mg/day.
TABLETS
Children age 6 and over. *Initial:* 5 mg daily or b.i.d. Increased by 5 mg/day every wk until desired response occurs. *Maximum:* 40 mg/day.
Children ages 3 to 6. *Initial:* 2.5 mg daily. Dosage increased by 2.5 mg/day every wk until desired response occurs. *Maximum:* 40 mg/day.
▶ *To treat narcolepsy*
TABLETS
Adults and children age 12 and over. *Initial:* 10 mg daily. Dosage increased by 10 mg/day every wk until desired response occurs. *Maximum:* 60 mg/day for adults.
Children ages 6 to 12. *Initial:* 5 mg daily. Dosage increased by 5 mg/day every wk until desired response occurs. *Maximum:* 40 mg/day.

Contraindications
Advanced arteriosclerosis; agitation; glaucoma; history of drug abuse; hypersensitivity to amphetamine, dextroamphetamine, or any of their components; hyperthyroidism; MAO inhibitor therapy within 14 days; moderate to severe hypertension; symptomatic CV disease; structural cardiac abnormalities

Interactions
DRUGS
anesthetics (inhaled): Increased risk of severe ventricular arrhythmias

antacids that contain calcium or magnesium, carbonic anhydrase inhibitors, citrates, sodium bicarbonate: Increased effects of amphetamine
antihypertensives, diuretics: Possibly decreased hypotensive effects
beta blockers: Increased risk of hypertension, excessive bradycardia, possibly heart block
CNS stimulants: Additive CNS stimulation
digoxin, levodopa: Possibly arrhythmias
ethosuximide, phenobarbital, phenytoin: Delayed intestinal absorption of these drugs
glutamic acid hydrochloride, urinary acidifiers (such as ammonium chloride and sodium acid phosphate): Increased excretion and decreased blood level and effects of amphetamine and dextroamphetamine
haloperidol, loxapine, molindone, phenothiazines, pimozide, thioxanthenes: Reduced antipsychotic efficacy of these drugs; inhibited CNS stimulant effects of amphetamine and dextroamphetamine
MAO inhibitors: Potentiated effects of amphetamine, possibly hypertensive crisis
meperidine: Increased analgesia
metrizamide: Increased risk of seizures
norepinephrine: Possibly increased adrenergic effect of norepinephrine
propoxyphene: Increased CNS stimulation, risk of fatal seizures
sympathomimetics: Increased CV effects of both drugs
thyroid replacement drugs: Enhanced effects of both drugs
tricyclic antidepressants: Possibly increased CV effects
FOODS
ascorbic acid, fruit juices: Decreased absorption and effects of amphetamine and dextroamphetamine

---

Mechanism of Action

Amphetamine and dextroamphetamine may produce its CNS stimulant effects by facilitating the release of norepinephrine at adrenergic nerve terminals and blocking its reuptake and by directly stimulating alpha and beta receptors in the peripheral nervous system. The drug also causes the release and blocks the reuptake of dopamine in limbic regions of the brain.

The main action of amphetamine and dextroamphetamine appears to be in the cerebral cortex and, possibly, the reticular activating system. Also, dextroamphetamine may stimulate inhibitory autoreceptors in the brain. These actions decrease drowsiness, fatigue, and motor restlessness and increase mental alertness. Peripheral actions include increased blood pressure, mild bronchodilation, and respiratory stimulation.

Adverse Reactions

CNS: Agitation, aggression, anxiety, depression, dizziness, drowsiness, emotional lability, fatigue, fever, headache, hostility, insomnia, irritability, light-headedness, mania, motor tics, nervousness, psychosis, seizures, somnolence, stroke, tremor
CV: Arrhythmias, hypertension, MI, sudden death, tachycardia
EENT: Accommodation abnormality, blurred vision, dry mouth, taste perversion
GI: Abdominal pain, anorexia, constipation, diarrhea, indigestion, nausea, vomiting
GU: Decreased libido, UTI
RESP: Dyspnea
SKIN: Diaphoresis, rash, Stevens-Johnson syndrome, toxic epidermal necrolysis
Other: Angioedema, anaphylaxis, infection, weight loss

Nursing Considerations

- Don't give amphetamine and dextroamphetamine to patients with serious heart conditions—such as cardiomyopathy, serious cardiac arrhythmias, coronary artery disease, structural cardiac abnormalities, or any other serious cardiac dysfunction—because the stimulatory effect of the drug may worsen these conditions or increase the risk of sudden death.
- Give first dose of tablet form when patient awakens and additional doses at 4- to 6-hour intervals. Give E.R. capsule form when patient awakens.
- If patient currently takes divided doses of tablet form, he may be switched to E.R. capsule form at the same daily dose, to be taken once in the morning.
- Monitor pulse rate and blood pressure in patients who have hypertension, even mild hypertension, because drug may increase blood pressure and cause arrhythmias, including tachycardia. Report abnormal findings to prescriber.
- Monitor patient for seizure activity because stimulants such as amphetamine and dextroamphetamine may lower the seizure threshold, even in patients with no history of seizures. If a seizure occurs, follow seizure protocol and expect to stop drug.
- **WARNING** If patient suddenly stops taking drug after long-term, high-dose therapy, watch for withdrawal signs and symptoms, such as abdominal pain, depression, fatigue, nausea, tremor, vomiting, and weakness. Anticipate restarting drug and gradually tapering dosage, as prescribed.
- Monitor growth and development in children because drug may

adversely affect growth.
- Assess patient for potential drug dependence, drug-seeking behavior, or drug tolerance. Be alert for signs and symptoms of long-term amphetamine abuse characterized by hyperactivity, irritability, marked insomnia, personality changes, and severe dermatoses.
- Monitor children and adolescents for onset of psychotic or manic symptoms, even patients with no history of such symptoms. If present, notify prescriber and expect to stop drug.
- Assess patient with history of Tourette syndrome, motor or vocal tics, or psychological disorders for exacerbation of these conditions during amphetamine therapy.

PATIENT TEACHING
- Advise patient to take amphetamine and dextroamphetamine with food or after a meal because anorexia may occur.
- Advise patient not to take drug with acidic fruit juice because it may decrease drug absorption.
- Tell patient or caregiver that E.R. capsules may be taken whole or opened and sprinkled on applesauce, then swallowed immediately without chewing.
- Stress the importance of taking drug exactly as prescribed because misuse may cause serious adverse cardiovascular reactions, including sudden death.
- Urge patient to avoid hazardous activities until he knows how drug affects him.
- Inform patient of abuse potential of drug, and stress the importance of not altering dosage unless prescribed.
- Inform parents or caregivers that child may be placed on drug-free weekend and holiday schedule, as prescribed, if signs and symptoms of ADHD are controlled.
- Monitor children and adolescents for first-time evidence of psychotic or manic symptoms. If they appear, notify prescriber and expect drug therapy to be stopped.

aspirin, caffeine, and dihydrocodeine bitartrate
Synalgos-DC

Class, Category, and Schedule
Chemical: Salicylate (aspirin), xanthine derivative (caffeine), opioid agonist (dihydrocodeine)

Therapeutic: Analagesic (aspirin, dihydrocodeine), CNS stimulant (caffeine)
Pregnancy category: D
Controlled substance schedule: III

Indications and Dosages

▶ *To relieve moderate to moderately severe pain*
CAPSULES
Adults. 712.8 mg aspirin, 60 mg caffeine, and 32 mg dihydrocodeine (2 capsules) every 4 hr, p.r.n.

Mechanism of Action

Aspirin blocks the activity of cyclooxygenase, the enzyme necessary for prostaglandin synthesis. By preventing prostaglandin synthesis, pain is relieved because prostaglandins play a role in pain transmission from the periphery to the spinal cord.

Caffeine is a potent, competitive inhibitor of phosphodiesterase, an enzyme that degrades c3'5' AMP. Increased cAMP mediates most of its actions, including CNS stimulation to counteract the sedative properties of dihydrocodeine.

Dihydrocodeine may produce analgesia through partial metabolism to the opioid, morphine. Opioids bind and interact with opiate receptors in the CNS, altering the perception of and emotional response to pain and causing generalized CNS depression.

Contraindications

Allergy to tartrazine dye; asthma; bleeding problems such as hemophilia; children under age 16 who have a viral illness; hypersensitivity to aspirin, dihydrocodeine, NSAIDs, other opioids, or their components; peptic ulcer disease; respiratory depression; severe vitamin K deficiency; upper airway obstruction

Interactions

DRUGS
aspirin, caffeine, and dihydrocodeine
CNS depressants: Additive CNS effects
aspirin
ACE inhibitors: Decreased antihypertensive effect
activated charcoal: Decreased aspirin absorption
antacids, urine alkalinizers: Decreased aspirin effectiveness
anticoagulants: Increased risk of bleeding; prolonged bleeding time
carbonic anhydrase inhibitors: Salicylism

corticosteroids: Increased excretion and decreased blood level of aspirin

heparin: Increased risk of bleeding

loop diuretics: Possibly decreased effectiveness of loop diuretics

methotrexate: Increased blood level and decreased excretion of methotrexate, causing toxicity

nizatidine: Increased blood aspirin level

NSAIDs: Possibly decreased blood NSAID level and increased risk of adverse GI effects

probenecid, sulfinpyrazone: Decreased effectiveness in treating gout

urine acidifiers, such as ammonium chloride and ascorbic acid: Decreased aspirin excretion

vancomycin: Increased risk of ototoxicity

caffeine

aspirin: Increased GI absorption of aspirin

beta-adrenergic agonists: Possibly enhanced cardiac inotropic effects of beta-adrenergic agonists

cimetidine, contraceptives (oral), disulfiram, fluoroquinolones: Decreased hepatic metabolism of caffeine and increased caffeine effect

clozapine: Possibly increased clozapine levels resulting in increased incidence of clozapine induced adverse reactions

lithium: Enhanced renal clearance of lithium

mexiletine: Decreased caffeine elimination resulting in increased caffeine effect

phenytoin: Increased caffeine clearance and decreased caffeine effect

theophylline: Reduced theophylline clearance with ingestion of more than 120 mg caffeine daily

dihydrocodeine

anticholinergics, paregoric: Increased risk of severe constipation

antihypertensives, diuretics: Potentiated hypotensive effects

buprenorphine: Decreased effectiveness of codeine

hydroxyzine: Increased codeine analgesic effect; increased CNS depressant and hypotensive effects

MAO inhibitors: Increased risk of unpredictable, severe, and sometimes fatal reactions

metoclopramide: Antagonized effect of metoclopramide on GI motility

naloxone: Antagonized dihydrocodeine analgesic effect

naltrexone: Precipitated withdrawal symptoms in dihydrocodeine-dependent patients

neuromuscular blockers: Additive respiratory depressant effects

opioids: Additive CNS and respiratory depressant effects and hypotensive effects
ACTIVITIES
aspirin, caffeine, and dihydrocodeine
alcohol use: Additive CNS effects
aspirin
alcohol use: Increased risk of ulcers
caffeine
smoking: Increased caffeine clearance resulting in decreased caffeine effect

Adverse Reactions

CNS: Coma, confusion, CNS depression, delirium, depression, disorientation, dizziness, drowsiness, euphoria, hallucinations, headache, lack of coordination
CV: Bradycardia, orthostatic hypotension, palpitations, tachycardia
EENT: Altered taste, blurred vision, diplopia, dry mouth, hearing loss, laryngeal edema, laryngospasm, miosis, tinnitus
GI: Abnormal cramps and pain, anorexia, constipation, diarrhea, flatulence, GI bleeding, gastroesophageal reflux, heartburn, hepatotoxicity, ileus, indigestion, nausea, stomach pain, vomiting
GU: Decreased libido, difficult ejaculation, dysuria, impotence, oliguria, ureteral spasm, urinary incontinence, urine retention
HEME: Decreased blood iron level, hemolytic anemia, leukopenia, prolonged bleeding time, shortened life span of RBCs, thrombocytopenia
RESP: Apnea, bronchoconstriction, bronchospasm, depressed cough reflex, respiratory depression
SKIN: Diaphoresis, ecchymosis, flushing, pallor, pruritus, rash, urticaria
Other: Anaphylaxis, angioedema, physical and psychological dependence, Reye's syndrome

Nursing Considerations

• Use cautiously in patients with head trauma or intracranial lesions because dihydrocodeine can cause an exaggerated respiratory depression and aspirin can increase the risk of bleeding.
• Use cautiously in elderly and debilitated patients as well as patients with severe renal or hepatic dysfunction, gallbladder disease, respiratory impairment, cardiac arrhythmias, inflammatory disorders of the GI tract, hypothyroidism, Addison's disease, prostatic hypertrophy or urethral stricture, coagulation disorders or acute abdominal conditions.

- **WARNING** Monitor patient closely for evidence of overdose, even at normal dosage, because some patients metabolize codeine quickly, leading to a sudden rise in blood codeine level. This metabolic defect occurs in about 0.5 to 1% of patients who are Chinese, Japanese, or Hispanic; 1 to 10% of Caucasians; 3% of African Americans; and 16 to 28% of North Africans, Ethiopians, and Arabs. Watch for extreme sleepiness, confusion and shallow breathing after giving drug. If present, notify prescriber and be prepared to provide supportive care and stop the drug, as ordered.
- Evaluate patient for therapeutic response, including report of decreased pain and body movements that would indicate pain relief has occurred.
- Take safety precautions, as needed.
- Monitor patient's respiratory depth, effort and rate. Notify prescriber immediately if respiratory rate drops below 10 breaths/minute.
- **WARNING** Monitor patient closely for allergic reaction. Be aware that anaphylactic shock and other severe allergic reactions can occur without a history of allergy.
- **WARNING** Assess patient for evidence of physical and psychological dependence.
- Monitor urine output; decreasing output may signal urine retention or renal failure.

PATIENT TEACHING
- Instruct patient to take aspirin, caffeine, and dihyrdocodeine with food or after meals to minimize stomach upset.
- Instruct patient to take drug exactly as prescribed and not to adjust dose or frequency without consulting prescriber.
- Instruct patient to notify prescriber about worsening or breakthrough pain.
- Advise patient to notify prescriber if he becomes short of breath, has trouble breathing, or has extreme sleepiness or confusion.
- Tell patient to consult with prescriber before taking drug with any prescription drug for blood disorder, diabetes, gout, or arthritis.
- Caution patient to avoid hazardous activities until drug's CNS effects are known.
- Caution patient to avoid alcohol or other CNS depressants while taking the drug.
- Advise patient to get up slowly from a sitting or lying position.

• To prevent constipation, urge patient to consume plenty of fluids and high-fiber foods, if not contraindicated.

aspirin and codeine phosphate
Empirin with Codeine No. 2, Empirin with Codeine No. 3, Empirin with Codeine No. 4

Class, Category, and Schedule
Chemical: Salicylate (aspirin), phenanthrene derivative (codeine)
Therapeutic: Analgesic (aspirin, codeine)
Pregnancy category: C
Controlled substance schedule: III

Indications and Dosages
▶ *To relieve mild, moderate, and moderate to severe pain*
TABLETS
Adults. 325 mg aspirin and 15 mg, 30 mg, or 60 mg codeine to 650 mg aspirin and 30 mg, 60 mg, or 120 mg codeine every 4 hr, p.r.n.

Mechanism of Action
Aspirin blocks the activity of cyclooxygenase, the enzyme needed for prostaglandin synthesis. Prostaglandins play a role in pain transmission from the periphery to the spinal cord. By preventing their synthesis, pain is relieved.

Codeine may produce analgesia through partial metabolism to the opioid, morphine. Opioids bind and interact with opiate receptors in the CNS, altering the perception of and emotional response to pain and causing generalized CNS depression.

Contraindications
Allergy to tartrazine dye; anticoagulant therapy; asthma; bleeding problems such as hemophilia; children under age 16 who have a viral illness; hypersensitivity to aspirin, codeine, NSAIDs, other opioids, or their components; peptic ulcer disease; respiratory depression; severe vitamin K deficiency; upper airway obstruction

Interactions
DRUGS
aspirin and codeine
penicillins, sulfonamides: Increased blood levels of penicillins and sulfonamides

aspirin

ACE inhibitors: Decreased antihypertensive effect

activated charcoal: Decreased aspirin absorption

antacids, urine alkalinizers: Decreased aspirin effectiveness

anticoagulants: Increased risk of bleeding; prolonged bleeding time

carbonic anhydrase inhibitors: Salicylism

corticosteroids: Increased excretion and decreased blood level of aspirin

heparin: Increased risk of bleeding

insulin, oral antidiabetics: Increased risk of hypoglycemia

loop diuretics: Possibly decreased effectiveness of loop diuretics

methotrexate: Increased blood level and decreased excretion of methotrexate, causing toxicity

nizatidine: Increased blood aspirin level

NSAIDs: Possibly decreased blood NSAID level and increased risk of adverse GI effects

probenecid, sulfinpyrazone: Decreased effectiveness in treating gout

urine acidifiers, such as ammonium chloride and ascorbic acid: Decreased aspirin excretion

vancomycin: Increased risk of ototoxicity

codeine

anticholinergics, paregoric: Increased risk of severe constipation

antihypertensives, diuretics: Potentiated hypotensive effects

buprenorphine: Decreased effectiveness of codeine

CNS depressants: Additive CNS effects

hydroxyzine: Increased codeine analgesic effect; increased CNS depressant and hypotensive effects

MAO inhibitors: Increased risk of unpredictable, severe, and sometimes fatal reactions

metoclopramide: Antagonized effect of metoclopramide on GI motility

naloxone: Antagonized codeine analgesic effect

naltrexone: Precipitated withdrawal symptoms in codeine-dependent patients

neuromuscular blockers: Additive respiratory depressant effects

opioids: Additive CNS and respiratory depressant effects and hypotensive effects

ACTIVITIES

aspirin

alcohol use: Increased risk of ulcers

codeine

alcohol use: Additive CNS effects

Adverse Reactions

CNS: Coma, confusion, CNS depression, delirium, depression, disorientation, dizziness, drowsiness, euphoria, hallucinations, headache, lack of coordination, lethargy, light-headedness, mental and physical impairment, mood changes, restlessness, sedation, seizures, tremor
CV: Bradycardia, heart block, orthostatic hypotension, palpitations, tachycardia
EENT: Altered taste, blurred vision, diplopia, dry mouth, hearing loss, laryngeal edema, laryngospasm, miosis, tinnitus
GI: Abdominal cramps and pain, anorexia, constipation, diarrhea, flatulence, GI bleeding, gastroesophageal reflux, heartburn, hepatotoxicity, ileus, indigestion, nausea, vomiting
GU: Decreased libido, difficult ejaculation, dysuria, impotence, nephrotoxicity, oliguria, ureteral spasm, urinary incontinence, urine retention
HEME: Decreased blood iron level, hemolytic anemia, leukopenia, prolonged bleeding time, shortened life span of RBCs, thrombocytopenia
MS: Muscle rigidity
RESP: Apnea, bronchoconstriction, bronchospasm, depressed cough reflex, respiratory depression
SKIN: Diaphoresis, ecchymosis, flushing, pallor, pruritus, rash, urticaria
Other: Anaphylaxis, angioedema, physical and psychological dependence, Reye's syndrome

Nursing Considerations

- Use cautiously in patients with head trauma or intracranial lesions because codeine can cause an exaggerated respiratory depression and aspirin can increase the risk of bleeding.
- Use cautiously in elderly and debilitated patients as well as patients with severe renal or hepatic dysfunction, gallbladder disease, respiratory impairment, cardiac arrhythmias, inflammatory disorders of the GI tract, hypothyroidism, Addison's disease, prostatic hypertrophy or urethral stricture, coagulation disorders or acute abdominal conditions.
- **WARNING** Monitor patient closely for evidence of overdose, even at normal dosage, because some patients metabolize codeine quickly, leading to a sudden rise in blood codeine level. This metabolic defect occurs in about 0.5 to 1% of patients who are Chinese, Japanese, or Hispanic; 1 to 10% of Caucasians; 3% of African Americans; and 16 to 28% of

North Africans, Ethiopians, and Arabs. Watch for extreme sleepiness, confusion and shallow breathing after giving drug. If present, notify prescriber and be prepared to provide supportive care and stop the drug, as ordered.

- Evaluate patient for therapeutic response using both patient reports of decreased pain and observation of body movements.
- Take safety precautions, as needed.
- Monitor respiratory depth, effort and rate. Notify prescriber immediately if respiratory rate drops below 10 breaths/minute.
- **WARNING** Monitor patient closely for allergic reaction. Be aware that anaphylactic shock and other severe allergic reactions can occur without a history of allergy.
- **WARNING** Assess patient for evidence of physical and psychological dependence.
- Monitor urine output; decreasing output may signal urine retention and renal failure.

PATIENT TEACHING

- Instruct patient to take aspirin and codeine with food or after meals to minimize stomach upset.
- Instruct patient to take drug exactly as prescribed and not to adjust dose or frequency without consulting prescriber.
- Instruct patient to report worsening or breakthrough pain.
- Advise patient to notify prescriber if he becomes short of breath or has trouble breathing or extreme sleepiness or confusion.
- Tell patient to consult prescriber before taking drug with any prescription drug for blood disorder, diabetes, gout, or arthritis.
- Caution patient to avoid hazardous activities until drug's CNS effects are known.
- Caution patient to avoid alcohol or other CNS depressants while taking aspirin and codeine.
- Advise patient to get up slowly from a sitting or lying position.
- To prevent constipation, encourage patient to consume plenty of fluids and high-fiber foods, if not contraindicated.

buprenorphine hydrochloride and naloxone hydrochloride
Suboxone

Class, Category, and Schedule
Chemical: Opioid as a thebaine derivative (buprenorphine), thebaine derivative (naloxone)

Therapeutic: Opioid analgesic (buprenorphine), opioid antagonist (naloxone)
Pregnancy category: C
Controlled substance schedule: III

Indications and Dosages

▶ *To treat opioid dependence*

S.L. TABLETS

Adults. 12 to 16 mg buprenorphine and 3 to 4 mg naloxone (6 to 8 tablets of 2-mg/0.5-mg strength or 2 tablets of 8/2-mg strength for highest dose) as a single dose daily.

Mechanism of Action

Buprenorphine may bind with CNS receptors to alter the perception of and emotional response to pain. Buprenorphine may act by displacing opioid agonists from their binding sites and competitively inhibiting their actions.

Naloxone briefly and competitively antagonizes mu, kappa, and sigma receptors in the CNS, thus reversing the analgesia, hypotension, respiratory depression, and sedation caused by most opioids. Mu receptors are responsible for analgesia, euphoria, miosis, and respiratory depression. Kappa receptors are responsible for analgesia and sedation. Sigma receptors control dysphoria and other delusional states.

Contraindications

Hypersensitivity to buprenorphine, naloxone, or their components

Interactions

DRUGS

buprenorphine and naloxone

antidepressants, benzodiazepines, sedatives, tranquilizers: Increased risk of serious overdose

buprenorphine

azole antifungals, such as ketoconazole; macrolide antibiotics, such as erythromycin; HIV protease inhibitors, such as indinavir, ritonavir and saquinavir: Possibly increased plasma levels of buprenorphine

CNS depressants, MAO inhibitors: Additive hypotensive and respiratory and CNS depressant effects of these drugs

opioid analgesics: Reduced therapeutic effects if buprenorphine is given before another opioid analgesic

naloxone

opioid analgesics: Reversal of the analgesic and adverse effects of

these drugs; possibly withdrawal symptoms in opioid-dependent patients
ACTIVITIES
buprenorphine and naloxone
alcohol use: Increased risk of serious overdose

Adverse Reactions

CNS: Anxiety, asthenia, chills, depression, dizziness, excitement, fever, headache, insomnia, irritability, nervousness, sedation, somnolence, tremors, vertigo
CV: Hypertension, hypotension, vasodilation, ventricular fibrillation or tachycardia
EENT: Excessive tearing, miosis, pharyngitis, rhinitis
GI: Abdominal pain, constipation, diarrhea, dyspepsia, nausea, vomiting
MS: Back pain
RESP: Bronchospasm, hypoventilation, increased cough, pulmonary edema
SKIN: Diaphoresis, pruritus, rash, urticaria
Other: Anaphylaxis, angioedema, flu syndrome, generalized pain, infection, withdrawal syndrome

Nursing Considerations

- Use buprenorphine and naloxone cautiously in patients with compromised respiratory function, severe hepatic or renal impairment, myxedema, hypothyroidism, adrenal insufficiency, CNS depression, coma, toxic psychosis, prostatic hypertrophy, urethral stricture, acute alcoholism, alcohol withdrawal syndrome, kyphoscoliosis, or biliary tract dysfunction.
- Because buprenorphine can increase cerebrospinal fluid (CSF) pressure, use cautiously in patients with head injury, intracranial lesions, or other conditions that increase CSF pressure.
- Obtain results of liver function studies, as ordered, before starting buprenorphine and naloxone therapy and then periodically throughout treatment because drug may contribute to the development of a hepatic abnormality. Expect patient with hepatic dysfunction to have increased circulating blood buprenorphine and naloxone levels, which may increase incidence and severity of adverse reactions.
- Frequently monitor vital signs and response to drug, and take safety precautions, especially after giving first dose.
- **WARNING** Monitor patient for withdrawal symptoms, especially when giving buprenorphine and naloxone to opioid-dependent patient. Symptoms may include abdominal

cramps, anorexia, anxiety, backache, bone or joint pain, confusion, depression, diaphoresis, dysphoria, erythema, fear, fever, irritability, labile blood pressure and pulse, lacrimation, muscle spasms, myalgia, mydriasis, nasal congestion, nausea, opioid craving, piloerection, restlessness, rhinorrhea, sensation of crawling skin, sleep disturbances, tremor, uneasiness, vomiting and yawning.

PATIENT TEACHING
- Tell patient, if prescribed, that he will receive only buprenorphine for 1 or 2 days and then be given the combination drug for maintenance therapy.
- Instruct patient to place the S.L. tablet under his tongue until it dissolves. Caution him not to swallow the tablet because it will be less effective. If patient is prescribed more than two tablets per dose, tell him to place all the tablets under his tongue at the same time if they will fit. If not, advise him to place two tablets at a time under his tongue until full dose has dissolved.
- WARNING Warn patient to avoid CNS depressants, such as alcohol or other opioids, while taking buprenorphine and naloxone because severe respiratory depression may occur.
- Instruct patient to rise slowly from a lying or sitting position to reduce dizziness.
- Caution patient to avoid hazardous activities until drug's CNS effects are known.
- Emphasize importance of wearing a medical alert item that in the event of an emergency, the emergency health team will know he is physically dependent on opioids and is being treated with buprenorphine and naloxone.
- Instruct patient to inform all prescribers that he takes buprenorphine and naloxone before taking any new prescriptions and to avoid OTC drugs that affect the nervous system to avoid potential overdose.

butalbital, acetaminophen, caffeine, and codeine phosphate

Fioricet with Codeine, Phrenilin with Caffeine and Codeine

Class, Category, and Schedule
Chemical: Barbiturate (butalbital), acetamide (acetaminophen), xanthine derivative (caffeine), phenanthrene derivative (codeine)
Therapeutic: Muscle relaxant (butalbital), analgesic (acetaminophen, codeine), CNS stimulant (caffeine)

Pregnancy category: C
Controlled substance schedule: III

Indications and Dosages

▶ *To relieve tension or muscle contraction headache*

CAPSULES

Adults. 50 mg butalbital, 325 mg acetaminophen, 40 mg caffeine, and 30 mg codeine (1 capsule) to 100 mg butalbital, 650 mg acetaminophen, 80 mg caffeine, and 60 mg codeine (2 capsules) every 4 hr, as needed. *Maximum:* 300 mg butalbital, 1,950 mg acetaminophen, 240 mg caffeine, and 180 mg codeine in 24 hr.

Mechanism of Action

Butalbital inhibits upward conduction of nerve impulses to the reticular formation of the brain, thereby disrupting impulse transmission to the cortex. This action depresses the CNS, producing drowsiness, hypnosis, and sedation.

Acetaminophen inhibits the enzyme cyclooxygenase, blocking prostaglandin production and disrupting peripheral pain impulse generation.

Caffeine is a potent, competitive inhibitor of phosphodiesterase, an enzyme that degrades c3'5' AMP. Increased cAMP mediates most of its actions, including CNS stimulation to counteract the sedative properties of butalbital and codeine and cerebral vasoconstriction to relieve headache caused by increased blood volume from vasodilation.

Codeine may produce analgesia through partial metabolism to the opioid, morphine. Opioids bind and interact with opiate receptors in the CNS, altering the perception of and emotional response to pain and causing generalized CNS depression.

Contraindications

History of barbiturate addiction; hypersensitivity to butalbital, other barbiturates, acetaminophen, caffeine, codeine, other opioids, or their components; porphyria; significant respiratory depression; upper airway obstruction

Interactions

DRUGS

butalbital, acetaminophen, caffeine, and codeine

CNS depressants, general anesthetics, opioids, tranquilizers: Additive CNS effects

butalbital

adrenocorticoids, oral anticoagulants, tricyclic antidepressants: Decreased effectiveness of these drugs *disulfiram:* Possibly increased risk of barbiturate (butalbital) toxicity

ketamine anesthesia: Increased risk of profound respiratory depression

MAO inhibitors: Increased CNS effects of butalbital

acetaminophen

anticholinergics: Decreased onset of action of acetaminophen

barbiturates (except butalbital or primidone), carbamazepine, hydantoins, isoniazid, rifampin, sulfinpyrazone: Decreased therapeutic effects and increased hepatotoxic effects of acetaminophen

lamotrigine, loop diuretics: Possibly decreased therapeutic effects of these drugs

oral contraceptives: Decreased effectiveness of acetaminophen

probenecid: Possibly increased therapeutic effects of acetaminophen

propranolol: Possibly increased action of acetaminophen

zidovudine: Possibly decreased effects of zidovudine

caffeine

aspirin: Increased GI absorption of aspirin

beta-adrenergic agonists: Possibly enhanced cardiac inotropic effects of beta-adrenergic agonists

cimetidine, contraceptives (oral), disulfiram, fluoroquinolones: Decreased hepatic metabolism of caffeine resulting in increased caffeine effect

clozapine: Possibly increased clozapine levels resulting in increased incidence of clozapine induced adverse reactions

lithium: Increased renal clearance of lithium

mexiletine: Decreased caffeine elimination resulting in increased caffeine effect

phenytoin: Increased caffeine clearance resulting in decreased caffeine effect

theophylline: Reduced theophylline clearance with ingestion of more than 120 mg caffeine daily

codeine

anticholinergics: Increased risk of paralytic ileus

antihypertensives, diuretics: Potentiated hypotensive effects

buprenorphine: Decreased effectiveness of codeine

hydroxyzine: Increased codeine analgesic effect; increased CNS depressant and hypotensive effects

MAO inhibitors: Increased risk of unpredictable, severe, and sometimes fatal reactions

metoclopramide: Antagonized effect of metoclopramide on GI motility

naloxone: Antagonized codeine analgesic effect
naltrexone: Precipitated withdrawal symptoms in codeine-dependent patients
neuromuscular blockers: Additive respiratory depressant effects
opioids: Additive CNS and respiratory depressant effects and hypotensive effects
paregoric: Increased risk of severe constipation

ACTIVITIES

butalbital, acetaminophen, caffeine, and codeine
alcohol use: Additive CNS effect; increased risk of hepatotoxicity

caffeine
smoking: Increased caffeine clearance resulting in decreased caffeine effect

Adverse Reactions

CNS: Anxiety, coma, confusion, delirium, depression, disorientation, dizziness, drowsiness, euphoria, excitement, hallucinations, headache, insomnia, intoxicated feeling, irritability, lack of coordination, lethargy light-headedness, mental and physical impairment, mood changes, nervousness, restlessness, sedation, seizures, tremor, twitching, vertigo

CV: Bradycardia, orthostatic hypotension, palpitations, tachycardia

EENT: Altered taste, blurred vision, diplopia, dry mouth, epistaxis, laryngeal edema, laryngospasm, miosis, salivation

ENDO: Altered blood glucose level

GI: Abdominal cramps and pain, anorexia, constipation, flatulence, gastroesophageal reflux, jaundice, hepatotoxicity, ileus, indigestion, nausea, vomiting

GU: Decreased libido, difficult ejaculation, dysuria, impotence, nephrotoxicity, oliguria, ureteral spasm, urinary incontinence, urine retention

HEME: Agranulocytosis, hemolytic anemia, leukopenia, neutropenia, pancytopenia, thrombocytopenia

MS: Muscle rigidity

RESP: Apnea, bronchoconstriction, bronchospasm, depressed cough reflex, respiratory depression, shortness of breath

SKIN: Diaphoresis, erythema multiforme, exfoliative dermatitis, flushing, pallor, pruritus, rash, toxic epidermal necrolysis, urticaria

Other: Angioedema, anaphylaxis, physical and psychological dependence

Nursing Considerations

- Use cautiously in patients with head trauma or intracranial lesions because codeine can cause an exaggerated respiratory depression.
- Use cautiously in elderly and debilitated patients as well as patients with severe renal or hepatic dysfunction, gallbladder disease, respiratory impairment, cardiac arrhythmias, inflammatory disorders of the GI tract, hypothyroidism, Addison's disease, prostatic hypertrophy or urethral stricture, coagulation disorders, or acute abdominal conditions.
- **WARNING** Monitor patient closely for evidence of overdose, even at normal dosage, because some patients metabolize codeine quickly, leading to a sudden rise in blood codeine level. This metabolic defect occurs in about 0.5 to 1% of patients who are Chinese, Japanese, or Hispanic; 1 to 10% of Caucasians; 3% of African Americans; and 16 to 28% of North Africans, Ethiopians, and Arabs. Watch for extreme sleepiness, confusion and shallow breathing after giving drug. If present, notify prescriber and be prepared to provide supportive care and stop the drug, as ordered.
- Before and during long-term therapy, monitor liver function test results, including AST, ALT, and bilirubin levels, as ordered.
- Evaluate patient for therapeutic response, including report of decreased pain that would indicate pain relief has occurred.
- Monitor renal function in patient on long-term therapy. Keep in mind that blood or albumin in urine may indicate nephritis and decreased urine output, renal failure. Expect to reduce dosage for patients with renal dysfunction.
- Take safety precautions, as needed.
- Monitor patient's respiratory depth, effort and rate. Notify prescriber immediately if respiratory rate drops below 10 breaths/ minute.
- **WARNING** Assess patient for evidence of physical and psychological dependence.
- Monitor urine output; decreasing output may signal urine retention or renal failure.

PATIENT TEACHING

- Instruct patient to take drug with food or after meals to minimize stomach upset.
- Instruct patient to take butalbital, acetaminophen, caffeine, and codeine exactly as prescribed and not to adjust dose or frequency without consulting prescriber.

- Instruct patient to notify prescriber about worsening or breakthrough pain.
- Advise patient to notify prescriber if he becomes short of breath or has trouble breathing or extreme sleepiness or confusion.
- Caution patient to avoid hazardous activities until drug's CNS effects are known.
- Caution patient to avoid alcohol or other CNS depressants while taking drug. Also to contact prescriber before taking other prescription or OTC drugs as they may contain acetaminophen and lead to toxicity.
- Advise patient to get up slowly from a sitting or lying position.
- To prevent constipation, urge patient to consume plenty of fluids and high-fiber foods, if not contraindicated.
- Teach patient to recognize signs of hepatotoxicity, such as bleeding, easy bruising, and chronic overdose.

butalbital, aspirin, and caffeine

Fiorinal, Fortabs

Class, Category, and Schedule

Chemical: Barbiturate (butalbital), salicylate (aspirin), and xanthine derivative (caffeine)
Therapeutic: Muscle relaxant (butalbital), analgesic (aspirin), CNS stimulant (caffeine)
Pregnancy category: C
Controlled substance schedule: III

Indications and Dosages

▶ *To relieve tension or muscle contraction headache*
CAPSULES
Adults. 50 mg butalbital, 325 mg aspirin, and 40 mg caffeine (1 capsule) to 100 mg butalbital, 650 mg aspirin, and 80 mg caffeine (2 capsules) every 4 hr, as needed. *Maximum:* 300 mg butalbital; 1,950 mg aspirin; and 240 mg caffeine in 24 hr.

Contraindications

Allergy to tartrazine dye; bleeding problems such as hemophilia; children under age 16 with a viral illness; history of barbiturate addiction; hypersensitivity to butalbital, other barbiturates, aspirin, caffeine, or their components; nephritis; peptic ulcer disease; porphyria; severe respiratory impairment; severe vitamin K deficiency; triad syndrome of angioedema, asthma, and nasal polyps

Mechanism of Action

Butalbital inhibits upward conduction of nerve impulses to the reticular formation of the brain, thereby disrupting impulse transmission to the cortex. This action depresses the CNS, producing drowsiness, hypnosis, and sedation.

Aspirin blocks the activity of cyclooxygenase, the enzyme necessary for prostaglandin synthesis. By preventing prostaglandin synthesis, pain is relieved because prostaglandins play a role in pain transmission from the periphery to the spinal cord.

Caffeine is a potent, competitive inhibitor of phosphodiesterase, an enzyme that degrades c3'5' AMP. Increased cAMP mediates most of its action, including CNS stimulation to counteract the sedative properties of butalbital.

Interactions

DRUGS

butalbital

adrenocorticoids, oral anticoagulants, tricyclic antidepressants: Decreased effectiveness of these drugs

CNS depressants: Increased CNS depressant effects

disulfiram: Possibly increased risk of barbiturate (butalbital) toxicity

ketamine anesthesia: Risk of profound respiratory depression

MAO inhibitors: Increased CNS effects of butalbital

aspirin

ACE inhibitors: Decreased antihypertensive effect

activated charcoal: Decreased aspirin absorption

antacids, urine alkalinizers: Decreased aspirin effectiveness

anticoagulants: Increased risk of bleeding; prolonged bleeding time

carbonic anhydrase inhibitors: Salicylism

corticosteroids: Increased excretion and decreased aspirin level

heparin: Increased risk of bleeding

loop diuretics: Possibly decreased effectiveness of loop diuretics

methotrexate: Increased blood level and decreased excretion of methotrexate, causing toxicity

nizatidine: Increased blood aspirin level

NSAIDs: Possibly decreased blood NSAID level and increased risk of adverse GI effects

oral antidiabetics and insulin: Increased risk of hypoglycemia

probenecid, sulfinpyrazone: Decreased effectiveness in treating gout

urine acidifiers, such as ammonium chloride and ascorbic acid: Decreased aspirin excretion

vancomycin: Increased risk of ototoxicity
caffeine
aspirin: Increased GI absorption of aspirin
beta-adrenergic agonists: Possibly enhanced cardiac inotropic effects of beta-adrenergic agonists
cimetidine, contraceptives (oral), disulfiram, fluoroquinolones: Decreased hepatic metabolism of caffeine and increased caffeine effect
clozapine: Possibly increased clozapine levels resulting in increased incidence of clozapine induced adverse reactions
lithium: Enhanced renal clearance of lithium
mexiletine: Decreased caffeine elimination resulting in increased caffeine effect
phenytoin: Increased caffeine clearance resulting in decreased caffeine effect
theophylline: Reduced theophylline clearance with ingestion of more than 120 mg caffeine daily
ACTIVITIES
butalbital
alcohol use: Increased CNS depression
aspirin
alcohol use: Increased risk of ulcers
caffeine
smoking: Increased caffeine clearance resulting in decreased caffeine effect

Adverse Reactions

CNS: Anxiety, clumsiness, confusion, CNS depression, dizziness, drowsiness, hangover, headache, insomnia, irritability, lethargy, light-headedness, nervousness, nightmares, paradoxical stimulation, syncope
CV: Hypotension
EENT: Hearing loss, laryngospasm, tinnitus
GI: Anorexia, constipation, diarrhea, flatulence, GI bleeding, heartburn, hepatotoxicity, jaundice, nausea, stomach pain, vomiting
HEME: Agranulocytosis, bone marrow suppression, decreased blood iron level, hemolytic anemia, leukopenia, megaloblastic anemia, prolonged bleeding time, shortened life span of RBCs, thrombocytopenia
MS: Arthralgia, muscle weakness
RESP: Apnea, bronchospasm, respiratory depression
SKIN: Ecchymosis, erythema multiforme, rash, toxic epidermal necrolysis, urticaria

Other: Angioedema, drug dependence, Reye's syndrome, weight loss

Nursing Considerations

- Use cautiously in patients with head trauma or intracranial lesions because aspirin can increase the risk of bleeding.
- Use cautiously in elderly and debilitated patients as well as patients with severe renal or hepatic dysfunction, gallbladder disease, respiratory impairment, cardiac arrhythmias, inflammatory disorders of the GI tract, hypothyroidism, Addison's disease, prostatic hypertrophy or urethral stricture, coagulation disorders or acute abdominal conditions.
- Evaluate patient for therapeutic response, including report of decreased pain that would indicate pain relief has occurred.
- Take safety precautions, as needed.
- Monitor patient for CNS depression.
- Monitor patient's respiratory depth, effort and rate. Notify prescriber immediately if rate drops below 10 breaths/minute.
- **WARNING** Monitor patient closely for allergic reaction. Be aware that anaphylactic shock and other severe allergic reactions can occur without a history of allergy.
- **WARNING** Assess patient for evidence of physical and psychological dependence.
- Monitor urine output; decreasing output may signal urine retention or renal failure.

PATIENT TEACHING

- Instruct patient to take butalbital, aspirin, and caffeine with food or after meals to minimize stomach upset.
- Instruct patient to take drug exactly as prescribed and not to adjust dose or frequency without consulting prescriber because drug can be habit forming.
- Instruct patient to notify prescriber about worsening or breakthrough pain.
- Advise patient to notify prescriber if he becomes short of breath or has difficulty breathing.
- Tell patient to consult prescriber before taking drug with any prescription drug for blood disorder, diabetes, gout, or arthritis.
- Caution patient to avoid hazardous activities until drug's CNS effects are known.
- Caution patient to avoid alcohol or other CNS depressants while taking drug.
- Advise patient to get up slowly from a sitting or lying position.
- To prevent constipation, encourage patient to consume plenty

of fluids and high-fiber foods, if not contraindicated by another condition.

butalbital, aspirin, caffeine, and codeine phosphate

Fiorinal with Codeine, Fiortal

Class, Category, and Schedule

Chemical: Barbiturate (butalbital) salicylate (aspirin), xanthine derivative (caffeine), phenanthrene derivative (codeine)
Therapeutic: Muscle relaxant (butalbital), analgesic (aspirin, codeine), CNS stimulant (caffeine)
Pregnancy category: C
Controlled substance schedule: III

Indications and Dosages

▶ *To relieve tension or muscle contraction headache*
CAPSULES
Adults. 50 mg butalbital, 325 mg aspirin, 40 mg caffeine, and 30 mg codeine (1 capsule) to 100 mg butalbital, 650 mg aspirin, 80 mg caffeine, and 60 mg codeine (2 capsules) every 4 hr, as needed. *Maximum:* 300 mg butalbital; 1,950 mg aspirin; 240 mg caffeine; 180 mg codeine in 24 hr.

Mechanism of Action

Butalbital inhibits upward conduction of nerve impulses to the reticular formation of the brain, thereby disrupting impulse transmission to the cortex. This action depresses the CNS, producing drowsiness, hypnosis, and sedation.

Aspirin blocks the activity of cyclooxygenase, the enzyme necessary for prostaglandin synthesis. By preventing prostaglandin synthesis, pain is relieved because prostaglandins play a role in pain transmission from the periphery to the spinal cord.

Caffeine is a potent, competitive inhibitor of phosphodiesterase, an enzyme that degrades c3'5' AMP. Increased cAMP mediates most of its action, including CNS stimulation to counteract the sedative properties of butalbital and codeine and cerebral vasoconstriction to relieve headache caused by increased blood volume from vasodilation.

Codeine may produce analgesia through partial metabolism to the opioid, morphine. Opioids bind and interact with opiate receptors in the CNS, altering the perception of and emotional response to pain and causing generalized CNS depression.

Contraindications

Allergy to tartrazine dye; asthma; bleeding problems such as hemophilia; children under age 16 with a viral illness; history of
barbiturate addiction; hypersensitivity to aspirin, butalbital, other
barbiturates, caffeine, codeine, other opioids, NSAIDs, or their
components; nephritis; peptic ulcer disease; porphyria; respiratory
depression; severe vitamin K deficiency; triad syndrome of angioedema, asthma, and nasal polyps; upper airway obstruction

Interactions

DRUGS

butalbital

adrenocorticoids, oral anticoagulants, tricyclic antidepressants: Decreased
effectiveness of these drugs

CNS depressants: Increased CNS depressant effects

disulfiram: Possibly increased risk of barbiturate (butalbital) toxicity

ketamine anesthesia: Increased risk of profound respiratory depression

MAO inhibitors: Increased CNS effects of butalbital

aspirin

ACE inhibitors: Decreased antihypertensive effect

activated charcoal: Decreased aspirin absorption

antacids, urine alkalinizers: Decreased aspirin effectiveness

anticoagulants: Increased risk of bleeding; prolonged bleeding time

carbonic anhydrase inhibitors: Salicylism

corticosteroids: Increased excretion and decreased blood level of aspirin

heparin: Increased risk of bleeding

loop diuretics: Possibly decreased effectiveness of loop diuretics

methotrexate: Increased blood level and decreased excretion of
methotrexate, causing toxicity

nizatidine: Increased blood aspirin level

NSAIDs: Possibly decreased blood NSAID level and increased risk
of adverse GI effects

oral antidiabetics and insulin: Increased risk of hypoglycemia

probenecid, sulfinpyrazone: Decreased effectiveness in treating gout

urine acidifiers, such as ammonium chloride and ascorbic acid: Decreased aspirin excretion

vancomycin: Increased risk of ototoxicity

caffeine

aspirin: Increased GI absorption of aspirin

beta-adrenergic agonists: Possibly enhanced cardiac inotropic effects of beta-adrenergic agonists

cimetidine, contraceptives (oral), disulfiram, fluoroquinolones: Decreased hepatic metabolism of caffeine resulting in increased caffeine effect

clozapine: Possibly increased clozapine levels resulting in increased incidence of clozapine induced adverse reactions

lithium: Enhanced renal clearance of lithium

mexiletine: Decreased caffeine elimination resulting in increased caffeine effect

phenytoin: Increased caffeine clearance resulting in decreased caffeine effect

theophylline: Reduced theophylline clearance with ingestion of more than 120 mg caffeine daily

codeine

anticholinergics, paregoric: Increased risk of severe constipation

antihypertensives, diuretics: Potentiated hypotensive effects

buprenorphine: Decreased effectiveness of codeine

CNS depressants: Additive CNS effects

hydroxyzine: Increased codeine analgesic effect; increased CNS depressant and hypotensive effects

MAO inhibitors: Increased risk of unpredictable, severe, and sometimes fatal reactions

metoclopramide: Antagonized effect of metoclopramide on GI motility

naloxone: Antagonized codeine analgesic effect

naltrexone: Precipitated withdrawal symptoms in codeine-dependent patients

neuromuscular blockers: Additive respiratory depressant effects

opioids: Additive CNS and respiratory depressant effects and hypotensive effects

ACTIVITIES

butalbital

alcohol use: Increased CNS depression

aspirin

alcohol use: Increased risk of ulcers

caffeine

smoking: Increased caffeine clearance and decreased caffeine effect

codeine

alcohol use: Additive CNS effects

Adverse Reactions

CNS: Anxiety, clumsiness, coma, confusion, CNS depression, delirium, disorientation, dizziness, drowsiness, euphoria, hallucinations, hangover, headache, insomnia, irritability, lack of coordination, lethargy, light-headedness, mental and physical impairment, mood changes, nervousness, nightmares, paradoxical stimulation, restlessness, sedation, seizures, syncope

CV: Bradycardia, orthostatic hypotension, palpitations, tachycardia

EENT: Altered taste, blurred vision, diplopia, dry mouth, hearing loss, laryngeal edema, laryngospasm, miosis, tinnitus

GI: Abdominal cramps and pain, anorexia, constipation, diarrhea, flatulence, gastroesphageal reflux, GI bleeding, heartburn, hepatotoxicity, ileus, indigestion, jaundice, nausea, stomach pain, vomiting

GU: Decreased libido, difficult ejaculation, dysuria, impotence, oliguria, ureteral spasm, urinary incontinence, urine retention

HEME: Agranulocytosis, bone marrow suppression, decreased blood iron level, hemolytic anemia, leukopenia, megaloblastic anemia, prolonged bleeding time, shortened life span of RBCs, thrombocytopenia

MS: Arthralgia, muscle weakness

RESP: Apnea, bronchospasm, respiratory depression

SKIN: Diaphoresis, ecchymosis, erythema multiforme, flushing, pallor, pruritus, rash, toxic epidermal necrolysis, urticaria

Other: Anaphylaxis, angioedema, physical and psychological dependence, Reye's syndrome, weight loss

Nursing Considerations

- Use cautiously in patients with head trauma or intracranial lesions because codeine can cause an exaggerated respiratory depression and aspirin can increase the risk of bleeding.
- Use cautiously in elderly and debilitated patients as well as patients with severe renal or hepatic dysfunction, gallbladder disease, respiratory impairment, cardiac arrhythmias, inflammatory disorders of the GI tract, hypothyroidism, Addison's disease, prostatic hypertrophy or urethral stricture, coagulation disorders or acute abdominal conditions.
- **WARNING** Monitor patient closely for evidence of overdose, even at normal dosage, because some patients metabolize codeine quickly, leading to a sudden rise in blood codeine level. This metabolic defect occurs in about 0.5 to 1% of patients who are Chinese, Japanese, or Hispanic; 1 to 10% of Caucasians; 3% of African Americans; and 16 to 28% of North Africans, Ethiopians, and Arabs. Watch for extreme

sleepiness, confusion and shallow breathing after giving drug. If present, notify prescriber and be prepared to provide supportive care and stop the drug, as ordered.

- Evaluate patient for therapeutic response, including report of decreased pain that would indicate pain relief has occurred.
- Take safety precautions, as needed.
- Monitor respiratory depth, effort and rate. Notify prescriber immediately if respiratory rate drops below 10 breaths/minute.
- **WARNING** Monitor patient closely for allergic reaction. Be aware that anaphylactic shock and other severe allergic reactions can occur without a history of allergy.
- **WARNING** Assess patient for evidence of physical and psychological dependence.
- Monitor urine output; decreasing output may signal urine retention or renal failure.

PATIENT TEACHING

- Instruct patient to take butalbital, aspirin, caffeine, and codeine with food or after meals to minimize stomach upset.
- Instruct patient to take drug exactly as prescribed and not to adjust dose or frequency without consulting prescriber because drug can be habit forming.
- Instruct patient to report worsening or breakthrough pain.
- Advise patient to notify prescriber if he becomes short of breath or has trouble breathing or extreme sleepiness or confusion.
- Tell patient to consult prescriber before taking drug with any prescription drug for blood disorder, diabetes, gout, or arthritis.
- Caution patient to avoid hazardous activities until drug's CNS effects are known.
- Caution patient to avoid alcohol or other CNS depressants while taking drug.
- Advise patient to get up slowly from a sitting or lying position.
- To prevent constipation, urge patient to consume plenty of fluids and high-fiber foods, if not contraindicated.

carisoprodol, aspirin, and codeine phosphate

Soma Compound with Codeine

Class, Category, and Schedule

Chemical: Dicarbamate (carisoprodol), salicylate (aspirin), phenanthrene derivative (codeine)

Therapeutic: Skeletal muscle relaxant (carisoprodol), analgesic (aspirin, codeine)
Pregnancy category: NR (carisoprodol C, aspirin D, codeine C)
Controlled substance schedule: III

Indications and Dosages

▶ *To treat acute painful musculoskeletal conditions*
TABLETS
Adults. 200 mg carisoprodol, 325 mg aspirin and 16 mg codeine (1 tablet) or 400 mg carisoprodol, 650 mg aspirin and 32 mg codeine (2 tablets) q.i.d.

Mechanism of Action

Carisoprodol blocks interneuronal activity in the descending reticular formation and spinal cord, producing muscle relaxation and sedation

Aspirin blocks the activity of cyclooxygenase, the enzyme necessary for prostaglandin synthesis. By preventing prostaglandin synthesis, pain is relieved because prostaglandins play a role in pain transmission from the periphery to the spinal cord.

Codeine may produce analgesia through partial metabolism to the opioid, morphine. Opioids bind and interact with opiate receptors in the CNS, altering the perception of and emotional response to pain and causing generalized CNS depression.

Contraindications

Allergy to tartrazine dye; asthma; bleeding problems such as hemophilia; children under age 16 with a viral illness; hypersensitivity to carisoprodol, aspirin, codeine, other opioids, NSAIDs, or their components; intermittent porphyria; peptic ulcer disease; respiratory depression; severe vitamin K deficiency; upper airway obstruction

Interactions

DRUGS
carisoprodol
CNS depressants, psychotropic drugs: Additive CNS depression
aspirin
ACE inhibitors: Decreased antihypertensive effect
activated charcoal: Decreased aspirin absorption
antacids, urine alkalinizers: Decreased aspirin effectiveness
anticoagulants: Increased risk of bleeding; prolonged bleeding time
carbonic anhydrase inhibitors: Salicylism

corticosteroids: Increased aspirin excretion and decreased blood level

heparin: Increased risk of bleeding

loop diuretics: Possibly decreased effectiveness of loop diuretics

methotrexate: Increased blood level and decreased excretion of methotrexate, causing toxicity

nizatidine: Increased blood aspirin level

NSAIDs: Possibly decreased blood NSAID level and increased risk of adverse GI effects

probenecid, sulfinpyrazone: Decreased effectiveness in treating gout

urine acidifiers, such as ammonium chloride and ascorbic acid: Decreased aspirin excretion

vancomycin: Increased risk of ototoxicity

codeine

anticholinergics, paregoric: Increased risk of severe constipation

antihypertensives, diuretics: Potentiated hypotensive effects

buprenorphine: Decreased effectiveness of codeine

CNS depressants: Additive CNS effects

hydroxyzine: Increased codeine analgesic effect; increased CNS depressant and hypotensive effects

MAO inhibitors: Increased risk of unpredictable, severe, and sometimes fatal reactions

metoclopramide: Antagonized effect of metoclopramide on GI motility

naloxone: Antagonized codeine analgesic effect

naltrexone: Precipitated withdrawal symptoms in codeine-dependent patients

neuromuscular blockers: Additive respiratory depressant effects

opioids: Additive CNS and respiratory depressant effects and hypotensive effects

ACTIVITIES

carisoprodol, aspirin, and codeine

alcohol use: Additive CNS effects and increased risk of adverse GI effects

Adverse Reactions

CNS: Agitation, ataxia, coma, confusion, CNS depression, delirium, depression, disorientation, dizziness, drowsiness, euphoria, fever, hallucinations, headache, insomnia, irritability, lack of coordination, syncope, tremor, vertigo

CV: Bradycardia, orthostatic hypotension, palpitations, tachycardia

EENT: Altered taste, blurred vision, diplopia, dry mouth, hearing loss, laryngeal edema, laryngospasm, miosis, tinnitus, transient vision loss

GI: Abnormal cramps and pain, anorexia, constipation, diarrhea, epigastric discomfort, flatulence, GI bleeding, gastroesophageal reflux, heartburn, hepatotoxicity, hiccups, ileus, indigestion, nausea, stomach pain, vomiting

GU: Decreased libido, difficult ejaculation, dysuria, impotence, oliguria, ureteral spasm, urinary incontinence, urine retention

HEME: Decreased blood iron level, eosinophilia, hemolytic anemia, leukopenia, prolonged bleeding time, shortened life span of RBCs, thrombocytopenia

MS: Muscle rigidity

RESP: Apnea, bronchoconstriction, bronchospasm, depressed cough reflex, respiratory depression

SKIN: Diaphoresis, ecchymosis, erythema multiforme, flushing, pallor, pruritus, rash, urticaria

Other: Anaphylaxis, angioedema, physical and psychological dependence, Reye's syndrome

Nursing Considerations

- Use cautiously in patients with drug addiction.
- Use cautiously in patients with head trauma or intracranial lesions because codeine can cause an exaggerated respiratory depression and aspirin can increase the risk of bleeding.
- Use cautiously in elderly and debilitated patients as well as patients with severe renal or hepatic dysfunction, gallbladder disease, respiratory impairment, cardiac arrhythmias, inflammatory disorders of the GI tract, hypothyroidism, Addison's disease, prostatic hypertrophy or urethral stricture, coagulation disorders or acute abdominal conditions.
- **WARNING** Monitor patient closely for evidence of overdose, even at normal dosage, because some patients metabolize codeine quickly, leading to a sudden rise in blood codeine level. This metabolic defect occurs in about 0.5 to 1% of patients who are Chinese, Japanese, or Hispanic; 1 to 10% of Caucasians; 3% of African Americans; and 16 to 28% of North Africans, Ethiopians, and Arabs. Watch for extreme sleepiness, confusion and shallow breathing after giving drug. If present, notify prescriber and be prepared to provide supportive care and stop the drug, as ordered.
- Evaluate patient for therapeutic response, including both patient reports and observation of body movements.
- Take safety precautions, as needed.
- Monitor respiratory depth, effort and rate. Notify prescriber immediately if respiratory rate drops below 10 breaths/minute.

- **WARNING** Monitor patient closely for allergic reaction. Be aware that anaphylactic shock and other severe allergic reactions can occur without a history of allergy.
- **WARNING** Assess patient for evidence of physical and psychological dependence.
- Monitor urine output; decreasing output may signal urine retention or renal failure.
- Expect prescriber to taper therapy rather than stopping it abruptly to avoid withdrawal symptoms.

PATIENT TEACHING
- Instruct patient to take carisoprodol, aspirin and codeine with food or after meals to minimize stomach upset.
- Instruct patient to take carisoprodol, aspirin, and codeine exactly as prescribed and not to adjust dose or frequency without consulting prescriber. Tell patient not to abruptly stop taking the drug to prevent withdrawal symptoms. Instead, expect prescriber to taper therapy when no longer needed.
- Instruct patient to report worsening or breakthrough pain.
- Advise patient to notify prescriber if he becomes short of breath or has trouble breathing or extreme sleepiness or confusion.
- Tell patient to consult prescriber before taking drug with any prescription drug for treating blood disorder, diabetes, gout, or arthritis.
- Urge patient to avoid hazardous activities until drug's CNS effects are known.
- Caution patient to avoid alcohol or other CNS depressants while taking carisoprodol, aspirin and codeine.
- Advise patient to get up slowly from a sitting or lying position.
- To prevent constipation, encourage patient to consume plenty of fluids and high-fiber foods, if not contraindicated.
- Inform patient that saliva, urine, and sweat may appear darker (red, brown, or black) because of the carisoprodol of the drug and reassure him that the color change is harmless.

chlordiazepoxide and amitriptyline hydrochloride

Limbitrol, Limbitrol DS 10-25

Class, Category, and Schedule

Chemical: Benzodiazepine (chlordiazepoxide), tertiary amine (amitriptyline)

Therapeutic: Antianxiety (chlordiazepoxide), antidepressant (amitriptyline)
Pregnancy category: D
Controlled substance schedule: IV

Indications and Dosages

▶ *To treat depression with moderate to severe anxiety*
TABLETS
Adults. *Initial:* 10 mg chlordiazepoxide and 25 mg amitriptyline (1 tablet) t.i.d. or q.i.d. *Maintenance:* Increase as needed to six times daily or decrease to twice daily or once daily at bedtime, as needed.

Mechanism of Action

Chlordiazepoxide may potentiate the effects of gamma-aminobutyric acid (GABA) and other inhibitory neurotransmitters by binding to specific benzodiazepine receptors in the limbic and cortical areas of the CNS. By binding to these receptors, chlordiazepoxide increases GABA's inhibitory effects and blocks cortical and limbic arousal, which helps control emotional behavior.

Amitriptyline blocks serotonin and norepinephrine reuptake by adrenergic nerves. By doing so, it raises serotonin and norepinephrine levels at nerve synapses. This action may elevate mood and reduce depression.

Contraindications

During acute recovery phrase after MI; hypersensitivity to chlordiazepoxide, other benzodiazepines, amitriptyline, other tricyclic antidepressants, or their components; use within 14 days of MAO inhibitor therapy

Interactions

DRUGS
chlordiazepoxide and amitriptyline
cimetidine, disulfiram, fluoxetine, fluvoxamine, haloperidol, H₂-receptor antagonists, isoniazid, ketoconazole, methylphenidate, metoprolol, oral contraceptives, paroxetine, phenothiazines, propoxyphene, propranolol, sertraline, valproic acid: Increased blood chlordiazepoxide or amitriptyline levels
chlordiazepoxide
antacids: Altered rate of chlordiazepoxide absorption
CNS depressants: Increased CNS effects
digoxin: Increased blood digoxin level and risk of digitalis toxicity
levodopa: Decreased efficacy of levodopa's antiparkinsonian effects

neuromuscular blockers: Potentiated, counteracted, or diminished effects of neuromuscular blockers

phenytoin: Possibly increased phenytoin toxicity

probenecid: Shortened onset of action or prolonged effect of chlordiazepoxide

rifampin: Decreased chlordiazepoxide effect

theophyllines: Antagonized sedative effects of chlordiazepoxide

amitriptyline

anticholinergics, epinephrine, norepinephrine: Increased effects of these drugs

barbiturates: Decreased serum amitriptyline level

carbamazepine: Decreased serum amitriptyline level and increased serum carbamazepine level, which increases therapeutic and toxic effects of carbamazepine

cisapride: Possibly prolonged QT interval and increased risk for arrhythmias

clonidine, guanethidine, other antihypertensives: Decreased antihypertensive effects

dicumarol: Increased anticoagulant effect od dicumarol

levodopa: Decreased levodopa absorption; sympathetic hyperactivity, sinus tachycardia, hypertension, agitation

MAO inhibitors: Possibly seizures and death

thyroid replacement drugs: Arrhythmias and increased antidepressant effects

ACTIVITIES

chlordiazepoxide and amitriptyline

alcohol use: Increased CNS effects

amitriptyline

smoking: Decreased amitriptyline effects

Adverse Reactions

CNS: Anxiety, ataxia, coma, confusion, chills, delusions, depression, disorientation, drowsiness, extrapyramidal reactions, fatigue, fever, headache, insomnia, nightmares, peripheral neuropathy, suicidal ideation, tremor

CV: Arrhythmias (including prolonged AV conduction, heart block, and tachycardia), cardiomyopathy, hypertension, MI, ECG changes, orthostatic hypotension, palpitations, tachycardia

EENT: Abnormal taste, black tongue, blurred vision, dry mouth, nasal congestion, tinnitus

ENDO: Gynecomastia, increased or decreased blood glucose level, increased prolactin level, syndrome of inappropriate antidiuretic hormone secretion

GI: Abdominal cramps, constipation, diarrhea, flatulence, hepatic dysfunction, ileus, increased appetite, jaundice, nausea, vomiting
GU: Impotence, libido changes, menstrual irregularities, testicular swelling, urinary hesitancy, urine retention
HEME: Agranulocytosis, bone marrow depression, eosinophilia, leukopenia, thrombocytopenia
SKIN: Alopecia, flushing, photosensitivity, purpura
Other: Physical and psychological dependence, weight gain

Nursing Considerations
- Use chlordiazepoxide and amitriptyline cautiously in patients with renal or hepatic impairment, porphyria, or thyroid disorders.
- Because amitriptyline has atropine-like effects, use caution when giving it to a patient with a history of seizures, urine retention, or angle-closure glaucoma.
- WARNING Don't give an MAO inhibitor within 14 days of chlordiazepoxide and amitriptyline therapy because of the risk of seizures and death.
- Closely monitor patient with a cardiovascular disorder because amitriptyline may cause arrhythmias, such as sinus tachycardia.
- Monitor blood pressure and assess patient for changes.
- Stay alert for behavior changes, such as hallucinations and decreased interest in personal appearance. Be aware that psychosis may develop in schizophrenic patients and symptoms may increase in paranoid patients.
- WARNING Be aware that prolonged use of therapeutic doses can lead to dependence.
- Avoid abrupt withdrawal of chlordiazepoxide and amitriptyline after prolonged therapy because nausea, headache, vertigo, and nightmares may occur.
- Monitor patient being treated for depression with chlordiazepoxide and amitriptyline closely for suicidal tendencies, especially at beginning of therapy and during dosage adjustments as depression may temporarily worsen during these times.
- Monitor patient's blood counts and liver function test results during therapy. Notify prescriber of any abnormalities.

PATIENT TEACHING
- Instruct patient to take drug exactly as prescribed.
- Advise patient to avoid performing hazardous activities until CNS effects of drug are known.
- Tell family or caregiver to observe patient closely for suicidal tendencies, especially when therapy starts or dosage changes.

- Instruct patient to avoid consuming alcohol or OTC drugs that contain alcohol during chlordiazepoxide and amitriptyline therapy because alcohol enhances the drug's CNS depressant effects.
- Warn patient not to take antacids with drug.
- Caution patient not to abruptly stop taking drug because withdrawal symptoms may occur.
- Inform female patients of childbearing age to report planned or suspected pregnancy immediately because drug may cause congenital abnormalities and will need to be stopped.
- Instruct patient to avoid direct sunlight as much as possible and to use sunscreen, protective clothing and sunglasses when exposure to sunlight can not be avoided.

choline salicylate and magnesium salicylate

Tricosal, Trilisate

Class and Category

Chemical: Salicylate
Therapeutic: Analgesic, anti-inflammatory, antipyretic
Pregnancy category: C (first trimester), NR (later trimesters)

Indications and Dosages

▶ *To treat osteoarthritis, rheumatoid arthritis, and acute painful shoulder*

LIQUID, TABLETS

Adults. 1,500 mg b.i.d. or 3,000 mg at bedtime.
Children weighing more than 37 kg (81 lb). 2,250 mg/day in equally divided doses b.i.d.
Children weighing 37 kg or less. 50 mg/kg/day in equally divided doses b.i.d.

▶ *To treat mild to moderate pain, reduce fever*

LIQUID, TABLETS

Adults. 2,000 to 3,000 mg/day in equally divided doses b.i.d.
DOSAGE ADJUSTMENT Dosage reduced to 750 mg t.i.d. for elderly patients.

Contraindications

Hypersensitivity to nonacetylated salicylates

Interactions

DRUGS

antacids: Increased salicylate clearance and decreased blood level

carbonic anhydrase inhibitors, phenytoin, valproic acid: Decreased blood levels and therapeutic effects of these drugs
corticosteroids: Decreased blood salicylate level, increased salicylate dosage requirements
insulin, sulfonylureas: Increased hypoglycemic response
methotrexate: Increased therapeutic and toxic effects of methotrexate, especially when given in chemotherapeutic doses
oral anticoagulants: Increased blood level of unbound anticoagulant and risk of bleeding
salicylate-containing products: Increased plasma salicylate level, possibly to toxic level
uricosuric drugs: Decreased uricosuric drug efficacy

Mechanism of Action

Choline and magnesium salicylates block the activity of cyclooxygenase, the enzyme needed for prostaglandin synthesis. As mediators in the inflammatory process, prostaglandins cause local vasodilation with swelling and pain. They also play a role in pain transmission from the periphery to the spinal cord. By blocking cyclooxygenase and inhibiting prostaglandins, this NSAID decreases inflammatory symptoms and relieves pain. It acts on the heat-regulating center in the hypothalamus and causes peripheral vasodilation, sweating, and heat loss.

Adverse Reactions

CNS: Dizziness, drowsiness, headache, lethargy, light-headedness
EENT: Hearing loss, tinnitus
GI: Constipation, diarrhea, epigastric pain, heartburn, indigestion, nausea, vomiting
HEME: Easy bruising, unusual bleeding

Nursing Considerations

- Use these salicylates cautiously in patients with gastritis, hepatic or renal dysfunction, or peptic ulcer disease.
- Don't give salicylates to children or adolescents with chickenpox or flu symptoms because of the risk of Reye's syndrome.
- **WARNING** During high-dose or long-term therapy, monitor for signs of salicylate intoxication, such as headache, dizziness, tinnitus, hearing loss, confusion, drowsiness, diaphoresis, vomiting, diarrhea, and hyperventilation. CNS disturbance, electrolyte imbalance, respiratory acidosis, hyperthermia, and dehydration also may occur. If intoxication occurs, prepare to induce vomiting, administer gastric lavage,

and give activated charcoal, as ordered. In extreme cases, prepare patient for peritoneal dialysis or hemodialysis.

PATIENT TEACHING

- Tell patient to store drug at room temperature, away from heat, light, and moisture.
- Instruct patient to take drug with food or after meals with a full glass of water.
- Tell patient to take a missed dose as soon as he remembers but to avoid double-dosing.
- Advise patient that optimal effects may take 2 to 3 weeks.
- Teach patient to recognize and immediately report signs of salicylate toxicity.
- Explain that drug is closely related to aspirin. Advise against taking aspirin-containing OTC remedies during therapy.

diclofenac sodium and misoprostol
Arthrotec

Class and Category
Chemical: Phenylacetic acid derivative (diclofenac), prostaglandin E1 analogue (misoprostol)
Therapeutic: Analgesic (diclofenac), antiulcer, gastric antisecretory (misoprostol)
Pregnancy category: X

Indications and Dosages
▶ *To treat signs and symptoms of osteoarthritis in patients at high risk of developing NSAID-induced gastric and duodenal ulcers and their complications*

TABLETS

Adults. 50 mg diclofenac and 200 mcg misoprostol (1 tablet) b.i.d. or t.i.d. Or, 75 mg diclofenac and 200 mcg misoprostol (1 tablet) b.i.d.

▶ *To treat signs and symptoms of rheumatoid arthritis in patients at high risk of developing NSAID-induced gastric and duodenal ulcers and their complications*

TABLETS

Adults. 50 mg diclofenac and 200 mcg misoprostol (1 tablet) b.i.d. to q.i.d. Or, 75 mg diclofenac and 200 mcg misoprostol (1 tablet) b.i.d.

Contraindications
History of asthma, urticaria, or other allergic-type reactions fol-

lowing aspirin or other NSAIDs use; hepatic porphyria; hypersensitivity to diclofenac, misoprostol, other prostaglandins, or their components; pregnancy; severe renal impairment; treatment of peri-operative pain during coronary artery bypass graft surgery

---

Mechanism of Action

Diclofenac blocks the activity of cyclooxygenase, the enzyme needed to synthesize prostaglandins, which mediate the inflammatory response and cause local vasodilation, swelling, and pain. By blocking cyclooxygenase and inhibiting prostaglandins, diclofenac reduces inflammatory symptoms. This mechanism also relieves pain because prostaglandins promote pain transmission from the periphery to the spinal cord.

Misoprostol may protect the stomach from NSAID-induced mucosal damage by increasing gastric mucus production and mucosal bicarbonate secretion. Misoprostol also inhibits gastric acid secretion caused by such stimuli as food, coffee, and histamine.

Interactions

DRUGS

diclofenac and misoprostol

antacids: Reduced bioavailability of misoprostol acid; delay absorption of diclofenac

diclofenac

ACE inhibitors, antihypertensives: Decreased antihypertensive effects

acetaminophen: Increased risk of adverse renal effects with long-term concurrent use

anticoagulants, thrombolytics: Prolonged PT, increased risk of bleeding

aspirin, other NSAIDs and salicylates: Increased GI irritability and bleeding, decreased diclofenac effectiveness

beta blockers: Impaired antihypertensive effects

cefamandole, cefoperazone, cefotetan, plicamycin, valproic acid: Increased risk of hypoprothrombinemia

cimetidine: Altered blood diclofenac level

colchicines, corticotropin (long-term use), glucocorticoids, potassium supplements: Increased GI irritability and bleeding

cyclosporine, gold compounds, nephrotoxic drugs: Increased risk of nephrotoxicity

digoxin: Increased serum digoxin level

insulin, oral antidiabetics: Decreased effects of these drugs

lithium: Increased risk of lithium toxicity

loop diuretics: Decreased loop diuretic effectiveness
methotrexate: Increased risk of methotrexate toxicity
phenytoin: Increased blood phenytoin level
potassium-sparing diuretics: Increased risk of hyperkalemia
probenecid: Increased diclofenac toxicity
warfarin: Increased risk of serious GI bleeding
misoprostol
magnesium-containing antacids: Increased misoprostol-caused diarrhea
ACTIVITIES
diclofenac
alcohol use: Increased risk of GI irritability and bleeding

Adverse Reactions

CNS: Aseptic meningitis, coma, dizziness, drowsiness, headache, paranoia, psychotic reaction, stroke, syncope
CV: Bradycardia and other arrhythmias, congestive heart failure, edema, hypertension, hypotension, MI, palpitations, phlebitis, seizures, thrombosis, vasculitis, vertigo
EENT: Glaucoma, hearing loss, laryngeal and pharyngeal edema, tinnitus
ENDO: Alterations in blood glucose level
GI: Abdominal pain, constipation, diarrhea, dyspepsia, dysphasia, elevated liver function test results, enteritis, esophageal ulceration, flatulence, gastritis, GI bleeding or ulceration, hepatic porphyria, hepatitis, hepatotoxicity, indigestion, intestinal perforation, jaundice, nausea, pancreatitis, peptic ulcer, vomiting
GU: Dysmenorrhea, hypermenorrhea, interstitial nephritis, menstrual irregularities, nephritic syndrome, papillary necrosis, renal failure, vaginal bleeding
HEME: Agranulocytosis, aplastic and hemolytic anemia, eosinophilia, increased coagulation time, leukopenia, leukocytosis, pancytopenia, thrombocytopenia
RESP: Asthma, dyspnea, pneumonia, pulmonary embolism, respiratory depression
SKIN: Blisters, exfoliative dermatitis, pruritus, rash, Stevens-Johnson Syndrome, toxic epidermal necrolysis, urticaria
Other: Anaphylaxis, angioedema, hyperuricemia, hyponatremia, lymphadenopathy, sepsis

Nursing Considerations

• **WARNING** Ask patient if she is or may be pregnant. If so, notify prescriber because misoprostol may cause uterine bleeding, contractions, and spontaneous abortion as well as teratogenic effects in the fetus.

- Rehydrate patient who is seriously dehydrated before starting diclofenac and misoprostol because drug may cause serious adverse renal effects in dehydrated patients.
- Use diclofenac and misoprostol with extreme caution in patients with a history of ulcer disease or GI bleeding because NSAIDs such as diclofenac increase the risk of GI bleeding and ulceration. Expect to use the drug for the shortest time possible.
- Also use diclofenac and misoprostol cautiously in patients with inflammatory bowel disease because drug may worsen intestinal inflammation and cause diarrhea. If diarrhea causes severe dehydration, drug may need to be stopped.
- Use diclofenac and misoprostol cautiously in patients with cerebrovascular disease, coronary artery disease, congestive heart failure, or uncontrolled epilepsy because of the risk of severe complications.
- Use drug cautiously in patients with hypertension, and monitor blood pressure closely throughout therapy. Drug may cause hypertension or worsen it.
- **WARNING** Monitor patient closely for thrombotic events, including MI and stroke, because NSAIDs increase the risk.
- Serious GI tract ulceration, bleeding, and perforation may occur without warning symptoms. Elderly patients are at greater risk. To minimize risk, give drug with food. If GI distress occurs, withhold drug and notify prescriber immediately.
- Monitor patient, especially if she's elderly or receiving long-term diclofenac and misoprostol therapy, for less common but serious adverse GI reactions, including anorexia, constipation, diverticulitis, dysphagia, esophagitis, gastritis, gastroenteritis, gastroesophageal reflux disease, hemorrhoids, hiatal hernia, melena, stomatitis, and vomiting.
- Monitor liver function test results and serum uric acid level. Liver enzyme elevations usually occur within 2 months of starting diclofenac and misoprostol therapy. If abnormal liver test results persist or worsen, if patient exhibits signs and symptoms consistent with liver disease, or if systemic manifestations such as eosinophilia or rash occur, discontinue drug immediately and notify prescriber.
- Monitor renal function in patients on long-term diclofenac and misoprostol therapy because they are at increased risk for renal papillary necrosis and other renal injury and in patients with existing renal disease, heart failure, liver dysfuction, those tak-

ing diuretics and ACE inhibitors, and the elderly. Notify prescriber if abnormalities develop and expect to discontinue drug.
- Be aware that although rare, aseptic meningitis with fever and coma has occurred in patients taking diclofenac, especially patients who have systemic lupus and related connective tissue disease. Notify prescriber immediately if patients develops fever and CNS dysfunction.
- Report weight gain of more than 1 kg (2 lb) in 24 hours, which suggests fluid retention.
- If patient takes a potassium-sparing diuretic, check for elevated serum potassium level, as ordered.
- Monitor patient's hemoglobin and hematocrit, as ordered, if receiving prolonged drug therapy because drug may cause anemia.
- **WARNING** If patient has bone marrow suppression or is receiving an antineoplastic drug, monitor laboratory results (including WBC count), and watch for evidence of infection because anti-inflammatory and antipyretic actions of diclofenac may mask signs and symptoms, such as fever and pain.
- Assess patient's skin regularly for signs of rash or other hypersensitivity reaction because diclofenac is an NSAID and may cause serious skin reactions without warning, even in patients with no history of NSAID sensitivity. At first sign of reaction, stop drug and notify prescriber.

PATIENT TEACHING
- Tell patient to alert prescriber before taking diclofenac and misoprostol if she has a history of ulcers, bleeding problems, hypertension, or heart or renal disease; if she takes a diuretic; or if she's over age 65.
- Advise patient to take drug exactly as prescribed and not to increase dosage because stomach bleeding may occur.
- Instruct patient to take drug with food to minimize GI distress.
- To decrease risk of esophageal ulceration, instruct patient to take drug with a full glass of water and not to lie down for 15 to 30 minutes after taking drug.
- **WARNING** Caution female patient about the risk of taking diclofenac and misoprostol during pregnancy, and urge her to use reliable contraception during therapy. Urge her to notify prescriber immediately if she is or could be pregnant. Also urge her not to breast-feed during therapy.
- Inform patient that diarrhea is dose-related and usually resolves after 8 days. Instruct her to avoid magnesium-containing

antacids because they may worsen diarrhea and to contact prescriber if diarrhea persists longer than 8 days.

- Urge female patient to notify prescriber immediately about postmenopausal bleeding; she may need diagnostic tests to rule out a gynecologic disorder.
- Caution patient to avoid hazardous activities until drug's CNS effects are known.
- Instruct patient to notify prescriber if she experiences ringing or buzzing in the ears, impaired hearing, dizziness, vision changes, swelling, or weight gain.
- Advise patient to avoid taking two different NSAIDs at the same time, unless directed, and to alert prescriber before taking drug if she has ever had an allergic reaction to an analgesic or fever-reducing drug. Also advise patient to consult prescriber before taking aspirin or other OTC analgesics or ingesting alcohol.
- Inform patient that drug increases the risk of inflammation, bleeding, ulceration, and perforation of the stomach and intestines, possibly without warning. If patient feels suddenly ill, she should seek medical attention.
- Warn patient of the possibility of hepatic injury. Instruct patient to notify prescriber if she experiences signs and symptoms of hepatotoxicity such as nausea, fatigue, lethargy, pruritus, jaundice, right upper quadrant tenderness, and flulike symptoms.
- Explain that drug may increase the risk of serious adverse cardiovascular reactions; urge patient to seek immediate medical attention if signs or symptoms arise, such as chest pain, shortness of breath, weakness, or slurring of speech.
- Alert patient to rare but serious skin reactions. Urge her to seek immediate medical attention for rash, blisters, itching, fever, or other indications of hypersensitivity.

edrophonium chloride and atropine sulfate
Enlon-Plus

Class and Category
Chemical: Anticholinesterase (edrophonium), belladonna alkoloid (atropine)
Therapeutic: Nondepolarizing neuromuscular blocker antagonist (edrophonium), parasympatholytic (atropine)
Pregnancy category: C

Indications and Dosages

▶ *To reverse the action of nondepolarizing neuromuscular blockers and as adjunct to treat respiratory depression caused by curare overdosage*
I.V. INJECTION
Adults. 0.5 to 1 mg/kg edrophonium and 0.007 to 0.014 mg/kg atropine (0.05 to 0.1 ml/kg) infused slowly over 45 to 60 seconds. *Maximum:* 1 mg/kg edrophonium total.

Mechanism of Action

Edrophonium acts mainly by inhibiting or inactivating the enzyme acetylcholinesterase. As a result, acetylcholine is not hydrolyzed as rapidly and accumulates at nicotinic cholinergic postjunctional receptors. The greater quantity of acetylcholine reaching these sites improves transmission of impulses across the myoneural junction, which reverses the effect of nondepolarizing neuromuscular blockers.

Atropine inhibits acetylcholine's muscarinic action at the neuroeffector junctions of smooth muscles, cardiac muscle, exocrine glands, sinoatrial and atrioventricular nodes, and urinary bladder. This counteracts the side effects of acetylcholine accumulation, such as bradycardia, bronchoconstriction, increased secretions, and other parasympathomimetic adverse effects.

Contraindications

Acute glaucoma; adhesions between the iris and lens of the eye; hypersensitivity to atropine, edrophonium, or their components; ileus; intestinal atony; intestinal or urinary obstruction; myasthenia gravis; myocardial ischemia; pyloric stenosis; severe ulcerative colitis; tachycardia; toxic megacolon; unstable cardiovascular status in acute hemorrhage or thyrotoxicosis

Interactions

DRUGS

edrophonium
beta blockers, opioid analgesics (except when combined with potent inhaled anesthetics): Increased frequency, duration, and severity of bradycardia
digoxin: Increased risk of bradycardia from edrophonium
succinylcholine: Prolonged or antagonized neuromuscular blockade
vecuronium and other muscle relaxants with no vagolytic effects: Possibly slight increased risk of bradycardia and first-degree heart block
atropine
amantadine; anticholinergics; antidyskinetics; glutethimide; meperidine;

muscle relaxants; phenothiazines; tricyclic antidepressants and other drugs with anticholinergic properties, including antiarrhythmics (disopyramide, procainamide, quinidine), antihistamines, buclizine, meclizine: Increased atropine effects

antimyasthenics: Reduced intestinal motility

cyclopropane: Risk of ventricular arrhythmias

haloperidol: Decreased antipsychotic effect

metoclopramide: Decreased effect on GI motility

opioid analgesics: Increased risk of ileus, severe constipation, and urine retention

potassium chloride, especially wax-matrix forms: Possibly GI ulcers

urinary alkalizers (calcium or magenesium antacids, carbonic anhydrase inhibitors, citrates, sodium bicarbonate): Delayed excretion and increased risk of adverse atropine effects

Adverse Reactions

CNS: Agitation, amnesia, anxiety, ataxia, Babinski's or Chaddock's reflex, behavioral changes, CNS stimulation (with high doses), coma, confusion, decreased concentration, decreased tendon reflexes, delirium, dizziness, drowsiness, fever, hallucinations, headache, hyperreflexia, insomnia, lethargy, loss of consciousness, mania, mental disorders, nervousness, paranoia, restlessness, seizures, somnolence, stupor, syncope, vertigo, weakness

CV: Arrhythmias, atrioventricular block, bradycardia, cardiac arrest or dilation, chest pain, hypertension, hypotension, left ventricular failure, MI, nodal rhythm, palpitations, premature atrial or ventricular contractions, tachycardia, weak or impalpable peripheral pulses

EENT: Acute angle-closure glaucoma, altered taste, blepharitis, blindness, blurred vision, conjunctivitis, conjunctival hyperemia, cyclophoria, cycloplegia, decreased visual acuity or accommodation, diplopia, dry eyes or conjunctiva, dry mucous membranes, dry mouth, dysphonia, eye irritation, eyelid crusting, heterophoria, increased intraocular pressure, increased salivation, keratoconjunctivitis, lacrimation, laryngitis, laryngospasm, miosis, mydriasis, nasal congestion, oral lesions, photophobia, pupils poorly reactive to light, spasm of accommodation, strabismus, tongue chewing

GI: Abdominal distention, abdominal pain, bloating, constipation, decreased bowel sounds or food absorption, delayed gastric emptying, diarrhea, dysphagia, flatulence, heartburn, ileus, increased peristalsis, nausea, vomiting

GU: Bladder distention; enuresis; impotence; incontinence; urinary frequency, hesitancy, urgency, and retention

MS: Dysarthria, hypertonia, muscle twitching

RESP: Bradypnea; bronchiolar constriction; bronchospasm; dyspnea; increased tracheobronchial secretions; inspiratory stridor; laryngospasm; pulmonary edema; respiratory arrest, depression, failure, and paralysis; shallow breathing; subcostal recession; tachypnea

SKIN: Cold skin, cyanosis, decreased sweating, dermatitis, flushing, rash, urticaria

Other: Anaphylaxis, dehydration, injection site reaction, polydipsia, sensations of warmth

Nursing Considerations

- Do not administer edrophonium and atropine before a nondepolarizing muscle relaxant.
- Use cautiously in patients with bronchial asthma, cardiac arrhythmias, or hepatic dysfunction because edrophonium and atropine have caused cardiac arrest in patients taking digoxin and patients with jaundice.
- To prevent severe bradycardia, patients with cardiovascular disease, given anesthesia with opioid and nitrous oxide without a potent inhalation agent, and patients receiving beta blockers should receive atropine sulfate alone, as prescribed, before administration of edrophonium and atropine.
- Have on hand additional atropine sulfate (1 mg) for immediate use, as prescribed, in the event of a severe cholinergic reaction after administration of edrophonium and atropine.
- WARNING Monitor patient closely for allergic reactions because drug contains sodium sulfite, which can produce anaphylaxis or other life-threatening adverse reactions in hypersensitive patients, especially those with asthma. Notify prescriber and provide supportive care, as indicated.
- Assess patient for symptoms of toxic doses of atropine, such as excitement, agitation, drowsiness, and confusion, which are likely to affect elderly patients even with low doses. If these symptoms occur, take safety precautions to prevent patient injury and notify prescriber.
- Monitor patient's cardiac rhythm closely during and after drug administration because arrhythmias usually appear within 2 minutes. Expect to treat arrhythmias related to increased vagal tone, bradycardia, and second- and third-degree heart block with atropine 0.2 to 0.4 mg intravenously, as prescribed. If pa-

tient develops bigeminy or ventricular ectopy, expect to administer lidocaine 50 mg intravenously, as prescribed.

- Assess bowel and bladder elimination. Notify prescriber if changes occur.
- Inspect the injection site for signs of tissue irritation that can result from extravascular seepage of drug.
- Provide frequent mouth care because dry mouth may be made worse when edrophonium and atropine administered with other drugs that also cause dry mouth.

PATIENT TEACHING

- Encourage patient to ask questions or discuss concerns before receiving drug.
- Reassure patient that he will be monitored closely when edrophonium and atropine is administered.

ergoloid mesylates (dihydrogenated ergot alkaloids)

Gerimal, Hydergine, Hydergine LC

Class and Category

Chemical: Dihydrogenated ergot alkaloid derivative
Therapeutic: Antidementia adjunct, cerebral metabolic enhancer
Pregnancy category: Not rated

Indications and Dosages

▶ *To treat age-related decline in mental capacity*

CAPSULES, ORAL SOLUTION, S.L. TABLETS, TABLETS

Adults. 1 to 2 mg t.i.d.

Mechanism of Action

Ergoloid mesylates may increase cerebral metabolism, blood flow, and oxygen uptake. These actions may increase neurotransmitter levels.

Contraindications

Acute or chronic psychosis, hypersensitivity to ergoloid mesylates or their components

Interactions

DRUGS

delavirdine, efavirenz, indinavir, nelfinavir, saquinavir: Increased risk of ergotism (blurred vision, dizziness, and headache) *dopamine:* Increased risk of gangrene

Adverse Reactions

CNS: Dizziness, headache, light-headedness, syncope
CV: Bradycardia, orthostatic hypotension
EENT: Blurred vision, nasal congestion, tongue soreness (with S.L. tablets)
GI: Abdominal cramps, anorexia, nausea, vomiting
SKIN: Flushing, rash

Nursing Considerations

- Expect ergoloid mesylates to be prescribed only after a pathophysiologic cause for mental decline has been ruled out.
- Measure patient's blood pressure and pulse rate and rhythm before therapy begins, and check them frequently during therapy.
- If bradycardia or hypotension develops, expect to discontinue drug permanently.

PATIENT TEACHING

- Stress the need to follow prescribed dosage and schedule.
- Teach caregiver to place S.L. tablet under patient's tongue and withhold food, fluids, and cigarettes until tablet dissolves.
- Instruct patient not to swallow S.L. tablets.
- Advise caregiver to skip a missed dose and resume the regular dosing schedule. Warn against doubling the dose, and urge caregiver to notify prescriber if patient misses two or more doses in a row.
- Instruct caregiver to store drug in a tightly closed, light-resistant container.
- Inform caregiver and family that drug may take 3 to 4 weeks to produce its effects.
- Stress the importance of follow-up care.

hydrocodone bitartrate and aspirin

Damason-P, Lortab ASA, Panasal 5/500

Class, Category, and Schedule

Chemical: Opioid and phenanthrene derivative (hydrocodone), salicylate (aspirin)
Therapeutic: Analgesic (hydrocodone, aspirin)
Pregnancy category: NR (hydrocodone C, aspirin D)
Controlled substance schedule: III

Indications and Dosages

▶ *To relieve moderate to severe pain*
TABLETS
Adults. 5 mg hydrocodone and 500 mg aspirin (1 tablet) to 10 mg hydrocodone and 1,000 mg aspirin (2 tablets) every 4 to 6 hr, as needed.

Mechanism of Action

Hydrocodone exerts a synergistic analgesic effect through two mechanisms of action. Hydrocodone, a mu opiate-receptor agonist, alters the perception of pain at the spinal cord and higher CNS levels by blocking the release of inhibitory neurotransmitters, such as gamma-aminobutyric acid and acetylcholine. It also alters the emotional response to pain.

Aspirin blocks cyclooxygenase, the enzyme needed for prostaglandin synthesis. Prostaglandins play a role in pain transmission from the periphery to the spinal cord.

Contraindications

Allergy to tartrazine dye; asthma; bleeding problems such as hemophilia; children under age 16 with a viral illness; hypersensitivity to aspirin, hydrocodone, other opioids, NSAIDs, or their components; peptic ulcer disease; respiratory depression; severe vitamin K deficiency; upper airway obstruction

Interactions

DRUGS
hydrocodone and aspirin
penicillins, sulfonamides: Increased blood levels of penicillins and sulfonamides
hydrocodone
anticholinergics, paregoric: Increased risk of severe constipation
antihypertensives, diuretics: Potentiated hypotensive effects
buprenorphine: Decreased effectiveness of codeine
CNS depressants: Additive CNS effects
hydroxyzine: Increased codeine analgesic effect; increased CNS depressant and hypotensive effects
MAO inhibitors: Increased risk of unpredictable, severe, and sometimes fatal reactions
metoclopramide: Antagonized effect of metoclopramide on GI motility
naloxone: Antagonized hydrocodone analgesic effect

naltrexone: Precipitated withdrawal symptoms in hydrocodone-dependent patients

neuromuscular blockers: Additive respiratory depressant effects

opioids: Additive CNS and respiratory depressant effects and hypotensive effects

aspirin

ACE inhibitors: Decreased antihypertensive effect

activated charcoal: Decreased aspirin absorption

antacids, urine alkalinizers: Decreased aspirin effectiveness

anticoagulants: Increased risk of bleeding and prolonged bleeding time

carbonic anhydrase inhibitors: Salicylism

corticosteroids: Increased excretion and decreased blood level of aspirin

heparin: Increased risk of bleeding

loop diuretics: Decreased effectiveness of loop diuretics

methotrexate: Increased blood level and decreased excretion of methotrexate, causing toxicity

nizatidine: Increased blood aspirin level

NSAIDs: Possibly decreased blood NSAID level and increased risk of adverse GI effects

oral antidiabetics, insulin: Increased risk of hypoglycemia

probenecid, sulfinpyrazone: Decreased effectiveness in treating gout

urine acidifiers, such as ammonium chloride and ascorbic acid: Decreased aspirin excretion

vancomycin: Increased risk of ototoxicity

ACTIVITIES

hydrocodone

alcohol use: Additive CNS effects

aspirin

alcohol use: Increased risk of ulcers

Adverse Reactions

CNS: Coma, confusion, CNS depression, delirium, depression, disorientation, dizziness, drowsiness, euphoria, hallucinations, headache, lack of coordination

CV: Bradycardia, orthostatic hypotension, palpitations, tachycardia

EENT: Altered taste, blurred vision, diplopia, dry mouth, hearing loss, laryngeal edema, laryngospasm, miosis, tinnitus

GI: Abnormal cramps and pain, anorexia, constipation, diarrhea, flatulence, GI bleeding, gastroesophageal reflux, heartburn, hepatotoxicity, ileus, indigestion, nausea, stomach pain, vomiting

GU: Decreased libido, difficult ejaculation, dysuria, impotence, oliguria, ureteral spasm, urinary incontinence, urine retention
HEME: Decreased blood iron level, hemolytic anemia, leukopenia, prolonged bleeding time, shortened life span of RBCs, thrombocytopenia
RESP: Apnea, bronchoconstriction, bronchospasm, depressed cough reflex, respiratory depression
SKIN: Diaphoresis, ecchymosis, flushing, pallor, pruritus, rash, urticaria
Other: Anaphylaxis, angioedema, physical and psychological dependence, Reye's syndrome

Nursing Considerations

- Use cautiously in patients with head trauma or intracranial lesions because hydrocodone can cause an exaggerated respiratory depression and aspirin can increase the risk of bleeding.
- Use cautiously in elderly and debilitated patients as well as patients with severe renal or hepatic dysfunction, gallbladder disease, respiratory impairment, cardiac arrhythmias, inflammatory disorders of the GI tract, hypothyroidism, Addison's disease, prostatic hypertrophy or urethral stricture, coagulation disorders or acute abdominal conditions.
- Evaluate patient for therapeutic response, including both patient reports and observatino of body movements.
- Take safety precautions, as needed.
- Monitor patient for evidence of CNS depression.
- Monitor respiratory depth, effort and rate. Notify prescriber immediately if respiratory rate drops below 10 breaths/min.
- **WARNING** Monitor patient closely for allergic reaction. Be aware that anaphylactic shock and other severe allergic reactions can occur without a history of allergy.
- **WARNING** Assess patient for evidence of physical and psychological dependence.
- Monitor urine output; decreasing output may signal urine retention or renal failure.

PATIENT TEACHING

- Instruct patient to take hydrocodone and aspirin with food or after meals to minimize stomach upset.
- Instruct patient to take hydrocodone and aspirin exactly as prescribed and not to adjust dose or frequency without consulting prescriber.
- Instruct patient to notify prescriber about worsening or breakthrough pain.

- Advise patient to notify prescriber if he becomes short of breath or has difficulty breathing.
- Tell patient to consult prescriber before taking drug with any prescription drug for blood disorder, diabetes, gout, or arthritis.
- Caution patient to avoid hazardous activities until drug's CNS effects are known.
- Caution patient to avoid alcohol and other CNS depressants while taking aspirin and codeine.
- Advise patient to get up slowly from a sitting or lying position.
- To prevent constipation, encourage patient to consume plenty of fluids and high-fiber foods, if not contraindicated.

hydrocodone and ibuprofen
Reprexain, Vicoprofen

Class, Category, and Schedule
Chemical: Opioid and phenanthrene derivative (hydrocodone), propionic acid derivative (ibuprofen)
Therapeutic: Analgesic
Pregnancy category: C
Controlled substance schedule: III

Indications and Dosages
▶ *To relieve acute pain*
TABLETS
Adults. 1 tablet (5 mg or 7.5 mg of hydrocodone and 200 mg of ibuprofen) every 4 to 6 hr, p.r.n., for up to 10 days. *Maximum:* 5 tablets (25 mg or 37.5 mg of hydrocodone and 1,000 mg of ibuprofen) daily.

Mechanism of Action
Exerts a synergistic analgesic effect through two mechanisms of action. Hydrocodone, a mu opiate-receptor agonist, alters the perception of pain at the spinal cord and higher CNS levels by blocking the release of inhibitory neurotransmitters, such as gamma-aminobutyric acid and acetylcholine. It also alters the emotional response to pain.

Ibuprofen blocks the activity of cyclooxygenase, the enzyme necessary for prostaglandin synthesis. Prostaglandins, important mediators in the inflammatory response, cause local vasodilation with swelling and pain. They also play a role in pain transmission from the periphery to the spinal cord. With the inhibition of cyclooxygenase and prostaglandin synthesis, inflammatory symptoms subside.

Contraindications

History of asthma, urticaria, or other allergic-type reactions following aspirin or other NSAID use; hypersensitivity to aspirin, hydrocodone, ibuprofen, opioids, other NSAIDs, or their components; respiratory depression; severe asthma; treatment of perioperative pain during coronary artery bypass graft surgery; upper airway obstruction

Interactions

DRUGS

hydrocodone

anticholinergics: Increased risk of paralytic ileus

CNS depressants: Increased CNS depression

MAO inhibitors, tricyclic antidepressants: Increased effect of either drug; increased risk of adverse reactions

Mixed agonist or antagonist analgesics, such as butorphanol, buprenorphine, nalbuphine, pentazocine: Possibly reduced analgesic effect of hydrocodone; possibly induced withdrawal symptoms

naloxone: Possibly withdrawal symptoms in physically dependent patients

naltrexone: Possibly prolonged respiratory depression and cardiac arrest

neuromuscular blocking agents: Possibly enhanced neuromuscular blocking action; increased degree of respiratory depression

ibuprofen

ACE inhibitors: Possibly decreased therapeutic effects of ACE inhibitors

aspirin, corticosteroids, NSAIDs: Possibly increased risk of GI ulceration and hemorrhage

diuretics: Possibly decreased diuresis, increased risk of renal failure

lithium: Increased blood lithium level, increased risk of lithium toxicity

methotrexate: Increased blood methotrexate level, increased risk of methotrexate toxicity

oral anticoagulants: Increased risk of GI bleeding

ACTIVITIES

alcohol use: Possibly increased CNS depression

Adverse Reactions

CNS: Anxiety, aseptic meningitis, asthenia, confusion, depression, dizziness, euphoria, fatigue, fever, headache, hypertonia, insomnia, irritability, lethargy, nervousness, paresthesia, sedation, slurred speech, somnolence, stroke, tremor, weakness

CV: Arrhythmias, congestive heart failure, peripheral edema, hy-

pertension, hypotension, orthostatic hypotension, MI, palpitations, tachycardia, thrombosis, vasodilation
EENT: Dry mouth, mouth ulcers, pharyngitis, rhinitis, sinusitis, tinnitus, vision changes
GI: Abdominal pain, anorexia, constipation, diarrhea, dyspepsia, dysphagia, esophagitis, elevated liver enzymes, flatulence, gastritis, gastroenteritis, GI bleeding or ulceration, hepatic failure or necrosis, hepatitis, indigestion, inflammation of GI tract, jaundice, melena, nausea, perforation of stomach or intestine, vomiting
GU: Impotence, renal papillary necrosis, renal toxicity, urinary frequency, urine retention
HEME: Anemia, prolonged bleeding time
RESP: Bronchitis, dyspnea, respiratory depression, suppressed cough reflex
SKIN: Blisters, diaphoresis, exfoliative dermatitis, flushing, pruritus, rash, Stevens-Johnson syndrome, toxic epidermal necrolysis, urticaria
Other: Anaphylaxis, angioedema, flu syndrome, physical and psychological dependence

Nursing Considerations

- Expect to give hydrocodone and ibuprofen for short-term pain relief only (no more than 10 days).
- Use hydrocodone and ibuprofen with extreme caution in patients with a history of ulcer disease or GI bleeding because NSAIDs such as ibuprofen increase the risk of GI bleeding and ulceration. Expect to use drug for the shortest time possible.
- Also use hydrocodone and ibuprofen cautiously in patients with inflammatory bowel disease because drug may worsen intestinal inflammation and cause diarrhea. If diarrhea causes severe dehydration, drug may need to be stopped.
- Use hydrocodone and ibuprofen cautiously in patients with cerebrovascular disease, coronary artery disease, congestive heart failure, or uncontrolled epilepsy because of the risk of severe complications.
- Use drug cautiously in patients with hypertension, and monitor blood pressure closely throughout therapy. Ibuprofen may cause hypertension or worsen it.
- **WARNING** Monitor patient closely for thrombotic events, including MI and stroke, because NSAIDs increase the risk.
- **WARNING** Stay alert for evidence of overdose, such as blurred vision; cold, clammy skin; confusion; dizziness; dyspnea; headache; hearing loss; malaise; mental or mood

changes; nausea; respiratory depression; sinus bradycardia; tinnitus; and vomiting. Notify prescriber immediately if they develop.

- Be aware that serious GI tract ulceration, bleeding, and perforation may occur without warning symptoms. Elderly patients are at greater risk. To minimize risk, give hydrocodone and ibuprofen with food. If GI distress occurs, withhold drug and notify prescriber immediately.
- Monitor patient, especially if elderly, for less common but serious adverse GI reactions, including anorexia, constipation, diverticulitis, dysphagia, esophagitis, gastritis, gastroenteritis, gastroesophageal reflux disease, hemorrhoids, hiatal hernia, melena, stomatitis, and vomiting.
- Monitor liver function test results and serum uric acid level. If abnormal liver test results persist or worsen, if patient has signs and symptoms consistent with liver disease, or if systemic changes such as eosinophilia or rash occur, discontinue drug immediately and notify prescriber.
- Monitor renal function—especially in patients with existing renal disease, heart failure, or liver dysfuction; those taking diuretics or ACE inhibitors; and the elderly—because patients are at increased risk for renal papillary necrosis and other renal injury. Notify prescriber if abnormalities develop, and expect to discontinue drug.
- Be aware that, although rare, aseptic meningitis with fever and coma has occurred in patients taking ibuprofen, especially patients who have systemic lupus and related connective tissue disease. Notify prescriber immediately if patient develops fever and CNS dysfunction.
- Report weight gain of more than 1 kg (2 lb) in 24 hours, which suggests fluid retention.
- If patient takes a potassium-sparing diuretic, check for elevated serum potassium level, as ordered.
- Monitor patient's hemoglobin and hematocrit, as ordered, during prolonged therapy because drug may cause anemia.
- WARNING If patient has bone marrow suppression or is receiving an antineoplastic drug, monitor laboratory results (including WBC count), and watch for evidence of infection because anti-inflammatory and antipyretic actions of ibuprofen may mask signs and symptoms, such as fever and pain.
- Assess patient's skin regularly for rash or other signs of hypersensitivity reaction because ibuprofen is an NSAID and may cause serious skin reactions without warning, even in patients

with no history of NSAID sensitivity. At first sign of reaction, stop drug and notify prescriber.

- **WARNING** Assess patient for evidence of physical and psychological dependence.

PATIENT TEACHING

- Tell patient to alert prescriber before taking hydrocodone and ibuprofen if she has a history of ulcers, bleeding problems, hypertension, or heart or renal disease; if she takes a diuretic; or if she's over age 65.
- Advise patient to take drug exactly as prescribed and not to increase dosage because stomach bleeding or physical or psychological dependence may occur.
- Instruct patient to take hydrocodone and ibuprofen with food to minimize GI distress.
- To decrease risk of esophageal ulceration, instruct patient to take drug with a full glass of water and not to lie down for 15 to 30 minutes afterward.
- Warn patient to avoid hazardous activities until drug's CNS effects are known.
- Instruct patient to notify prescriber if she has ringing or buzzing in the ears, impaired hearing, dizziness, vision changes, swelling, or weight gain.
- Advise patient to avoid taking two different NSAIDs at the same time, unless directed, and to alert prescriber before taking drug if she has ever had an allergic reaction to an analgesic or fever-reducing drug. Also advise patient to consult prescriber before taking aspirin or other OTC analgesics or ingesting alcohol.
- Inform patient that drug increases the risk of inflammation, bleeding, ulceration, and perforation of the stomach and intestine, possibly without warning. If patient feels suddenly ill, she should seek medical attention.
- Warn patient of the possibility of hepatic injury. Instruct her to notify prescriber if she has signs and symptoms of hepatotoxicity, such as nausea, fatigue, lethargy, pruritus, jaundice, right upper quadrant tenderness, and flulike symptoms.
- Explain that drug may increase the risk of serious adverse cardiovascular reactions; urge patient to seek immediate medical attention if signs or symptoms arise, such as chest pain, shortness of breath, weakness, and slurring of speech.
- Alert patient to rare but serious skin reactions. Urge her to seek immediate medical attention for rash, blisters, itching, fever, or other indications of hypersensitivity.
- Urge patient to avoid consuming alcohol during drug therapy.

- Advise patient to change positions slowly to minimize effects of orthostatic hypotension.
- Advise woman of childbearing age to alert prescriber if she is or could be pregnant.

levodopa and carbidopa

Apo-Levocarb (CAN), Atamet, Parcopa, Sinemet, Sinemet CR

Class and Category

Chemical: Hydralazine analogue of levodopa (carbidopa), levorotatory isomer of dihydroxyphenylalanine (levodopa)
Therapeutic: Antidyskinetic
Pregnancy category: C

Indications and Dosages

▶ *To relieve symptoms of Parkinson's disease*
E.R. TABLETS

Adults not taking levodopa. *Initial:* 1 tablet of 100 mg levodopa and 25 mg carbidopa b.i.d. or 1 tablet of 200 mg levodopa and 50 mg carbidopa b.i.d. with doses spaced at least 6 hr apart. Dose increased or decreased every 3 days or more, if needed, based on response. *Maintenance:* 400 to 1,600 mg levodopa daily in divided doses every 4 to 8 hr. *Maximum:* 2,400 mg levodopa daily.

Adults taking levodopa regardless of dose. 1 tablet of 100 mg levodopa and 25 mg carbidopa b.i.d. or 1 tablet of 200 mg levodopa and 50 mg carbidopa b.i.d. at least 12 hr after levodopa is stopped. *Maximum:* 2,400 mg levodopa daily.

Adults taking conventional carbidopa-levodopa. If patient takes 300 to 400 mg of levodopa in combination product, regimen switched to 1 E.R. tablet (200 mg levodopa) b.i.d. given 4 to 8 hr apart. If patient takes 500 to 600 mg of levodopa in combination product, regimen switched to 1 E.R. tablet (300 mg levodopa) b.i.d. or t.i.d. given 4 to 8 hr apart. If patient takes 700 to 800 mg of levodopa in combination product, regimen switched to 4 E.R. tablets (800 mg levodopa) daily divided into three doses and given 4 to 8 hr apart. *Maximum:* 2,400 mg levodopa daily.
TABLETS

Adults not taking levodopa. *Initial:* 1 tablet of 100 mg levodopa and 25 mg carbidopa t.i.d., or 1 tablet of 100 mg levodopa and 10 mg carbidopa t.i.d. or q.i.d. Increased by 1 tablet daily or every other day, if needed, up to maximum. *Maximum:* 2,000 mg levodopa and 200 mg carbidopa daily.

Adults taking more than 1,500 mg of levodopa. 1 tablet of 250 mg levodopa and 25 mg carbidopa t.i.d. or q.i.d. at least 12 hr after levodopa stops. *Maximum:* 2,000 mg levodopa and 200 mg carbidopa daily.

Adults taking less than 1,500 mg of levodopa. 1 tablet of 100 mg levodopa and 25 mg carbidopa t.i.d. or q.i.d. or 1 tablet of 100 mg levodopa and 10 mg carbidopa t.i.d. or q.i.d. at least 12 hr after levodopa stops. *Maximum:* 2,000 mg levodopa and 200 mg carbidopa daily.

ORALLY DISINTEGRATING TABLETS

Adults. *Initial:* 1 tablet of 100 mg levodopa and 25 mg carbidopa t.i.d., increased as needed by 1 tablet daily or every other day. Or 1 tablet of 100 mg levodopa and 10 mg carbidopa t.i.d. or q.i.d., increased as needed by 1 tablet daily or every other day. *Maximum:* 8 tablets of 100 mg levodopa and 25 mg carbidopa or 100 mg levodopa and 10 mg carbidopa daily.

Mechanism of Action

In extracerebral tissues, levodopa is converted to dopamine and moves to the CNS, where it replenishes dopamine, thus helping to improve muscle control and normalize body movements.

Carbidopa inhibits peripheral distribution of levodopa, making more levodopa available to the brain.

Contraindications

Concurrent MAO inhibitor therapy; history of melanoma; hypersensitivity to carbidopa, levodopa, or their components; narrow-angle glaucoma; suspicious undiagnosed skin lesions

Interactions

DRUGS

antihypertensives: Increased risk of symptomatic orthostatic hypotension

benzodiazepines, droperidol, haloperidol, hydantoin anticonvulsants, loxapine, metoclopramide, metyrosine, molindone, papaverine, phenothiazines, rauwolfia alkaloids, thioxanthenes: Decreased carbidopa-levodopa effects

bromocriptine: Additive levodopa and carbidopa effects

iron salts: Decreased absorption, blood level, and effectiveness of levodopa

MAO inhibitors: Increased risk of severe orthostatic hypotension

methyldopa: Altered antiparkinsonian effects of levodopa, additive toxic CNS effects

pyridoxine: Reversed levodopa effects

tricyclic antidepressants: Increased risk of adverse reactions to levodopa and carbidopa

FOODS

high-protein food: Possibly delayed or reduced drug absorption

Adverse Reactions

CNS: Anxiety, confusion, depression, headache, insomnia, mood or mental changes, nervousness, neuroleptic malignant syndrome, nightmares, tiredness, uncontrolled movements, weakness

CV: Arrhythmias, orthostatic hypotension

EENT: Blurred vision, darkened saliva, dry mouth, eyelid spasm, ptosis

GI: Anorexia, constipation, diarrhea, nausea, vomiting

GU: Darkened urine, dysuria

MS: Muscle twitching

SKIN: Darkened sweat, flushing

Nursing Considerations

- Use drug cautiously in patients with history of psychosis. Monitor all patients for depression and suicidal tendencies.
- Administer cautiously to patients with severe CV or pulmonary disease; bronchial asthma; renal, hepatic, or endocrine disease; history of MI and residual atrial, nodal, or ventricular arrhythmias; or history of peptic ulcer. Monitor patient closely, especially when therapy begins and dosage is adjusted.
- **WARNING** Avoid giving levodopa and carbidopa within 2 weeks of an MAO inhibitor because sudden, extreme hypertension may occur.
- Assess patient for neuroleptic malignant syndrome if drug is stopped or dose reduced, especially if patient also takes a neuroleptic drug. Rare but life-threatening, the syndrome causes altered level of consciousness, autonomic dysfunction, diaphoresis, fever, altered blood pressure, involuntary movement, muscle rigidity, tachycardia, and tachypnea. If these changes occur, notify prescriber immediately.

PATIENT TEACHING

- If patient can't swallow E.R. tablet whole, tell him to break it in half for swallowing but not to crush or chew it.
- If patient takes orally disintegrating form, tell him to gently remove tab from bottle with dry hands, place it on top of his

tongue, let it dissolve (which takes seconds), and swallow it with saliva. Explain that no other liquids are needed.

- Remind patient that it may take several weeks or months to feel full drug effects.
- Stress the need to take levodopa and carbidopa regularly and exactly as prescribed. Altering the dose or interval may increase the risk of adverse reactions or decrease drug effectiveness.
- Tell patient to notify prescriber if involuntary movements appear or worsen during therapy; dose may need to be adjusted.
- Inform patient being switched from regular to E.R. tablets that effect may be delayed for up to 1 hour after the first morning dose, compared with the effect from the regular tablet. If delay poses a problem, tell patient to notify prescriber.

levodopa, carbidopa, and entacapone
Stalevo

Class and Category
Chemical: Levorotatory isomer of dihydroxyphenylalanine (levodopa), hydralazine analogue of levodopa (carbidopa), catechol-O-methyltransferase (COMT) inhibitor (entacapone)
Therapeutic: Antidyskinetic
Pregnancy category: C

Indications and Dosages
▶ *To treat idiopathic Parkinson's disease*
TABLETS
Adults. Highly individualized and used only as a substitute for patients already stabilized on equivalent doses of levodopa, carbidopa, and entacapone. *Maintenance:* Highly individualized. When less levodopa is needed, strength or frequency of dosage can be decreased; when more levodopa is needed, frequency can be increased or next higher strength can be given. *Maximum:* 1 tablet of equivalent strength (50 mg levodopa, 12.5 mg carbidopa, and 200 mg entacapone; 100 mg levodopa, 25 mg carbidopa, and 200 mg entacapone; or 150 mg levodopa, 37.5 mg carbidopa, and 200 mg entacapone) per dosing interval; 8 tablets daily.

Contraindications
Angle-closure glaucoma; history of melanoma; hypersensitivity to levodopa, carbidopa, entacapone, or their components; suspicious, undiagnosed skin lesions; use within 14 days of an MAO inhibitor

Mechanism of Action

In extracerebral tissues, levodopa is converted to dopamine and transported to the CNS, where it replenishes depleted dopamine (which is thought to cause Parkinson's disease), thus helping to improve muscle control and normalize body movements.

Carbidopa inhibits peripheral distribution of levodopa, making more levodopa available in the brain.

Entacapone inhibits peripheral COMT, the major metabolizing enzyme for levodopa. During levodopa metabolism, COMT produces a levodopa metabolite that reduces levodopa effectiveness. By inhibiting COMT, entacapone increases levodopa level, making more available for diffusion into the CNS.

Interactions

DRUGS

levodopa, carbidopa, and entacapone

alpha-methyldopa, apomorphine, bitolterol, dobutamine, dopamine, epinephrine, isoetharine, isoproterenol, norepinephrine, other COMT metabolizers: Possibly increased heart rate, arrhythmias, and extreme changes in blood pressure

anti-hypertensives: Possibly symptomatic orthostatic hypotension

iron salts: Possibly reduced bioavailability of carbidopa, levodopa, and entacapone

MAO inhibitors: Possibly inhibited catecholamine metabolism

selegiline: Possibly severe orthostatic hypotension

tricyclic antidepressants: Possibly hypertension and dyskinesia

levodopa

dopamine D2-receptor antagonists (such as butyrophenones, isoniazid, phenothiazines, and risperidone): Possible reduced effectiveness of levodopa

metoclopramide: Increased bioavailability but decreased effectiveness of levodopa

papaverine, phenytoin: Possible reversed effects of levodopa in Parkinson's disease

entacapone

ampicillin, cholestyramine, erythromycin, probenecid, rifampin: Possible interference with biliary excretion of entacapone

FOODS

high-protein food: Possibly delayed or reduced drug absorption

Adverse Reactions

CNS: Activation of latent Horner's syndrome, aggravation of Parkinson's disease symptoms, agitation, anxiety, asthenia, ataxia, bradykinetic episodes, confusion, decreased mental acuity, delusions, dementia, depression, disorientation, dizziness, dyskinesia, euphoria, fatigue, gait abnormalities, hallucinations, headache, hyperkinesia, hypokinesia, insomnia, malaise, memory loss, nervousness, neuroleptic malignant syndrome, nightmares, paranoia, paresthesia, peripheral neuropathy, sense of stimulation, somnolence, syncope, tremor increase, trismus

CV: Arrhythmias; chest pain; edema; hypotension, including orthostatic; hypertension; MI; palpitations; phlebitis

EENT: Blepharospasm, blurred vision, darkened saliva, dilated pupils, diplopia, dry mouth, excessive salivation, hoarseness, oculogyric crisis, taste disturbance, tongue burning

ENDO: Hyperglycemia

GI: Abdominal pain, elevated function test results, anorexia, bruxism, constipation, diarrhea, duodenal ulcer, dysphagia, flatulence, gastritis, GI bleeding, GI pain, hiccups, indigestion, nausea, vomiting

GU: Bacteria, blood, glucose, or protein in urine, darkened urine; elevated BUN and serum creatinine levels; elevated uric acid levels; elevated WBC count in urine; increased libido; urinary frequency, incontinence, or retention; UTI

HEME: Agranulocytosis, decreased hemoglobin and hematocrit, hemolytic and nonhemolytic anemia, leukopenia, positive Coombs' test, thrombocytopenia

MS: Back, leg, and shoulder pain; muscle cramps or twitching; rhabdomyolysis

RESP: Abnormal breathing patterns, dyspnea, upper respiratory tract infection

SKIN: Alopecia, bullous lesions, darkened sweat, diaphoresis, flushing, malignant melanoma, pruritus, purpura, rash, urticaria

Other: Angioedema, hot flashes, hypokalemia, weight gain or loss

Nursing Considerations

- Use drug cautiously in patients with past or current psychosis because drug may cause depression and suicidal tendencies.
- Use cautiously in patients with severe CV or pulmonary disease; biliary obstruction; bronchial asthma; or renal, hepatic, or endocrine disease.
- If patient has chronic open-angle glaucoma, make sure intraocular pressure is well controlled because drug may lead to increased intraocular pressure.

- If patient has a history of MI with residual atrial, nodal, or ventricular arrhythmias, expect to make initial dosage adjustment in a facility with intensive cardiac care.
- Monitor patient closely for adverse CNS effects. Such adverse effects as dyskinesia may occur at lower dosages and more quickly with the use of carbidopa, levodopa, and entacapone tablets than when levodopa is used alone. If dyskinesia occurs, notify prescriber and expect to decrease dosage.
- Closely monitor patient with a history of peptic ulcer because drug may increase risk of GI hemorrhage.
- If drug must be stopped, taper it slowly to prevent high fever or severe rigidity.
- Assess patient for neuroleptic malignant syndrome during dosage reduction or drug discontinuation, especially in a patient who also receives a neuroleptic drug. This uncommon syndrome is life-threatening and causes altered level of consciousness, autonomic dysfunction, diaphoresis, fever, high or low blood pressure, involuntary movement, muscle rigidity, tachycardia, and tachypnea. If these occur, notify prescriber immediately.

PATIENT TEACHING

- To provide uniform drug effect, stress importance of taking carbidopa, levodopa, and entacapone at regular intervals according to the prescribed schedule.
- Advise patient to avoid a high-protein diet and iron salts (such as those found in many multi-vitamin tablets) because protein and iron may delay levodopa absorption and reduce the amount available for the body to use to control Parkinson's disease symptoms.
- Alert patient to the possibility of nausea, especially at the beginning of therapy. Tell him that this adverse reaction usually resolves with continued therapy.
- Tell patient to notify prescriber if he's taking any other medication, including OTC and herbal preparations, because of potential drug interactions.
- Inform patient that drug's effect may sometimes appear to wear off at the end of a dosing interval. If this occurs, instruct him to notify his prescriber to determine if a dosage adjustment is needed.
- Caution patient that hallucinations may occur, and advise him to avoid hazardous activities until drug's CNS effects are known.

- Advise patient to rise slowly after sitting or lying down to avoid a sudden drop in blood pressure.
- Instruct patient to notify prescriber if dyskinesia occurs.
- Tell patient that body fluids, such as saliva, urine and sweat, may turn a dark color, such as red, brown, or black. Reassure him that this effect is harmless but that fluids may stain clothing.
- Advise female patients of childbearing age to notify prescriber immediately about known or suspected pregnancy because changes to drug therapy may be required.
- Inform patient with diabetes that drug may cause a false-positive result for urinary ketones when a test tape product is used to check for ketonuria and a false-negative result for urine glucose when a glucose-oxidase method is used. Encourage patient to monitor blood glucose levels and seek medical attention if he suspects ketonuria.

meperidine hydrochloride and promethazine hydrochloride
Mepergan, Mepergan Forte

Class, Category, and Schedule
Chemical: Phenylpiperidine derivative opioid (merperidine), phenothiazine derivative (promethazine)
Therapeutic: Analgesic (meperidine), antiemetic (promethazine)
Pregnancy category: C (D for prolonged use or high dose at term)
Controlled substance schedule: II

Indications and Dosages
▶ *To relieve moderate to severe pain*
CAPSULES
Adults. 50 mg meperidine and 25 mg promethazine (1 capsule) every 4 to 6 hr, as needed.
I.M. INJECTION
Adults. 25 mg meperidine and 25 mg promethazine every 4 to 6 hr, as needed.

Contraindications
Acute asthma, angle-closure glaucoma; benign prostatic hyperplasia; bladder neck obstruction; bone marrow depression; breastfeeding; coma; hypersensitivity or history of idiosyncratic reaction to meperidine, other opioids, promethazine, other phenothiazines, or their components; hypertensive crisis; increased in-

tracranial pressure; pyloroduodenal obstruction; severe respiratory depression; stenosing peptic ulcer; upper respiratory tract obstruction; use of large quantities of CNS depressants or within 14 days of MAO inhibitor therapy

---

Mechanism of Action

Meperidine binds with opiate receptors in the spinal cord and higher levels of the CNS. In this way, meperidine stimulates mu and kappa receptors, which alters the perception of and emotional response to pain.

Promethazine may prevent nausea and vertigo by acting centrally on the medullary chemoreceptive trigger zone and by decreasing vestibular stimulation and labyrinthine function in the inner ear. In addition, it promotes sedation and relieves anxiety by blocking receptor sites within the CNS, directly reducing stimuli to the brain.

Interactions

DRUGS

meperidine and promethazine

amphetamines, MAO inhibitors: Risk of increased CNS excitation or depression with possibly fatal reactions

anticholinergics: Increased risk of intensified anticholinergic adverse effects

meperidine

acyclovir, ritonavir: Possibly increased blood meperidine level

alfentanil, CNS depressants, fentanyl, sufentanil: Increased risk of CNS and respiratory depression and hypotension

antidiarrheals (such as loperamide and difenoxin and atropine): Increased risk of severe constipation and increased CNS depression

antihypertensives: Increased risk of hypotension

buprenorphine: Possibly decreased therapeutic effects of meperidine and increased risk of respiratory depression

cimetidine: Reduced clearance and volume of distribution of meperidine

hydroxyzine: Increased risk of CNS depression and hypotension

metoclopramide: Possibly decreased effects of metoclopramide

naloxone, naltrexone: Decreased pharmacologic effects of meperidine

neuromuscular blockers: Increased risk of prolonged respiratory and CNS depression

oral anticoagulants: Possibly increased anticoagulant effect and risk of bleeding

phenytoin: Possibly enhanced hepatic metabolism of meperidine
promethazine
anticonvulsants: Lowered seizure threshold
appetite suppressants: Possibly antagonized anorectic effect of appetite suppressants
beta blockers: Increased risk of additive hypotensive effects, irreversible retinopathy, arrhythmias, and tardive dyskinesia
bromocriptine: Decreased effectiveness of bromocriptine
CNS depressants: Additive CNS depression
dopamine: Possibly antagonized peripheral vasoconstriction (with high doses of dopamine)
ephedrine, metaraminol, methoxamine: Decreased vasopressor response to these drugs
epinephrine: Blocked alpha-adrenergic effects of epinephrine, increased risk of hypotension
guanadrel, guanethidine: Decreased antihypertensive effects of these drugs
hepatotoxic drugs: Increased risk of hepatotoxicity
hypotension-producing drugs: Possibly severe hypotension with syncope
levodopa: Inhibitied antidyskinetic effects of levodopa
metrizamide: Increased risk of seizures
ototoxic drugs: Possibly masking of some symptoms of ototoxicity, such as dizziness, tinnitus, and vertigo
quinidine: Additive cardiac effects
riboflavin: Increased riboflavin requirements
ACTIVITIES
meperidine and promethazine
alcohol use: Possibly increased CNS and respiratory depression and hypotension

Adverse Reactions
CNS: Akathisia, CNS stimulation, confusion, depression, dizziness, drowsiness, dystonia, euphoria, excitation, fatigue, hallucinations, headache, hysteria, increased intracranial pressure, insomnia, irritability, lack of coordination, malaise, nervousness, neuroleptic malignant syndrome, nightmares, paradoxical stimulation, pseudoparkinsonism, restlessness, sedation, seizures, syncope, tardive dyskinesia, tremor
CV: Bradycardia, hypertension, hypotension, orthostatic hypotension, tachycardia
EENT: Blurred vision; diplopia; dry mouth, nose, and throat; nasal congestion; tinnitus; vision changes

ENDO: Hyperglycemia

GI: Abdominal cramps, pain, or spasms; anorexia; cholestatic jaundice; constipation; ileus; nausea; vomiting

GU: Dysuria, urinary frequency, urine retention

HEME: Agranulocytosis, leukopenia, thrombocytopenia, thrombocytopenic purpura

RESP: Apnea, dyspnea, respiratory arrest or depression, tenacious bronchial secretions, wheezing

SKIN: Dermatitis, diaphoresis, flushing, photosensitivity, rash, urticaria

Other: Angioedema; injection site pain, redness, and swelling; paradoxical reactions; physical and psychological dependence

Nursing Considerations

- Use with extreme caution in patients with acute abdominal conditions, hepatic or renal disorders, hypothyroidism, prostatic hyperplasia, seizures, or supraventricular tachycardia. Be aware that multiple doses are not recommended for these patients.
- Also use cautiously in patients with asthma because of its anticholinergic effects and in patients with seizure disorders or those who use medication that may affect seizure threshold because meperidine and promethazine may lower patient's seizure threshold.
- Know that meperidine and promethazine should not be used longer than 48 hours to manage acute pain.
- Inject I.M. form deep into large muscle mass and rotate sites. Never inject the drug subcutaneously.
- **WARNING** Avoid inadvertent intra-arterial injection of promethazine because it can cause arteriospasm; gangrene may develop from impaired circulation.
- **WARNING** Monitor respiratory function because drug may suppress cough reflex and cause thickening of bronchial secretions, aggravating such conditions as asthma and COPD, and, in rare cases, may depress respirations and induce apnea. Notify prescriber immediately and expect to discontinue drug if respiratory rate falls to less than 12 breaths/minute or if respiratory depth decreases.
- Evaluate for therapeutic response, including report of decreased pain and body movements that would indicate pain relief has occurred.
- Monitor bowel function to detect constipation and assess the need for stool softeners.
- Monitor patient's hematologic status as ordered because

promethazine may cause bone marrow depression, especially when used with other known marrow-toxic agents. Assess patient for signs and symptoms of infection or bleeding.

• **WARNING** Monitor patient for evidence of neuroleptic malignant syndrome, such as fever, hypertension or hypotension, involuntary motor activity, mental changes, muscle rigidity, tachycardia, and tachypnea. Be prepared to provide supportive treatment and additional drug therapy as prescribed.

• Assess for signs of physical and psychological dependence and abuse.

• Expect withdrawal symptoms to occur if drug is abruptly stopped after long-term use.

• Be aware that patient shouldn't have intradermal allergen tests within 72 hours of receiving promethazine because drug may significantly alter flare response.

PATIENT TEACHING

• Inform patient that meperidine and promethazine is a controlled substance and is habit forming if taken long-term.

• Advise patient to take drug exactly as prescribed.

• Instruct patient to report constipation, severe nausea, and shortness of breath and to notify prescriber immediately if he experiences involuntary movements and restlessness.

• Instruct patient to notify prescriber about worsening or breakthrough pain

• Caution patient to avoid hazardous activities until drug's CNS effects are known.

• Urge patient to avoid alcohol, OTC drugs, sedatives, and tranquilizers during meperidine and promethazine use unless approved by prescriber.

• Suggest frequent rinsing and use of sugarless gum or hard candy to relieve dry mouth.

• Advise patient to avoid excessive sun exposure and to use sunscreen when outdoors.

meprobamate and aspirin
Equagesic, Micrainin

Class, Category, and Schedule
Chemical: Carbamate derivative (meprobamate), salicylate (aspirin)
Therapeutic: Antianxiety (meprobamate), analgesic (aspirin)
Pregnancy category: X
Controlled substance schedule: IV

Mechanism of Action

Meprobamate is an anxiolytic that may act at multiple sites in the CNS, including the thalamus and limbic system. Meprobamate inhibits spinal reflexes, causing CNS relaxation. It also has muscle relaxant properties.

Aspirin blocks the activity of cyclooxygenase, the enzyme necessary for prostaglandin synthesis. By preventing prostaglandin synthesis, pain is relieved because prostaglandins play a role in pain transmission from the periphery to the spinal cord.

Indications and Dosages

▶ *To relieve pain accompanied by tension or anxiety in patients with musculoskeletal disease.*

TABLETS

Adults. 200 mg meprobamate and 325 mg aspirin (1 tablet) or 400 mg meprobamate and 650 mg aspirin (2 tablets) t.i.d. or q.i.d., as needed

Contraindications

Acute intermittent porphyria; allergy to tartrazine dye; asthma; bleeding problems such as hemophilia; breast-feeding; children under age 16 with a viral illness; hypersensitivity to meprobamate, aspirin or their components; peptic ulcer disease; pregnancy; triad syndrome of asthma, rhinitis, and nasal polyps

Interactions

DRUGS

meprobamate

CNS depressants: Increased CNS depression

aspirin

acetazolamide: Increased serum acetazolamide level and risk of toxicity

ACE inhibitors: Decreased antihypertensive effect

activated charcoal: Decreased aspirin absorption

antacids, urine alkalinizers: Decreased aspirin effectiveness

anticoagulants: Increased risk of bleeding; prolonged bleeding time

beta blockers: Diminished hypotensive effect of beta blockers

carbonic anhydrase inhibitors: Salicylism

corticosteroids: Increased excretion and decreased blood level of aspirin

heparin: Increased risk of bleeding

loop diuretics: Decreased effectiveness of loop diuretics

methotrexate: Increased blood level and decreased excretion of

methotrexate, causing toxicity
nizatidine: Increased blood aspirin level
NSAIDs: Possibly decreased blood NSAID level and increased risk of adverse GI effects
oral hypoglycemics: Increased effectiveness of oral hypoglycemics increasing risk of hypoglycemia
phenytoin, valproic acid: Decreased phenytoin level; increased serum valproic acid levels
probenecid, sulfinpyrazone: Decreased effectiveness in treating gout
urine acidifiers, such as ammonium chloride and ascorbic acid: Decreased aspirin excretion
vancomycin: Increased risk of ototoxicity

ACTIVITIES

meprobamate and aspirin
alcohol use: Increased CNS depression; increased risk of ulcers

Adverse Reactions

CNS: Ataxia, confusion, CNS depression, dizziness, drowsiness, euphoria, headache, light-headedness, paradoxical stimulation, paresthesia, slurred speech, syncope, vertigo, weakness
CV: Arrhythmias, including tachycardia; hypotension; palpitations
EENT: Blurred vision, hearing loss, impaired visual accommodation, tinnitus
GI: Diarrhea, GI bleeding, heartburn, hepatotoxicity, nausea, stomach pain, vomiting
GU: Nephrotoxicity
HEME: Decreased blood iron level, hemolytic anemia, leukopenia, prolonged bleeding time, shortened life span of RBCs, thrombocytopenia
SKIN: Ecchymosis, erythematous maculopapular rash, pruritus, Stevens-Johnson syndrome, urticaria
Other: Anaphylaxis, angioedema, physical dependence, Reye's syndrome

Nursing Considerations

- Use cautiously in elderly and debilitated patients as well as patients with severe renal or hepatic dysfunction, seizure disorder, gallbladder disease, respiratory impairment, cardiac arrhythmias, inflammatory disorders of the GI tract, hypothyroidism, Addison's disease, prostatic hypertrophy or urethral stricture, coagulation disorders or acute abdominal conditions.
- Also use drug cautiously in patients with suicidal tendencies or a history of drug dependence or abuse because meprobamate can lead to physical dependence and abuse.

- Evaluate for therapeutic response, including report of decreased pain and body movements that would indicate pain relief has occurred.
- Observe for signs of chronic drug intoxication, such as ataxia, slurred speech, and vertigo or CNS depression.
- Be aware that meprobamate and aspirin should be used for no longer than 10 days. If drug is used longer, expect to taper dosage gradually when discontinuing because abrupt discontinuation could exacerbate previous symptoms, such as anxiety, or cause withdrawal symptoms, such as confusion, hallucinations, muscle twitching, tremor, and vomiting.

PATIENT TEACHING
- Instruct patient to take meprobamate and aspirin exactly as directed and not to stop taking it abruptly.
- Tell patient to take drug with food or after meals because it may cause GI upset if taken on an empty stomach.
- Instruct patient to notify prescriber about worsening or breakthrough pain.
- Advise patient to consult prescriber before taking drug with any prescription drug for blood disorder, diabetes, gout, or arthritis.
- Advise patient to avoid hazardous activities until drug's CNS effects are known.
- Direct patient to avoid alcohol, sedatives, and other CNS depressants while taking drug.
- Instruct patient to report rash.
- Urge female patients of childbearing age to use effective contraception during drug therapy and to notify prescriber immediately if pregnancy is suspected.

olanzapine and fluoxetine hydrochloride
Symbyax

Class and Category
Chemical: Thienobenzodiazepine derivative (olanzapine) and selective serotonin reuptake inhibitor (fluoxetine)
Therapeutic: Antipsychotic
Pregnancy category: C

Indications and Dosages
▶ *To treat depression associated with bipolar disorder*
CAPSULES
Adults. *Initial:* 6 mg olanzapine and 25 mg fluoxetine daily in

the evening and then dosage increased as needed. *Maximum:* 12 mg olanzapine and 50 mg fluoxetine.

Mechanism of Action

Olanzapine may achieve its antipsychotic effects by antagonizing dopamine and serotonin receptors. Anticholinergic effects may result from competitive binding to and antagonism of the muscarinic receptors M_1 through M_3.

Fluoxetine selectively inhibits reuptake of the neurotransmitter serotonin by CNS neurons and increases the amount of serotonin available in synsapses.

Together, these drugs may activate monoaminergic neural system's serotonin, norepinephrine, and dopamine release in the prefrontal cortex to increase antidepressant effect.

Contraindications

Concurrent therapy with pimozide; hypersensitivity to olanzapine, fluoxetine, or other selective serotonin reuptake inhibitors or their components; use within 14 days of an MAO inhibitor or within 5 weeks of thioridazine

Interactions

DRUGS

olanzapine

anticholinergics: Increased anticholinergic effects, altered thermoregulation

antihypertensives: Increased effects of both drugs, increased risk of hypotension

benzodiazepines (parenteral): Increased risk of excessive sedation and cardiorespiratory depression

carbamazepine, omeprazole, rifampin: Increased olanzapine clearance

CNS depressants: Additive CNS depression, potentiated orthostatic hypotension

diazepam: Increased CNS depressant effects

fluvoxamine: Decreased olanzapine clearance

levodopa: Decreased levodopa efficacy

lorazepam (parenteral): Possibly increased somnolence with I.M. injection of olanzapine

fluoxetine

alprazolam, diazepam: Possibly prolonged half-life of these drugs

aspirin, NSAIDs, warfarin: Increased anticoagulant activity and risk of bleeding

astemizole: Increased risk of serious arrhythmias

buspirone: Decreased buspirone effects
clozapine, fluphenazine, haloperidol, maprotiline, trazodone: Increased risk of adverse effects
CYP2D6-metabolized drugs, such as antiarrhythmics (especially flecainide, propafenone), selected antidepressants (tricyclics), antipyschotics (phenothiazines and most atypicals), thioridazine, and vinblastine: Increased plasma levels of these drugs and increased risk of serious adverse reactions
linezolid, lithium, serotonergics (such as amphetamines and other psychostimulants, antidepressants, and dopamine agonists), St. John's wort, tramadol, triptans: Increased risk of serotonin syndrome
MAO inhibitors: Possibly severe and life-threatening adverse effects
phenytoin: Increased blood phenytoin level and risk of toxicity
pimozide: Possibly prolonged QT interval
sumatriptan: Possibly increased risk of weakness, hyperreflexia, and incoordination
tryptophan: Increased risk of central and peripheral toxicity
ACTIVITIES
olanzapine
alcohol use: Additive CNS depression, potentiated orthostatic hypotension
smoking: Decreased blood olanzapine level

Adverse Reactions

CNS: Amnesia, asthenia, chills, fever, hyperkinesia, migraine, neuroleptic malignant syndrome, personality changes, seizures, serotonin syndrome, sleep disturbance, somnolence, speech alteration, suicidal ideation, tardive dyskinesia, tremor
CV: Bradycardia, chest pain, edema, hyperlipidemia, hypertension, orthostatic hypotension, tachycardia, vasodilation
EENT: Abnormal vision, amblyopia, dry mouth, ear pain, increased salivation, otitis media, pharyngitis, taste perversion, tinnitus
ENDO: Breast pain, hyperglycemia, increased prolactin level, menorrhagia
GI: Diarrhea, elevated liver function test results, hepatitis, increased appetite, jaundice, thirst
GU: Abnormal ejaculation, anorgasmia, decreased libido, impotence, urinary frequency or incontinence, UTI
MS: Arthralgia, muscle twitching, neck pain or rigidity,
RESP: Bronchitis, dyspnea
SKIN: Ecchymosis, erythema multiforme, photosensitivity, rash, urticaria

Other: Anaphylaxis, angioedema, hyponatremia, infection, weight gain or loss

Nursing Considerations

- Use with caution in patients with cardiovascular or cerebrovascular disease or conditions that would predispose patients to hypotension because of olanzapine and fluoxetine's potential to cause orthostatic hypotension.
- Be aware that olanzapine in this combination drug should not be used in patients with dementia-related psychosis because of an increased risk of death.
- Obtain a baseline evaluation of patient's lipid status before starting therapy and periodically thereafter, as ordered, because drug can cause significant and sometimes very high lipid elevations.
- Monitor patient's blood glucose level routinely because drug may increase risk of hyperglycemia and, in rare cases, ketoacidosis or hyperosmolar coma.
- Monitor patient closely for neuroleptic malignant syndrome (hyperthermia, muscle rigidity, altered level of consciousness, irregular pulse or blood pressure, tachycardia, diaphoresis, and arrhythmias), a rare but potentially fatal adverse effect.
- Monitor hepatic function, as ordered, in patients with hepatic disease because olanzapine and fluoxetine combination can elevate hepatic enzyme levels.
- Monitor patient being treated for depression with olanzapine and fluoxetine closely for suicidal tendencies, especially when therapy starts or dosage is adjusted, because depression may temporarily worsen during these times.

PATIENT TEACHING

- Advise patient to avoid exercise in hot weather to reduce the risk of dehydration and hypotension. Also instruct him to notify prescriber about prolonged diarrhea, nausea, or vomiting.
- Caution patient to avoid hazardous activities until drug's CNS effects are known.
- Instruct patient to change position slowly to minimize effects of orthostatic hypotension.
- Caution patient to avoid using aspirin or NSAIDs while taking olanzapine and fluoxetine because concomitant use can increase the risk of bleeding.
- Advise patient to notify all prescribers about olanzapine and fluoxetine therapy because of potentially dangerous drug interactions.
- Advise patient to avoid alcohol and smoking during therapy be-

cause of increased risk of adverse effects.
- Instruct patient to notify prescriber about a rash or hives.
- Tell family or caregiver to watch patient closely for suicidal tendencies, especially when therapy starts or dosage changes
- Advise patient with diabetes to monitor blood glucose level closely.

oxycodone and acetaminophen
Endocet, Oxycocet (CAN), Percocet, Percocet-Demi (CAN), Roxicet, Roxilox, Tylox

Class, Category, and Schedule
Chemical: Phenanthrene derivative (oxycodone), aminophenyl derivative (acetaminophen)
Therapeutic: Analgesic
Pregnancy category: Not rated
Controlled substance schedule: II

Indications and Dosages
▶ *To control moderate to moderately severe pain*
CAPSULES, TABLETS
Adults. 5 mg of oxycodone and 325 to 500 mg of acetaminophen (1 tablet or capsule) every 4 to 6 hr, p.r.n. *Maximum:* 4,000 mg/day of acetaminophen.
ORAL SOLUTION
Adults. 5 mg (5 ml) of oxycodone and 325 mg of acetaminophen every 4 to 6 hr, p.r.n. *Maximum:* 4,000 mg/day of acetaminophen.

Mechanism of Action
Produces a synergistic analgesic effect through two mechanisms of action. Oxycodone, a mu receptor agonist, alters the perception of and emotional response to pain at the spinal cord and higher levels of the CNS by blocking the release of inhibitory neurotransmitters, such as gamma-aminobutyric acid and acetylcholine.

Acetaminophen blocks the activity of cyclooxygenase, an enzyme necessary for prostaglandin synthesis. Prostaglandins, important mediators in the inflammatory response, cause local vasodilation with swelling and pain.

Contraindications
Hypercapnia; hypersensitivity to oxycodone, acetaminophen, or

their components; ileus; use within 14 days of MAO inhibitor therapy

Interactions

DRUGS

antacids: Decreased and delayed acetaminophen absorption

antianxiety drugs, benzodiazepines, brompheniramine, carbinoxamine, chlorpheniramine, clemastine, dimenhydrinate, diphenhydramine, doxylamine, general anesthetics, hypnotics, methdilazine, opioid antagonists, phenothiazines, promethazine, sedatives, skeletal muscle relaxants, tramadol, tricyclic antidepressants, trimeprazine: Potentiated respiratory depression from these drugs and oxycodone

anticholinergics: Possibly severe constipation and paralytic ileus

antidiarrheals: Possibly severe constipation and additive CNS depression

antihypertensives: Possibly exaggerated antihypertensive effects and risk of orthostatic hypotension

antineoplastics, immunosuppressants: Risk of masking signs of infection, such as fever and pain

barbiturates: Additive CNS depression

butorphanol, pentazocine: Possibly acute withdrawal symptoms in opioid-dependent patients, decreased analgesic effect

carbamazepine, phenobarbital, phenytoin, primidone, rifampin: Possibly a need for increased oxycodone dosage to achieve analgesia and prevent withdrawal symptoms in opioid-dependent patients; possibly an increased risk of acetaminophen-induced hepatotoxicity

cimetidine, ritonavir: Possibly apnea, confusion, disorientation, and seizures from respiratory depression and impaired CNS function, increased risk of acetaminophen-induced hepatotoxicity (ritonavir)

MAO inhibitors: Possibly fatal reactions, including cardiac arrest, coma, respiratory depression, seizures, and severe hypertension

nalbuphine, nalmefene, naloxone, naltrexone: Blocked oxycodone effects, withdrawal symptoms in opioid-dependent patients

verapamil: Increased constipation

warfarin: Increased INR and risk of bleeding

FOODS

all foods: Decreased and delayed acetaminophen absorption

ACTIVITIES

alcohol use: Additive CNS depression; increased risk of acetaminophen-induced hepatotoxicity

Adverse Reactions

CNS: Confusion, dizziness, drowsiness, euphoria, excitation, hallucinations, headache, restlessness, sedation, somnolence
CV: Bradycardia, hypotension, orthostatic hypotension, palpitations
EENT: Blurred vision, dry eyes, lens opacities, miosis
GI: Abdominal pain, constipation, elevated liver function test results, hepatotoxicity, nausea, vomiting
GU: Amenorrhea, decreased libido, erectile dysfunction, oliguria, renal tubular necrosis, urinary hesitancy, urine retention
RESP: Respiratory depression
SKIN: Erythema, flushing, pruritus, urticaria
Other: Drug tolerance, hypoprothrombinemia, physical and psychological dependence, withdrawal symptoms

Nursing Considerations

- **WARNING** Be aware that oxycodone has a high potential for abuse.
- Use drug cautiously in patients with head injury because drug may alter neurologic findings.
- Assess pain level regularly, and give drug as prescribed before pain becomes severe.
- Administer drug with a full glass of water or, to minimize GI distress, with food or milk.
- Adjust dosage to relieve pain as prescribed, keeping in mind the maximum daily dose of acetaminophen. Be prepared to adjust dosage for patient who hasn't previously received opioids until he can tolerate drug's effects.
- Avoid giving drug within 1 to 2 hours of antacids or food because of risk of decreased drug effectiveness.
- Assess for possible respiratory depression or paradoxical excitation during dosage titration.
- Assess for abdominal pain because oxycodone may mask signs and symptoms of underlying GI disorders.
- Increase patient's dietary fiber intake if needed to prevent constipation.
- Anticipate an increased risk of falling during therapy. Institute safety precautions according to facility policy.

PATIENT TEACHING
- Instruct patient not to take oxycodone and acetaminophen more often than prescribed and not to stop taking drug abruptly after long-term use.

- Encourage patient to take drug with a full glass of water and with food, if possible.
- Suggest that patient change position slowly to minimize effects of orthostatic hypotension.
- Caution patient to avoid alcohol and hazardous activities during therapy.
- Advise patient to notify prescriber about possible signs of toxicity or hypersensitivity, such as excessive light-headedness, extreme dizziness, itching, swelling, and trouble breathing.

oxycodone hydrochloride, oxycodone terephthalate, and aspirin
Endodan, Percodan, Percodan-Demi, Roxiprin

Class, Category, and Schedule
Chemical: Phenanthrene derivative (oxycodone), salicylate (aspirin)
Therapeutic: Anaglesic (oxycodone, aspirin)
Pregnancy category: Not rated (oxycodone C, aspirin D)
Controlled substance schedule: II

Indications and Dosages
▶ *To manage acute, moderate to moderately severe pain short term*
TABLETS
Adults. 2.25 mg oxycodone hydrodrochloride, 0.19 mg oxycodone terephthalate and 325 mg aspirin (1 tablet) to 4.5 mg oxycodone hydrochloride, 0.38 mg oxycodone terephthalate and 325 mg aspirin (1 tablet) every 4 to 6 hr, as needed.

Mechanism of Action
Oxycodone alters the perception of and emotional response to pain at the spinal cord and higher levels of the CNS by blocking the release of inhibitory neurotransmitters, such as gamma-aminobutyric acid and acetylcholine.

Aspirin blocks the activity of cyclooxygenase, the enzyme necessary for prostaglandin synthesis. By preventing prostaglandin synthesis, pain is relieved because prostaglandins play a role in pain transmission from the periphery to the spinal cord.

Contraindications
Allergy to tartrazine dye; asthma; bleeding problems such as hemophilia; children under age 16 with a viral illness; hypercapnia;

hypersensitivity to oxycodone, other opioids, aspirin, or their components; ileus; peptic ulcer disease; respiratory depression; severe vitamin K deficiency; upper airway obstruction; use within 14 days of MAO inhibitor therapy

Interactions
DRUGS

oxycodone
anticholinergics: Possibly severe constipation and ileus
antidiarrheals: Possibly severe constipation and additive CNS depression
antihypertensives: Possibly exaggerated antihypertensive effects and risk of orthostatic hypotension
butorphanol, pentazocine: Possibly acute withdrawal symptoms in opioid-dependent patients, decreased analgesic effects
CNS depressants: Possibly increased CNS and respiratory depression and orthostatic hypotension
MAO inhibitors: Possibly fatal reactions, including cardiac arrest, coma, respiratory depression, seizures, and severe hypertension
nalbuphine, nalmefene, naloxone, naltrexone: Blocked oxycodone effects, withdrawal symptoms in opioid-dependent patients

aspirin
ACE inhibitors: Decreased antihypertensive effect
activated charcoal: Decreased aspirin absorption
antacids, urine alkalinizers: Decreased aspirin effectiveness
anticoagulants: Increased risk of bleeding; prolonged bleeding time
carbonic anhydrase inhibitors: Salicylism
corticosteroids: Increased aspirin excretion and decreased blood level
heparin: Increased risk of bleeding
loop diuretics: Decreased effectiveness of loop diuretics
methotrexate: Increased blood level and decreased excretion of methotrexate, causing toxicity
nizatidine: Increased blood aspirin level
NSAIDs: Possibly decreased blood NSAID level and increased risk of adverse GI effects
probenecid, sulfinpyrazone: Decreased effectiveness in treating gout
urine acidifiers, such as ammonium chloride and ascorbic acid: Decreased aspirin excretion
vancomycin: Increased risk of ototoxicity
ACTIVIITES

oxycodone and aspirin
alcohol use: Additive CNS effects and increased risk of adverse GI effects

Adverse Reactions

CNS: Confusion, CNS depression, dizziness, drowsiness, euphoria, excitation, headache, sedation, somnolence

CV: Braydcardia, chest pain, hypotension, orthostatic hypotension, palpitations, tachycardia

EENT: Blurred vision, dry eyes, hearing loss, lens opacitites, miosis, tinnitus

GI: Constipation, diarrhea, elevated liver function tests results, GI bleeding, heartburn, hepatotoxicity, nausea, stomach pain, vomiting

GU: Amenorrhea, decreased libido, erectile dysfunction, oliguria, urinary hesitancy, urine retention

HEME: Decreased blood iron level, hemolytic anemia, leukopenia, prolonged bleeding time, shortened life span of RBCs, thrombocytopenia

RESP: Apnea, bronchoconstriction, bronchospasm, respiratory depression

SKIN: Ecchymosis, pruritus, rash, urticaria

Other: Anaphylaxis, angioedema, drug tolerance, physical and psychological dependence, Reye's syndrome

Nursing Considerations

- Use with extreme caution in patients with significant chronic obstructive pulmonary disease or cor pulmonale and in patients who have substantially decreased respiratory reserve, hypoxia, or hypercapnia because oxycodone can depress respiratory drive.
- Use with caution in elderly or debilitated patients and in those with severe impairment of hepatic or renal function, hypothyroidism, Addison's disease, acute alcoholism, convulsive disorders, CNS depression or coma, delirium tremens, kyphoscoliosis associated with respiratory depression, toxic psychosis, prostatic hypertrophy or urethral stricture because drug can cause hypotension, alter mental state, or depress respirations.
- Monitor patient's blood pressure because opioid analgesics such as the oxycodone-aspirin combination can cause severe hypotension.
- Monitor patients with biliary tract disease including pancreatitis for pain because the drug may cause spasm of the sphincter of Oddi.
- **WARNING** Be aware that oxycodone and aspirin combination has a high potential for abuse because of oxycodone.

- Assess pain level regularly and give drug as prescribed before pain becomes severe.
- Be prepared to adjust the oxycodone and aspirin dosage for a patient who hasn't previously received opioids until he can tolerate drug's effects.
- Assess patient for possible respiratory depression or paradoxical excitation during dosage titration.
- Monitor patient for evidence of CNS depression.
- Assess patient for abdominal pain because oxycodone may mask signs and symptoms of underlying GI disorders.
- Be aware that aspirin's anti-inflammatory and antipyretic actions may mask signs and symptoms of infection.

PATIENT TEACHING
- Tell patient to take oxycodone and aspirin with food or after meals to reduce GI distress that may occur because of aspirin. Also tell patient to take with a full glass of water and to avoid lying down for 15 to 30 minutes afterward to prevent esophageal irritation.
- Warn patient to take drug only as prescribed and needed because it can become habit-forming.
- Instruct patient to notify prescriber about worsening or breakthrough pain.
- Advise patient to avoid taking another NSAID at the same time, unless directed by prescriber because of increased risk of adverse reactions.
- Caution patient to avoid alcohol and hazardous activities during oxycodone and aspirin therapy.
- Advise patient to notify prescriber right away about possible signs of toxicity or hypersensitivity, such as excessive lightheadedness, extreme dizziness, itching, swelling, and trouble breathing.

oxycodone hydrochloride and ibuprofen
Combunox

Class, Category, and Schedule
Chemical: Phenanthrene derivative (oxycodone), propionic acid derivative (ibuprofen)
Therapeutic: Anaglesic
Pregnancy category: C
Controlled substance schedule: II

Indications and Dosages

▶ *To manage acute, moderate to severe pain short term*

TABLETS

Adults. 5 mg oxycodone and 400 mg ibuprofen (1 tablet) every 6 hr for no longer than 7 days.

Mechanism of Action

Oxycodone alters the perception of and emotional response to pain at the spinal cord and higher levels of the CNS by blocking the release of inhibitory neurotransmitters, such as gamma-aminobutyric acid and acetylcholine.

Ibuprofen blocks the activity of cyclooxygenase, the enzyme needed to synthesize prostaglandins, which mediate the inflammatory response and cause local vasodilation, swelling, and pain. By blocking cyclooxygenase and inhibiting prostaglandins, this NSAID reduces inflammatory symptoms and relieves pain.

Contraindications

Angioedema; asthma; bronchospasm; hypercapnia; hypersensitivity to oxycodone, other opioids, ibuprofen, other NSAIDs, or their components; paralytic ileus; previously experienced allergic reactions after taking aspirin or other NSAIDs; respiratory depression; treatment of perioperative pain with coronary artery bypass graft surgery; use within 14 days of MAO inhibitor therapy

Interactions

DRUGS

oxycodone and ibuprofen

antihypertensives: Possibly exaggerated antihypertensive effects and risk of orthostatic hypotension

oxycodone

anticholinergics: Possibly severe constipation and ileus

antidiarrheals: Possibly severe constipation and additive CNS depression

butorphanol, pentazocine: Possibly acute withdrawal symptoms in opioid-dependent patients, decreased analgesic effects

CNS depressants: Possibly increased CNS and respiratory depression and orthostatic hypotension

MAO inhibitors: Possibly fatal reactions, including cardiac arrest, coma, respiratory depression, seizures, and severe hypertension

nalbuphine, nalmefene, naloxone, naltrexone: Blocked oxycodone effects, withdrawal symptoms in opioid-dependent patients

ibuprofen

ACE inhibitors: Possibly decreased antihypertensive effect of ACE inhibitors

acetaminophen: Possibly increased renal effects with long-term use of both drugs

aspirin, other NSAIDs: Increased risk of bleeding and adverse GI effects

bone marrow depressants: Possibly increased leukopenic and thrombocytopenic effects of bone marrow depressants

cefamandole, cefoperazone, cefotetan: Increased risk of hypoprothrombinemia and bleeding

colchicines, platelet aggregation inhibitors: Increased risk of GI bleeding, hemorrhage, and ulcers

corticosteroids, potassium supplements: Increased risk of adverse GI effects

cyclosporine: Increased risk of nehprotoxicity from both drugs, increased blood cyclosporine level

digoxin: Increased blood digoxin level and risk of digitalis toxicity

diuretics (loop, potassium-sparing, and thiazide): Decreased diuretic and antihypertensive effects

gold compounds, nephrotoxic drugs: Increased risk of adverse renal effects

heparin, oral anticoagulants, thrombolytics: Increased anticoagulant effects, increased risk of hemorrhage

insulin, oral antidiabetics: Possibly increased hypoglycemic effects of these drugs

lithium: Increased blood lithium level

methotrexate: Decreased methotrexate clearance, increased risk of methotrexate toxicity

plicamycin, valproic acid: Increased risk of hypoprothrombinemia and GI bleeding, hemorrhage, and ulcers

probenecid: Possibly increased blood level, effectiveness, and risk of toxicity of ibuprofen

warfarin: Increased risk of serious GI bleeding because of synergistic effects

ACTIVITIES

oxycodone and ibuprofen

alcohol use: Additive CNS effects and increased risk of adverse GI effects

Adverse Reactions

CNS: Abnormal thinking, anxiety, aseptic meningitis, asthenia, chills, dizziness, drowsiness, euphoria, excitation, fever, headache, hyperkinesias, hypertonia, nervousness, sedation, somnolence, stroke

CV: Bradycardia, chest pain, fluid retention, heart failure, hypertension, hypotension, left ventricular dysfunction, MI, palpitations, peripheral edema, thrombophlebitis, thromboembolism, vasodilation

EENT: Amblyopia, blurred vision, dry eyes, epistaxis, lens opacities, miosis, stomatitis, taste perversion, tinnitus

GI: Abdominal cramps or pain, anorexia, constipation, diarrhea, distention, dyspepsia, elevated liver function test results, epigastric discomfort, flatulence, gastritis, GI bleeding or ulceration, heartburn, hepatic failure, hepatitis, indigestion, inflammation of GI tract, jaundice, melena, nausea, perforation of stomach or intestine, vomiting

GU: Acute renal failure, amenorrhea, cystitis, decreased libido, erectile dysfunction, hematuria, oliguria, renal papillary necrosis, renal toxicity, urinary frequency or hesitancy, urine retention

HEME: Agranulocytosis, anemia, aplastic anemia, eosinophilia, hemolytic anemia, neutropenia, prolonged bleeding time, thromboctopenia

RESP: Bronchospasm, dyspnea, respiratory depression, wheezing

MS: Arthritis, back pain

SKIN: Blisters, diaphoresis, ecchymosis, erythema multiforme, exfoliative dermatitis, photosensitivity, pruritus, rash, Stevens-Johnson syndrome, toxic epidermal necrolysis, urticaria

Other: Anaphylaxis, angioedema, drug tolerance, flulike symptoms, hypokalemia, infection, physical and psychological dependence, weight gain, withdrawal symptoms

Nursing Considerations

- Use with extreme caution in patients with significant chronic obstructive pulmonary disease or cor pulmonale and in patients who have substantially decreased respiratory reserve, hypoxia, or hypercapnia because oxycodone can depress respiratory drive.
- Use oxycodone and ibuprofen with extreme caution in patients with a history of ulcer disease or GI bleeding because NSAIDs such as ibuprofen increase the risk of GI bleeding and ulceration. Expect to use oxycodone and ibuprofen for the shortest time possible.
- Also use oxycodone and ibuprofen cautiously in patients with inflammatory bowel disease because drug may worsen intestinal

inflammation and cause diarrhea. If diarrhea causes severe dehydration, drug may need to be stopped.

- Use oxycodone and ibuprofen cautiously in patients with cerebrovascular disease, coronary artery disease, congestive heart failure, or uncontrolled epilepsy because of the risk of severe complications.

- Use drug cautiously in patients with hypertension, and monitor blood pressure closely throughout therapy. Ibuprofen may cause hypertension or worsen it.

- Use oxycodone and ibuprofen with caution in elderly or debilitated patients and in those with severe impairment of hepatic or renal function, hypothyroidism, Addison's disease, acute alcoholism, convulsive disorders, CNS depression or coma, delirium tremens, kyphoscoliosis associated with respiratory depression, toxic psychosis, prostatic hypertrophy or urethral stricture because drug can cause hypotension, alter mental state, or depress respirations.

- Monitor patient's cardiovascular status closely because use of NSAIDs such as ibuprofen increases the risk of serious cardiovascular adverse effects. Also be aware that opioid analgesics such as oxycodone can cause severe hypotension.

- Be aware that serious GI tract ulceration, bleeding, and perforation may occur without warning symptoms. Elderly patients are at greater risk. To minimize risk, give oxycodone and ibuprofen with food. If GI distress occurs, withhold drug and notify prescriber immediately.

- Monitor patient, especially if elderly, for less common but serious adverse GI reactions, including anorexia, constipation, diverticulitis, dysphagia, esophagitis, gastritis, gastroenteritis, gastroesophageal reflux disease, hemorrhoids, hiatal hernia, melena, stomatitis, and vomiting.

- Monitor liver function test results and serum uric acid level. If abnormal liver test results persist or worsen, if patient has signs and symptoms consistent with liver disease, or if systemic changes such as eosinophilia or rash occur, discontinue drug immediately and notify prescriber.

- Monitor renal function—especially in patients with existing renal disease, heart failure, or liver dysfuction; those taking diuretics or ACE inhibitors; and the elderly—because patients are at increased risk for renal papillary necrosis and other renal injury. Notify prescriber if abnormalities develop, and expect to discontinue drug.

- Be aware that, although rare, aseptic meningitis with fever and coma has occurred in patients taking ibuprofen, especially patients who have systemic lupus and related connective tissue disease. Notify prescriber immediately if patient develops fever and CNS dysfunction.
- Report weight gain of more than 1 kg (2 lb) in 24 hours, which suggests fluid retention.
- If patient takes a potassium-sparing diuretic, check for elevated serum potassium level, as ordered.
- Monitor patient's hemoglobin and hematocrit, as ordered, during prolonged therapy because oxycodone and ibuprofen may cause anemia.
- **WARNING** If patient has bone marrow suppression or is receiving an antineoplastic drug, monitor laboratory results (including WBC count), and watch for signs and symptoms of infection because anti-inflammatory and antipyretic actions of ibuprofen may mask signs and symptoms, such as fever and pain.
- Assess patient's skin regularly for rash or other signs of hypersensitivity reaction because ibuprofen is an NSAID and may cause serious skin reactions without warning, even in patients with no history of NSAID sensitivity. At first sign of reaction, stop drug and notify prescriber.
- Monitor patients with biliary tract disease including pancreatitis for pain because the drug may cause spasm of the sphincter of Oddi.
- **WARNING** Be aware that oxycodone and ibuprofen have a high potential for abuse. Assess patient for evidence of physical and psychological dependence.
- Assess pain level regularly and give drug as prescribed before pain becomes severe.
- Monitor patient for evidence of CNS depression caused by oxycodone.
- Be prepared to adjust dosage for patient who hasn't previously received opioids until he can tolerate drug's effects.
- Assess patient for possible respiratory depression or paradoxical excitation during dosage titration.
- Assess patient for abdominal pain because oxycodone may mask signs and symptoms of underlying GI disorders.
- Be aware that the anti-inflammatory and antipyretic actions of ibuprofen may mask signs and symptoms of infection in the patient.

PATIENT TEACHING

- Tell patient to alert prescriber before taking hydrocodone and ibuprofen if he has a history of ulcers, bleeding problems, hypertension, or heart or renal disease; if he takes a diuretic; or if he's over age 65.
- Tell patient to take oxycodone and ibuprofen with food or after meals to reduce GI distress that may occur as a result of ibuprofen. Also advise patient to take the drug with a full glass of water and to avoid lying down for 15 to 30 minutes afterward to prevent esophageal irritation.
- Instruct patient not to take oxycodone and ibuprofen more often than prescribed and that drug should not be used longer than 7 days.
- Instruct patient to notify prescriber about worsening or breakthrough pain
- Advise patient to avoid taking another NSAID at the same time, unless directed by prescriber because of increased risk of adverse reactions.
- Tell patient to avoid alcohol and aspirin during oxycodone and ibuprofen therapy.
- Advise patient to notify prescriber about possible signs of toxicity or hypersensitivity, such as excessive light-headedness, extreme dizziness, itching, swelling of any body area and trouble breathing.
- Encourage the patient wear sunscreen and protective clothing when going outdoors to minimize the possible effects of photosensitivity.
- Warn patient to avoid hazardous activities until drug's CNS effects are known.
- Instruct patient to notify prescriber if he has ringing or buzzing in the ears, impaired hearing, dizziness, vision changes, swelling, or weight gain.
- Advise patient to avoid taking two different NSAIDs at the same time, unless directed, and to alert prescriber before taking oxycodone and ibuprofen if he has ever had an allergic reaction to an analgesic or fever-reducing drug. Also advise patient to consult prescriber before taking aspirin or other OTC analgesics or ingesting alcohol.
- Inform patient that drug increases the risk of inflammation, bleeding, ulceration, and perforation of the stomach and intestine, possibly without warning. If patient feels suddenly ill, he should seek medical attention.

- Warn patient of the possibility of hepatic injury, and instruct patient to notify prescriber if he develops signs and symptoms of hepatotoxicity such as nausea, fatigue, lethargy, pruritus, jaundice, right upper quadrant tenderness, and flulike symptoms.
- Explain that oxycodone and ibuprofen may increase the risk of serious adverse cardiovascular reactions; urge patient to seek immediate medical attention if signs or symptoms arise, such as chest pain, shortness of breath, weakness, and slurring of speech.
- Alert patient to the possibility of rare but serious skin reactions. Encourage him to seek immediate medical attention if he develops rash, blisters, itching, fever, or other indications of hypersensitivity.
- Advise patient to change position slowly to minimize effects of orthostatic hypotension.
- Advise women of childbearing age to consult with prescriber if she becomes pregnant or thinks she could be pregnant.

pentazocine hydrochloride and acetaminophen

Talacen

Class, Category, and Schedule

Chemical: Benzaocine (pentazocine), acetamide (acetaminophen)
Therapeutic: Analgesic (pentazocine, acetaminophen)
Pregnancy category: C
Controlled substance schedule: IV

Indications and Dosages

▶ *To relieve mild to moderate pain*

CAPLETS

Adults. 25 mg pentazocine and 650 mg acetaminophen (1 caplet) every 4 hr, as needed. *Maximum:* 150 mg pentazocine and 3,900 mg acetaminophen every 24 hr.

Contraindications

Hypersensitivity to pentazocine, acetaminophen or their components; severe hepatic impairment

Mechanism of Action

Pentazocine binds with opioid receptors, primarily kappa and sigma receptors, at many CNS sites to alter the perception of and emotional response to pain.

Acetaminophen inhibits the enzyme cyclooxygenase, thereby blocking prostaglandin production and interfering with pain impulse generation in the peripheral nervous system.

Interactions
DRUGS

pentazocine and acetaminophen
anticholinergics: Increased risk of urine retention and severe constipation

pentazocine
antidiarrheals, antiperistaltics: Increased risk of severe constipation and CNS depression
antihypertensives, diuretics, other hypotension-producing drugs: Additive hypotensive effects
buprenorphine: Increased respiratory depression
CNS depressants: Increased CNS depression, increased risk of habituation
MAO inhibitors: Increased risk of unpredictable, severe, and sometimes fatal adverse reactions
metoclopramide: Antagonized effects of metoclopramide on GI motility
naloxone: Antagonized analgesic, CNS, and respiratory depressant effects of pentazocine
naltrexone: Withdrawal symptoms in patients who are physically dependent on pentazocine
neuromuscular blockers: Increased respiratory depression
opioid analgesics: Increased analgesia, CNS depression, and hypotensive effects; possibly withdrawal symptoms

acetaminophen
barbiturates, carbamazepine, hydantoins, isoniazid, rifampin, sulfinpyrazone: Decreased therapeutic effects and increased hepatotoxic effects of acetaminophen
lamotrigine, loop diuretics: Possibly decreased therapeutic effects of these drugs
oral contraceptives: Decreased effectiveness of acetaminophen

probenecid: Possibly increased therapeutic effects of acetaminophen
propranolol: Possibly increased action of acetaminophen
zidovudine: Possibly decreased effects of zidovudine
ACTIVITIES
pentazocine and acetaminophen
alcohol use: Additive CNS depression and increased risk of habituation (pentazocine); increased risk of hepatotoxicity (acetaminophen)

Adverse Reactions

CNS: Dizziness, drowsiness, euphoria, fatigue, headache, lightheadedness, nervousness, nightmares, restlessness, weakness
CV: Hypotension, tachycardia
EENT: Blurred vision, diplopia, dry mouth, laryngeal edema, larngospasm
ENDO: Hypoglycemic coma
GI: Abdominal pain, constipation, hepatotoxicity, jaundice, nausea, vomiting
GU: Decreased urine output, dysuria, urinary frequency
HEME: Hemolytic anemia, leukopenia, neutropenia, pancytopenia, thrombocytopenia
RESP: Atelectasis, bronchospasm, dyspnea, hypoventilation, wheezing
SKIN: Diaphoresis, facial flushing, pruritus, rash, toxic epidermal necrolysis, urticaria
Other: Angioedema, physical and psychological dependence

Nursing Considerations

• Use pentazocine and acetaminophen with extreme caution in patients who have a head injury, an intracranial lesion, or increased intracranial pressure because drug may mask neurologic signs and symptoms.
• Use pentazocine and acetaminophen cautiously in patients who are physically dependent on opioid agonists because drug may prompt withdrawal symptoms; in patients with acute MI because drug's cardiovascular effects can increase cardiac workload; in patients with renal or hepatic dysfunction because drug is metabolized in the liver and excreted in urine; and in patients with respiratory conditions because drug depresses the respiratory system.
• Monitor patient for evidence of CNS depression.
• Before and during long-term therapy, monitor patient's liver function test results, including AST, ALT, and bilirubin levels, as ordered.

- Evaluate for therapeutic response, including report of decreased pain and body movements that would indicate pain relief has occurred.
- Monitor renal function in patient on long-term therapy. Keep in mind that blood or albumin in urine may indicate nephritis; decreased urine output may indicate renal failure.
- Expect to reduce dosage for patients with renal dysfunction.

PATIENT TEACHING
- Instruct patient to take pentazocine and acetaminophen exactly as prescribed and not to increase dosage or frequency without consulting prescriber.
- Caution patient that prolonged use of pentazocine and acetaminophen may result in drug dependence.
- Inform patient about possible dizziness, drowsiness, and other adverse CNS effects. Advise her to avoid hazardous activities until drug's CNS effects are known.
- Caution patient not to use alcohol or OTC drugs without consulting prescriber.
- Instruct patient to notify prescriber about worsening or breakthrough pain.
- Advise patient to notify prescriber if she notices signs of an allergic reaction, such as a rash or itching.
- Teach patient to recognize signs of hepatotoxicity, such as bleeding, easy bruising, and malaise, which commonly occurs with chronic overdose.

pentazocine hydrochloride and naloxone hydrochloride
Talwin NX

Class, Category, and Schedule
Chemical: Benzaocine (pentazocine), thebaine derivative (naloxone)
Therapeutic: Analgesic (pentazocine), opioid antagonist (naloxone)
Pregnancy category: C
Controlled substance schedule: IV

Indications and Dosages
▶ *To relieve mild to moderate pain*
TABLETS
Adults. 50 mg pentazocine and 0.5 mg naloxone (1 tablet) every 3 to 4 hr, increased to 100 mg pentazocine and 1 mg naloxone

(2 tablets), as needed. *Maximum:* 600 mg pentazocine and 6 mg naloxone daily.

Mechanism of Action

Pentazocine binds with opioid receptors, primarily kappa and sigma receptors, at many CNS sites to alter the perception of and emotional response to pain.

While naloxone briefly and competitively antagonizes mu, kappa, and sigma receptors in the CNS, thus reversing the analgesia, hypotension, respiratory depression, and sedation caused by most opioids, this effect is negligible in this combination product because oral bioavailability is poor and is used instead to decrease risk of physical dependence on pentazocine.

Contraindications

Hypersensitivity to pentazocine, naloxone, or their components

Interactions

DRUGS

pentazocine

antidiarrheals, antiperistaltics: Increased risk of severe constipation and CNS depression

antihypertensives, diuretics, other hypotension-producing drugs: Additive hypotensive effects

buprenorphine: Decreased pentazocine effectiveness, increased respiratory depression

CNS depressants: Increased CNS depression, increased risk of habituation

hydroxyzine, other opioid analgesics: Increased analgesia, CNS depression, and hypotensive effects

MAO inhibitors: Increased risk of unpredictable, severe, and sometimes fatal adverse reactions

metoclopramide: Antagonized metoclopramide effects on GI motility

naloxone: Antagonized analgesic, CNS, and respiratory depressant effects of pentazocine

naltrexone: Withdrawal symptoms in patients who are physically dependent on pentazocine

neuromuscular blockers: Increased respiratory depression

naloxone

butorphanol, nalbuphine, pentazocine: Reversal of these drugs' analgesic and adverse effects

opioid analgesics: Reversal of these drugs' analgesic and adverse effects, and possibly withdrawal symptoms in opioid-dependent patients

Adverse Reactions

CNS: Chills, dizziness, drowsiness, excitement, euphoria, fatigue, headache, insomnia, irritability, light-headedness, nervousness, nightmares, paresthesia, restlessness, weakness

CV: Hypertension, hypotension, tachycardia

EENT: Blurred vision, diplopia, dry mouth, laryngeal edema, laryngospasm

GI: Constipation, hepatotoxicity, nausea, vomiting

GU: Decreased urine output, dysuria, urinary frequency, urinary retention

RESP: Atelectasis, bronchospasm, dyspnea, hypoventilation, wheezing

SKIN: Diaphoresis, erythema multiforme, facial flushing, pruritus, rash, Stevens-Johnson syndrome, toxic epidermal necrolysis, urticaria

Other: Angioedema, physical and psychological dependence

Nursing Considerations

- Use with extreme caution in patients who have a head injury, an intracranial lesion, or increased intracranial pressure because drug may mask neurologic signs and symptoms.
- Use drug cautiously in patients who are physically dependent on opioid agonists because drug may prompt withdrawal symptoms and in patients with acute MI because drug's cardiovascular effects can increase cardiac workload.
- Evaluate for therapeutic response, including report of decreased pain and body movements that would indicate pain relief has occurred.

PATIENT TEACHING

- Instruct patient to take pentazocine and naloxone exactly as prescribed and not to increase dosage or frequency without consulting prescriber.
- Caution patient that prolonged use of pentazocine and naloxone may result in drug dependence because pentazocine may overcome naloxone effect with increased doses.
- Inform patient about possible dizziness, drowsiness, and other adverse CNS effects. Advise her to avoid hazardous activities until drug's CNS effects are known.
- Caution patient not to use alcohol or OTC drugs without consulting prescriber.

- Instruct patient to notify prescriber about worsening or breakthrough pain.
- Advise patient to notify prescriber if she notices signs of an allergic reaction, such as a rash or itching.

perphenazine and amitriptyline hydrochloride

Etrafon 2-10, Etrafon-A, Etrafon Forte, Triavil, Triavil 2-10, Triavil 2-25, Triavil 4-10, Triavil 4-25

Class and Category

Chemical: Piperazine phenothiazine (perphenazine), tertiary amine (amitriptyline)

Therapeutic: Antipyschotic (perphenazine), antianxiety, antidepressant (amitriptyline)

Pregnancy category: Not rated (perphenazine not rated, amitriptyline D)

Indications and Dosages

▶ *To treat moderate to severe anxiety or agitation and depression associated with chronic disease or when anxiety and depression cannot be clearly differentiated; to treat depression in schizophrenic patients*

TABLETS

Adults. 2 to 4 mg perphenazine and 10 to 50 mg amitriptyline (1 to 2 tablets depending on strength used) t.i.d. or q.i.d.

Mechanism of Action

Perphenazine depresses areas of the brain that governs activity and aggression, including the cerebral cortex, hypothalamus, and limbic system through an unknown mechanism. This action may be responsible for controlling agitation and aggression seen in schizophenia.

Amitriptyline blocks serotonin and norepinephrine reuptake by adrenergic nerves. By doing so, it raises serotonin and norepinephrine levels at nerve synapses. This action may elevate mood and reduce depression.

Contraindications

Blood dysrasias; bone marrow depression; cerebral arteriosclerosis; coma; concurrent use of CNS depressants (large doses); coronary artery disease; acute recovery phase after MI; hepatic impairment; hypersensitivity to perphenazine, amitriptyline, other phenothiazines, or their components; myeloproliferative disorders; severe CNS depression; severe hypertension or hypotension; subcortical brain damage; use of MAO inhibitor within 14 days

Interactions

DRUGS

perphenazine and amitriptyline
anticholinergics: Increased adverse anticholinergic effects

perphenazine
aluminum- and magnesium-containing antacids, antidiarrheals (adsorbent): Decreased absorption of oral perphenazine
amantadine, antidyskinetics, antihistamines: Increased adverse anticholinergic effects
amphetamines: Decreased therapeutic effects of both drugs
anticonvulsants: Decreased seizure threshold, inhibited metabolism and toxicity of anticonvulsant
antithyroid drugs: Increased risk of agranulocytosis
apomorphine: Additive CNS depression, decreased emetic response to apomorphine if perphenazine is given first
appetite suppressants (except phenmetrazine): Antagonized anorectic effect of appetite suppressants
beta blockers: Increased blood levels of both drugs and risk of arrhythmias, hypotension, irreversible retinopathy, and tardive dyskinesia
bromocriptine: Possibly interference with bromocriptine's effects
CNS depressants: Increased CNS and respiratory depression and hypotensive effects
dopamine: Antagonized peripheral vasoconstriction with high doses of dopamin
ephedrine: Decreased vasopressor response to ephedrine
epinephrine: Blocked alpha-adrenergic effects of epinephrine, possibly causing severe hypotension and tachycardia
hepatotoxic drugs: Increased risk of hepatotoxicity
hypotension-causing drugs: Increased risk of severe orthostatic hypotension
levodopa: Inhibited antidyskinetic effects of levodopa
lithium: Possibly neurotoxicity (disorientation, extrapyramidal symptoms, unconsciousness)
maprotiline, selective serotonin reuptake inhibitors, tricyclic antidepressants: Prolonged and intensified sedative and anticholinergic effects of these drugs or perphenazine
metrizamide: Decreased seizure threshold
opioid analgesics: Increased CNS and respiratory depression, and

increased risk of orthostatic hypotension and severe constipation

ototoxic drugs, especially antibiotics: Possibly masking of some symptoms of ototoxicity, such as dizziness, tinnitus, and vertigo

probucol, other drugs that prolong the QT interval: Prolonged QT interval, which may increase risk of ventricular tachycardia

thiazide diuretics: Possibly hyponatremia and water intoxication

amitriptyline

antihypertensives, clonidine, guanethidine: Decreased antihypertensive effects

barbiturates: Decreased serum amitriptyline level

carbamazepine: Decreased serum amitriptyline level and increased serum carbamazepine level, which increases therapeutic and toxic effects of carbamazepine

cimetidine, disulfiram, fluoxetine, fluvoxamine, haloperidol, H₂-receptor antagonists, methylphenidate, oral contraceptives, paroxetine, phenothiazines, sertraline: Increased serum amitriptyline level

cisapride: Possibly prolonged QT interval and risk of arrhythmias

dicumarol: Increased anticoagulant effect of dicumarol

epinephrine, norepinephrine: Increased effects of these drugs

levodopa: Decreased levodopa absorption; sympathetic hyperactivity, sinus tachycardia, hypertension, agitation

MAO inhibitors: Possibly seizures and death

thyroid replacement drugs: Arrhythmias and increased antidepressant effects

ACTIVITIES

perphenazine

alcohol use: Increased CNS and respiratory depression, hypotensive effects, and risk of heatstroke

amitriptyline

smoking: Decreased amitriptyline effects

Adverse Reactions

CNS: Anxiety, ataxia, behavioral changes, cerebral edema, chills, coma, delusions, disorientation, dizziness, drowsiness, extrapyramidal reactions, fatigue, fever, headache, insomnia, neuroleptic malignant syndrome, nightmares, peripheral neuropathy, seizures, suicidal ideation, syncope, tardive dyskinesia (persistent), tremor

CV: Arrhythmias (including prolonged AV conduction and heart block), bradycardia, cardiac arrest, cardiomyopathy, hypertension, hypotension, MI, nonspecific ECG changes, orthostatic hypotension, palpitations, tachycardia

EENT: Abnormal taste, black tongue, blurred vision, dry mouth, glaucoma, increased salivation, laryngeal edema, miosis, mydraisis, nasal congestion, ocular changes (corneal opacification, retinopathy), tinnitus

ENDO: Decreased libido, galactorrhea, gynecomastia, hyperglycemia, hypoglycemia, syndrome of inappropriate ADH secretion

GI: Abnormal cramps, anorexia, constipation, diarrhea, fecal impaction, flatulence, ileus, increased appetite, nausea, vomiting

GU: Bladder paralysis, ejaculation failure, impotence, libido changes, menstrual irregularities, polyuria, testicular swelling, urinary frequency, urinary hesitancy, urinary incontinence, urine retention

HEME: Agranulocytosis, bone marrow depression, eosinophilia, hemolytic anemia, leukopenia, pancytopenia, thrombocytopenic purpura

RESP: Asthma

SKIN: Alopecia, diaphoresis, eczema, erythema, exfoliative dermatitis, flushing, hyperpigmentation, jaundice, pallor, photosensitivity, pruritus, purpura, urticaria

Other: Anaphylaxis, angioedema, weight gain

Nursing Considerations

- Use cautiously in patient with a history of seizures, urine retention, or angle-closure glaucoma because of amitriptyline's atropine-like effects.
- Use cautiously in patient with hepatic, pulmonary or renal dysfunction and in elderly patients who are at increased risk for increased plasma concentrations and tardive dyskinesia from perphenazine.
- **WARNING** Don't give an MAO inhibitor within 14 days of perphenazine and amitriptyline therapy because of the risk of seizures and death.
- Be aware that elderly patients with dementia-related psychosis are at increased risk for death when treated with antipsychotic drugs such as perphenazine. Monitor patient closely.
- Closely monitor patient with cardiovascular disorder because perphenazine and amitriptyline may cause arrhythmias, such as conduction abnormalities or sinus tachycardia.
- Monitor blood pressure and assess patient for hypotension or hypertension.
- Avoid abrupt withdrawal of drug after prolonged therapy; otherwise withdrawal symptoms such as nausea, headache, vertigo, and nightmares may occur.

- Monitor patient being treated for depression with perphenazine and amitriptyline closely for suicidal tendencies, especially when therapy starts or dosage changes; depression may worsen temporarily during these times.
- Monitor patient's blood counts and liver and renal function test results during therapy. Notify prescriber of any abnormalities.
- Monitor patient's temperature frequently and notify prescriber if it rises; a significant increase suggests drug intolerance to perphenazine.
- Stay alert for behavior changes, such as hallucinations and decreased interest in personal appearance. Be aware that psychosis may develop in schizophrenic patients and symptoms may increase in paranoid patients.
- Assess patient regularly to determine effectiveness of perphenazine and amitriptyline therapy.

PATIENT TEACHING

- Instruct patient to take perphenazine and amitriptyline exactly as prescribed to ensure optimal effectiveness and minimize adverse reactions.
- Instruct patient to avoid using alcohol, OTC drugs that contain alcohol or to smoke during perphenazine and amitriptyline therapy because of potential adverse effects.
- Caution patient to avoid hazardous activities until drug's CNS effects are known.
- Tell family or caregiver to observe patient closely for evidence of suicidal tendencies, especially when therapy starts or dosage changes.
- Advise patient to avoid excessive sun exposure and to protect skin when outdoors.
- Instruct patient to notify prescriber about persistent or severe adverse reactions.
- Urge patient to comply with long-term follow up to detect adverse reactions and need for dosage adjustments.

propoxyphene hydrochloride and acetaminophen

E-Lor, Wygesic

propoxyphene napsylate and acetaminophen

Darvocet-N 50, Darvocet-N 100, Propacet 100

Class, Category, and Schedule
Chemical: Synthetic opioid (propoxyphene), acetamide (acetaminophen)
Therapeutic: Analgesic (propoxyphene, acetaminophen)
Pregnancy category: C
Controlled substance schedule: IV

Indications and Dosages
▶ *To relieve mild to moderate pain*
TABLETS (PROPOXYPHENE HYDROCHLORIDE AND ACETAMINOPHEN)
Adults. 65 mg propoxyphene and 650 mg acetaminophen
(1 tablet) every 4 hr, p.r.n.
TABLETS (PROPOXYPHENE NAPSYLATE AND ACETAMINOPHEN)
Adults. 100 mg propoxyphene and 650 mg acetaminophen (1 or
2 tablets depending on strength prescribed) every 4 hr, p.r.n.

Mechanism of Action
Propoxyphene strongly antagonizes mu receptors, blocking release of such inhibitory neurotransmitters as gamma-aminobutyric acid (GABA) and acetylcholine. It also mediates analgesia by changing pain perception at the spinal
cord and higher CNS levels and by altering the emotional response to pain.
   Acetaminophen acts centrally to increase the pain threshold by inhibiting
cyclooxygenase, an enzyme involved in prostaglandin synthesis.

Contraindications
Hypersensitivity to propoxyphene, acetaminophen or their components, respiratory depression, severe asthma, upper airway obstruction, use within 14 days of MAO inhibitor therapy

Interactions
DRUGS
propoxyphene and acetaminophen
anticholinergics: Decreased onset of action of acetaminophen; increased risk of severe constipation and urine retention
carbamazepine: Decreased therapeutic effects and increased hepatotoxic effects of acetaminophen; possibly carbamazepine toxicity
from propoxyphene use
propoxyphene
amphetamines: Possibly fatal seizures (with propoxyphene overdose)
antidiarrheals: Severe constipation, possibly increased CNS depression

antihypertensives: Possibly exaggerated antihypertensive response
buprenorphine: Possibly decreased propoxyphene effectiveness, increased respiratory depression
CNS depressants: Increased CNS and respiratory depression, hypotensive effects, and risk of habituation
hydroxyzine: Increased analgesic, CNS depressant, and hypotensive effects of propoxyphene
MAO inhibitors: Severe, possibly fatal reactions, including hypertensive crisis
metoclopramide: Possibly antagonized effects of metoclopramide on GI motility
naloxone: Antagonized analgesic and CNS and respiratory depressant effects of propoxyphene
naltrexone: Risk of withdrawal symptoms in patients who are dependent on propoxyphene, possibly decreased analgesic effect of propoxyphene
neuromuscular blockers: Additive respiratory depressant effects
opioid analgesics: Additive CNS and respiratory depressant and hypotensive effects
warfarin: Increased anticoagulation effects
acetaminophen
barbiturates, hydantoins, isoniazid, rifampin, sulfinpyrazone: Decreased therapeutic effects and increased hepatotoxic effects of acetaminophen
lamotrigine, loop diuretics: Possibly decreased therapeutic effects of these drugs
oral contraceptives: Decreased effectiveness of acetaminophen
probenecid: Possibly increased therapeutic effects of acetaminophen
propranolol: Possibly increased action of acetaminophen
zidovudine: Possibly decreased effects of zidovudine
ACTIVITIES
propoxyphene
alcohol use: Increased CNS and respiratory depression, hypotensive effects, and risk of habituation
nicotine chewing gum, other smoking deterrents, smoking cessation: Decreased effectiveness of propoxyphene

Adverse Reactions
CNS: Dizziness, drowsiness, fatigue, insomnia, light-headedness, malaise, nervousness, sedation, tremor
CV: Orthostatic hypotension, tachycardia
EENT: Blurred vision, diplopia, dry mouth, tinnitus
ENDO: Hypoglycemic coma

GI: Abdominal cramps or pain, anorexia, constipation, jaundice, hepatotoxicity, nausea, vomiting
GU: Decreased urine output
HEME: Hemolytic anemia (with long-term use), leukopenia, neutropenia, pancytopenia, thrombocytopenia
MS: Muscle weakness
RESP: Dyspnea, respiratory depression, wheezing
SKIN: Facial flushing, pruritus, rash, urticaria
Other: Angioedema, psychological dependence

Nursing Considerations

• Use propoxyphene and acetaminophen cautiously in patients with hepatic or renal dysfunction because delayed elimination may occur. Monitor hepatic and renal function test results.
• Monitor patient's response to drug for pain relief.
• **WARNING** Be aware that long-term, high dose propoxyphene and acetaminophen therapy may lead to psychological dependence in some patients. Assess for opioid and alcohol use, which increase the risk of drug abuse or dependence.
• Be aware that abruptly discontinuing drug can result in withdrawal symptoms.
• Know that the dosage of acetaminophen in the combination drug should not exceed 4 g/day to reduce the risk of acetaminophen-induced hepatotoxicity.

PATIENT TEACHING
• Inform patient she may take propoxyphene and acetaminophen with food if she experiences GI distress.
• Instruct patient not to take more than the prescribed amount because drug may be addictive.
• Caution patient to avoid hazardous activities until drug's CNS effects are known.
• Instruct patient to avoid alcohol and other sedatives while taking drug.
• Advise smokers to inform prescriber if they try to stop smoking during propoxyphene and acetaminophen therapy because increased drug dosage may be required for effective analgesia.
• Urge patient to notify prescriber immediately if pain isn't relieved or worsens.
• Advise her to contact prescriber before taking other prescription or OTC drugs; they may contain acetaminophen and lead to toxicity.
• Teach patient to recognize signs of hepatotoxicity, such as bleeding, easy bruising, and chronic overdose.

propoxyphene hydrochloride, aspirin, and caffeine
Darvon Compound-65, PC-Cap, Propoxyphene Compound-65
propoxyphene napsylate and aspirin
Darvon-N (CAN)
propoxyphene napsylate, aspirin and caffeine
Darvon-N Compound (CAN)

Class, Category, and Schedule
Chemical: Synthetic opioid (propoxyphene), salicylate (aspirin), xanthine derivative (caffeine)
Therapeutic: Analgesic (propoxyphene, aspirin), CNS stimulant (caffeine)
Pregnancy category: NR
Controlled substance schedule: IV

Indications and Dosages
▶ *To relieve mild to moderate pain*
CAPSULES (PROPOXYPHENE HYDROCHLORIDE, ASPIRIN AND CAFFEINE)
Adults. 65 mg propoxyphene, 389 mg aspirin, and 32.4 mg caffeine (1 capsule) every 4 hr, p.r.n. *Maximum:* 390 mg propoxyphene hydrochloride daily
TABLETS (PROPOXYPHENE HYDROCHLORIDE, ASPIRIN, AND CAFFEINE)
Adults. 65 mg propoxyphene, 375 mg aspirin, and 30 mg caffeine (1 tablet) every 4 hr, p.r.n. *Maximum:* 390 mg propoxyphene hydrochloride daily
CAPSULES (PROPOXYPHENE NAPSYLATE AND ASPIRIN)
Adults. 100 mg propoxyphene and 325 mg aspirin (1 capsule) every 4 hr, p.rn. *Maximum:* 600 mg of propoxyphene napsylate daily.
CAPSULES (PROPOXYPHENE NAPSYLATE, ASPIRIN, AND CAFFEINE)
Adults. 100 mg propoxyphene napsylate, 375 mg aspirin, and 30 mg caffeine (1 capsule) every 4 hr, p.rn. *Maximum:* 600 mg propoxyphene napsylate daily.

Contraindications
Allergy to tartrazine dye; asthma; bleeding problems such as hemophilia; hypersensitivity to propoxyphene, aspirin, caffeine or their components; peptic ulcer disease; respiratory depression; upper airway obstruction; use within 14 days of MAO inhibitor therapy

Mechanism of Action

Propoxyphene strongly antagonizes mu receptors, blocking release of such inhibitory neurotransmitters as gamma-aminobutyric acid (GABA) and acetylcholine. It also mediates analgesia by changing pain perception at the spinal cord and higher CNS levels and by altering the emotional response to pain.

Aspirin blocks the activity of cyclooxygenase, the enzyme necessary for prostaglandin synthesis. By preventing prostaglandin synthesis, pain is relieved because prostaglandins play a role in pain transmission from the periphery to the spinal cord.

Caffeine is a competitive, nonselective antagonist of adenosine receptor sites, which results in stimulation of the central nervous system to counteract the sedative properties of propoxyphene.

Interactions

DRUGS

propoxyphene

amphetamines: Possibly fatal seizures (with propoxyphene overdose)

anticholinergics: Increased risk of severe constipation and urine retention

antidiarrheals: Severe constipation, possibly increased CNS depression

antihypertensives: Possibly exaggerated antihypertensive response

buprenorphine: Possibly decreased propoxyphene effectiveness, increased respiratory depression

carbamazepine: Possibly carbamazepine toxicity from propoxyphene use

CNS depressants: Increased CNS and respiratory depression, hypotensive effects, and risk of habituation

hydroxyzine: Increased analgesic, CNS depressant, and hypotensive effects of propoxyphene

MAO inhibitors: Severe, possibly fatal reactions, including hypertensive crisis

metoclopramide: Possibly antagonized effects of metoclopramide on GI motility

naloxone: Antagonized analgesic and CNS and respiratory depressant effects of propoxyphene

naltrexone: Risk of withdrawal symptoms in patients who are dependent on propoxyphene, possibly decreased analgesic effect of propoxyphene

neuromuscular blockers: Additive respiratory depressant effects

opioid analgesics: Additive CNS and respiratory depressant and hypotensive effects

warfarin: Increased anticoagulation effects

aspirin

ACE inhibitors: Decreased antihypertensive effect

activated charcoal: Decreased aspirin absorption

antacids, urine alkalinizers: Decreased aspirin effectiveness

anticoagulants: Increased risk of bleeding; prolonged bleeding time

carbonic anhydrase inhibitors: Salicylism

corticosteroids: Increased excretion and decreased blood level of aspirin

heparin: Increased risk of bleeding

loop diuretics: Decreased effectiveness of loop diuretics

methotrexate: Increased blood level and decreased excretion of methotrexate, causing toxicity

nizatidine: Increased blood aspirin level

NSAIDs: Possibly decreased blood NSAID level and increased risk of adverse GI effects

probenecid, sulfinpyrazone: Decreased effectiveness in treating gout

urine acidifiers, such as ammonium chloride and ascorbic acid: Decreased aspirin excretion

vancomycin: Increased risk of ototoxicity

caffeine

aspirin: Increased GI absorption of aspirin

beta-adrenergic agonists: Possibly enhanced cardiac inotropic effects of beta-adrenergic agonists

cimetidine, contraceptives (oral), disulfiram, fluoroquinolones: Decreased hepatic metabolism of caffeine resulting in increased caffeine effect

clozapine: Possibly increased clozapine levels resulting in increased incidence of clozapine induced adverse reactions

lithium: Enhanced renal clearance of lithium

mexiletine: Decreased caffeine elimination resulting in increased caffeine effect

phenytoin: Increased caffeine clearance resulting in decreased caffeine effect

theophylline: Reduced theophylline clearance with ingestion of more than 120 mg caffeine daily

ACTIVITIES

propoxyphene, aspirin and caffeine

alcohol use: Increased risk of ulcers (aspirin, caffeine); increased CNS and respiratory depression, hypotensive effects, and risk of habituation (propoxyphene)

propoxyphene

nicotine chewing gum, other smoking deterrents, smoking cessation: Decreased effectiveness of propoxyphene

Adverse Reactions

CNS: Confusion, CNS depression, dizziness, drowsiness, fatigue, insomnia, light-headedness, malaise, nervousness, sedation, tremor

CV: Orthostatic hypotension, tachycardia

EENT: Blurred vision, diplopia, dry mouth, hearing loss, tinnitus

ENDO: Hypoglycemic coma

GI: Abdominal cramps or pain, anorexia, constipation, diarrhea, GI bleeding, heartburn, nausea, vomiting

GU: Decreased urine output

HEME: Decreased blood iron level, leukopenia, prolonged bleeding time, shortened life span of RBCs, thrombocytopenia

MS: Muscle weakness

RESP: Dyspnea, respiratory depression, wheezing

SKIN: Ecchymosis, facial flushing, pruritus, rash, urticaria

Other: Angioedema, Reye's syndrome, psychological dependence

Nursing Considerations

- Be aware that drug should not be taken by patients who are suicidal or prone to addiction.
- Use drug cautiously in patients with hepatic or renal dysfunction because delayed elimination may occur. Monitor hepatic and renal function test results.
- Monitor patient's response to drug for pain relief.
- **WARNING** Be aware that long-term, high-dose propoxyphene therapy may lead to psychological dependence in some patients. Assess for opioid and alcohol use, which increase the risk of drug abuse or dependence.
- Be aware that abruptly discontinuing drug can result in withdrawal symptoms.
- Question patient taking drug regularly about presence of tinnitus. This reaction usually occurs when blood aspirin level reaches or exceeds maximum for therapeutic effect.

PATIENT TEACHING

- Tell patient to take this drug with food to minimize stomach upset.
- Instruct patient not to take more than the prescribed amount because drug may be addictive.
- Caution patient to avoid hazardous activities until drug's CNS effects are known.

- Instruct patient to avoid alcohol and other sedatives while taking drug.
- Advise smokers to inform prescriber if they attempt to stop smoking during propoxyphene and aspirin or propoxyphene, aspirin and caffeine therapy because increased drug dosage may be required for effective analgesia.
- Urge patient to notify prescriber immediately if pain isn't relieved or worsens.
- Tell patient to consult prescriber before taking drug with any prescription or OTC preparation that may contain aspirin to avoid aspirin overdose.

sumatriptan and naproxen sodium
Treximet

Class and Category
Chemical: Serotonin 5-HT₁ receptor agonist (sumatriptan), propionic acid derivative, NSAID (naproxen)
Therapeutic: Antimigraine (sumatriptan, naproxen)
Pregnancy category: C, D (3rd trimester)

Indications and Dosages
▶ *To relieve acute migraine attacks, with or without aura*
TABLETS
Adults. *Initial:* 85 mg sumatriptan and 500 mg naproxen
(1 tablet) as soon as possible after onset of migraine symptoms, repeated, if needed and prescribed, after 2 hours. *Maximum:*
170 mg sumatriptan and 1,000 mg naproxen (2 tablets) in
24 hours.

Mechanism of Action
Sumatriptan may stimulate 5-HT₁ receptors, causing selective vasoconstriction of inflamed and dilated cranial blood vessels in carotid circulation, thus decreasing carotid artery blood flow and relieving acute migraines.

Naproxen blocks cyclooxygenase, the enzyme needed to synthesize prostaglandins, which mediate the inflammatory response and cause local vasodilation, swelling, and pain. Thus, naproxen, an NSAID, reduces symptoms of inflammation and relieves migraine pain.

Contraindications
Angioedema, asthma, bronchospasm, nasal polyps, rhinitis, or

urticaria induced by aspirin, iodides, or other NSAIDs; basilar or hemiplegic migraine; cardiovascular disease; hepatic impairment; history of coronary artery bypass surgery; hypersensitivity to sumatriptan, naproxen, or their components; ischemic cerebrovascular, heart, or peripheral vascular disease; uncontrolled hypertension; use within 14 days of an MAO inhibitor; use within 24 hours of another serotonin 5-HT$_1$ receptor agonist or an ergotamine-containing or ergot-type drug

Interactions
DRUGS

sumatriptan and naproxen
lithium: Increased risk of lithium toxicity
sumatriptan
antidepressants: Increased risk of serious adverse effects
citalopram, duloxetine, escitalopram, fluoxetine, fluvoxamine, paroxetine, sertraline, venlafaxine: Increased risk of life-threatening serotonin syndrome
ergotamine-containing drugs: Possibly additive or prolonged vasoconstrictive effects
MAO inhibitors: Risk of decreased sumatriptan clearance; increased risk of serious adverse effects
naproxen
ACE inhibitors: Decreased antihypertensive effects; increased risk of renal dysfunction
antacids containing aluminum hydroxide or magnesium oxide, cholestyramine, sucralfate: Possibly delayed absorption of naproxen
anticoagulants, thrombolytics: Prolonged PT, increased risk of bleeding
antihypertensives: Decreased effectiveness of antihypertensive
aspirin: Decreased aspirin effectiveness
beta blockers: Decreased antihypertensive effects of these drugs
bone marrow depressants, such as aldesleukin and cisplatin: Increased risk of leukopenia and thrombocytopenia
cefamandole, cefoperazone, cefotetan, plicamycin, valproic acid: Increased risk of hypoprothrombinemia and bleeding
cimetidine: Altered blood naproxen level
colchicine, glucocorticoids, NSAIDs, potassium supplements, salicylates: Increased GI irritability and bleeding
cyclosporine, gold compounds, nephrotoxic drugs: Increased risk of nephrotoxicity
digoxin: Increased blood digoxin level and increased risk of digitalis toxicity

diuretics: Decreased diuretic effectiveness
furosemide: Decreased natriuretic effect
insulin, oral antidiabetic drugs: Increased effectiveness of these drugs; risk of hypoglycemia
methotrexate: Increased risk of methotrexate toxicity
phenytoin: Increased blood phenytoin level
probenecid: Increased risk of naproxen toxicity
ACTIVITIES
naproxen
alcohol use, smoking: Increased risk of naproxen-induced GI ulceration

Adverse Reactions

CNS: Anxiety, aseptic meningitis, atypical depression, chills, cognitive impairment, decreased concentration, depression, dizziness, dream disturbances, drowsiness, fatigue, fever, headache, insomnia, light-headedness, malaise, sedation, seizures, stroke, vertigo, weakness

CV: Arrhythmias; chest heaviness, pain, pressure, or tightness; coronary artery vasospasm; ECG changes; edema; heart failure; hypertension; hypotension; MI; palpitations; tachycardia; vasculitis

EENT: Abnormal vision; mouth, nose, or throat discomfort; papilledema; papillitis; photophobia; retrobulbar optic neuritis; stomatitis; tinnitus; tongue soreness or numbness; vision or hearing changes

ENDO: Hyperglycemia, hypoglycemia

GI: Abdominal pain, anorexia, colitis, constipation, diarrhea, diverticulitis, dyspepsia, dysphagia, elevated liver enzyme levels, esophagitis, flatulence, gastritis, gastroenteritis, gastroesophageal reflux disease, GI bleeding and ulceration, heartburn, hematemesis, hepatitis, indigestion, melena, nausea, pancreatitis, peptic ulceration, perforation of stomach or intestines, stomatitis, vomiting

GU: Elevated serum creatinine level, glomerulonephritis, hematuria, infertility (in women), interstitial nephritis, menstrual irregularities, nephrotic syndrome, renal failure, renal papillary necrosis

HEME: Agranulocytosis, anemia, aplastic anemia, eosinophilia, granulocytopenia, hemolytic anemia, leukopenia, neutropenia, pancytopenia, thrombocytopenia

MS: Jaw discomfort, muscle cramps or weakness, myalgia, neck pain or stiffness

RESP: Asthma, dyspnea, eosinophilic pneumonitis, respiratory depression
SKIN: Alopecia, dermatitis, diaphoresis, ecchymosis, erythema multiforme, flushing, pallor, photosensitivity, pruritus, pseudoporphyria, purpura, rash, Stevens-Johnson syndrome, systemic lupus erythematosus, toxic epidermal necrolysis, urticaria
Other: Anaphylaxis, angioedema, hyperkalemia

Nursing Considerations

- Sumatriptan and naproxen isn't recommended for patients with advanced renal disease and shouldn't be given to elderly patients because they're more likely to have decreased hepatic function, coronary artery disease, and more pronounced blood pressure increases.
- Use sumatriptan and naproxen with extreme caution in patients with a history of ulcer disease or GI bleeding because NSAIDs such as naproxen increase the risk of GI bleeding and ulceration.
- Use sumatriptan and naproxen cautiously in patients with hypertension, and monitor blood pressure closely. Drug may cause hypertension or worsen it.
- Assess patient for chest pain. Also, monitor blood pressure in patients who have coronary artery disease before, during, and for at least 1 hour after sumatriptan and naproxen administration.
- Don't give sumatriptan and naproxen within 24 hours of another 5-HT_1 receptor agonist, such as naratriptan, rizatriptan, or zolmitriptan.
- Serious GI tract ulceration, bleeding, and perforation may occur without warning symptoms. Elderly patients and patients taking oral anticoagulants are at greater risk. If GI distress occurs, withhold drug and notify prescriber immediately.
- If patient has renal disease, monitor renal function closely during therapy with sumatriptan and naproxen. Usually, NSAIDs are avoided in these patients.
- **WARNING** Monitor patient closely for thrombotic events, including MI and stroke, because NSAIDs such as naproxen increase the risk.
- Monitor patient—especially if elderly—for less common but serious adverse GI reactions, including anorexia, constipation, diverticulitis, dysphagia, esophagitis, gastritis, gastroenteritis, gastroesophageal reflux disease, hemorrhoids, hiatal hernia, melena, stomatitis, and vomiting.

- Monitor patient's liver function test results because, in rare cases, elevated enzyme levels may progress to severe hepatic reactions, including fatal hepatitis, liver necrosis, and hepatic failure.
- Monitor BUN and serum creatinine levels in elderly patients, patients taking diuretics or ACE inhibitors, and patients with heart failure, impaired renal function, or hepatic dysfunction. Naproxen may cause renal failure.
- Monitor CBC for decreased hemoglobin and hematocrit because drug may worsen anemia.
- **WARNING** If patient has bone marrow suppression or is receiving treatment with an antineoplastic drug, monitor laboratory results (including WBC count), and watch for evidence of infection. Anti-inflammatory and antipyretic actions of naproxen may mask signs and symptoms, such as fever and pain.
- Assess patient's skin regularly for rash or other hypersensitivity reaction because naproxen may cause serious skin reactions without warning, even in patients with no history of NSAID sensitivity. At first sign of reaction, stop drug and notify prescriber.
- Tell prescriber if patient complains of vision changes; patient may need ophthalmic exam.
- For patients with seizure disorder, institute seizure precautions according to facility policy because sumatriptan of drug may lower seizure threshold.

PATIENT TEACHING
- Advise patient to take sumatriptan and naproxen as soon as possible after onset of migraine symptoms.
- Urge patient to contact prescriber and avoid taking drug if headache symptoms aren't typical.
- Caution patient not to exceed recommended dose because serious adverse reactions may occur.
- Stress importance of waiting 2 hours before taking second dose, if prescribed.
- Tell patient to swallow tablets whole and not to break, crush, or chew them.
- Tell patient to take sumatriptan and naproxen with a full glass of water and to remain upright for 15 to 30 minutes afterward to prevent drug from lodging in esophagus and causing irritation.

- Caution patient to avoid hazardous activities until drug's CNS effects are known.
- Tell pregnant patient to avoid naproxen-containing products such as sumatriptan and naproxen late in pregnancy.
- Encourage patient to lie down in a dark, quiet room after taking drug to help relieve migraine.
- Instruct patient to seek emergency care for chest, jaw, or neck tightness after taking sumatriptan and naproxen because drug may cause coronary artery vasospasm. Later doses may require ECG monitoring.
- Urge patient to notify prescriber about palpitations or rash.
- Advise patient with seizure disorder that drug may lower seizure threshold.

tramadol hydrochloride and acetaminophen
Ultracet

Class and Category
Chemical: Cyclohexanol (tramadol), aminophenol derivative (acetaminophen)
Therapeutic: Opioid analgesic (tramadol), non-opioid analgesic (acetaminophen)
Pregnancy category: C

Indications and Dosages
▶ *To provide short-term management of acute pain*
TABLETS
Adults. Initial: 75 mg tramadol and 650 mg acetaminophen every 4 to 6 hr, p.r.n. *Maximum:* 300 mg tramadol and 2,600 mg acetaminophen/day for up to 5 days.
DOSAGE ADJUSTMENT Dosing interval increased to 12 hr and maximum dose reduced to 75 mg tramadol and 650 mg acetaminophen/dose in patients with creatinine clearance of less than 30 ml/min/1.73 m².

Contraindications
Acute intoxication with alcohol, centrally acting analgesics, hypnotics, opioids, or psychotropic drugs; hypersensitivity to tramadol, other opioids, acetaminophen, or components of these drugs

Mechanism of Action

Tramadol binds with mu receptors and also inhibits the reuptake of norepinephrine and serotonin. These actions may account for the drug's analgesic effect.

Acetaminophen blocks the activity of cyclooxygenase, an enzyme needed for prostaglandin synthesis. Prostaglandins are important mediators of the inflammatory response that cause local vasodilation, swelling, and pain.

Interactions

DRUGS

acetaminophen-containing products: Increased risk of hepatotoxicity

carbamazepine: Increased metabolism of tramadol and increased risk of seizures; possibly significantly reduced analgesic effect of tramadol

CNS depressants: Increased risk of CNS and respiratory depression

CYP 2D6 inhibitors, such as amitriptyline, fluoxetine, and paroxetine: Possibly inhibited tramadol metabolism

digoxin: Possibly digitalis toxicity, although rare

MAO inhibitors, selective serotonin reuptake inhibitors: Increased risk of seizures and serotonin syndrome

neuroleptics, opioids, tricyclic antidepressants: Increased risk of seizures

quinidine: Increased blood tramadol level

warfarin: Possibly elevated PT and altered effects of warfarin

FOODS

any food: Possibly delayed peak plasma time

ACTIVITIES

alcohol use: Increased risk of CNS and respiratory depression

Adverse Reactions

CNS: Dizziness, insomnia, seizures, somnolence
EENT: Dry mouth
GI: Anorexia, constipation, diarrhea, hepatotoxicity, nausea
GU: Prostate disorder
RESP: Respiratory depression
SKIN: Increased sweating, pruritus
Other: Hypersensitivity, physical and psychological dependence

Nursing Considerations

• Be aware that tramadol and acetaminophen shouldn't be given to patients with a history of anaphylactoid reactions to codeine or other opioid analgesics.

• Avoid giving tramadol and acetaminophen to patients with acute abdominal conditions because drug may mask signs and symptoms and disrupt assessment of the abdomen.

• Monitor liver function test results, as appropriate, and notify prescriber of abnormal results. This drug combination isn't recommended for patients with hepatic impairment.

• After patient receives first dose of tramadol and acetaminophen, watch for allergic reactions, including angioedema, bronchospasm, pruritus, Stevens-Johnson syndrome, toxic epidermal necrolysis, and urticaria. Also watch for evidence of anaphylaxis, such as dyspnea and hypotension.

• If patient has respiratory depression, assess respiratory status often, and expect to give a nonopioid analgesic—not tramadol and acetaminophen.

• If patient develops respiratory depression, expect to give naloxone. Watch for seizures, because naloxone may increase this risk. Take seizure precautions.

• Assess respiratory status often if patient has increased intracranial pressure or head injury because of possible increased carbon dioxide retention and CSF pressure, either of which may cause respiratory depression. Also, be aware that tramadol may constrict pupils, obscuring evidence of intracranial complications.

• **WARNING** Watch for seizures in patients with epilepsy, a history of seizures, or an increased risk of seizures, such as those with head injury, metabolic disorders, alcohol or drug withdrawal, or CNS infection.

• Expect to taper tramadol and acetaminophen dosage rather than stopping drug abruptly to avoid such acute withdrawal symptoms as anxiety, diarrhea, insomnia, nausea, pain, panic attacks, paresthesia, piloerection, rigors, sweating, tremor, and upper respiratory symptoms.

• Because tramadol and acetaminophen may lead to physical and psychological dependence and abuse, assess patient for evidence of dependence or abuse, such as drug-seeking behavior. Be aware that this drug shouldn't be used in patients with a history of dependence on other opioids because dependence may recur.

PATIENT TEACHING

• Caution patient that taking more of this drug than prescribed or taking it more often than prescribed can lead to serious adverse reactions, including respiratory depression, seizures, hepatotoxicity, and death.

- Caution patient not to stop drug abruptly.
- Caution patient to avoid hazardous activities until drug's adverse effects are known.
- Warn patient to avoid alcohol while taking tramadol and acetaminophen.
- Warn patient to avoid other drugs that contain tramadol or acetaminophen, including OTC preparations.
- Urge patient to notify prescriber if she becomes pregnant, thinks she might be pregnant, or is trying to become pregnant.

Dermatologic Drugs

adapalene 0.1% and benzoyl peroxide 2.5%

Epiduo

Class and Category

Chemical: Naphthoic acid derivative (adapalene), benzoic acid (benzoyl peroxide)
Therapeutic: Antiacne and keratolytic (adapalene, benzoic acid)
Pregnancy category: C

Indications and Dosages

▶ *To treat acne vulgaris*

GEL

Adults and adolescents age 12 and over. Applied as a thin layer to affected areas once daily after skin has been washed, rinsed, and patted dry.

Mechanism of Action

Adapalene binds to specific retinoic acid nuclear receptors to modulate cell differentiation, keratinization, and inflammation. These actions help improve acne vulgaris.

Benzoyl peroxide works against *Propionibacterium acnes* by releasing active oxygen to cause cell death. It also has some keratolytic effect, which produces comedone lysis and drying and also desquamative effects.

Contraindications

Hypersensitivity to adapalene, benzoyl peroxide, other benzoic acid derivatives, or their components

Interactions

DRUGS

resorcinol, salicyclic acid, sulfur-containing drugs: Possibly cumulative irritant effect

Adverse Reactions

SKIN: Burning, contact dermatitis, dryness, erythema, irritation, photosensitivity, pruritus, scaling

Nursing Considerations

- Wash hands before and after application.
- When applying drug, avoid contact with patient's eyes, mucous membranes, and open wounds.
- Assess skin for drug effectiveness and localized adverse effects.
- If adverse effects are troublesome to patient, notify prescriber and expect application frequency to be decreased or drug discontinued.

PATIENT TEACHING

- Instruct patient to place a pea-size portion of gel on his fingertip and then dab it onto his chin, cheeks, nose, and forehead before blending over face.
- Tell patient to apply gel exactly as prescribed and to avoid contact with eyes, inside the nose or mouth, and all mucous membranes. Remind him that using more than the recommended amount will not produce faster results but may increase the severity of adverse reactions.
- Instruct patient not to apply to cuts, abrasions, or eczematous or sunburned skin. Tell him to rinse the drug immediately with water if it contacts these areas.
- Caution patient not to use waxing as a depilatory method on skin being treated with drug.
- Warn patient not to use any other topical acne preparation unless instructed by prescriber and to avoid other potentially irritating topical products such as medicated or abrasive soaps and cleansers, soaps and cosmetics that have strong skin-drying effect, and products that contain high concentrations of alcohol, astringent, spices, or lime.
- Reassure patient that adverse skin reactions most likely will occur during the first 4 weeks of therapy and usually will lessen over time. If adverse effects are troublesome, encourage patient to use a moisturizer or notify prescriber.
- Urge patient to avoid exposure to sunlight, including sunlamps, and to take precautions when outdoors by wearing a hat and protective clothing and using a sunscreen of SPF 15 or higher.
- Alert patient that weather extremes, such as wind or cold, may be irritating to skin areas being treated with adapalene and benzoyl peroxide.
- Warn patient that drug may bleach hair and colored fabric.

benzocaine 14%, butyl aminobenzoate 2%, and tetracaine hydrochloride 2%
Cetacaine

Class and Category
Chemical: Aminobenzoate (benzocaine, butyl aminobenzoate), amethocaine (tetracaine)
Therapeutic: Local anesthetic (benzocaine, butyl aminobenzoate, tetracaine)
Pregnancy category: NR

Indications and Dosages
▶ *To anesthetize all accessible mucous membranes except eyes*
GEL, LIQUID, OINTMENT, SPRAY
Adults. Sprayed or applied with cotton applicator to affected area for 1 second or less at needed time.

Mechanism of Action
Benzocaine, butyl aminobenzoate, and tetracaine act by reversibly blocking nerve conduction to prevent pain perception.

Contraindications
Application to eyes or large denuded or inflamed areas; cholinesterase deficiencies; hypersensitivity to benzocaine, butyl aminobenzoate, tetracaine, or their components

Adverse Reactions
SKIN: Local site reactions such as dehydration of epithelium, edema, erythema, pruritus, rash, urticaria, vesiculation, oozing
Other: Anaphylaxis, methemoglobinemia

Nursing Considerations
• Ask any female patient of childbearing age whether she is or could be pregnant. Notify prescriber before applying benzocaine, butyl aminobenzoate, and tetracaine because drug isn't recommended during early pregnancy.
• Apply directly to the site where pain control is needed. There's no need to dry the area before applying the drug. If applying to the face, avoid contact with patient's eyes.
• Don't spray or apply under dentures or on cotton rolls because doing so increases the risk of an escharotic effect. Never spray or apply for more than 2 seconds because doing so increases

the risk of serious, local adverse reactions and may induce methemoglobinemia.

- **WARNING** If application exceeds 2 seconds, notify prescriber and monitor patient for cyanosis. If if occurs, be prepared to provide supportive care and counteract drug with methylene blue, if prescribed.
- In debilitated, elderly, or acutely ill patients, reduce dosage.
- Assess patient's response, and notify prescriber if it's less than optimal; tolerance varies among patients.

PATIENT TEACHING

- Warn patient to follow application directions exactly to prevent serious local skin reactions at application site.
- Instruct patient to alert prescriber if pain control is inadequate.

benzoyl peroxide 5% and sulfur 2%
Sulfoxyl Lotion Regular
benzoyl peroxide 10% and sulfur 5%
Sulfoxyl Lotion Strong

Class and Category

Chemical: Benzoic acid derivative (benzoyl peroxide), nonmetal element (sulfur)
Therapeutic: Antiacne and keratolyitc (benzoyl peroxide, sulfur)
Pregnancy category: C

Indications and Dosages

▶ *To treat acne vulgaris*

LOTION

Adults and adolescents. Applied to affected areas once daily for 1 wk and then b.i.d. thereafter, as tolerated and needed.

Mechanism of Action

Benzoyl peroxide exerts antibacterial action against *Propionibacerium acnes*, an anaerobe found in sebaceous follicles and comedones of acne, by releasing active oxygen to cause cell death. It also has some keratolytic effect, which produces comedone lysis and drying and desquamative effects. These contribute to the improvement of acne vulgaris.

Sulfur is thought to also inhibit *Propionibacerium acnes* and the formation of fatty acids through unknown mechanisms. It relieves the plugging and rupturing of follicles, easing the evacuation of comedones and promoting peeling of the skin to reduce acne vulgaris symptoms.

Contraindications

Hypersensitivity to benzoyl peroxide, other benzoic acid derivatives, sulfur, or their components

Adverse Reactions

SKIN: Excessive erythema and peeling

Nursing Considerations

- Be aware that benzoyl peroxide 5% and sulfur 2% (Sulfoxyl Lotion Regular) is recommended for use first; if tolerated, patient may be advanced to benzoyl peroxide 10% and sulfur 5% (Sulfoxyl Lotion Strong).

PATIENT TEACHING

- Stress the importance of continuous use to obtain maximum effectiveness of benzoyl peroxide and sulfur lotion.
- Instruct patient to shake container well before applying and to cleanse affected area with a non-medicated soap before application.
- Inform patient that visible improvement may take up to 3 weeks and that maximum improvement may take up to 12 weeks of drug use.
- Tell patient to notify prescriber about excessive erythema and peeling because strength or frequency of benzoyl peroxide and sulfur lotion may need to be decreased.

calcipotriene hydrate 0.005% and betamethasone dipropionate 0.064%

Taclonex, Taclonex Scalp

Class and Category

Chemical: Synthetic vitamin D_3 analogue (calcipotrine), synethetic corticosteroid (betamethasone)
Therapeutic: Skin cell growth inhibitor (calcipotriene), anti-inflammatory (betamethasone)
Pregnancy category: C

Indications and Dosages

▶ *To treat psoriasis vulgaris*
OINTMENT
Adults. Applied to affected skin areas and rubbed in gently and completely once daily for up to 4 weeks. *Maximum:* 100 grams per week.

▶ *To treat moderate to severe psoriasis vulgaris of the scalp*

SUSPENSION
Adults. Applied to affected areas of scalp and rubbed in gently once daily for 2 to 8 weeks or until scalp areas clear. *Maximum:* 100 grams per week.

Mechanism of Action

Calcipotriene, a synthetic vitamin D_3 derivative, is a seco-steroid hormone that works locally in an unknown manner to control overproduction of skin cells in areas affected by psoriasis.

Betamethasone, a corticosteroid, may decrease the number and activity of cells involved in the inflammatory response (such as mast cells, eosinophils, basophils, lymphocytes, macrophages, and neutrophils) to relieve psoriasis symptoms.

Contraindications

Calcium metabolism disorders; erythrodermic, exfoliative, and pustular psoriasis; hypersensitivity to calcipotriene, betamethasone, other corticosteroids, or their components

Interactions

DRUGS

calcipotriene
anticonvulsants, cimetidine, thiazide diuretics: Increased vitamin D catabolism
betamethasone
corticosteroids: Increased risk of adverse reactions

Adverse Reactions

CNS: Headache
EENT: Nasopharyngitis, upper respiratory tract infection
ENDO: Cushing syndrome, hyperglycemia, hypothalamic-pituitary-adrenal (HPA) axis suppression
SKIN: Burning senstation, ecchymosis, erythema, folliculitis, hand dermatitis, irritation, pustular psoriasis, pruritus, scaly rash, skin atrophy or hypopigmentation, worsening of psoriasis
Other: Hypercalcemia

Nursing Considerations

- Do not apply calcipotriene and betamethasone ointment to face, axillae, or groin.
- Do not apply drug to any area with pre-existing skin atrophy because it could become worse.
- Monitor patient's serum calcium level, as ordered, because cal-

cipotriene and betamethasone may cause hypocalcemia.

- Monitor patient for HPA axis suppression, especially if using drug over a large body surface area. No more than 30% of total body surface should be treated with calcipotriene and betamethasone at any one time to help prevent HPA axis suppression. If suppression is suspected, contact prescriber and prepare patient for adrenocorticotropic hormone stimulation, morning plasma cortisol, and urine free-cortisol tests, as ordered. If confirmed, expect to withdraw the drug and substitute a less potent drug, as prescribed.
- Don't use calcipotriene and betamethasone under occlusive dressings because of the increased risk of systemic absorption.
- Report infection at application site because drug will need to be discontinued until infection clears.

PATIENT TEACHING
- Instruct patient to use calcipotriene and betamethasone ointment or suspension exactly as prescribed and for the length of time prescribed, even when symptoms improve.
- Teach patient to wash her hands before and after applying drug.
- Tell patient to shake suspension well before applying and to store container at room temperature.
- Inform patient that it may be helpful to part hair before applying suspension to scalp. Instruct patient not to wash her hair right after applying drug to scalp. Also tell her to discuss safety of chemical hair treatments with prescriber before having them done and, if approved by prescriber, to avoid chemical hair treatment for 12 hours before or after drug application.
- Remind patient that drug should not be applied to unaffected areas or to face, axillae, or groin. Also remind her to avoid contact with eyes, mouth, or open wounds, including cuts and scrapes.
- Tell patient not to cover treated area with dressing unless instructed to do so by prescriber.
- Inform female patients that drug is not for vaginal use.
- Instruct patient to notify prescriber if symptoms don't improve during treatment or if they become worse.
- Urge patient to notify prescriber about adverse reactions at application site.
- Advise patient to check with prescriber before using any other products that contain calipotriene or a cortiscosteroid.
- Warn patient to avoid excessive exposure of treated areas to sunlight, including tanning booths and sun lamps.

clindamycin phosphate 1% and benzoyl peroxide 5%
BenzaClin, Duac

clindamycin phosphate 1.2% and benzoyl peroxide 2.5%
Acanya

Class and Category
Chemical: Lincosamide (clindamycin), benzoic acid derivative (benzoyl peroxide)
Therapeutic: Antiacne, antibiotic (clindamycin, benzoyl peroxide), keratolytic (benzoyl peroxide)
Pregnancy category: C

Indications and Dosages
▶ *To treat acne vulgaris*
GEL (BENZACLIN)
Adults and adolescents. Applied to affected areas b.i.d., morning and evening, after skin has been washed, rinsed with warm water, and patted dry.
GEL (ACANYA, DUAC)
Adults and adolescents. Applied as pea-size amount to affected areas once daily in evening, after skin has been washed, rinsed with warm water, and patted dry.

Mechanism of Action
Clindamycin inhibits protein synthesis against *Propionibacerium acnes,* an anaerobe found in sebaceous follicles and comedones of acne, by binding to the 50S subunits of bacterial ribosomes and preventing peptide bond formation, which causes bacterial cells to die. This eradicates the bacterial infection present in acne vulgaris.

Benzoyl peroxide exerts antibacterial action against *Propionibacerium acnes* by releasing active oxygen to cause cell death. It also has some keratolytic effect, which produces comedone lysis and drying and desquamative effects. These contribute to the improvement of acne vulgaris.

Contraindications
History of regional enteritis, ulcerative colitis, or antibiotic-related colitis; hypersensitivity to clindamycin, benzoyl peroxide, other benzoic acid derivatives, lincomycin, or their components

Interactions
DRUGS
clindamycin
erythromycin: Possibly blocked access of clindamycin to its site of action

neuromuscular blockers: Increased neuromuscular blockade

Adverse Reactions
EENT: Mouth ulcerations

GI: Abdominal cramps, diarrhea (including bloody diarrhea), pseudomembranous colitis, severe colitis

GU: Vagnitis

SKIN: Dry or peeling skin, erythema, photosensitivity, pruritus

Other: Anaphylaxis, angioedema

Nursing Considerations
• Be aware that clindamycin and benzoyl peroxide should be used cautiously in patients using topical acne therapy because of possible cumulative irritation, especially if the patient uses peeling, desquamating, or abrasive agents.

• Don't give drug with products that contain erythromycin because clindamycin and erythromycin may inactivate each other. Notify prescriber if patient is using an erythromycin product.

• When applying drug, avoid contact with patient's eyes and mucous membranes.

• Observe patient for signs of superinfection, such as vaginal itching and sore mouth. If present, notify prescriber.

• Monitor patient closely for diarrhea, which may herald pseudomembranous colitis because clindamycin is absorbed systemically. If diarrhea occurs, notify prescriber and expect to stop topical application of drug. If pseudomembranous colitis occurs, expect to stop drug and possibly administer fluids, electrolytes, protein, and an antibiotic effective against *Clostridium difficile.*

• **WARNING** Monitor patient closely for severe allergic reactions such as angioedema and anaphylaxis. Discontinue drug immediately and provide supportive care, as appropriate.

PATIENT TEACHING

• Instruct patient to wash the affected area, rinse with warm water, and gently pat area dry before applying clindamycin and benzolyl peroxide gel.

• Tell patient to apply gel exactly as prescribed and to avoid contact with eyes, inside the nose, mouth, and all mucous membranes.

- Warn patient not to use any other topical acne preparation unless instructed by prescriber.
- Urge patient to minimize exposure to sunlight and to take precautions when outdoors, such as wearing a hat and protective clothing and using a sunscreen that's SPF 15 or higher.
- Tell patient to report adverse reactions to prescriber, especially abdominal cramps, diarrhea, and signs of superinfection, such as vaginal itching or sore mouth. If patient develops an allergic reaction, such as severe swelling of any part of body or shortness of breath, instruct him to discontinue drug immediately and seek emergency care.
- Warn patient that drug may bleach hair or colored fabric.
- Tell patient to discard any unused product after 3 months.

clindamycin phosphate 1.2% and tretinoin 0.025%

Ziana

Class and Category

Chemical: Lincosamide (clindamycin), retinoid (tretinoin)
Therapeutic: Antiacne, antibiotic (clindamycin), keratolytic (tretinoin)
Pregnancy category: C

Indications and Dosages

▶ *To treat acne vulgaris*
GEL
Adults and adolescents age 12 and over. Pea-size amount applied to fingertip and then dotted onto chin, cheeks, nose, and forehead and gently rubbed over entire face at bedtime.

Mechanism of Action

Clindamycin inhibits protein synthesis against *Propionibacterium acnes,* an anaerobe found in sebaceous follicles and comedones of acne, by binding to the 50S subunits of bacterial ribosomes and preventing peptide bond formation, which causes bacterial cells to die. This eradicates the bacterial infection present in acne vulgaris.

Tretinoin decreases cohesiveness of follicular epithelial cells with decreased microcomedo formation. It also stimulates mitotic activity and increased turnover of follicular epithelial cells, causing extrusion of comedones.

Contraindications

History of regional enteritis, ulcerative colitis, or antibiotic-related colitis; hypersensitivity to clindamycin, tretinoin, or their components

Interactions

DRUGS

clindamycin

erythromycin: Possibly blocked access of clindamycin to its site of action

ACTIVITIES

clindamycin and tretinoin

topical products with strong skin-drying effect or high concentrations of alcohol, astringent, spices, or lime: Increased risk of skin dryness or irritation

Adverse Reactions

EENT: Nasopharyngitis, pharynolaryngeal pain, sinusitis
GI: Abdominal cramps, diarrhea (including bloody diarrhea), pseudomembranous colitis, severe colitis
RESP: Cough
SKIN: Burning, dryness, erythema, photosensitivity, pruritus, scaling, stinging

Nursing Considerations

- Don't give drug with products that contain erythromycin because clindamycin and erythromycin may inactive each other.
- When applying drug, avoid contact with patient's eyes, mucous membranes, and open wounds.
- **WARNING** Monitor patient closely for diarrhea, which may herald pseudomembranous colitis because clindamycin is absorbed systemically. If diarrhea occurs, notify prescriber and expect to stop topical application of drug. If pseudomembranous colitis occurs, expect to stop drug and possibly administer fluids, electrolytes, protein, and an antibiotic effective against *Clostridium difficile.*

PATIENT TEACHING

- Instruct patient to apply a pea-size portion of gel to a fingertip and then dab onto chin, cheeks, nose, and forehead before blending over face at bedtime.
- Tell patient to apply gel exactly as prescribed and to avoid contact with eyes, inside the nose, mouth, mucous membranes, and open wounds, including cuts and scratches.

- Warn patient not to use any other topical acne preparation unless instructed by prescriber.
- Tell patient to report adverse reactions to prescriber, especially abdominal cramps and diarrhea.
- Urge patient to avoid exposure to sunlight, including sunlamps, and to take precautions when outdoors by wearing a hat and protective clothing and using a sunscreen of SPF 15 or higher.

clotrimazole 1% and betamethasone dipropionate 0.05%

Lotrisone

Class and Category

Chemical: Imidazole (clotrimazole), corticosteroid (betamethasone)
Therapeutic: Antifungal (clotrimazole), anti-inflammatory (betamethasone)
Pregnancy category: C

Indications and Dosages

▶ *To treat symptomatic inflammatory tinea pedis, tinea cruris, or tinea corporis caused by* Epidermophyton floccosum, Trichophyton mentagrophytes, *or* Trichophyton rubrum

CREAM, LOTION

Adults. Sufficient amount applied to affected skin areas b.i.d. in the morning and evening. *Maximum:* 45 grams (cream) or 45 ml (lotion) per week for 2 wk (tinea corporis or cruris) or 4 wk (tinea pedis).

Contraindications

Hypersensitivity to clotrimazole, betamethasone, other corticosteroids or imidazoles, or their components

---

Mechanism of Action

Clotrimazole binds to one of the cytochrome P-450 enzymes inhibiting 14-alpha-demethylation of lanosterol in fungi. This leads to an accumulation of 14-alpha-methysterols and reduced concentrations of ergosterol, a sterol essential for the development of fungal cytoplasmic membrane. Clotrimazole also may affect the electron transport system to inhibit fungal growth.

Betamethasone may decrease the number and activity of cells involved in the inflammatory response, such as mast cells, eosinophils, basophils, lymphocytes, macrophages, and neutrophils.

Interactions
DRUGS
betamethasone
other corticosteroids: Increased risk of adverse reactions

Adverse Reactions
CNS: Paresthesia
EENT: Perioral dermatitis
ENDO: Cushing's syndrome, hyperglycemia, hypothalamic-pituitary-adrenal (HPA) axis suppression
SKIN: Acneiform eruptions, allergic contact dermatitis, atrophy or maceration of the skin, blisters, burning, dryness, ecchymoses, erythema, folliculitis, hypertrichosis, hypopigmentation, increased sensitization, irritation, localized edema, miliaria, peeling, pruritus, rash, secondary infection, stinging, striae, urticaria

Nursing Considerations
- Monitor patient for HPA axis suppression, especially if using clotrimazole and betamethasone cream or lotion over a large surface, for longer than recommended time (2 weeks for tinea corporis or cruris or 4 weeks for tinea pedis), or with other corticosteroids. If suppression is suspected, contact prescriber and prepare patient for ACTH stimulation, morning plasma cortisol, and urine free-cortisol tests, as ordered. If confirmed, expect to withdraw the drug, reduce the frequency of application, or substitute a less potent corticosteroid, as prescribed.
- Don't use clotrimazole and betamethasone under occlusive dressings because of the increased risk of systemic absorption.

PATIENT TEACHING
- Instruct patient to use clotrimazole and betamethasone cream or lotion exactly as prescribed and for the length of time prescribed, even when symptoms improve.
- Teach patient to wash her hands before and after applying drug.
- Tell patient to shake lotion well before applying and to store container in an upright position.
- Instruct patient to store clotrimazole and betamethasone cream or lotion at room temperature.
- Remind patient that drug is for topical use only and to avoid contact with eyes or mouth during application.
- Instruct patient with groin involvement to use drug sparingly in the groin area and to wear loose-fitting clothes during treatment.
- Tell patient not to cover treated area after applying drug unless instructed to do so by prescriber.

- Inform female patients that drug is not for intravaginal use.
- Instruct patient to notify prescriber if symptoms don't improve after 1 week (tinea cruris or tinea corporis) or 2 weeks (tinea pedis).
- Caution patient to avoid anyone with an infection and to avoid re-infecting herself.
- Urge patient to notify prescriber about adverse reactions at application site.

erythromycin 3% and benzoyl peroxide 5%

Benzamycin, Benzamycin Pak

Class and Category

Chemical: Macrolide (erythromycin), benzoic acid derivative (benzoyl peroxide)
Therapeutic: Antiacne, antibotic (erythromycin, benzoyl peroxide)
Pregnancy category: C

Indications and Dosages

▶ *To treat acne vulgaris*
GEL
Adults and adolescents. Applied to affected areas b.i.d., morning and evening, after skin has been washed, rinsed with warm water, and patted gently dry.

Mechanism of Action

Erythromycin inhibits protein synthesis in susceptible organisms by reversibly binding to 50S ribosomal subunits, thereby inhibiting translocation of aminoacyl transfer-RNA and inhibiting polypeptide synthesis. This eradicates the bacterial infection in acne vulgaris.

Benzoyl peroxide exerts antibacterial action against *Propionibacerium acnes*, an anaerobe found in sebaceous follicles and comedones of acne, by releasing active oxygen to cause cell death. It also has some keratolytic effect, which produces comedone lysis and drying and desquamative effects. These contribute to the improvement of acne vulgaris.

Contraindications

Hypersensitivity to erythromycin, benzoyl peroxide, other benzoic acid derivatives, or their components

Interactions
DRUGS
erythromycin
chloramphenicol, clindamycin, lincomycin: Antagonized actions between both drugs

Adverse Reactions
EENT: Mouth ulcerations
GI: Diarrhea
GU: Vaginitis
SKIN: Application site reaction such as stinging, erythema, and burning; blepharitis; dry skin; photosensitivity; pruritus

Nursing Considerations
- Use erythromycin and benzoyl peroxide cautiously in patients using other topical acne therapy (especially peeling, desquamating, or abrasive agents) because of possible cumulative irritation.
- Don't give drug with any product that contains clindamycin because erythromcyin and clindamycin may inactivate each other. Notify prescriber if patient is using a clindamycin product.
- Avoid contact with eyes and mucous membranes when applying drug.
- Observe patient for signs of superinfection, such as diarrhea, vaginal itching, and sore mouth. If present, notify prescriber.

PATIENT TEACHING
- Instruct patient to wash the affected area, rinse with warm water, and gently pat dry before applying erythromycin and benzoyl peroxide gel.
- Teach patient how to thoroughly mix drug in the palm of her hand immediately before each application. Drug comes in a two-compartment foil pouch.
- Tell patient to apply erythromycin and benzoyl peroxide exactly as prescribed and to avoid contact with eyes, inside the nose, mouth, and all mucous membranes.
- Instruct patient to wash hands thoroughly after mixing and applying drug.
- Caution patient not to apply drug near an open flame and to store it away from heat.
- Warn patient not to use any other topical acne preparation unless instructed by prescriber.
- Instruct patient to minimize exposure to sunlight and to take precautions when outdoors, such as wearing a hat and protective clothing and using a sunscreen of SPF 15 or higher.

- Tell patient to report adverse reactions to prescriber, especially severe skin reactions and signs of superinfection, such as diarrhea, vaginal itching, or sore mouth.
- Warn patient that drug may bleach hair or colored fabric.

fluocinolone acetonide 0.01%, hydroquinone 4%, and tretinoin 0.05%

Tri-Luma

Class and Category

Chemical: Florinated corticosteroid (fluocinolone), benzoquinone (hydroquinone), retinoid (tretinoin)

Therapeutic: Anti-inflammatory (fluocinolone), depigmenting agent (hydroquinone), keratolytic (tretinoin)

Pregnancy category: C

Indications and Dosages

▶ *To treat moderate to severe melasma of the face with measures for sun avoidance*

CREAM

Adults. Thin film applied and then gently rubbed into hyperpigmented areas of melasma including about ½ inch of normal-looking skin around each lesion daily, 30 minutes before bedtime.

Contraindications

Hypersensitivity to fluocinolone, hydroquinone, tretinoin, or their components

---

Mechanism of Action

Absorbed through the skin, fluocinolone binds to intracellular glucocorticoid receptors and suppresses the inflammatory and immune responses by:

- inhibiting neutrophil and monocyte accumulation at the inflammation site and suppressing their phagocytic and bactericidal activity
- stabilizing lysosomal membranes
- suppressing the antigen response of macrophages and helper T cells
- inhibiting synthesis of cellular mediators of the inflammatory response, such as cytokines, interleukins, and prostaglandins

Hydroquinone may interrupt one or more steps in the tyrosine-tyrosinase pathway of melanin synthesis to reduce skin color.

Tretinoin increases the number and activity of fibroblasts in photo-damaged skin, which disperses melanin granules and decreases melanin content to lighten dark spots caused by excessive sun exposure.

Interactions
DRUGS
fluocinolone, hydroquinone, and tretinoin
photosensitizers (such as fluoroquinolones, phenothiazines, sulfonamides, tetracyclines, and thiazides): Increased risk of phototoxicity
ACTIVITIES
hair depilatories or waxes; medicated soaps or shampoos; permanent wave solutions; topical products with strong skin-drying effect or high concentrations of alcohol, astringent, spices, or lime: Increased risk of skin dryness or irritation

Adverse Reactions
EENT: Dry mouth
ENDO: Cushing's syndrome, hyperglycemia, hypothalamic-pituitary-adrenal (HPA) axis suppression
SKIN: Acne, allergic contact dermatitis, blistering, burning, crusting, desquamation, dryness, erythema, exogenous ochronosis, hypopigmentation, irritation, localized hyperesthesia or paresthesia, peeling, pruritus, rash, rosacea, swelling, telangiectasia, vesicles

Nursing Considerations
• Monitor patient for HPA axis suppression, especially if using fluocinolone, hydroquinolone, and tretinoin cream with other corticosteroids.
• Contact prescriber if HPA axis suppression is suspected, and prepare patient for ACTH stimulation, morning plasma cortisol, and urine free-cortisol tests, as ordered. If confirmed, expect to withdraw the drug.
• Regularly assess effectiveness of fluocinolone, hydroquinolone, and tretinoin cream in lightening dark spots.
• Discontinue topical fluocinolone, hydroquinolone, and tretinoin and notoify prescriber if serious irritation or a gradual blue-black skin darkening develops at application sites.
PATIENT TEACHING
• Inform patient that results may be seen in as little as 4 weeks, but that drug may need to be used for months or therapy repeated if melasma returns.
• Instruct patient to wash her face with a mild soapless cleanser, pat dry, apply cream to hyperpigmented areas and about ½ inch of normal-looking skin around each lesion, and then lightly and uniformly rub into the skin.
• Tell patient not to cover treated areas with any type of dressing.
• Advise patient to avoid applying excessive cream to affected ar-

eas because it may cause marked redness, peeling, or discomfort.
- Caution patient not to get solution into her eyes or on mucous membranes inside her nose or mouth.
- Advise patient to apply a moisturizer after washing her face in the morning, and tell her she may use cosmetics.
- Warn patient to avoid exposing her face to sunlight and ultraviolet light (including sunlamp), to use a daily sunscreen of at least SPF 30, and to wear protective clothing during therapy.
- Tell patient that skin reddening or mild burning sensation may occur. Urge her to notify prescriber if local irritation persists or becomes severe or skin undergoes a gradual blue-black darkening. The drug will need to be discontinued.
- Warn patient that extremes of hot or cold weather may cause discomfort.
- Instruct patient to stop treatment when melasma is resolved.

hydrocortisone acetate 1% and iodoquinol 1%

Hydrocortisone and Iodoquinol 1% Cream, Vytone

Class and Category

Chemical: Glucocorticoid (hydrocortisone), halogenated 8-hydroxyquinoline (iodoquinol)
Therapeutic: Anti-inflammatory (hydrocortisone), antifungal and antibacterial (iodoquinol)
Pregnancy category: C

Indications and Dosages

▶ *To treat chronic and subacute dermatoses*

CREAM

Adults and adolescents. Applied to affected areas t.i.d. or q.i.d.

Contraindications

Hypersensitivity to hydrocortisone, other corticosteroids, iodoquinol, other 8-hydroxyquinolines, or their components

Adverse Reactions

EENT: Perioral dermatitis
ENDO: Cushing's syndrome, hyperglycemia, hypothalamic-pituitary-adrenal (HPA) axis suppression
SKIN: Allergic contact dermatitis; acneiform eruptions; folliculitis; hypertrichosis; hypopigmentation; localized atrophy, burning, dryness, irritation, maceration, miliaria, pruritus, and striae

Mechanism of Action
Absorbed through the skin, hydrocortisone binds to intracellular glucocorti-coid receptors and suppresses the inflammatory and immune responses by:
- inhibiting neutrophil and monocyte accumulation at the inflammation site and suppressing their phagocytic and bactericidal activity
- stabilizing lysosomal membranes
- suppressing the antigen response of macrophages and helper T cells
- inhibiting the synthesis of cellular mediators of the inflammatory response, such as cytokines, interleukins, and prostaglandins.
Combined, these actions alleviate inflammation.

Iodoquinol destroys trace metals on bacterial surfaces essential for bacte-rial growth. It also has slight antifungal activity, although the exact mecha-nism is unknown. These actions irradiate underlying bacterial and fungal in-fections in dermatoses.

Nursing Considerations
- Monitor patient for HPA axis suppression, especially if using topical hydrocortisone and iodoquinol over a large surface, ap-plying occlusive dressings over application sites, or using other corticosteroid products. Also monitor adolescents closely for HPA suppression because they may absorb proportionally larger amounts of drug.
- If HPA suppression is suspected, contact prescriber and prepare patient for ACTH stimulation, morning plasma cortisol, and urine free-cortisol tests, as ordered. If confirmed, expect to withdraw the drug, reduce frequency of application, or substi-tute a less potent corticosteroid, as prescribed.
- Assess effectiveness of topical hydrocortisone and iodoquinol regularly.
- Notify prescriber and stop topical hydrocortisone and iodo-quinol if irritation develops at application sites.
- High iodine content in iodoquinol may alter thyroid function test results; they shouldn't be done until at least 1 month after hydrocortisone and iodoquinol therapy has stopped.

PATIENT TEACHING
- Instruct patient to use topical hydrocortisone and iodoquinol exactly as prescribed.
- Advise patient to keep drug away from her eyes, and remind her that drug is for external use only.
- Tell patient to wash her hands before and after applying drug.
- Instruct patient not to bandage, cover, or wrap affected area

unless directed to do so by prescriber.

- Instruct patient to notify prescriber if about local adverse reactions and symptoms that worsen or do not improve.
- Warn patient that hydrocortisone and iodoquinol cream may alter color of skin and clothing.
- Advise patient to wait at least 1 month before having any thyroid function studies performed.

hydrocortisone acetate 1% and pramoxine hydrochloride 1%

Analpram-HC, Enzone, Epifoam, Pramosone, ProctoCream-HC, ProctoFoam-HC, Zone-A

hydrocortisone acetate 2.5% and pramoxine hydrochloride 1%

Analpram-HC, Enzone, Epifoam, Pramosone, Proctocream HC, ProctoFoam HC, Rectocort HC, Zone-A Forte

Class and Category

Chemical: Glucocortoid (hydrocortisone), unclassified (pramoxine)
Therapeutic: Anti-inflammatory (hydrocortisone), local anesthetic (pramoxine)
Pregnancy category: C

Indications and Dosages

▶ *To relieve inflammation, pruritus, and pain from dermatoses*
CREAM, LOTION, OINTMENT
Adults and children. Thin layer applied to affected area and rubbed in gently t.i.d. or q.i.d.
FOAM
Adults and children. Foam dispensed onto tissue or cloth and gently rubbed into affected area or applicator used to instill foam into the rectum t.i.d. or q.i.d.

Contraindications

Hypersensitivity to hydrocortisone, other corticosteroids, pramoxine or their components

Adverse Reactions

EENT: Perioral dermatitis
ENDO: Cushing's syndrome, hyperglycemia, hypothalamic-pituitary-adrenal (HPA) axis suppression
SKIN: Allergic contact dermatitis; acneiform eruptions; folliculitis; hypertrichosis; hypopigmentation; localized atrophy, burning, dry-

ness, irritation, maceration, miliaria, pruritus and striae; secondary dermatologic infection

---

Mechanism of Action
Absorbed through the skin, hydrocortisone binds to intracellular glucocorticoid receptors and suppresses the inflammatory and immune responses by:
- inhibiting neutrophil and monocyte accumulation at the inflammation site and suppressing their phagocytic and bactericidal activity
- stabilizing lysosomal membranes
- suppressing the antigen response of macrophages and helper T cells
- inhibiting synthesis of cellular mediators of the inflammatory response, such as cytokines, interleukins, and prostaglandins.

Pramoxine, once absorbed through the skin, provides temporary relief from itching and pain by stabilizing the neuronal membrane of nerve endings it contacts.

Nursing Considerations
- Monitor patient for HPA axis suppression, especially if using topical hydrocortisone and pramoxine over a large surface, applying occlusive dressings over application sites, or using other corticosteroid products. Also monitor children closely for HPA suppression because they may absorb proportionally larger amounts of drug.
- Contact prescriber if HPA suppression is suspected, and prepare patient for ACTH stimulation, morning plasma cortisol, and urine free-cortisol tests, as ordered. If confirmed, expect to withdraw the drug, reduce frequency of application, or substitute a less potent corticosteroid, as prescribed.
- Assess effectiveness of topical hydrocortisone and pramoxine regularly.
- If irritation develops at application sites, stop topical hydrocortisone and pramoxine and notify prescriber.
- Monitor patient for development of dermatologic infections. If present, notify prescriber and expect to use an appropriate antifungal or antibacterial agent, as prescribed. If infection isn't resolved promptly, expect topical hydrocortisone and pramoxine to be stopped.

PATIENT TEACHING
- Instruct patient to use topical hydrocortisone and pramoxine exactly as prescribed and for no more than 14 days unless instructed by prescriber.

- Advise patient to avoid getting the drug in her eyes, and remind her that drug is for external use only.
- Urge patient to wash her hands before and after applying the drug.
- If cream, ointment, or lotion is prescribed, advise patient to use her fingers or a tissue to apply a thin film to the affected area and rub in gently.
- If foam is prescribed, instruct her to shake the container vigorously for 5 to 10 seconds before each use. Tell her to press down on the top several times until foam appears and then dispense it onto a tissue or cloth and gently rub into the affected area. Caution her not to use her fingers to apply the foam and not to inhale its vapors. Tell her to rinse the container and cap after applying the drug.
- If foam is prescribed for rectal use, give patient these instructions: Hold the container upright and gently place the tip of the applicator onto the nose of the container cap. Then pull the applicator plunger past the fill line on the applicator barrel. Holding the container and applicator at eye level, place your index and middle fingers on the arms of the container cap and your thumb beneath container. Support the applicator with your other hand. Prime the container by pressing down firmly on the arms of the cap, and then release. It usually takes one or two pumps for the foam to appear. To fill the applicator, press down firmly on the cap flanges, hold for 1 or 2 seconds, and then release. Wait 5 to 10 seconds to let the foam expand in the applicator. Repeat until the foam reaches the fill line, which may take three or four pumps. Then remove the applicator from the container. Holding the applicator firmly, place your index finger over the plunger. Gently insert the tip of the applicator into your anus. Once it's in place, push the plunger to expel the foam, and then withdraw the applicator. After each use, disassemble the applicator parts, container, and cap, and rinse with warm water.
- Alert patient that foam is flammable, and instruct her not to use it near heat or while smoking.
- Tell patient not to bandage, cover, or wrap affected area unless directed by prescriber. Advise parents of young children not to use tight-fitting diapers or plastic pants if child is being treated in the diapered area.
- Instruct patient to notify prescriber about local adverse reactions and about symptoms that worsen or don't improve in 7 days.

lidocaine hydrochloride 3% and hydrocortisone acetate 0.5%
AnaMantle HC, LidaMantle HC

Class and Category
Chemical: Aminoacyamide (lidocaine), glucocorticoid (hydrocortisone)
Therapeutic: Local anesthetic (lidocaine), anti-inflammatory (hydrocortisone)
Pregnancy category: C

Indications and Dosages
▶ *To relieve inflammation, itching, pain and soreness from hemorrhoids, anal fissures, pruritus ani, and other anal conditions*
CREAM, LOTION
Adults. Thin film applied externally to affected area or 1 applicatorful inserted into rectum b.i.d.

Mechanism of Action
Lidocaine blocks nerve impulses by decreasing the permeability of neuronal membranes to sodium. This action produces local anesthesia.

Hydrocortisone, absorbed through the skin, binds to intracellular glucocorticoid receptors and suppresses inflammatory and immune responses by:
- inhibiting neutrophil and monocyte accumulation at the inflammation site and suppressing their phagocytic and bactericidal activity
- stabilizing lysosomal membranes
- suppressing the antigen response of macrophages and helper T cells
- inhibiting synthesis of cellular mediators of the inflammatory response, such as cytokines, interleukins, and prostaglandins.

Contraindications
Hypersensitivity to lidocaine, other amide anesthetics, hydrocortisone, or their components; presence of tuberculous, fungal, or viral lesions of the skin (herpes simplex, vaccinia, and varicella)

Interactions
DRUGS
lidocaine
class I antiarrhythmic drugs: Additive and synergistic adverse effects

Adverse Reactions
ENDO: Cushing's syndrome, hyperglycemia, hypothalamic-pituitary-adrenal (HPA) axis suppression

SKIN: Transient blanching, burning, erythema, or stinging at application site

Nursing Considerations

- Use cautiously in patients with impaired liver function, those who are seriously ill or elderly, and those who are taking antiarrhythmic class I drugs.
- Monitor patient for HPA axis suppression, especially if using topical lidocaine and hydrocortisone over a large surface, using for a prolonged period, using occlusive dressings over application sites, or using other corticosteroid products.
- Contact prescriber if HPA suppression is suspected, and prepare patient for ACTH stimulation, morning plasma cortisol, and urine free cortisol tests, as ordered. If confirmed, expect to withdraw the drug, reduce frequency of application, or substitute a less potent corticosteroid, as prescribed.
- Assess effectiveness of topical lidocaine and hydrocortisone to relieve dermatoses regularly.
- Discontinue use of topical lidocaine and hydrocortisone if irritation develops at application sites and notify prescriber.

PATIENT TEACHING

- Instruct patient to use topical lidocaine and hydrocortisone exactly as prescribed.
- Instruct patient to wash her hands before and after applying drug.
- Instruct patient how to administer lidocaine and hydrocortisone when prescribed for rectal administration. Tell patient, after screwing the applicator tip unto the end of the tube tightly, to squeeze the tube to fill the applicator until a small amount of cream shows and lubricates the end of the tip with cream. Then she should gently insert the applicator tip with attached tube into anal area and continue squeezing the body of the tube as it is moved around the areas of discomfort and lastly around and in the anal opening, if directed to do so by prescriber. Warn patient not to completely insert the applicator and tube into the anus or insert deep into the rectum. When administration is finished, instruct patient to gently remove the applicator and tube from the area and dispose.
- Advise patient to avoid drug contact with her eyes and other mucus membranes such as inside of nose or mouth. If eye contact accidentally occurs, instruct patient to rinse eye immediately with saline or water and protect the eye surface until sensation is restored.

- Tell patient not to bandage, cover or wrap affected area unless directed to do so by prescriber.
- Instruct patient to notify prescriber if any signs of local adverse reactions or infection occurs and if symptoms worsen or do not improve.
- Warn patients with small children that individual tubes are not child resistant and so should be left inside the child-resistant blister unit until ready to use.

lidocaine 2.5% and prilocaine 2.5%
EMLA

Class and Category
Chemical: Acetamide (lidocaine), propanamide (prilocaine)
Therapeutic: Local anesthetics (lidocaine, prilocaine)
Pregnancy category: B

Indications and Dosages
▶ *To provide local analgesia on normal intact skin before minor dermal procedures*
CREAM
Adults and adolescents. 2.5 grams (half of 5-gram tube) applied at selected site to cover 20 to 25 cm² of skin surface at least 1 hour before procedure.
Children ages 7 to 12 weighing more than 20 kg (44 lb). Up to 20 grams applied to maximum skin surface of 200 cm² for no longer than 4 hr.
Children ages 1 to 7 weighing more than 10 kg (22 lb). Up to 10 grams applied to maximum skin surface of 100 cm² for no longer than 4 hr.
Children ages 3 months to 12 months weighing more than 5 kg (11 lb). Up to 2 grams applied to maximum skin surface of 20 cm² for no longer than 4 hr.
Newborns (at least 37 wk gestational age) to age 3 months weighing less than 5 kg. Up to 1 gram applied to maximum skin surface of 10 cm² for no longer than 1 hr.
▶ *To provide local analgesia on normal intact skin before major dermal procedure*
CREAM
Adults and adolescents. 2 grams (slightly less than half of 5-gram tube) applied at selected site to cover 10 cm² of skin surface at least 2 hr before procedure.

Children ages 7 to 12 weighing more than 20 kg. Up to 20 grams applied to maximum skin surface of 200 cm^2 for no longer than 4 hr.

Children ages 1 to 7 weighing more than 10 kg. Up to 10 grams applied to maximum skin surface of 100 cm^2 for no longer than 4 hr.

Children ages 3 months to 12 months weighing more than 5 kg. Up to 2 grams applied to maximum skin surface of 20 cm^2 for no longer than 4 hr.

Newborns (at least 37 wk gestational age) to age 3 months weighing less than 5 kg. Up to 1 gram applied to maximum skin surface of 10 cm^2 for no longer than 1 hr.

▶ *To provide adjunct local analgesia to male genital skin before infiltration of local anesthetic*
CREAM
Male adults. 1 g/10 cm^2 applied to genital skin 15 minutes before infiltration of local anesthetic.

▶ *To provide local analgesia to female genital mucous membranes*
CREAM
Female adults. 5 to 10 grams applied to site for 5 to 10 minutes before procedure or infiltration of local anesthetic.

Mechanism of Action
Lidocaine and prilocaine are released from cream into the epidermal and dermal layers of the skin, where they accumulate in the vicinity of dermal pain receptors and nerve endings. There they inhibit the ionic fluxes needed for initiation and conduction of pain impulses, thus producing local anesthesia.

Contraindications
Congenital or idiopathic methemoglobinemia; hypersensitivity to lidocaine, prilocaine, other local anesthetics of the amide type, or their components; infants under age 12 months who are receiving treatment with methemoglobin-inducing agents

Interactions
DRUGS
lidocaine and prilocaine
acetaminophen, acetanilide, aniline dyes, benzocaine, chloroquine, dapsone, naphthalene, nitrates and nitrites, nitrofurantoin, nitroglycerin, nitroprusside, pamaquine, para-aminosalicylic acid, phenacetin, phenobarbital, phenytoin, primaquine, quinine, sulfonamides: Increased risk for developing methemoglobinemia

Class I antiarrhythmics (such as tocainide and mexiletine), class III antiarrhythmics (such as amiodarone, bretylium, dofetilide, and sotalol): Additive toxic effects and potentially synergistic activity

drugs containing lidocaine or prilocaine: Increased risk of drug accumulation in the body, with potentially serious adverse reactions

Adverse Reactions

CNS: Apprehension, confusion, dizziness, drowsiness, euphoria, light-headedness, nervousness, seizures, tremors, unconsciousness

CV: Bradycardia, circulatory collapse, hypotension, shock

EENT: Blurred or double vision, tinnitus

GI: Vomiting

GU: Blistering on foreskin (neonates); burning, edema or erythema of female genital mucous membranes

HEME: Methemoglobinemia

RESP: Bronchospasm, respiratory depression or arrest

SKIN: Alteration of temperature sensation; edema, erythema, pallor, pruritus, purpuric or petechial reactions, rash, or swelling at application site; urticaria

Other: Allergic reaction, angioedema

Nursing Considerations

- Use cautiously in patients who may be more sensitive to absorbed lidocaine and prilocaine, such as those who are acutely ill, debilitated, or elderly; those with a history of drug sensitivities; and those with severe hepatic disease because drug metabolism may be impaired, leading to possibly toxic plasma levels of lidocaine and prilocaine.
- Don't apply more cream or leave it on longer than prescribed because excessive absorption may cause serious adverse reactions, such as methemoglobinemia. Also don't apply to open wounds because doing so increases systematic absorption.
- Wipe off lidocaine and prilocaine cream at the prescribed time, and clean the entire area with an antiseptic solution. Effective skin anesthesia will last at least 1 hour after removal.
- Avoid getting rug in eye during application because severe eye irritation may occur. If eye contact occurs, immediately wash out the eye with water or saline and protect the eye from injury until sensation returns.
- Lidocaine and prilocaine cream shouldn't be used for any condition in which its penetration or migration beyond the tympanic membrane into the middle ear is possible because it may have an ototoxic effect.
- Monitor patients, especially young patients, patients with glu-

cose-6-phosphate dehydrogenase deficiencies, and patients taking drugs linked to drug-induced methemoglobinemia, closely for methemoglobinemia throughout therapy. If suspected, discontinue lidocaine and prilocaine immediately and notify prescriber. Although most patients recover spontaneously after removal of cream, be prepared to give I.V. methylene blue, if needed and prescribed.

• Monitor neonates and infants up to age 3 months for Met-Hb levels before, during, and after application of lidocaine and prilocaine cream, as ordered, provided test results can be obtained quickly.

• **WARNING** Especially when applying cream over large areas and for longer than 2 hours, monitor patient for systemic adverse effects from drug absorption. Although unlikely, they can be severe and lead to cardiac or respiratory arrest.

PATIENT TEACHING

• Stress need to apply cream carefully and exactly as prescribed.

• Demonstrate how to measure dose using supplied dosing strips. Explain that cream should be contained within the lines of the strip to ensure accurate an dose (1 gram is 1.5 inches long and 0.2 inches wide) and to use the number of strips needed to obtain correct the dose.

• Caution patient to avoid getting drug into his eyes. If he does, tell him to immediately wash the affected eye with water or saline solution and protect it until sensation returns.

• Warn patient never to apply drug to an open wound.

• Until normal sensation returns, urge patient to avoid inadvertent trauma to the treated area by not scratching, rubbing, or exposing it to extreme hot or cold.

• Advise patient to avoid hazardous activities until CNS effects of drug are known.

• Caution patient or parents to remove drug immediately and to seek emergency medical care if application causes dizziness, excessive sleepiness, or duskiness of face or lips.

lidocaine 7% and tetracaine 7%
S-Caine, Synera

Class and Category
Chemical: Aminoacyamide (lidociane), amethocaine (tetracaine)
Therapeutic: Local anesthetic (lidocaine, tetracaine)
Pregnancy category: B

Indications and Dosages

▶ *To provide local dermal analgesia for superficial dermatological procedures such as dermal filler injection, pulsed dye laser therapy, facial laser resurfacing, and laser-assisted tattoo removal*

CREAM (S-CAINE)

Adults. Applied to intact skin in amount specified by manufacturer for size of area to be treated, 20 to 30 minutes before procedure (such as dermal filler injection, pulsed dye laser therapy, or facial laser resurfacing), and spread evenly and thinly across treatment area using a flat-surfaced tool such as a metal spatula or tongue depressor. May be applied 60 minutes before laser-assisted tattoo removal. Drug removed before procedure by grasping a free edge with gloved fingers and pulling away from skin.

▶ *To provide local dermal analgesia for superficial venous access and superficial dermatologic procedures such as excision, electrodessication, and shave biopsy of skin lesions.*

TOPICAL PATCH (SYNERA)

Adults and children age 3 and older. Applied to intact skin 20 to 30 minutes before venipuncture or intravenous cannulation or 30 minutes before superficial dermatologic procedure. One additional patch may be applied to new area if venous access fails at original site. Patch removed immediately before procedure.

Mechanism of Action

Lidocaine blocks nerve impulses by decreasing the permeability of neuronal membranes to sodium. This action produces local anesthesia.

Tetracaine acts by reversibly blocking nerve conduction to produce local anesthesia and prevent pain perception.

Contraindications

Hypersensitivity to lidocaine, tetracaine, local anesthetics of the amide or ester types, para-aminobenzoic acid, or their components

Interactions

DRUGS

lidocaine and tetracaine

class 1 antiarrhythmics, such as mexiletine and tocainide: Possibly increased risk of adverse effects

local anesthetics: Possibly additive and potentiated synergistic analgesia and adverse reactions

Adverse Reactions

CNS: Confusion, dizziness, fever, headache, nervousness, neurologic excitation or depression, paresthesia, somnolence, stupor, syncope
CV: Bradycardia, hypotension
EENT: Pharyngitis
GI: Nausea, vomiting
HEME: Methemoglobinemia
RESP: Bronchospasm, hyperventilation
SKIN: Abnormal sensation, blanching, edema, erythema, or purpura at application site; blister formation; contact dermatitis; diaphoresis; dryness; pallor; pruitus; rash; urticaria
Other: Anaphylaxis, angioedema, dehydration

Nursing Considerations

- Use cautionsly in patients who may be more sensitive to systemic effects of lidocaine and tetracaine, such as acutely ill or debilitated patients.
- Observe patient closely for adverse reactions after applying drug. Although uncommon, serious allergic reactions including anaphylaxis may occur. If a reaction occurs, remove drug from skin, notify prescriber, and be prepared to provide supportive treatment, as indicated and ordered.
- Apply drug immediately after removing cap from tube or opening pouch containing a patch.
- Don't let drug contact your skin. Even used patches may contain enough drug to alter sensation.
- Don't leave drug on patient's skin longer than ordered because systematic absorption could cause serious adverse reactions.
- Remove patch or hardened cream with gloved hands, and wash your hands immediately after handling.
- Discard patch immediately after removing by folding in half, adhesive side together. To remove cream, grasp a free edge of the hardened cream with your fingers and peel away from the skin.
- Keep drug away from eyes. If eye contact occurs, immediately wash it with water or saline solution and protect the eye until sensation returns.
- Never apply drug to mucous membranes or broken or inflamed skin. Doing aso could increase absorption and lead to serious systemic adverse effects.
- Monitor patients with severe hepatic disease or pseudo-cholinesterase deficiency closely for adverse effects. These pa-

tients are at greater risk of serious systemic adverse effects.
- **WARNING** Topical patch must be removed before patient undergoes magnetic resonance imaging because the patch contains iron powder and could cause burns.

PATIENT TEACHING
- Tell patient to expect changes in sensation at application site but to report bothersome or severe reactions. Explain that, if irritation or a burning sensation occurs, drug will need to be removed.
- Warn patient to protect treatment area from trauma until sensation returns.
- Urge patient to immediately report serious adverse reactions, such as trouble breathing or development of hives, because further supportive care may be needed.

mequinol 2% and tretinoin 0.01%
Solage

Class and Category
Chemical: 4-hydroxyanisole (mequinol), retinoid (tretinoin)
Therapeutic: Depigmentor (mequinol, tretinoin)
Pregnancy category: X

Indications and Dosages
▶ *To treat solar lentigines*
SOLUTION
Adults. Applied to affected areas using the applicator tip b.i.d., morning and evening, with at least 8 hr between applications.

Mechanism of Action
Mequinol acts competitively to inhibit formation of melania precursors, which decreases melanin pigmentation in melanocytes and keratinocytes to lighten or irradiate brown spots on the skin caused by prolonged sun exposure.

Tretinoin increases the number and activity of fibroblasts in photo-damaged skin, which disperses melanin granules and decreases melanin content to lighten dark spots on skin.

Contraindications
Hypersensitivity to mequinol, tretinoin, or their components; pregnancy

Interactions
DRUGS
mequinol and tretinoin
photosensitizers (such as fluoroquinolones, phenothiazines, sulfonamides, tetracyclines, and thiazides): Increased risk of phototoxicity
ACTIVITIES
mequinol and tretinoin
electrolysis; hair depilatories or waxes; medicated soaps or shampoos; permanent wave solutions; topical products with strong skin-drying effect or high concentrations of alcohol, astringents, spices, or lime: Increased risk of skin dryness or irritation

Adverse Reactions
SKIN: Burning sensation, crusting, dermatitis, desquamation, dryness, erythema, halo hypopigmentation, hypopigmentation, irritation, pruritus, rash, stinging, tingling

Nursing Considerations
• Use with extreme caution in patients with eczema because mequinol and tretinoin can be highly irritating when applied to eczematous skin.
• Use mequinol and tretinoin cautiously in patients with a personal or family history of vitiligo because hypopigmentation may occur even in areas not exposed to drug.
• When applying drug, avoid getting solution on surrounding normal-pigmented skin because hypopigmentation may occur.
• Before therapy starts, make sure female patient of childbearing age isn't pregnant. The drug may cause fetal harm.
PATIENT TEACHING
• Warn patient to avoid getting mequinol and tretinoin on surrounding normal-pigmented skin during application and to apply just enough solution to each spot to make it moist.
• Caution patient to avoid getting drug in eyes, mouth, paranasal creases, and any mucous membrane. If it does, instruct patient to wash area liberally with water and to notify the prescriber.
• Tell patient to stop applying drug to lesions that have become the same color as surrounding skin.
• Explain that drug therapy may last up to 6 months and that some repigmentation of lesions may occur after drug is stopped.
• Tell patient not to shower or bathe the treatment areas for at least 6 hours after applying drug. Tell patient to wait at least 30 minutes after applying drug before applying cosmetics.
• Explain that using more solution than prescribed will not cause faster or better results and may cause serious adverse reactions.

- Instruct patient to notify prescriber if adverse reactions occur. Dosage frequency or amount applied may need to be decreased or drug may need to be withheld temporarily or permanently.
- Warn female patients of childbearing age to use adequate birth control measures during therapy and to stop the drug and notify the prescriber immediately if pregnancy is suspected.
- Caution patient to wear protective clothing outdoors and to avoid exposing treated areas to sunlight, including sunlamps. If sunburn occurs, instruct patient to notify prescriber and temporarily withhold drug until sunburn is completely gone.
- Alert patient that weather conditions such as wind or cold may be more irritating during mequinol and tretinoin therapy.
- Warn patient that drug solution is flammable; urge her to store it away from heat.
- Yrge patient to avoid topical products that contain strong skin-drying effects or large amounts of alcohol, astringent, spices, or lime; medicated soaps or shampoos; permanent wave solutions; electrolysis; and hair depilatories or waxes during therapy.

neomycin sulfate 0.5%, polymyxin B sulfate, bacitracin zinc, and hydrocortisone acetate 1%

Cortisporin Ointment

Class and Category

Chemical: *Streptomyces fradiae Waksman* derivative (neomycin), *Bacillus polymyxa* derivative (polymyxin B), *Bacillus subtilis* derivative (bacitracin), glucocorticoid (hydrocortisone)
Therapeutic: Antibiotic (neomycin, polymyxin B, bacitracin), anti-inflammatory (hydrocortisone)
Pregnancy category: C

Indications and Dosages

▶ *To treat corticosteroid-responsive dermatoses with secondary infection*
CREAM
Adults. Small quantity applied to affected areas and gently rubbed in, if appropriate, b.i.d. to q.i.d. for no longer than 7 days.

Contraindications

Hypersensitivity to neomycin, polymyxin B, bacitracin, hydrocortisone, or their components; presence of tuberculous, fungal, or viral lesions of the skin (herpes simplex, vaccinia, and varicella)

Mechanism of Action

Neomycin is transported into bacterial cells, where it competes with messenger RNA to bind with a specific receptor protein on the 30S ribosomal subunit of DNA. This action causes abnormal, nonfunctioning proteins to form. A lack of functional proteins causes bacterial cells to die.

Polymyxin B binds to cell membrane phospholipids in gram-negative bacteria, increasing cell membrane permeability. Polymyxin B also acts as a cationic detergent, altering the membrane's osmotic barrier and causing essential intracellular metabolites to leak out. Both actions lead to cell death.

Bacitracin interferes with bacterial cell-wall synthesis by binding with isoprenyl pyrophosphate (a lipid-carrying molecule that transports substances out of bacterial cells to help build new cell walls), forming an unusable complex in bacterial cells. This weakens cell walls and causes lysis and death.

Hydrocortisone, absorbed through the skin, binds to intracellular glucocorticoid receptors and suppresses inflammatory and immune responses by:

- inhibiting neutrophil and monocyte accumulation at the inflammation site and suppressing their phagocytic and bactericidal activity
- stabilizing lysosomal membranes
- suppressing the antigen response of macrophages and helper T cells
- inhibiting the synthesis of cellular mediators of the inflammatory response, such as cytokines, interleukins, and prostaglandins.

Adverse Reactions

EENT: Hearing loss, mouth ulcerations, tinnitus
ENDO: Cushing's syndrome, hyperglycemia, hypothalamic-pituitary-adrenal (HPA) axis suppression
GI: Diarrhea
GU: Nephrotoxicity, vaginitis
SKIN: Allergic contact dermatitis; acneiform eruptions; folliculitis; hypertrichosis; hypopigmentation; localized atrophy, burning, dryness, irritation, maceration, miliaria, pruritus and striae; secondary dermatologic infection

Nursing Considerations

- Because of neomycin, ointment shouldn't be used over a wide area or for extended time to avoid nephrotoxicity and ototoxicity. Expect to monitor BUN and serum creatinine levels and patient's hearing before and during topical therapy. If nephrotoxicity or ototoxicity (hearing loss or tinnitus) develops, expect to decrease or discontinue drug as ordered.
- Watch for HPA axis suppression, especially in patients who use

neomycin, polymyxin B, bacitracin, and hydrocortisone ointment for a prolonged period or over a large surface, those who use occlusive dressings over application sites, and those who use other corticosteroid products.

- Contact prescriber if HPA suppression is suspected, and prepare patient for ACTH stimulation, morning plasma cortisol, and urine free-cortisol tests, as ordered. If confirmed, expect to withdraw the drug, reduce frequency of application, or substitute a less potent corticosteroid, as prescribed.
- Assess drug's effectiveness regularly.
- If irritation develops at application sites, stop use of drug and notify prescriber.
- Observe patient for signs of superinfection, such as diarrhea, vaginal itching, and sore mouth. If present, notify prescriber.

PATIENT TEACHING
- Urge patient to use drug exactly as prescribed, for length of time prescribed.
- Advise patient to avoid getting drug in her eyes, and remind her that drug is for external use only.
- Instruct patient to wash hands before and after applying drug.
- Instruct patient to notify prescriber if local adverse reactions such as redness, irritation, swelling, or pain persist or increase.
- Tell patient to notify prescriber immediately about diarrhea, mouth sores, or vaginitis, possible early signs of superinfection.

neomycin sulfate 0.5%, polymyxin B sulfate, and hydrocortisone acetate 1%
Cortisporin Cream

Class and Category
Chemical: Streptomyces fradiae Waksman derivative (neomycin), *Bacillus polymyxa* derivative (polymyxin B), glucocorticoid (hydrocortisone)
Therapeutic: Antibiotic (neomycin, polymyxin B), anti-inflammatory (hydrocortisone)
Pregnancy category: C

Indications and Dosages
▶ *To treat corticosteroid-responsive dermatoses with secondary infection*
CREAM
Adults. Small quantity applied to affected areas and gently rubbed in, if appropriate, b.i.d. to q.i.d.

Contraindications

Hypersensitivity to neomycin, polymyxin B or hydrocortisone, and their components; presence of tuberculous, fungal, or viral lesions of the skin (herpes simplex, vaccinia, and varicella)

Mechanism of Action

Neomycin is transported into bacterial cells, where it competes with messenger RNA to bind with a specific receptor protein on the 30S ribosomal subunit of DNA. This action causes abnormal, nonfunctioning proteins to form. A lack of functional proteins causes bacterial cells to die.

Polymyxin B binds to cell membrane phospholipids in gram-negative bacteria, increasing the permeability of the cell membrane. Polymyxin B also acts as a cationic detergent, altering the osmotic barrier of the membrane and causing essential intracellular metabolites to leak out. Both actions lead to cell death.

Hydrocortisone, absorbed through the skin, binds to intracellular glucocorticoid receptors and suppresses the inflammatory and immune responses by:
- inhibiting neutrophil and monocyte accumulation at the inflammation site and suppressing their phagocytic and bactericidal activity
- stabilizing lysosomal membranes
- suppressing the antigen response of macrophages and helper T cells
- inhibiting the synthesis of cellular mediators of the inflammatory response, such as cytokines, interleukins, and prostaglandins.

Adverse Reactions

EENT: Hearing loss, mouth ulcerations, tinnitus
ENDO: Cushing's syndrome, hyperglycemia, hypothalamic-pituitary-adrenal (HPA) axis suppression
GI: Diarrhea
GU: Nephrotoxicity, vaginitis
SKIN: Allergic contact dermatitis; acneiform eruptions; folliculitis; hypertrichosis; hypopigmentation; localized atrophy, burning, dryness, irritation, maceration, miliaria, pruritus and striae; secondary dermatologic infection

Nursing Considerations

- Because of neomycin, cream shouldn't be used over a wide area or for extended periods of time to avoid nephrotoxicity and ototoxicity. If use is necessary, expect to monitor BUN and serum creatinine levels to assess renal function and patient's hearing before and during topical drug therapy. If nephrotoxicity or ototoxicity (hearing loss or tinnitus) develops, expect to decrease frequency of use or stop drug, as ordered.

• Watch for HPA axis suppression, especially in patients using drug for a prolonged period or over a large body surface, using occlusive dressings over application sites, or using other corticosteroid products.

• Contact prescriber if HPA suppression is suspected, and prepare patient for ACTH stimulation, morning plasma cortisol, and urine free-cortisol tests, as ordered. If confirmed, expect to withdraw the drug, reduce frequency of application, or substitute a less potent corticosteroid, as prescribed.

• Assess drug's effectiveness regularly.

• If irritation develops at application sites, stop drug and notify prescriber.

• Observe patient for signs of superinfection, such as diarrhea, vaginal itching, and sore mouth. Notify prescriber, if present.

PATIENT TEACHING

• Instruct patient to use cream exactly as prescribed, for as long as prescribed.

• Advise patient to avoid getting drug in her eyes, and remind her that drug is for external use only.

• Urge patient to wash her hands before and after applying neomycin, polymyxin B, and hydrocortisone.

• Instruct patient to notify prescriber if local adverse reactions such as redness, irritation, swelling, or pain persist or increase.

• Tell patient to notify prescriber immediately about diarrhea, mouth sores, or vaginitis; they may be signs of superinfection.

nystatin and triamcinolone acetonide 0.1%

Mycogen, Mycolog, Mycolog-II, Myconel, Myco-Triacet II, Mytrex, Tri-Statin

Class and Category

Chemical: Amphoteric polyene macrolide (nystatin), glucocorticoid (triamcinolone)

Therapeutic: Antifungal (nystatin), anti-inflammatory (triamcinolone)

Pregnancy category: NR

Indications and Dosages

▶ *To treat skin infection caused by candidiasis*

CREAM, OINTMENT
Adults and children. Applied to affected areas b.i.d., morning and evening.

Mechanism of Action
Nystatin binds to sterols in fungal cell membranes, thereby impairing membrane integrity. As a result, fungal cells lose intracellular potassium and other cellular contents and eventually die.

Triamcinolone, absorbed through the skin, binds to intracellular glucocorticoid receptors and suppresses the inflammatory and immune responses by:
- inhibiting neutrophil and monocyte accumulation at the inflammation site and suppressing their phagocytic and bactericidal activity
- stabilizing lysosomal membranes
- suppressing the antigen response of macrophages and helper T cells
- inhibiting the synthesis of cellular mediators of the inflammatory response, such as cytokines, interleukins, and prostaglandins.

Contraindications
Hypersensitivity to nystatin, triamcinolone, acetonide, other antifungals or steroids, or their components

Adverse Reactions
ENDO: Cushing's syndrome, hyperglycemia, hypothalamic-pituitary-adrenal (HPA) axis suppression
SKIN: Alopecia; blistering; burning; dryness; eruptions resembling acne; excessive discoloring of the skin; excessive hair growth; inflammation around mouth or hair follicles; irritation; itching; peeling; prickly heat; reddish purple lines on skin; secondary infection; severe inflammation, softening, stretching or thinning of skin; stretch marks

Nursing Considerations
- Watch for HPA axis suppression, especially in patients using nystatin and triamcinolone cream or ointment for a prolonged period or over a large body surface, using occlusive dressings over application sites, or using other corticosteroid products because of absorption of triamcinolone.
- Contact prescriber if HPA suppression is suspected, and prepare patient for ACTH stimulation, morning plasma cortisol, and urine free-cortisol tests, as ordered. If confirmed, expect to withdraw the drug, reduce frequency of application or substi-

tute a less potent corticosteroid, as prescribed.
• Assess drug's effectiveness regularly.
• Be aware that drug shouldn't be used longer than 25 days.
• If irritation develops at application sites, stop drug and notify prescriber.

PATIENT TEACHING
• Tell patient to use topical nystatin and triamcinolone cream or ointment exactly as prescribed, for the length of time prescribed.
• Urge patient to wash her hands before and after applying nystatin and triamcinolone cream.
• Inform patient that drug shouldn't be used longer than 25 days.
• Advise patient to avoid drug contact with her eyes and remind her that drug is for external use only. Tell her to immediately wash her eye(s) with water and notify prescriber if accidental drug contact occurs with either of her eyes.
• Tell patient or parent not to wrap or bandage the affected areas after applying drug. If patient is being treated in the groin area, advise wearing loose-fitting clothing. Tight-fitting clothing, including diapers or plastic pants for young children, are not recommended because these garments act like airtight dressings and increase the risk of adverse reactions from drug absorption through the skin.
• Instruct patient to notify prescriber if local adverse reactions, such as redness, irritation, swelling, or pain, persist or increase or if condition persists or worsens after 2 to 3 weeks of therapy with nystatin and triamcinolone.

papain and urea 10%
Accuzyme, Ethezyme 830, Gladase, Panafil

Class and Category
Chemical: Carica papaya fruit enzyme (papain), diamide of carbonic acid (urea)
Therapeutic: Debriding agent (papain), denaturant of proteins (urea)
Pregnancy category: NR

Indications and Dosages
▶ *For debridement of necrotic tissue and liquefaction of slough in acute and chronic lesions, such as pressure ulcers, varicose and diabetic ulcers, burns, postoperative wounds, pilonidal cyst wounds, carbuncles, and traumatic or infected wounds*

OINTMENT

Adults. Applied directly to wound and then covered with appropriate dressing once or twice daily.

Contraindications
Hypersensitivity to papain, urea, or their components

Mechanism of Action
Papain is the proteolytic enzyme from the fruit of carica papaya, which digests nonviable protein matter when the surrounding pH is 3 to 12.

Urea doubles the action of papain by releasing papain activators through a solvent action and denaturing nonviable protein matter in lesions. This makes necrotic tissue and slough more susceptible to enzymatic digestion.

Adverse Reactions
SKIN: Irritation of surrounding area, transient burning on application

Nursing Considerations
- Cleanse wound with prescribed wound cleanser or saline solution before applying drug. Avoid using hydrogen peroxide solution because it may inactivate papain.
- Apply papain and urea ointment directly to wound, cover with an appropriate dressing, and secure the dressing.
- Irrigate the wound at each redressing to remove any accumulation of liquefied necrotic material.
- Avoid contact between the drug and the salts of heavy metals, such as lead, silver, and mercury, because they can inactivate drug.
- Assess effectiveness of papain and urea regularly.
- If profuse exudate causes skin irritation, increase the frequency of dressing changes to reduce discomfort until exudate decreases.

PATIENT TEACHING
- Warn patient that papain and urea may cause a transient burning sensation.
- Show caregiver how to apply ointment to wound.
- Teach caregiver how to irrigate wound before reapplying ointment. Tell caregiver to use a prescribed cleanser or saline solution to irrigate the wound but not hydrogen peroxide.
- Tell caregiver to keep wound covered with an appropriate dressing between drug applications.

sodium sulfacetamide 10% and sulfur 5%

Rosac Cream, Rosula, Zetacet

Class and Category

Chemical: Sulfonamide (sodium sulfacetamide), nonmetal element (sulfur)

Therapeutic: Antiacne and antibacterial (sodium sulfacetamide), antiacne and keratolytic (sulfur)

Pregnancy category: C

Indications and Dosages

▶ *To treat acne vulgaris, acne rosacea, and seborrheic dermatitis*

CREAM, GEL, LOTION, TOPICAL SUSPENSION

Adults and adolescents. Thin film applied to affected areas once daily to t.i.d.

ACQUEOUS CLEANSER, WASH

Adults and adolescents. Applied to affected areas after wetting skin, massaging into skin gently for 10 to 20 seconds to work into a full lather, and then rinsed off thoroughly and skin patted dry once daily or b.i.d.

Mechanism of Action

Sodium sulfacetamide acts as a competitive antagonist to para-aminobenzoic acid (PABA), which is an essential component in bacterial growth. By disrupting bacterial ability to grow, symptoms of acne, such as pus formation and inflammation, improve.

Sulfur is thought to inhibit growth of *Propionibacerium acnes* and formation of fatty acids through unknown mechanisms that help relieve plugging and rupturing of follicles. By easing evacuation of comedones and promoting peeling of the skin, it helps eradicate the symptoms of acne and dermatitis.

Contraindications

Hypersensitivity to sodium sulfacetamide, other sulfonamides, sulfur or their components, renal disease

Adverse Reactions

HEME: Acute hemolytic anemia, agranulocytosis, purpura hemorrhagica

SKIN: Contact dermatitis, dry skin, erythema, jaundice, scaling of epidermis

Other: Drug fever

Nursing Considerations

- Observe patient closely for local irritation, such as contact dermatitis or sensitization, during long-term therapy. Notify prescriber and expect to stop therapy.
- **WARNING** Monitor patient for systemic hypersensitivity reactions, such as acute hemolytic anemia, agranulocytosis, and purpura hemorrhagica, especially if applying drug to denuded or abraded skin. Although rare, toxic reactions may occur because sodium sulfacetamide can induce toxic hypersensitivity reactions in susceptible patients after being absorbed.

PATIENT TEACHING

- Instruct patient to wash the affected area, rinse with warm water, and pat gently dry before applying sodium sulfacetamide and sulfur cream, lotion, or topical suspension.
- For lotion form, tell patient to shake container well before using and to lightly massage into skin.
- For wash form, tell patient to wet application site, apply wash liberally, massage it gently into skin for 10 to 20 seconds, work into a full lather, rinse the area thoroughly, and pat dry. If dryness occurs, urge patient to notify prescriber; rinsing the wash off more quickly or using it less often may control the dryness.
- Tell patient to apply drug exactly as prescribed and to avoid getting it in eyes, nose, mouth, and all mucous membranes.

sodium thiosulfate and salicylic acid

Versiclear

Class and Category

Chemical: Sulfate derivative (sodium thiosulfate), salicylate (salicylic acid)
Therapeutic: Antiacne and antifungal (sodium thiosulfate), antiacne and keratolytic (salicylic acid)
Pregnancy category: C

Indications and Dosages

▶ *To treat tinea versicolor (*Malassezia furfur *infection)*
LOTION
Adults. Thin film of lotion applied to affected and susceptible areas b.i.d.

Contraindications

Hypersensitivity to sodium thiosulfate, salicylic acid, or their components

Mechanism of Action

Sodium thiosulfate damages fungal cells by interfering with a cytochrome P-450 enzyme needed to convert lanosterol to ergosterol, an essential part of the fungal cell membrane. Decreased ergosterol synthesis causes increased cell permeability, which allows cell contents to leak. Sodium thiosulfate also may lead to fungal cell death by inhibiting fungal respiration under aerobic conditions. Removing fungal activity alleviates source of acne formation.

Salicylic acid softens and destroys the stratum corneum by increasing endogenous hydration, probably because of decreased pH, which causes the cornified epithelium of the skin to swell, soften, and then desquamate. Maceration and desquamation of epidermal tissue reduces the number and severity of acne lesions.

Adverse Reactions

SKIN: Dry or peeling skin, erythema, pruritus

Nursing Considerations

- Monitor effectiveness of sodium thiosulfate and salicylic acid therapy to reduce number and severity of acne lesions.
- Notify prescriber if local skin reactions develop; drug may need to be stopped.

PATIENT TEACHING

- Tell patient to thoroughly wash, rinse, and dry affected and susceptible areas before applying drug.
- Caution patient to avoid getting sodium thiosulfate and salicylic acid in or around eye area.
- To prevent relapse, stress importance of using drug exactly as prescribed and not stopping, even after acne improves, until directed by prescriber.

trypsin and balsam peru

Granulderm, Granulex

Class and Category

Chemical: Enzyme (trypsin), *Myroxolon balsamum* derivative (balsam peru)
Therapeutic: Debriding agent (trypsin), circulatory stimulant, odor reducer (balsam peru)
Pregnancy category: NR

Indications and Dosages

▶ *To promote wound healing of varicose ulcers, dehiscent wounds, and decubital ulcers; to promote debridement of eschar; to reduce odor from necrotic wounds*

AEROSOL

Adults. Sprayed rapidly, holding can about 12 inches from affected areas to coat wound completely b.i.d.

Mechanism of Action

Trypsin promotes wound healing by stimulating the vascular bed and improving epithelization by reducing premature epithelial desiccation and cornification. It also digests nonviable protein matter.

Balsam peru stimulates the capillary bed to increase circulation to the wound site, which promotes healing. Its vanilla scent helps to lessen odor from necrotic wounds.

Contraindications

Hypersensitivity to trypsin, balsam peru, or their components; use on fresh arterial clots

Adverse Reactions

SKIN: Transient stinging at application site

Nursing Considerations

- Shake can well before spraying. Hold can upright, about 12 inches from affected area, and spray to cover wound rapidly with trypsin and balsam peru.
- Leave wound unbandaged or apply a wet dressing, as ordered.
- Before reapplication, wash area gently with water to remove residual drug.
- Evaluate effectiveness of drug regularly.

PATIENT TEACHING

- Warn patient that drug may cause temporary stinging when applied to a sensitive area.
- Teach patient or caregiver how to administer drug. Tell him to avoid getting drug in eyes. If it does, tell patient to wash his eyes with water immediately and to notify prescriber.
- Warn patient or caregiver that drug is flammable and should be kept away from fire or open flame.
- Instruct patient or caregiver not to puncture or incinerate the can because it could explode.

Endocrine Drugs

alendronate sodium and cholecalciferol
Fosamax Plus D

Class and Category
Chemical: Bisphosphonate (alendronate), vitamin D analogue (cholecalciferol)
Therapeutic: Antiosteoporotic (alendronate), antihypocalcemic (cholecalciferol)
Pregnancy category: C

Indications and Dosages
▶ *To treat postmenopausal osteoporosis; to increase bone mass in men with osteoporosis*
TABLETS
Adults. 70 mg alendronate and 2,800 international units cholecalciferol (1 tablet) or 70 mg alendronate and 5,600 international units cholecalciferol (1 tablet) with 6 to 8 ounces of plain water every wk at least 30 min before the first food, beverage, or medication of the day.

Contraindications
Esophageal abnormalities that delay esophageal emptying, such as stricture or achalasia; hypersensitivity to alendronate, cholecalciferol, or their components; hypocalcemia; inability to stand or sit upright for at least 30 minutes

Interactions
DRUGS
alendronate and cholecalciferol
estrogen-progestin combinations: Increased suppression of bone turnover, enhancing effectiveness of alendronate and cholecalciferol
alendronate
antacids, calcium, iron, multivalent cations: Decreased alendronate absorption

aspirin: Increased risk of GI distress
rantidine (I.V. form): Doubled alendronate bioavailability
cholecalciferol
anticonvulsants, cimetidine, thiazide diuretics: Increased vitamin D catabolism
cholestyramine, colestipol, mineral oil, olestra, orlistat: Decreased calcitriol absorption
FOODS
alendronate
any food: Delayed absorption and decreased serum level of alendronate

---

Mechanism of Action

Alendronate binds to bone hydroxyapatite and reduces the activity of cells that cause bone loss, slows the rate of bone loss after menopause, and increases the amount of bone mass. It may act by inhibiting osteoclast activity on newly formed bone resorption surfaces, which reduces the number of sites where bone is remodeled. Bone formation then exceeds bone resorption at these remodeling sites, and bone mass gradually increases.

Cholecalciferol is the natural precursor of the calcium-regulating hormone calcitriol and is converted to calcitriol in the kidneys under the influence of parathyroid hormone and hypophosphatemia. Calcitriol binds to specific receptors in the intestinal mucosa to increase intestinal absorption of calcium and phosphate and to regulate serum calcium, renal excretion of calcium and phosphate, bone formation, and bone resorption.

Adverse Reactions

CNS: Asthenia, dizziness, headache, vertigo
CV: Peripheral edema
EENT: Episcleritis, localized osteonecrosis of the jaw, oropharyngeal ulceration, scleritis, uveitis
GI: Abdominal distention and pain, constipation, diarrhea, dysphagia, esophageal perforation or ulceration, esophagitis, fever, flatulence, gastric or duodenal ulcers, gastritis, heartburn, indigestion, malaise, melena, nausea, vomiting
MS: Arthralgia; bone, joint, and muscle pain; joint swelling; muscle spasms; myalgia; osteonecrosis of jaw
SKIN: Photosensitivity, pruritus, rash, Stevens-Johnson syndrome, toxic epidermal necrolysis
Other: Angioedema, hypocalcemia

Nursing Considerations

- Be aware that alendronate and cholecalciferol therapy isn't recommended for patients with renal insufficiency and a creatinine clearance less than 35 ml/minute.
- Use alendronate and cholecalciferol cautiously in patients with active upper GI problems such as dysphagia, esophageal diseases, gastritis, duodenitis, or ulcers.
- Monitor serum calcium level before, during, and after treatment. If patient has hypocalcemia or vitamin D deficiency, expect prescriber to order a calcium supplement and vitamin D replacement before therapy begins.
- Administer alendronate and cholecalciferol with 6 to 8 ounces of plain water at least 30 minutes before the patient's first food, beverage, or other medication of the day to prevent decreased absorption of the drug.
- Ensure adequate dietary intake of calcium and vitamin D before, during, and after treatment.
- Be aware that alendronate and cholecalciferol shouldn't be used alone to treat vitamin D deficiency. Patients at risk for vitamin D deficiency (such as those who are homebound, chronically ill or over age 70) also should receive vitamin D supplementation, as ordered.
- Expect to give higher doses of vitamin D supplement and to measure 25-hydroxyvitamin D level, as ordered, in patients with GI malabsorption syndromes who receive alendronate and cholecalciferol.
- Check to determine if patient has had a dental examination before starting alendronate and cholecalciferol therapy, especially if patient has cancer; is receiving chemotherapy, head or neck radiation, or corticosteroids; or has poor oral hygiene. The risk of osteonecrosis is higher in these patients and invasive dental procedures and alendronate can worsen osteonecrosis.
- **WARNING** Alendronate may irritate upper GI mucosa, causing such adverse reactions as esophageal ulceration. To help minimize these reactions, have patient remain upright for at least 30 minutes after taking drug and until he has eaten.
- If patient receives long-term alendronate and cholecalciferol therapy, be alert for vitamin D toxicity. Early signs and symptoms include bone pain, constipation, dry mouth, headache, metallic taste, myalgia, nausea, somnolence, vomiting, and weakness. Late signs and symptoms include albuminuria, anorexia, arrhythmias, azotemia, conjunctivitis, decreased li-

bido, elevated AST and ALT levels, elevated BUN level, generalized vascular calcification, hypercholesterolemia, hypertension, hyperthermia, irritability, mild acidosis, nephrocalcinosis, nocturia, pancreatitis, photophobia, polydipsia, polyuria, pruritus, rhinorrhea, and weight loss.

PATIENT TEACHING

- Advise patient to take alendronate and cholecaliferol in the morning with a full glass of water at least 30 minutes before he takes any food, medication, or other fluids. Explain that such beverages as orange juice, coffee, and mineral water reduce alendronate's effects.
- To help reduce esophageal irritation, tell patient not to chew or suck on tablet.
- Instruct patient to wait at least 30 minutes after taking alendronate to eat, drink, or take other drugs. Teach patient to remain upright for 30 minutes after taking alendronate and cholecaliferol and until he has eaten the first food of the day.
- Advise patient that if he misses a dose, he should take 1 tablet on the morning after he remembers and then return to his originally scheduled weekly dose. Tell him never to take 2 tablets on the same day.
- Tell patient to stop taking alendronate and cholecaliferol and to notify prescriber if he develops difficulty swallowing or talking, retrosternal pain, or new or worsening heartburn.
- Warn patient not to take other forms of vitamin D while taking alendronate and cholecalciferol unless otherwise prescribed.
- Advise patient to notify prescriber immediately if he develops signs or symptoms of vitamin D toxicity, such as headache, irritability, nausea, photophobia, vomiting, weakness, and weight loss.
- Instruct patient on proper oral hygiene and to notify prescriber before having any invasive dental procedure performed.

17 beta-estradiol and norgestimate
Prefest

Class and Category
Chemical: Estrogen steroid hormone derivative (17 beta-estradiol), progesterone derivative (norgestimate)
Therapeutic: Antiosteoporotic, ovarian hormone replacement (17 beta-estradiol, norgestimate)

Pregnancy category: X

Indications and Dosages

▶ *To treat menopausal symptoms and vaginal and vulvar atrophy in postmenopausal women with an intact uterus; to prevent osteoporosis from estrogen deficiency in postmenopausal women with an intact uterus*

TABLETS

Adult women. 1 mg 17 beta-estradiol (1 tablet) daily for 3 days followed by 1 mg 17 beta-estradiol and 0.09 mg norgestimate (1 tablet) for 3 days. Cycle repeated continuously.

Mechanism of Action

Estrogens such as 17 beta-estradiol increase the rate of DNA and RNA synthesis in the cells of female reproductive organs, pituitary gland, hypothalamus, and other target organs. In the hypothalamus, estrogens decrease release of gonadotropin-releasing hormone, which reduces pituitary release of follicle-stimulating hormone and luteinizing hormone. In women, these hormones are needed for normal GU and other essential body functions. At the cellular level, estrogens increase cervical secretions, cause endometrial cell proliferation, and improve uterine tone. Estrogen replacement helps maintain GU function and reduces vasomotor symptoms when estrogen production declines from menopause, surgical removal of ovaries, or other estrogen deficiency. Estrogen replacement also helps prevent osteoporosis by inhibiting bone resorption.

Progestins such as norgestimate prolong some positive effects of estrogens on HDL cholesterol. Norgestimate diffuses freely into target cells of the female reproductive tract, mammary glands, hypothalamus, and pituitary gland and binds to the progesterone cell receptor. It converts a proliferative endometrium into a secretory one in women with adequate estrogen replacement, reducing endometrial growth and the risk of endometrial cancer compared with women who have an intact uterus and take unopposed estrogens. Norgestimate also decreases nuclear estradiol receptors and suppresses epithelial DNA synthesis in endometrial tissues.

Contraindications

Active thrombophlebitis or thromboembolic disorders; hepatic disorders; hypersensitivity to 17 beta-estradiol, norgestimate, or their components; jaundice; known or suspected breast cancer or history of breast cancer from estrogen use; known or suspected estrogen-dependent cancer; pregnancy; undiagnosed abnormal genital bleeding; vaginal disorders

Interactions

DRUGS

17 beta-estradiol and norgestimate

corticosteroids: Increased therapeutic and toxic effects of corticosteroids

cyclosporine: Increased risk of hepatotoxicity and nephrotoxicity

hepatotoxic drugs, such as isoniazid: Increased risk of hepatitis and hepatotoxicity

oral antidiabetics: Decreased therapeutic effects of these drugs

thyroid hormones: Decreased effectiveness of thyroid hormones

warfarin: Altered anticoagulant effect

FOODS

17 beta-estradiol

grapefruit juice: Decreased metabolism and possibly increased adverse effects of 17 beta-estradiol

ACTIVITIES

17 beta-estradiol and norgestimate

smoking: Increased risk of stroke, pulmonary embolism, thrombophlebitis, and transient ischemic attack

Adverse Reactions

CNS: Chorea, dementia, depression, dizziness, exacerbation of epilepsy, headache, irritability, migraine headache, mood disturbances, nervousness, porphyria, stroke

CV: Hypertension, increased triglycerides, MI, peripheral edema, pulmonary embolism, thromboembolism, thrombophlebitis

EENT: Diplopia, intolerance of contact lenses, retinal vascular thrombosis, sinusitis, vision changes or loss

ENDO: Breast enlargement, pain, tenderness, or tumors; endometrial hyperplasia, galactorrhea; gynecomastia; hyperglycemia; nipple discharge

GI: Abdominal cramps or pain, aggravation of hepatic porphyria, anorexia, bloating, constipation, diarrhea, elevated liver function test results, enlargement of hepatic hemangiomas, flatulence, gallbladder obstruction, hepatitis, increased appetite, nausea, pancreatitis, vomiting

GU: Amenorrhea, breakthrough bleeding, cervical erosion, clear vaginal discharge, dysmenorrhea, endometiral or ovarian tumors, increased libido, increased size of uterine leiomyomata, leukorrhea, prolonged or heavy menstrual bleeding, urinary tract infection, vaginitis including vaginal candidiasis

MS: Arthralgias, back or extremity pain, leg cramps

RESP: Bronchitis, exacerbation of asthma, upper respiratory infection

SKIN: Alopecia, application site irritation, chloasma, erythema multiforme or nodosum, hirsutism, jaundice, melasma, pruritus, purpura, rash, urticaria

Other: Anaphylaxis, angioedema, flulike syndrome, folic acid deficiency, hypercalcemia (with bone metastases), hypocalcemia, hyperkalemia, hyponatremia, weight gain or loss

Nursing Considerations

- Use 17 beta-estradiol and norgestimate cautiously in women with asthma, diabetes mellitus, epilepsy, migraine headaches, porphyria, systemic lupus erythematosus, or hepatic hemangiomas because estradiol can worsen these conditions.

- Verify that patient has an intact uterus before starting 17 beta-estradiol and norgestimate therapy. If not, patient doesn't need a product that contains a progestin, such as norgestimate.

- **WARNING** Assess patient for possible contact lens intolerance or changes in vision or visual acuity because estrogens can cause keratoconus. Be prepared to stop therapy immediately, as prescribed, if patient has sudden partial or complete loss of vision or sudden onset of diplopia or migraine.

- Monitor PT in patients taking warfarin. Estrogens such as 17 beta-estradiol increase production of clotting factors VII, VIII, IX, and X and promote platelet aggregation and thus may lead to loss of anticoagulant effect.

- Monitor patient for elevated liver function test results because estrogens and progestins such as 17 beta-estradiol and norgestimate may worsen such conditions as acute intermittent or variegate hepatic porphyria.

- Closely monitor patient's blood pressure. Some patients may have a substantial increase in blood pressure as an indiosyncratic reaction to estrogens such as 17 beta-estradiol. Monitor patients who already have hypertension for increases in blood pressure because estrogens may cause fluid retention. Also monitor patients who have asthma, heart disease, migraines, renal disease, or seizure disorder for worsening of these conditions.

- Monitor blood glucose level often in patients who have diabetes mellitus because 17 beta-estradiol may decrease insulin sensitivity and alter glucose tolerance.

- **WARNING** Expect to stop 17 beta-estradiol and norgestimate therapy in any woman who develops signs or symptoms of dementia or cardiovascular disease, such as MI, pulmonary embolism, stroke, or venous thrombosis.

- Be aware that 17 beta-estradiol and norgestimate may worsen mood disorders, including depression. Monitor patient for depression, mood changes, anxiety, fatigue, dizziness, or insomnia.
- **WARNING** Be aware that patients with bone metastasis from breast cancer may develop severe hypercalcemia because estrogens such as 17 beta-estradiol influence calcium and phosphorus metabolism. Watch for toxic effects of increased calcium absorption in patients predisposed to hypercalcemia or nephrolithiasis.
- Assess patient's skin for melasma (tan or brown patches), which may develop on forehead, cheeks, temples, and upper lip. These patches may persist after drug is stopped.
- Monitor thyroid function test results in patients with hypothyroidism because long-term use of 17 beta-estradiol may decrease effectiveness of thyroid therapy.
- Expect to stop 17 beta-estradiol and norgestimate therapy several weeks before patient undergoes major surgery, as prescribed, because prolonged immobilization poses a risk of thromboembolism.

PATIENT TEACHING
- Before 17 beta-estradiol and norgestimate therapy starts, inform patient of risks involved in taking 17 beta-estradiol and norgestimate therapy, such as increased risk of cardiovascular disease, breast or endometrial cancer, dementia, gallbladder disease, and vision abnormalities.
- Urge patient to notify prescriber immediately if vaginal bleeding or any other abnormal signs and symptoms occur while taking 17 beta-estradiol and norgestimate.
- Advise patient to avoid smoking while taking an estrogen-progestin product such as 17 beta-estradiol and norgestimate.
- Stress importance of having follow-up visits every 3 to 6 months to determine effectiveness of 17 beta-estradiol and norgestimate in relieving menopausal symptoms and osteoporosis. Also stress importance of having scheduled diagnostic tests to detect adverse reactions.
- Emphasize importance of good dental hygiene and regular dental checkups because an elevated progestin (norgestimate) blood level increases growth of normal oral flora, which may lead to gum tenderness, bleeding, or swelling.

drospirenone and estradiol
Angeliq
drospirenone and ethinyl estradiol
Yaz

Class and Category
Chemical: Synthetic progestin and spironolactone analogue (drospirenone), estrogenic steroid hormone derivative (estradiol)
Therapeutic: Ovarian hormone replacement (drospirenone and estradiol)
Pregnancy category: X

Indications and Dosages
▶ *To treat moderate to severe vasomotor symptoms of menopause; to treat moderate to severe vulvar and vaginal atrophy in menopause*
TABLETS (ANGELIQ)
Adult women. 0.5 mg drospirenone and 1 mg estradiol (1 tablet) daily.
▶ *To treat premenstrual dysphoric disorder (PMDD) in women who also use an oral contraceptive*
TABLETS (YAZ)
Adult women. 3 mg drospirenone and 0.02 mg ethinyl estradiol (1 pink tablet) daily for 24 days followed by 1 inert white tablet daily for 4 days. Cycle repeated every 28 days.
▶ *To treat moderate acne vulgaris in women who also chose to use an oral contraceptive*
TABLETS (YAZ)
Adult women and adolescents age 14 and older. 3 mg drospirenone and 0.02 mg ethinyl estradiol (1 pink tablet) daily for 24 days followed by 1 inert white tablet daily for 4 days. Cycle repeated every 28 days.

Contraindications
Active deep vein thrombosis, pulmonary embolism, or history of these conditions; adrenal insufficiency; hepatic disorders; hypersensitivity to drospirenone, estradiol, or their components; known or suspected breast cancer or history of breast cancer from estrogen use; known or suspected estrogen-dependent cancer; new or recent (within past year) stroke or MI; hysterectomy; pregnancy; renal insufficiency; undiagnosed abnormal genital bleeding

Interactions
DRUGS
drospirenone

ACE inhibitors, angiotensin receptor blockers, heparin, NSAIDs, potassium-sparing diuretics, potassium supplements: Increased risk of hyperkalemia

estradiol

barbiturates, carbamazepine, hydantoins, rifabutin, rifampin: Possibly reduced activity of estradiol

corticosteroids: Increased therapeutic and toxic effects of corticosteroids

cyclosporine: Increased risk of hepatotoxicity and nephrotoxicity

didanosine, lamivudine, zalcitabine: Possibly pancreatitis

clarithromycin, erythromycin, itraconazole, ketoconazole, ritonivir: Decreased metabolism and possible increased adverse effects of estradiol

hepatotoxic drugs (such as isoniazid): Increased risk of hepatitis and hepatotoxicity

oral antidiabetics: Decreased therapeutic effects of these drugs

thyroid hormone replacement: Decreased effectiveness of thyroid hormone

warfarin: Decreased or increased anticoagulant effect

FOODS

estradiol

grapefruit juice: Decreased metabolism and possibly increased adverse effects of estradiol

ACTIVITIES

estradiol

smoking: Increased risk of pulmonary embolism, stroke, thrombophlebitis, and transient ischemic attack

Adverse Reactions

CNS: Chorea, dementia, depression, dizziness, exacerbation of epilepsy, headache, insomnia, irritability, migraine headache, mood disturbances, nervousness, porphyria, stroke, worsening of epilepsy

CV: Deep and superficial venous thrombosis, hypertension, increased triglycerides, MI, peripheral edema, pulmonary embolism, thromboembolism, thrombophlebitis

EENT: Diplopia, intolerance of contact lenses, retinal vascular thrombosis, sinusitis, vision changes or loss

ENDO: Breast enlargement, pain, tenderness, or tumors; endometrial hyperplasia, galactorrhea; gynecomastia; hyperglycemia; nipple discharge

GI: Abdominal cramps or pain, anorexia, bloating, constipation, diarrhea, elevated liver function test results, enlargement of hepatic hemangiomas, gallbladder obstruction, hepatitis, increased appetite, nausea, pancreatitis, vomiting

GU: Amenorrhea, breakthrough bleeding, cervical erosion, clear vaginal discharge, dysmenorrhea, endometiral or ovarian tumors, increased libido, leukorrhea, prolonged or heavy menstrual bleeding, vaginal candidiasis

MS: Arthralgias, back or extremity pain, leg cramps

RESP: Exacerbation of asthma, respiratory distress, upper respiratory infection

SKIN: Alopecia, chloasma, erythema multiforme or nodosum, hirsutism, jaundice, melasma, pruritus, purpura, rash, urticaria

Other: Anaphylaxis, angioedema, flulike syndrome, folic acid deficiency, hypercalcemia (with bone metastases), hypocalcemia, hyperkalemia, hyponatremia, weight gain or loss, worsening of systemic lupus erythematosus

---

Mechanism of Action

Drospirenone counters estrogenic effects in menopause by decreasing the number of nuclear estradiol receptors and suppressing epithelial DNA synthesis in endometrial tissue. It also is an aldosterone antagonist, which increases excretion of sodium and water.

Estradiol increases the rate of DNA and RNA synthesis in the cells of female reproductive organs, pituitary gland, hypothalamus, and other target organs. In the hypothalamus, estrogens reduce the release of gonadotropin-releasing hormone, which decreases pituitary release of follicle-stimulating hormone and luteinizing hormone. In women, these hormones are required for normal GU and other essential body functions. At the cellular level, estrogens increase cervical secretions, cause endometrial cell proliferation, and improve uterine tone. Estrogen replacement helps maintain GU function and reduces vasomotor symptoms when estrogen production declines from menopause, surgical removal of ovaries, or other estrogen deficiency.

Nursing Considerations

- Use drospirenone and estradiol cautiously in women with asthma, diabetes mellitus, epilepsy, migraine headaches, porphyria, systemic lupus erythematosus, and hepatic hemangiomas because estrogens may worsen these conditions.
- Give drospirenone and estradiol with or immediately after food to decrease nausea.
- **WARNING** Assess patient for possible contact lens intolerance or changes in vision or visual acuity because estrogens

can cause keratoconus. Be prepared to stop therapy immediately, as prescribed, if patient has sudden partial or complete loss of vision or sudden onset of diplopia or migraine.

- Monitor PT in patients taking warfarin. Estrogens increase production of clotting factors VII, VIII, IX, and X and promote platelet aggregation and thus may cause loss of anticoagulant effect.

- Monitor patient for elevated liver function test results because estrogens and progestins may worsen such conditions as acute intermittent or variegate hepatic porphyria.

- Monitor patient's electrolyte levels as ordered, especially early in therapy, because drospirenone has antialdosterone activity, which may increase serum potassium and decrease serum sodium levels in high-risk patients.

- Closely monitor patient's blood pressure. Some patients may have a substantial increase in blood pressure as an indiosyncratic reaction to estrogen. Monitor patients who already have hypertension for increased blood pressure because estrogens may cause fluid retention. Also monitor patients with asthma, heart disease, migraines, renal disease, or seizure disorder for exacerbation of these conditions.

- Monitor blood glucose level often in patients who have diabetes mellitus because estrogens may decrease insulin sensitivity and alter glucose tolerance.

- Expect to stop drospirenone and estradiol in any woman who develops signs or symptoms of dementia or cardiovascular disease, such as MI, pulmonary embolism, stroke, or venous thrombosis.

- Be aware that drospirenone and estradiol may worsen mood disorders, including depression. Monitor patient for depression, mood changes, anxiety, fatigue, dizziness, or insomnia.

- **WARNING** Be aware that patients with breast cancer and bone metastasis may develop severe hypercalcemia because estrogens influence calcium and phosphorus metabolism. Watch for toxic effects of increased calcium absorption in patients predisposed to hypercalcemia or nephrolithiasis.

- Assess skin for melasma (tan or brown patches), which may develop on forehead, cheeks, temples, and upper lip. These patches may persist after drug is stopped.

- Monitor thyroid function test results in patients with hypothyroidism because long-term use of estradiol may decrease effectiveness of thyroid therapy.

- Expect to stop drospirenone and estradiol therapy several weeks before patient undergoes major surgery, as prescribed, because prolonged immobilization increases the risk of thromboembolism.

PATIENT TEACHING

- Before therapy starts, inform patient of the risks of estrogen-progestin therapy, such as increased risk of cardiovascular disease, breast or endometrial cancer, dementia, gallbladder disease, and vision abnormalities.
- Inform patient that a cyclic regimen of drospirenone and estradiol may cause monthly withdrawal bleeding.
- Instruct patient to avoid eating large quantities of foods high in potassium (such as bananas, oranges, or spinach) or using salt substitutes that contain potassium.
- Instruct patient to report any abnormal signs and symptoms to prescriber.
- Stress importance of having follow-up visits every 3 to 6 months to determine effectiveness of drospirenone and estradiol in relieving menopausal symptoms and having scheduled diagnostic tests to detect adverse reactions.
- Advise patient taking drospirenone and estradiol not to smoke because smoking increases the risk of deep vein thrombosis, MI, and other thromboembolic disorders.

estradiol and levonorgestrel
Climara Pro

Class and Category
Chemical: Estrogenic steroid hormone derivative (estradiol), progesterone steroid hormone derivative (levonorgestrel),
Therapeutic: Ovarian hormone replacement (estradiol, levonorgestrel)
Pregnancy category: X

Indications and Dosages
▶ *To treat moderate to severe vasomotor symptoms of menopause in women who have an intact uterus; to prevent postmenopausal osteoporosis*
PATCH
Adult women. 1 patch (4.4 mg estradiol and 1.39 mg levonorgestrel) applied weekly to lower abdomen, which delivers 0.045 mg estradiol and 0.015 mg levonorgestrel daily.

Mechanism of Action

Estrogens like estradiol increases the rate of DNA and RNA synthesis in the cells of female reproductive organs, pituitary gland, hypothalamus, and other target organs. In the hypothalamus, estrogens reduce the release of gonadotropin-releasing hormone, which decreases pituitary release of follicle-stimulating hormone and luteinizing hormone. In women, these hormones are required for normal GU and other essential body functions. At the cellular level, estrogens increase cervical secretions, cause endometrial cell proliferation, and improve uterine tone. Estrogen replacement helps maintain GU function and reduces vasomotor symptoms when estrogen production declines as a result of menopause, surgical removal of ovaries, or other estrogen deficiency states.

Levonorgestrel inhibits gonadotropin production resulting in retardation of follicular growth and inhibition of ovulation. It also counteracts the proliferative effects of estrogens on the endometrium.

Contraindications

Active deep vein thrombosis, pulmonary embolism, or history of these conditions; adrenal insufficiency; hepatic disorders; hypersensitivity to estradiol, levonorgestrel, or their components; known or suspected breast cancer or history of breast cancer from estrogen use; known or suspected estrogen-dependent cancer, new or recent (within past year) stroke or MI; hysterectomy; pregnancy; renal insufficiency; undiagnosed abnormal genital bleeding

Interactions
DRUGS

estradiol and levonorgestrel
barbiturates, carbamazepine, phenytoin, rifabutin, rifampin: Possibly reduced activity of estradiol and levonorgestrel
estradiol
corticosteroids: Increased therapeutic and toxic corticosteroid effects
hepatotoxic drugs (such as isoniazid): Increased risk of hepatitis and hepatotoxicity
oral antidiabetics: Decreased therapeutic effects of these drugs
warfarin: Decreased anticoagulant effect
FOODS
estradiol
grapefruit juice: Decreased metabolism and possibly increased adverse effects of estradiol

ACTIVITIES
estradiol
smoking: Increased risk of pulmonary embolism, stroke, thrombophlebitis, and transient ischemic attack

Adverse Reactions
CNS: Chorea, dementia, depression, dizziness, exacerbation of epilepsy, headache, irritability, migraine headache, mood disturbances, nervousness, porphyria, stroke
CV: Hypertension, increased triglycerides, MI, peripheral edema, pulmonary embolism, thromboembolism, thrombophlebitis
EENT: Diplopia, intolerance of contact lenses, retinal vascular thrombosis, sinusitis, vision changes or loss
ENDO: Breast enlargement, pain, tenderness, or tumors; endometrial hyperplasia, fibrocystic breast changes; galactorrhea; hyperglycemia; nipple discharge
GI: Abdominal cramps or pain, aggravation of porphyria, anorexia, bloating, cholestatic jaundice, constipation, diarrhea, elevated liver function test results, enlargement of hepatic hemangiomas, flatulence, gallbladder obstruction, hepatitis, increased appetite or incidence of gallbladder disease, nausea, pancreatitis, vomiting
GU: Amenorrhea, breakthrough bleeding, cervical erosion, clear vaginal discharge, dysmenorrhea, endometiral or ovarian tumors, increased libido, increased size of uterine leiomyomata, leukorrhea, prolonged or heavy menstrual bleeding, urinary tract infection, vaginitis including vaginal candidiasis
MS: Arthralgias, back or extremity pain, leg cramps
RESP: Bronchitis, exacerbation of asthma, upper respiratory infection
SKIN: Alopecia, application site irritation, chloasma, erythema multiforme or nodosum, hirsutism, jaundice, melasma, pruritus, purpura, rash, urticaria
Other: Anaphylaxis, angioedema, flulike syndrome, folic acid deficiency, hypercalcemia (with bone metastases), hypocalcemia, hyperkalemia, hyponatremia, weight gain or loss

Nursing Considerations
- Use estradiol and levonorgestrel cautiously in women with asthma, diabetes mellitus, epilepsy, migraine headaches, porphyria, systemic lupus erythematosus, and hepatic hemangiomas because estrogens may worsen these conditions.
- Women using continuous estrogen or combination estrogen-

progestin therapy should complete the current cycle of therapy before starting estradiol and levonorgestrel. Those not using continuous estrogen or combination estrogen-progestin therapy may start estradiol and levonorgestrel immediately.

- Verify that patient has an intact uterus before starting estradiol and levonorgestrel. If not, she doesn't need a product that contains a progestin such as levonorgestrel.
- **WARNING** Assess patient for possible contact lens intolerance or changes in vision or visual acuity because estrogens can cause keratoconus. Be prepared to stop therapy immediately, as prescribed, if patient has sudden partial or complete loss of vision or sudden onset of diplopia or migraine.
- Monitor PT in patients taking warfarin. Estrogens increase production of clotting factors VII, VIII, IX, and X and promote platelet aggregation and thus may cause loss of anticoagulant effect.
- Watch for elevated liver function test results because estrogens and progestins may worsen such conditions as acute intermittent or variegate hepatic porphyria.
- Closely monitor patient's blood pressure. Some patients may have a substantial increase in blood pressure as an indiosyncratic reaction to estrogen. Monitor patients who already have hypertension for increased blood pressure because estrogens may cause fluid retention. Also monitor patients with asthma, heart disease, migraines, renal disease, or seizure disorder for worsening of these conditions.
- Monitor blood glucose level often in patients who have diabetes mellitus because estrogens may decrease insulin sensitivity and alter glucose tolerance.
- **WARNING** Expect to stop estradiol and levonorgestrel in any woman who develops signs or symptoms of dementia or cardiovascular disease, such as MI, pulmonary embolism, stroke, or venous thrombosis.
- Be aware that estradiol and levonorgestrel may worsen mood disorders, including depression. Monitor patient for depression, mood changes, anxiety, fatigue, dizziness, or insomnia.
- **WARNING** Be aware that patients with breast cancer and bone metastasis may develop severe hypercalcemia because estrogens influence calcium and phosphorus metabolism. Watch for toxic effects of increased calcium absorption in patients predisposed to hypercalcemia or nephrolithiasis.
- Assess skin for melasma (tan or brown patches), which may de-

velop on forehead, cheeks, temples, and upper lip. These patches may persist after drug is stopped.

• Monitor thyroid function test results in patients with hypothyroidism because long-term use of estradiol may decrease effectiveness of thyroid therapy.

• Expect to stop estradiol and levonorgestrel therapy several weeks before patient undergoes major surgery, as prescribed, because prolonged immobilization poses a risk of thromboembolism.

PATIENT TEACHING

• Before therapy starts, inform patient of the risks of estrogen-progestin therapy, such as increased risk of cardiovascular disease, breast or endometrial cancer, dementia, gallbladder disease, and vision abnormalities.

• Instruct patient to select application site on lower abdomen but not to use a site that's oily, scarred, irritated, or at the waistline.

• Teach patient how to apply the transdermal patch. Tell patient to remove one side of the protective liner, being careful not to touch the adhesive part of the patch, and immediately apply to a smooth area of skin. She should then remove the second side of the protective liner and press the patch firmly in place for at least 10 seconds, ensuring good contact, especially at the edges.

• Caution patient never to apply patch on or near the breasts.

• Instruct patient to apply a new patch once a week, rotating sites in the lower abdomen after carefully and gently removing the previous patch. If any adhesive remains on the skin, instruct patient to let the area dry for 15 minutes and then gently rub it with an oil-based cream or lotion to remove the adhesive residue. Tell her to fold the used patch carefully in half so that it sticks to itself before discarding it.

• Tell patient that if patch is dislodged, it can be reapplied to another area of the lower abdomen or a new patch applied, keeping the original treatment schedule.

• Stress importance of wearing only one patch at a time.

• Caution patient to avoid exposing patch to sun for long periods.

• Urge patient to notify prescriber immediately about vaginal bleeding or any other abnormal signs and symptoms while using estradiol and levonorgestrel.

• Advise patient to avoid smoking while using an estrogen-progestin product such as estradiol and levonorgestrel.

• Stress importance of having follow-up visits every 3 to 6 months to determine effectiveness of estradiol and levonorgestrel at re-

lieving menopausal symptoms. Also stress need to have scheduled diagnostic tests to detect adverse reactions.
• Emphasize importance of good dental hygiene and regular dental checkups because an elevated progestin blood level increases the growth of normal oral flora, which may lead to gum tenderness, bleeding, or swelling.

estradiol and norethindrone acetate
Activella, CombiPatch
estradiol, norethindrone acetate, and ferrous fumarate
Estrostep Fe

Class and Category
Chemical: Estrogen derivative (estradiol), steroid hormone (norethindrone)
Therapeutic: Antiosteoporotic agent, ovarian hormone replacement
Pregnancy category: X

Indications and Dosages
▶ *To treat estrogen deficiency caused by hypogonadism, oophorectomy, or primary ovarian failure in patients with an intact uterus*
TRANSDERMAL (COMBIPATCH)
Adult women. For continuous combined regimen in women who don't want to resume menses: 9-cm^2 CombiPatch (0.05 mg estradiol and 0.14 mg norethindrone acetate daily) worn continuously on lower abdomen; may be increased to 16-cm^2 CombiPatch (0.05 mg estradiol and 0.25 mg norethindrone acetate daily), as prescribed, if a larger progestin dose is desired. New patch is applied twice weekly (every 3 to 4 days) during a 28-day cycle.

For continuous sequential regimen in combination with transdermal estradiol-only system: Vivelle (0.05 mg daily) estradiol transdermal system is worn for the first 14 days of a 28-day cycle, replaced twice weekly according to product directions. For the remaining 14 days of the 28-day cycle, 9-cm^2 CombiPatch (0.05 mg estradiol and 0.14 mg norethindrone acetate daily) is worn on the lower abdomen; may be increased to 16-cm^2 CombiPatch (0.05 mg estradiol and 0.25-mg norethindrone acetate daily), as prescribed, if a larger progestin dose is desired. CombiPatch should be replaced twice weekly (every 3 to 4 days) during this period in the cycle.

▶ *To treat menopausal symptoms and prevent osteoporosis from estrogen deficiency in postmenopausal women with an intact uterus*

TRANSDERMAL (COMBIPATCH)

Adult women. For continuous combined regimen in women who don't want to resume menses: 9-cm^2 CombiPatch (0.05 mg estradiol and 0.14 mg norethindrone acetate daily) worn continuously on lower abdomen; may be increased to 16-cm^2 Combi-Patch (0.05 mg estradiol and 0.25 mg norethindrone acetate daily), as prescribed, if a larger progestin dose is desired. New patch is applied twice weekly (every 3 to 4 days) during a 28-day cycle.

For continuous sequential regimen in combination with transdermal estradiol-only system: Vivelle (0.05 mg daily) estradiol transdermal system is worn for the first 14 days of a 28-day cycle, replaced twice weekly according to product directions. For the remaining 14 days of the 28-day cycle, 9-cm^2 CombiPatch (0.05 mg estradiol and 0.14 mg norethindrone acetate daily) is worn on the lower abdomen; may be increased to 16-cm^2 Combi-Patch (0.05 mg estradiol and 0.25-mg norethindrone acetate daily), as prescribed, if a larger progestin dose is desired. Combi-Patch should be replaced twice weekly (every 3 to 4 days) during this period in the cycle.

▶ *To treat moderate to severe vasomotor symptoms of meonopause; to prevent postmenopausal osteoporosis*

TABLETS (ACTIVELLA)

Adult women. 0.5 to 1 mg estradiol and 0.1 to 0.5 mg norethindrone acetate (1 tablet of appropriate strength) daily.

▶ *To treat moderate to severe symptoms of vulvar and vaginal atrophy*

TABLETS (ACTIVELLA)

Adult women. 1 mg estradiol and 0.5 mg norethindrone acetate (1 tablet) daily.

▶ *To treat moderate acne vulgaris in women who also desire oral contraceptive therapy for at least 6 months*

TABLETS (ESTROSTEP FE)

Adult women and adolescents age 15 and older. 20 mcg ethinyl estradiol and 1 mg norethindrone (1 triangle white tablet) once daily for 5 days; then, 30 mcg ethinyl estradiol and 1 mg norethindrone (1 square white tablet) once daily for 7 days; then, 35 mcg ethinyl estradiol and 1 mg norethindrone (1 round white tablet) once daily for nine days; then, 75 mg ferrous fumarate (1 brown tablet) once daily for 7 days. Cycle repeated every 28 days.

Mechanism of Action

Estradiol increases the rate of DNA and RNA synthesis in the cells of female reproductive organs, pituitary gland, hypothalamus, and other target organs. In the hypothalamus, estrogens decrease release of gonadotropin-releasing hormone, which reduces pituitary release of follicle-stimulating hormone and luteinizing hormone. In women, these hormones are required for normal GU and other essential body functions. At the cellular level, estrogens increase cervical secretions, cause endometrial cell proliferation, and improve uterine tone. Estrogen replacement helps maintain GU function and reduces vasomotor symptoms when estrogen production declines from menopause, removal of ovaries, or estrogen deficiency. Estrogen replacement also helps prevent osteoporosis by inhibiting bone resorption.

Norethindrone is a progestin. Progestins prolong some positive effects of estrogens on high-density lipoprotein cholesterol. Norethindrone diffuses freely into target cells of the female reproductive tract, mammary glands, hypothalamus, and pituitary gland and binds to the progesterone cell receptor. It converts a proliferative endometrium into a secretory one in women with adequate estrogen replacement, reducing endometrial growth and the risk of endometrial cancer compared with women who have an intact uterus and take unopposed estrogens. Norethindrone also decreases nuclear estradiol receptors and suppresses epithelial DNA synthesis in endometrial tissues.

Contraindications

Active deep vein thrombosis, pulmonary embolism, or history of these conditions; endometrial hyperplasia; hepatic disorders; hypersensitivity to estradiol, norethindrone, or their components; jaundice; known or suspected breast cancer or history of breast cancer from estrogen use; known or suspected estrogen-dependent cancer; new or recent (within past year) stroke or MI; pregnancy; undiagnosed abnormal genital bleeding; vaginal disorders

Interactions

DRUGS

estradiol and norethindrone

aminocaproic acid: Possibly an increase in hypercoagulability caused by aminocaproic acid

barbiturates, carbamazepine, hydantoins, rifabutin, rifampin: Possibly reduced activity of estradiol and norethindrone

bromocriptine: Possibly decreased bromocriptine effects

calcium: Possibly increased calcium absorption

corticosteroids: Increased therapeutic and toxic effects of corticosteroids

cyclosporine: Increased risk of hepatotoxicity and nephrotoxicity

didanosine, lamivudine, zalcitabine: Possibly pancreatitis

hepatotoxic drugs (such as isoniazid): Increased risk of hepatitis and hepatotoxicity

oral antidiabetics: Decreased therapeutic effects of these drugs

somatrem, somatropin: Possibly accelerated epiphyseal maturation

tamoxifen: Possibly decreased therapeutic effects of tamoxifen

vitamin C: Decreased metabolism and possibly increased adverse effects of estradiol and norethindrone

warfarin: Decreased anticoagulant effect

estradiol

thyroid hormone replacement: Decreased effectiveness of thyroid hormone

FOODS

estradiol and norethindrone

grapefruit juice: Decreased metabolism and possibly increased adverse effects of estradiol and norethindrone

ACTIVITIES

estradiol and norethindrone

smoking: Increased risk of pulmonary embolism, stroke, thrombophlebitis, and transient ischemic attack

Adverse Reactions

CNS: Dementia, depression, dizziness, headache, irritability, migraine headache, insomnia, mood swings, stroke, worsening of epilepsy

CV: Deep and superficial venous thrombosis, hypertension, hypertriglyceridemia, MI, peripheral edema, pulmonary embolism, thromboembolism, thrombophlebitis

EENT: Intolerance of contact lenses, retinal vascular thrombosis, sinusitis, vision changes

ENDO: Breast enlargement, pain, tenderness, or tumors; gynecomastia; hyperglycemia; nipple discharge

GI: Abdominal cramps or pain, anorexia, constipation, diarrhea, elevated liver function test results, enlargement of hepatic hemangiomas, gallbladder obstruction, gastroenteritis, hepatitis, increased appetite, nausea, pancreatitis, vomiting

GU: Amenorrhea, breakthrough bleeding, cervical erosion, clear vaginal discharge, decreased libido (men), dysmenorrhea, endometrial hyperplasia or cancer, impotence, increased libido

(women), ovarian cancer or cyst, prolonged or heavy menstrual bleeding, testicular atrophy, uterine fibroid, vaginal candidiasis
MS: Back pain, leg cramps
RESP: Worsening of asthma
SKIN: Acne, alopecia, hirsutism, jaundice, melasma, oily skin, purpura, rash, seborrhea, urticaria
Other: Anaphylaxis, folic acid deficiency, hypercalcemia (in metastatic bone disease), hypocalcemia, weight gain, worsening of systemic lupus erythematosus

Nursing Considerations

- Use estradiol and norethindrone cautiously in patients with asthma, diabetes mellitus, epilepsy, migraine, porphyria, systemic lupus erythematosus, or hepatic hemangioma because drug may worsen these conditions.
- **WARNING** Be aware that patients with breast cancer and bone metastasis may develop severe hypercalcemia because estrogens influence calcium and phosphorus metabolism. Watch for toxic effects of increased calcium absorption in patients predisposed to hypercalcemia or nephrolithiasis.
- **WARNING** Assess patient for contact lens intolerance or changes in vision or visual acuity because estrogens can cause keratoconus. Be prepared to stop drug immediately, as prescribed, if patient has sudden partial or complete loss of vision or sudden onset of diplopia, migraine, or proptosis.
- Monitor PT in patients receiving warfarin for loss of anticoagulant effect because estrogens increase production of clotting factors VII, VIII, IX, and X and promote platelet aggregation.
- Watch for elevated liver function test results because estrogen and progestins may worsen such conditions as acute intermittent or variegate hepatic porphyria.
- Closely monitor patient's blood pressure. Some patients may have a substantial increase in blood pressure as an idiosyncratic reaction to estrogen. Monitor patients who already have hypertension for increases in blood pressure because estrogens may cause fluid retention. Also monitor patients with asthma, heart disease, migraines, renal disease, or seizure disorder for worsening of these conditions.
- Watch for peripheral edema or mild weight gain because estrogens can cause sodium and fluid retention.
- Check triglyceride levels routinely because, in patients with hypertriglyceridemia, estrogen may increase serum triglyceride level enough to cause pancreatitis and other complications.

- Monitor blood glucose level often in patients who have diabetes mellitus because conjugated estrogens may decrease insulin sensitivity and alter glucose tolerance.
- Be aware that exogenous estradiol and norethindrone may worsen mood disorders, including depression. Monitor patient for anxiety, depression, dizziness, fatigue, insomnia, or mood changes. If significant depression occurs, expect to stop hormone replacement therapy.
- Assess skin for melasma (tan or brown patches), which may develop on forehead, cheeks, temples, and upper lip. These patches may persist after drug is stopped.
- Expect to stop estrogen combination therapy in any woman with evidence of dementia, cancer, or cardiovascular disease, such as MI pulmonary embolism, stroke, or venous thrombosis.
- Monitor thyroid function test results in patients with hypothyroidism because long-term estradiol use may decrease effectiveness of thyroid replacement therapy.
- **WARNING** Expect to stop estrogen combination therapy in any woman with evidence of dementia, cancer, or cardiovascular disease, such as MI, pulmonary embolism, stroke, or venous thrombosis.
- Expect to stop estrogen therapy several weeks before major surgery, as prescribed, because prolonged immobilization increases the risk of thromboembolism.

PATIENT TEACHING
- Before therapy starts, explain the risks of estrogen-progestin therapy, such as increased risk of breast, endometrial, or ovarian cancer; cardiovascular disease; gallbladder disease; and vision abnormalities.
- Instruct patient taking oral drug for acne vulgaris and contraception to take the tablet at the same time every day. If a tablet is missed, tell her to take the missed dose as soon as she remembers and to use an alternate birth control method for 7 days.
- Teach patient proper application and use of CombiPatch. Instruct her to tear pouch open, rather than cutting it with scissors, and to remove stiff protective liner covering adhesive without touching adhesive. Tell her not to cut or trim the patch. Advise her to apply patch to a clean, dry, hairless part of lower abdomen. Caution her not to apply patch to breasts; to injured, irritated, callused, or scarred areas; or to areas where it may not adhere properly, such as the waistline.

- Advise patient to rotate application sites at least weekly and to remove old patch before applying new one. If patch falls off, instruct her to reapply it to another area or to apply a new patch and continue the original treatment schedule. Caution her not to expose patch to sun for prolonged periods. Explain that she may bathe while wearing the patch.
- Advise patient taking estradiol and norethindrone not to smoke because smoking increases the risk of deep vein thrombosis, MI, and other thromboembolic disorders.
- Explain that estradiol and norethindrone may cause monthly withdrawal bleeding.
- Advise patient receiving estradiol treatment to have an annual pelvic examination, including a Papanicolaou smear, to screen for cervical dysplasia.
- Emphasize the importance of good dental hygiene and regular dental checkups because an elevated serum progestin (norethindrone) level increases the growth of normal oral flora, which may lead to gum tenderness, bleeding, or swelling.

estrogens (conjugated) and medroxyprogesterone
Premphase, Prempro

Class and Category
Chemical: Estrogen steroid hormone derivative (conjugated estrogens), progesterone steroid hormone derivative (medroxyprogesterone)
Therapeutic: Antiosteoporotic, ovarian hormone replacement (conjugated estrogens, medroxyprogesterone)
Pregnancy category: X

Indications and Dosages
▶ *To treat moderate to severe vasomotor menopausal symptoms and vaginal and vulvar atrophy*
TABLETS (PREMPRO)
Adult women. 0.3 mg conjugated estrogens and 1.5 mg medroxyprogesterone (1 tablet) daily. Increased to 0.625 mg conjugated estrogens and 5 mg medroxyprogesterone (1 tablet) daily as needed.
TABLETS (PREMPHASE)
Adult women. 0.625 mg conjugated estrogen (1 tablet) daily on days 1 through day 14 and 0.625 mg conjugated estrogens and

5 mg medroxyprogesterone (1 tablet) on days 15 through 28. Cycle repeated every 28 days.

▶ *To prevent postmenopausal osteoporosis*

TABLETS (PREMPRO)

Adult women. 0.3 mg conjugated estrogens and 1.5 mg medroxyprogesterone (1 tablet) daily. Increased to 0.625 mg conjugated estrogens and 5 mg medroxyprogesterone (1 tablet) daily as needed.

TABLETS (PREMPHASE)

Adult women. 0.625 mg conjugated estrogen (1 tablet) daily on days 1 through 14. Then 0.625 mg conjugated estrogens and 5 mg medroxyprogesterone (1 tablet) on days 15 through 28.

Mechanism of Action

Conjugated estrogens increase DNA and RNA synthesis in the cells of female reproductive organs, hypothalamus, pituitary glands, and other target organs. In the hypothalamus, estrogens reduce release of gonadotropin-releasing hormone, which decreases pituitary release of follicle-stimulating hormone and luteinizing hormone. In women, these hormones are required for normal GU and other essential body functions. At the cellular level, estrogens increase cervical secretions, cause endometrial cell proliferation, and increase uterine tone. Estrogen replacement helps maintain GU function and reduce vasomotor symptoms when estrogen production declines from menopause, surgical removal of ovaries, or other estrogen deficiency states. Estrogen replacement also helps prevent osteoporosis by inhibiting bone resorption so that resorption doesn't exceed bone formation.

Medroxyprogesterone, a progestin, may achieve its beneficial effect on the endometrium in part by decreasing nuclear estrogen receptors and suppression of epithelial DNA synthesis in endometrial tissue.

Contraindications

Abnormal or undiagnosed vaginal bleeding; breast, endometrial, or estrogen-dependent cancer; hypersensitivity to conjugated estrogens, medroxyprogesterone, other progestins, peanuts or their components; pregnancy; thromboembolic disorders

Interactions

DRUGS

conjugated estrogens and medroxyprogesterone

barbiturates, carbamazepine, hydantoins, rifabutin, rifampin: Possibly reduced activity of estrogen and medroxyprogesterone

conjugated estrogens
corticosteroids: Increased therapeutic and toxic effects of corticosteroids
cyclosporine: Increased risk of hepatotoxicity and nephrotoxicity
oral antidiabetics: Decreased therapeutic effects of these drugs
warfarin: Decreased anticoagulant effect

medroxyprogesterone
aminoglutethimide: Possibly increased hepatic metabolism of medroxyprogesterone, decreasing its therapeutic effects

ACTIVITIES

conjugated estrogens
smoking: Increased risk of pulmonary embolism, stroke, thrombophlebitis, and transient ischemic attack

Adverse Reactions

CNS: Anxiety, chorea, dementia, depression, dizziness, exacerbation of epilepsy, fatigue, fever, headache, insomnia, irritability, migraine headache, mood disturbances, nervousness, somnolence, stroke

CV: Edema, increased triglycerides, MI, peripheral edema, hypertension, thromboembolism, thrombophlebitis

EENT: Diplopia, intolerance of contact lenses, neuro-ocular lesions, optic neuritis, retinal vascular thrombosis, vision change or loss

ENDO: Breast enlargement, pain, tenderness, or tumors; fibrocystic breast changes; galactorrhea; hyperglycemia; nipple discharge

GI: Abdominal cramps or pain, aggravation of porphyria, anorexia, bloating, cholestatic jaundice, constipation, diarrhea, enlargment of hepatic hemangiomas, gallbladder obstruction, hepatitis, increased or decreased appetite, increased incidence of gallbladder disease, nausea, pancreatitis, vomiting

GU: Amenorrhea, breakthrough bleeding, change in cervical erosion, change in amount of cervical secretions, clear vaginal discharge, cystitislike syndrome, changes in libido, dysmenorrhea, endometrial hyperplasia or cancer, increase in size of uterine leiomyomata, ovarian cancer, premenstruallike syndrome, prolonged or heavy menstrual bleeding, vaginal candidiasis, worsening of endometriosis

MS: Backache

RESP: Exacerbation of asthma, pulmonary embolism

SKIN: Acne, alopecia, chloasma, erythema multiforme, erythema nodosum, hemorrhagic eruption, hirsutism, jaundice, melasma,

oily skin, purpura, pruritus, rash, seborrhea, urticaria
Other: Anaphylaxis, angioedema, folic acid deficiency, hypercalcemia (in metastatic bone disease), hypocalcemia, weight gain or loss

Nursing Considerations

- Use conjugated estrogens and medroxyprogesterone cautiously in patients with severe hypocalcemia because a sudden increase in serum calcium level may cause adverse effects.
- Monitor women age 75 or older closely during therapy with estrogens (conjugated) and medroxyprogesterone because they have an increased risk of stroke and invasive breast cancer.
- Monitor serum calcium level in patients with breast cancer and bone metastasis for severe hypercalcemia because conjugated estrogens influence calcium and phosphorus metabolism.
- Assess for peripheral edema, a sign of fluid retention, and evaluate patient's fluid intake and output, watching for positive fluid balance.
- Assess hypertensive patients for increases in blood pressure because conjugated estrogens may cause fluid retention.
- Monitor patients with asthma, diabetes mellitus, endometriosis, heart disease, renal disease, migraine headaches, seizure disorder, or lupus erythematosus for worsening of these conditions.
- **WARNING** Assess patient for possible contact lens intolerance or changes in vision or visual acuity because estrogens can cause keratoconus. Be prepared to stop drug immediately, as prescribed, if patient has sudden partial or complete loss of vision or sudden onset of diplopia or migraine.
- If patient takes warfarin, assess PT for loss of anticoagulant effects because conjugated estrogens increase production of clotting factors and promote platelet aggregation.
- Monitor blood glucose level often in patients who have diabetes mellitus because conjugated estrogens may decrease insulin sensitivity and alter glucose tolerance.
- Assess skin for melasma (tan or brown patches), which may develop on forehead, cheeks, temples, and upper lip. These patches may persist after drug is stopped.
- **WARNING** Expect to stop conjugated estrogens and medroxyprogesterone in any woman who develops dementia or has cardiovascular disease, such as MI, pulmonary embolism, srtoke, or venous thrombosis.
- Assess patient for evidence of depression, such as changes in mental status, affect, and mood.

- Watch for elevated liver function test values because conjugated estrogen and medroxyprogesterone may worsen such conditions as acute intermittent or variegate hepatic porphyria.
- Expect to stop therapy during periods of immobilization, 4 weeks before elective surgery, and if jaundice develops.

PATIENT TEACHING

- Before therapy starts, explain the risks of conjugated estrogens and medoxyprogesterone, such as an increased risk of cardio-vascular disease, breast or endometrial cancer, dementia, and gallbladder disease.
- Urge patient to immediately report breakthrough bleeding.
- Instruct patient to perform monthly breast self-examination and comply with all prescribed follow-up examinations, especially endometrial tests, because conjugated estrogens increase the risk of breast and endometrial cancer.
- Encourage patient to stay active to reduce the risk of throm-bophlebitis.
- Warn women that long-term use may increase risk of heart dis-ease, stroke, dementia, and breast or endometrial cancer.
- Urge patient to avoid smoking while using conjugated estrogens and medroxyprogesterone.
- Emphasize importance of good dental hygiene and regular den-tal checkups because an elevated progestin level increases growth of normal oral flora, which may lead to gum tender-ness, bleeding, or swelling.

estrogens (esterified) and methyltestosterone
Estratest, Estratest H.S.

Class and Category
Chemical: Sodium salts of sulfate esters of estrogenic substances (esterified estrogens), synthetic androgen (methyltestosterone)
Therapeutic: Hormone replacement (esterified estrogens, methyl-testosterone)
Pregnancy category: X

Indications and Dosages
▶ *To treat moderate to severe vasomotor symptoms of menopause in patients who haven't responded to estrogen alone*
TABLETS
Adult women. 0.625 mg to 1.25 mg esterified estrogens and

1.25 to 2.5 mg methyltestosterone (1 or 2 tablets Estratest H.S., 1 tablet Estratest) daily for 21 days, followed by 7 days without therapy. Cycle repeated as often as needed.

Mechanism of Action

Esterified estrogens increase DNA and RNA synthesis in the cells of female reproductive organs, pituitary gland, hypothalamus, and other target organs. In the hypothalamus, estrogens reduce release of gonadotropin-releasing hormone, which reduces pituitary release of follicle-stimulating hormone and luteinizing hormone. In women, these hormones are required for normal GU and other essential body functions. At the cellular level, estrogens increase cervical secretions, cause endometrial cell proliferation, and improve uterine tone. Estrogen replacement helps maintain GU function and reduces vasomotor symptoms when estrogen production declines from menopause, surgical removal of ovaries, or other estrogen deficiency.

Methyltestosterone is a synthetic form of testosterone. Testosterone first undergoes hydrolysis to the active form, free testosterone in the liver. Free testosterone is further converted into two of the major active metabolites, DHT and estradiol. Thus, testosterone can produce estrogenic effects as a result of its conversion to estradiol to help maintain GU function and reduce vasomotor symptoms when estrogen production declines from menopause, surgical removal of ovaries, or other estrogen deficiency.

Contraindications

Active thrombophlebitis or thromboembolic disorders; breast-feeding; hypersensitivity to estrogens, methyltestosterone, or their components; known or suspected breast cancer (except in select patients being treated for metastatic disease); known or suspected estrogen-dependent cancer; pregnancy; severe liver damage; undiagnosed abnormal genital bleeding

Interactions

DRUGS

esterified estrogens and methyltestosterone
oral antidiabetics: Decreased or increased therapeutic effects of these drugs with risk of hyperglycemia or hypoglycemia
warfarin: Altered anticoagulant effect
esterified estrogens
barbiturates, carbamazepine, hydantoins, rifabutin, rifampin: Possibly reduced activity of esterified estrogens
clarithromycin, erythromycin, intraconazole, ketoconazole, ritonivir: Pos-

sibly increased plasma estrogen concentration

hepatotoxic drugs (such as isoniazid): Increased risk of hepatitis and hepatotoxicity

methyltestosterone

cyclosporine: Possibly increased risk of nephrotoxicity

estradiol, estrogens: Enhanced estrogenic effects

oxyphenbutazone: Increased serum oxyphenbutazone levels

FOODS

esterified estrogens

grapefruit juice: Decreased metabolism and possibly increased adverse effects of esterified estrogens

ACTIVITIES

esterified estrogens and methyltestosterone

smoking: Increased risk of pulmonary embolism, stroke, thrombophlebitis, and transient ischemic attack

Adverse Reactions

CNS: Anxiety, chorea, dementia, depression, dizziness, exacerbation of epilepsy, generalized parasthesia, headache, irritability, migraine headache, mood disturbances, nervousness, stroke

CV: Edema, elevated cholesterol and triglyceride levels, hypertension, MI, peripheral edema, thromboembolism, thrombophlebitis

EENT: Diplopia, intolerance of contact lenses, retinal vascular thrombosis, steepening of corneal curvature, vision changes or loss

ENDO: Breast enlargement, pain, tenderness or tumors; fibrocystic breast changes; galactorrhea; hypercalcemia; hyperglycemia; hypocalcemia; hypoglycemia; nipple discharge; virilization

GI: Abdominal cramps or pain, aggravation of porphyria, anorexia, bloating, cholestatic jaundice, constipation, diarrhea, elevated liver function test results, gallbladder obstruction, hepatitis including increased appetite, jaundice, nausea, pancreatitis, vomiting

GU: Alteration in amount of cervical secretions, amenorrhea, breakthrough bleeding, cervical erosion, changes in cervical ectropion, clear vaginal discharge, cystitis-like syndrome, dysmenorrhea, changes in libido, increased size of uterine leiomyomata, ovarian cancer, prolonged or heavy menstrual bleeding, vaginitis including vaginal candidiasis

HEME: Polycythemia

MS: Arthralgias, leg cramps

RESP: Exacerbation of asthma, pulmonary embolism

SKIN: Acne, alopecia, chloasma, erythema multiforme or no-

dosum, hemorrhagic eruption, hirsutism, jaundice, melasma, oily skin, pruritus, purpura, rash, seborrhea, urticaria
Other: Anaphylaxis, angioedema, fluid and electrolyte imbalance, folic acid deficiency, weight gain or loss

Nursing Considerations

- Use cautiously in patients with mild to moderate hepatic dysfunction because estrogens such as esterified estrogens are poorly metabolized in patients with hepatic dysfunction. Do not administer the drug to patients with severe hepatic dysfunction.
- Also use cautiously in patients with renal insufficiency or patients with metabolic bone diseases because estrogens influence the metabolism of calcium and phosphorus.
- **WARNING** Be aware that patients with breast cancer and bone metastasis may develop severe hypercalcemia because esterified estrogens influence calcium and phosphorus metabolism and methyltestosterone stimulates osteolysis. Watch for toxic effects of increased calcium levels in patients predisposed to hypercalcemia or nephrolithiasis.
- Monitor PT in patients receiving warfarin for altered anticoagulant effect because estrogens increase production of clotting factors VII, VIII, IX, and X and promote platelet aggregation.
- Watch for elevated liver function test results because esterified estrogens and methyltestosterone may worsen such conditions as acute intermittent or variegate hepatic porphyria as well as cause peliosis hepatis, cholestatic hepatitis, and hepatocellular carcinoma. If jaundice develops, stop drug and notify prescriber.
- **WARNING** Assess patient for possible contact lens intolerance or changes in vision or visual acuity because estrogens can cause keratoconus. Be prepared to stop drug immediately, as prescribed, if patient has sudden partial or complete loss of vision or sudden onset of diplopia or migraine.
- Closely monitor patient's blood pressure. Some patients may have a substantial increase in blood pressure as an indiosyncratic reaction to estrogens. Monitor patients who already have hypertension for increases in blood pressure because estrogens may cause fluid retention. Also monitor patients with asthma, heart disease, migraines, renal disease, or seizure disorder for exacerbation of these conditions.
- Watch for peripheral edema or mild weight gain because esterified estrogens and methyltestosterone can cause sodium and fluid retention.
- Monitor blood glucose level often in patients with diabetes mel-

litus because estrogens may decrease insulin sensitivity and alter glucose tolerance.

• **WARNING** Expect to stop esterified estrogens and methyltestosterone therapy in any woman who develops signs or symptoms of cardiovascular disease, such as MI, pulmonary embolism, stroke, or venous thrombosis.

• Be aware that exogenous estrogens may worsen mood disorders, including depression. Monitor patient for depression, mood changes, anxiety, fatigue, dizziness, or insomnia.

• Assess skin for melasma (tan or brown patches), which may develop on forehead, cheeks, temples, and upper lip. These patches may persist after drug is stopped.

• Monitor thyroid function test results in patients with hypothyroidism because long-term use of esterified estrogens may decrease effectiveness of thyroid therapy.

• Expect to stop therapy several weeks before patient undergoes major surgery, as prescribed, because prolonged immobilization poses a risk of thromboembolism.

PATIENT TEACHING

• Before therapy starts, inform patient of risks involved in esterified estrogens and methyltestosterone therapy, such as increased risk of cardiovascular disease, breast or endometrial cancer, dementia, gallbladder disease, and vision abnormalities.

• Inform patient that she should have an annual physical examination including a pelvic examination to screen for adverse effects such as cervical dysplasia.

• Inform patient that a cyclic combination regimen may cause monthly withdrawal bleeding.

• Instruct patient to notify prescriber if masculine changes appear, such as a deepening of the voice or facial hair growth.

• Also tell patient to notify prescriber of any unusual signs and symptoms because drug can cause serious adverse effects.

• Urge patient taking esterified estrogens and methyltestosterone not to smoke because smoking increases the risk of deep vein thrombosis, heart attack, and other thromboemolic disorders.

glipizide and metformin hydrochloride
Metaglip

Class and Category

Chemical: Sulfonylurea (glipizide), dimethylbiguanide (metformin)

Therapeutic: Antidiabetic
Pregnancy category: C

Indications and Dosages

▶ *To reduce blood glucose level as initial therapy in patients with type 2 diabetes mellitus*
TABLETS
Adults. *Initial:* If fasting blood glucose is 280 to 320 mg/dl, give 2.5 mg glipizide and 250 mg metformin daily with morning meal or 2.5 mg glipizide and 500 mg metformin b.i.d. with morning and evening meals. Dosage increased by initial dosage strength every 2 wk, as needed. *Maximum:* 10 mg glipizde and 1,000 mg metformin, or 10 mg glipizide and 2,000 mg metformin daily in divided doses if initial fasting glucose level is 280 to 320 mg/dl.

▶ *To reduce blood glucose level in patients with type 2 diabetes mellitus who aren't adequately controlled with either a sulfonylurea or metformin*
TABLETS
Adults. *Initial:* 2.5 mg glipizide and 500 mg metformin or 5 mg glipizide and 500 mg metformin b.i.d. with morning and evening meals. Dosage increased by no more than 5 mg glipizide and 500 mg metformin as needed. *Maximum:* 20 mg glipizide and 2,000 mg metformin daily.

DOSAGE ADJUSTMENT For patients taking glipizide or another sulfonylurea, metformin, or a combination of these drugs, expect initial dosage of combination drug to be equal to or less than that currently being taken individually.

Mechanism of Action

Glipizide and metformin hydrochloride work in complementary ways to improve glucose control. Glipizide stimulates insulin release from beta cells in the pancreas. It also increases peripheral tissue sensitivity to insulin, either by enhancing insulin binding to cellular receptors or by increasing the number of insulin receptors.

Metformin may promote storage of excess glucose as glycogen in the liver, thus reducing glucose production. It also may improve glucose use by skeletal muscle and adipose tissue by facilitating glucose transport, increasing insulin receptors, and making them more sensitive to insulin.

Contraindications

Acute or chronic metabolic acidosis; diabetic coma; heart failure requiring drug treatment; hypersensitivity to glipizide, metformin, or their components; ketoacidosis; pregnancy; renal disease or dysfunction (serum creatinine level 1.5 mg/dl or more in men or 1.4 mg/dl or more in women or abnormal creatinine clearance)

Interactions
DRUGS
glipizide and metformin hydrochloride
calcium channel blockers, corticosteroids, diuretics, estrogens, isoniazid, nicotinic acid, oral contraceptives, phenothiazine, phenytoin, sympathomimetics, thiazide diuretics, thyroid hormones: Possibly hyperglycemia or hypoglycemia when these drugs are withdrawn
vitamin B_{12}: Probably decreased vitamin B_{12} absorption
glipizide
ACE inhibitors, anabolic steroids, androgens, azole antifungals, bromocriptine, chloramphenicol, disopyramide, fibric acid derivatives, guanethidine, H_2-receptor antagonists, insulin, magnesium salts, MAO inhibitors, methyldopa, octreotide, oral anticoagulants, oxyphenbutazone, phenylbutazone, probenecid, quinidine, salicylates, sulfonamides, tetracycline, theophylline, tricyclic antidepressants, urinary acidifiers: Increased risk of hypoglycemia
asparaginase, calcium channel blockers, cholestyramine, clonidine, corticosteroids, danazol, diazoxide, estrogen, glucagons, hydantoins, isoniazid, lithium, morphine, nicotinic acid, oral contraceptives, phenothiazines, rifabutin, rifampin, sympathomimetics, thiazide diuretics, thyroid drugs, urinary alkalinizers: Increased risk of hyperglycemia
beta blockers: Possibly hyperglycemia or masking of hypoglycemia
cardiac glycosides: Increased risk of digitalis toxicity
pentamidine: Initially hypoglycemia and then hyperglycemia if beta cell damage occurs
metformin
calcium channel blockers, corticosteroids, estrogens, hormonal contraceptives, isoniazid, nicotinic acid, phenothiazines, phenytoin, sympathomimetics, thiazide and other diuretics, thyroid drugs: Possibly hyperglycemia
clofibrate, MAO inhibitors, probenecid, propranolol, rifabutin, rifampin, salicylates, sulfonamides, sulfonylureas: Increased risk of hypoglycemia
cationic drugs (such as amiloride, cimetidine, digoxin, morphine, procainamide, quinidine, quinine, ranitidine, triamterene, trimethoprim, vancomycin) nifedipine: Increased blood metformin level
ACTIVITIES
metformin
alcohol use: Possibly increased risk of hypoglycemia; possibly po-

tentiated lactate metabolism by metformin

Adverse Reactions

CNS: Dizziness, headache
CV: Hypertension
ENDO: Hypoglycemia
GI: Abdominal pain, diarrhea, nausea, vomiting
GU: UTI
MS: Pain
RESP: Upper respiratory tract infection

Nursing Considerations

- **WARNING** Monitor renal function, as ordered, before starting glipizide and metformin therapy and at least annually thereafter because renal impairment can result in tissue hypoperfusion and hypoxemia, leading to lactic acidosis.
- **WARNING** Monitor patient closely for signs and symptoms of lactic acidosis or ketoacidosis (changes in level of consciousness, fruity breath, Kussmaul's respirations, restlessness), especially during new onset of illness or trauma. If acidosis or ketoacidosis is suspected, obtain blood samples to evaluate serum electrolyte, ketone, glucose, possibly blood pH, lactate, pyruvate, and metformin levels, as ordered. If acidosis is confirmed, expect to stop drug immediately and provide corrective care, as prescribed.
- Expect to stop drug, as ordered, if patient develops cardiovascular collapse, acute heart failure, acute MI, or other conditions that include hypoxemia, or if patient develops hepatic insufficiency, because lactic acidosis may develop.
- **WARNING** Monitor patients—especially those who are malnourished or debilitated; those with renal, pituitary or adrenal insufficiency; and those with alcohol intoxication—for hypoglycemia because the drug increases the risk.
- Check vitamin B_{12} levels at least every 2 to 3 years in patients with inadequate vitamin B_{12} or calcium intake or absorption because prolonged drug use may result in decreased vitamin B_{12} response.
- Drug should be temporarily withheld for any surgical procedure that requires restricted intake of food and fluids and should not be restarted until the patient can eat and drink and renal function is normal.
- Expect to stop glipizide and metformin for 48 hours before and after radiographic tests involving I.V. administration of iodinated contrast materials because iodinated media increase the risk of

renal failure and lactic acidosis during drug therapy. Check patient's renal function before restarting glipizide and metform 48 hours after radiographic tests are completed, as ordered.

- Monitor patient's blood glucose level to determine response to drug. Expect to monitor glycosylated hemoglobin level every 3 to 6 months, as ordered, to evaluate long-term blood glucose control.
- Monitor blood glucose level often to detect hyperglycemia and to assess the need for supplemental insulin during circumstances of increased stress, such as infection, surgery, or trauma.
- Arrange for instruction about diabetes and consultation with a dietitian or certified diabetes educator, if possible.

PATIENT TEACHING

- Instruct patient to take glipizide and metformin with morning meal if taking once a day or morning and evening meals if taking twice a day. Caution against skipping meals after taking drug.
- Advise patient not to skip doses, stop therapy, or take OTC drugs without first consulting prescriber because of a risk of hyperglycemia.
- Advise patient to report signs or symptoms of hypoglycemia (anxiety, confusion, dizziness, excessive sweating, headache, nausea), and teach him how to respond to hypoglycemia if it occurs.
- Tell patient to stop drug and notify prescriber immediately if he develops an increased respiratory rate unexplained by exercise or other activities, myalgia, malaise, unusual somnolence, or other nonspecific symptoms.
- Instruct patient to carry identification showing that he has diabetes.
- Caution patient to avoid alcohol because it increases the risk of hypoglycemia.
- Tell patient to inform all prescribers that he is taking glipizide and metformin.

glyburide and metformin hydrochloride
Glucovance

Class and Category
Chemical: Sulfonylurea (glyburide), dimethylbiguanide (metformin)
Therapeutic: Antidiabetic
Pregnancy category: B

Indications and Dosages

▶ *To reduce blood glucose level as initial therapy in patients with type 2 diabetes mellitus or in those receiving glyburide and metformin combination therapy who need addition of a thiazolidinedione*
TABLETS
Adults. *Initial:* 1.25 mg glyburide and 250 mg metformin daily or b.i.d. Dosage increased by 1.25 mg glyburide and 250 mg metformin daily every 2 wk as needed.

▶ *To reduce blood glucose level in patients with type 2 diabetes mellitus who aren't adequately controlled by a sulfonylurea or metformin alone*
TABLETS
Adults. *Initial:* 2.5 mg glyburide and 500 mg metformin or 5 mg glyburide and 500 mg metformin b.i.d. Dosage increased, as prescribed, by 5 mg glyburide and 500 mg metformin daily. *Maximum:* 20 mg glyburide and 2,000 mg metformin daily.

DOSAGE ADJUSTMENT For patients currently receiving glyburide or another sulfonylurea, metformin, or a combination of these drugs, expect initial dosage to be equal to or less than that currently being taken. For patients receiving a combination of glyburide and metformin who also need a thiazolidinedione, expect dosage of glyburide and metformin combination to be unchanged when the thiazolidinedione is added.

Mechanism of Action

Glyburide and metformin work in complementary ways to improve glucose control. Glyburide stimulates insulin release from beta cells in the pancreas. It also increases peripheral tissue sensitivity to insulin either by enhancing insulin binding to cellular receptors or by increasing the number of insulin receptors.

Metformin hydrochloride may promote the storage of excess glucose as glycogen in the liver, thus reducing glucose production. Metformin also may improve glucose use by skeletal muscle and adipose tissue by facilitating glucose transport across cell membranes. It also may increase the number of insulin receptors on cell membranes and make them more sensitive to insulin.

Contraindications

Acute or chronic metabolic acidosis; diabetes complicated by pregnancy; diabetic coma; heart failure requiring drug treatment; hypersensitivity to glyburide, metformin, biguanides, sulfonylureas, or their components; ketoacidosis; renal disease or dysfunction (serum creatinine level of 1.5 mg/dl or more in men or 1.4 mg/dl or more in women); type 1 diabetes

Interactions
DRUGS
glyburide and metformin hydrochloride
calcium channel blockers, corticosteroids, diuretics, estrogens, hormonal contraceptives, isoniazid, nicotinic acid, phenothiazine, phenytoin, sympathomimetics, thiazide diuretics, thyroid hormones: Possibly hyperglycemia; possibly hypoglycemia when these drugs are withdrawn
vitamin B_{12}: Probably decreased vitamin B_{12} absorption
glyburide
beta blockers, chloramphenicol, highly protein-bound drugs, MAO inhibitors, NSAIDs, oral anticoagulants, probenecid, salicylates, sulfonamides: Potentiated hypoglycemic action of glyburide; possibly hyperglycemia when these drugs are withdrawn
ciprofloxacin: Potentiated hypoglycemic action of glyburide
miconazole (oral): Possibly severe hypoglycemia
metformin hydrochloride
cimetidine: Increased blood metformin level and possibly increased risk of hypoglycemia
furosemide: Increased blood metformin level and decreased blood furosemide level
nifedipine: Enhanced metformin absorption
FOODS
metformin hydrochloride
all foods: Delayed and reduced metformin absorption
ACTIVITIES
metformin hydrochloride
alcohol use: Altered blood glucose control (usually hyperglycemia); possibly potentiated effect of metformin on lactate metabolism

Adverse Reactions
CNS: Headache
ENDO: Hypoglycemia
GI: Abdominal pain, diarrhea, indigestion, nausea, vomiting
HEME: Megaloblastic anemia, thrombocytopenia
RESP: Upper respiratory tract infection
Other: Lactic acidosis

Nursing Considerations
• Administer glyburide and metformin as a single dose before first meal of the day. If patient takes more than 10 mg of glyburide

daily or if severe GI distress occurs, expect to divide dose and give b.i.d. before morning and evening meals.

- **WARNING** Monitor renal function, as ordered, before beginning therapy and at least annually thereafter because significant renal impairment can result in tissue hypoperfusion and hypoxemia, leading to lactic acidosis.
- **WARNING** Expect to stop glyburide and metformin for 48 hours before and after radiographic tests involving I.V. administration of iodinated contrast materials because iodinated media increase the risk of renal failure and lactic acidosis during drug therapy.
- **WARNING** Monitor malnourished or debilitated patients; those with renal, hepatic, pituitary, or adrenal insufficiency; and those who are also prescribed a thiazolidinedione because they're at increased risk for hypoglycemia. Expect to monitor vitamin B_{12} blood levels at least every 2 to 3 years in patients with inadequate vitamin B_{12} or calcium intake or absorption because prolonged drug use may result in decreased vitamin B_{12} absorption.
- Monitor fasting blood glucose level to determine patient's response to drug. Expect to monitor glycosylated hemoglobin (HbA_{1c}) level every 3 to 6 months, as ordered, to evaluate long-term blood glucose control.
- Monitor blood glucose level often to detect hyperglycemia and to assess the need for supplemental insulin during circumstances of increased stress, such as infection, surgery, and trauma.
- When patient switches from insulin to glyburide and metformin, expect to increase frequency of blood glucose monitoring to t.i.d. before meals.
- In pregnant women, expect to stop drug at least 2 weeks before expected delivery date, as prescribed, to avoid profound hypoglycemia in neonate.
- Arrange for diabetes teaching and consultation with a dietitian or certified diabetes educator, if possible.

PATIENT TEACHING
- Instruct patient to take glyburide and metformin with morning meal if taking once a day, or with morning and evening meals if taking twice a day. Caution him not to skip meal after taking drug.
- Advise patient not to skip doses, stop drug, or take OTC drugs without asking prescriber because hyperglycemia may result.

- Inform patient that most common adverse effects are minor, including diarrhea, nausea, and upset stomach, and typically occur during first few weeks of therapy; explain that taking drug with meals reduces these effects.
- Teach patient how to monitor his blood glucose level and when to notify prescriber.
- Advise patient to expect laboratory monitoring of HbA$_{1c}$ level every 3 months until blood glucose level is controlled.
- Instruct patient to report signs of hypoglycemia, such as anxiety, confusion, dizziness, excessive sweating, headache, and nausea.
- Advise patient to carry identification showing that he has diabetes, and suggest carrying candy to treat mild hypoglycemia.
- Teach patient about exercise, diet, signs of hyperglycemia and hypoglycemia, hygiene, foot care, and ways to avoid infection.
- Urge patient to notify prescriber if he develops easy bruising, unusual bleeding, fever, hypoglycemia or hyperglycemia, rash, or sore throat because drug may need to be stopped.
- Advise patient to avoid alcohol because it increases the risk of hypoglycemia.
- Inform pregnant patient that she may be taken off glyburide and metformin and switched to insulin therapy, as prescribed, at least 2 weeks before expected delivery date.

70% insulin aspart protamine suspension and 30% insulin aspart injection
NovoLog Mix 70/30

50% insulin aspart protamine suspension and 50% insulin aspart injection
NovoLog Mix 50/50

Class and Category
Chemical: Human insulin analogue (insulin aspart protamine suspension, insulin aspart injection)
Therapeutic: Antidiabetic (insulin aspart protamine suspension, insulin aspart injection)
Pregnancy category: C

Indications and Dosages
▶ *To control hyperglycemia in patients with diabetes mellitus*

SUBCUTANEOUS INJECTION

Adults. Dosage highly individualized based on patient's metabolic needs, eating habits, and other lifestyle variables. Injected b.i.d. within 15 minutes of breakfast and dinner.

DOSAGE ADJUSTMENT Dosage reduced in patients with renal impairment and possibly those with hepatic impairment

---

Mechanism of Action

Insulin aspart protamine suspension and insulin aspart injection bind to insulin receptors in muscle and other tissues (except the brain) causing rapid intracellular transport of glucose and amino acids, promoting anabolism, and inhibiting protein catabolism. In the liver, insulin promotes uptake and storage of glucose as glycogen, inhibits gluconeogenesis, and promotes conversion of excess glucose into fat. As a result, the blood glucose level declines.

Contraindications

Episodes of hypoglycemia, diabetic coma, diabetic ketoacidosis, hyperosmolar hyperglycemic state, hypersensitivity to insulin aspart or its components

Interactions

DRUGS

insulin aspart protamine suspension and insulin aspart injection

anabolic steroids, baclofen, beta blockers, clonidine, corticosteroids, danazol, diuretics, estrogens, hormonal contraceptives, isoniazid, lithium salts, phenothiazines, some lipid-lowering drugs (such as niacin), somatropin, sympathomimetics, thyroid hormone: Possibly increased risk of hyperglycemia

ACE inhibitors, androgens, beta blockers, clonidine, disopyramide, fibrates, fluoxetine, inhibitors of pancreatic function (such as octreotide), lithium salts, MAO inhibitors, oral antidiabetics, propoxyphene, salicylates, sulfa antibiotics: Increased risk of hypoglycemia

beta blockers, clonidine, guanethidine, reserpine: Possibly masked symptoms of hypoglycemia

pentamidine: Possibly hypoglycemia, sometimes followed by hyperglycemia

ACTIVITIES

insulin aspart protamine suspension and insulin aspart injection

alcohol use: Possibly increased or decreased blood glucose–lowering effect of insulin

Adverse Reactions
CNS: Headache, hypreflexia, sensory disturbance
CV: Chest pain, hypotension, tachycardia
EENT: Sinusitis
ENDO: Hypoglycemia, insulin resistance
GI: Abdominal pain, diarrhea, nausea
GU: UTI
RESP: Dyspnea, wheezing
SKIN: Diaphoresis, injection site reaction, such as redness, swelling, or pruritus; lipodystrophy; whole-body pruritus or rash
Other: Anaphylaxis, hypokalemia, weight gain

Nursing Considerations
- Give insulin aspart protamine suspension and insulin aspart injection by subcutaneous injection, never intravenously. Rotate injection site within selected anatomical site.
- Be aware that 1 unit of insulin aspart protamine suspension and insulin aspart injection has the same glucose-lowering effect as 1 unit of regular human insulin, but its effect is more rapid and of shorter duration.
- **WARNING** Monitor patient closely for hypoglycemia, the most common adverse effect of insulin therapy. Evidence includes sudden fatigue or weakness, irritability, shakiness, trouble concentrating, diaphoresis, headache, or change in mental status that may progress to coma, seizure, or neurologic impairment if treatment is delayed. Know that early warning symptoms may be different or less pronounced under certain conditions, such as the patient having been diabetic for a long time, presence of diabetic neuropathy, or use of beta blockers. More intensified diabetes control also increases risk of hypoglycemia.
- If hypoglycemia is suspected, obtain blood glucose level to confirm, and treat according to severity.
- For mild hypoglycemia, give 10 to 15 grams of a fast-acting carbohydrate such as 4 ounces of orange juice, 6 ounces of regular soda, 6 to 8 ounces of skim or 1% milk, 2 large lumps or teaspoons of sugar, 5 to 7 Lifesavers, or 2 to 5 glucose tablets. Wait 15 minutes; then retest patient's blood glucose level. If it's still low, treat again. If the patient's next meal or snack is more than 30 minutes away, also provide a follow-up snack. Determine the cause of hypoglycemia to prevent future episodes, if possible, and notify prescriber to determine next insulin dose.

- For severe hypoglycemia, expect to give subcutaneous or intramuscular glucagon or concentrated intravenous glucose, as ordered. If glucagon is given, keep patient's head turned to the side and elevated because vomiting may occur. If patient doesn't respond within 5 to 20 minutes, repeat glucagon injection. Once the patient is awake enough to swallow, provide some clear liquids such as regular non-cola soda followed by a substantial snack, such as a roll with peanut butter or half of a cheese sandwich. Determine the cause of hypoglycemia to prevent future episodes, if possible, and notify prescriber to determine next insulin dose.
- Monitor patient's blood glucose level and glycosylated hemoglobin level, as ordered to determine insulin dosage needs.
- Inspect patient's injection site regularly for adverse reactions, such as localized redness, swelling, pruritus, or lipodystrophy.
- Monitor patient's serum potassium level because hypokalemia may occur with insulin use, especially in patients with autonomic neuropathy, patients who are fasting (always check with prescriber before administering insulin in a patient who is fasting), or patients who are using potassium-lowering drugs or taking drugs known to alter serum potassium level.
- **WARNING** Monitor patient closely for hypersensitivity reactions, which may be life-threatening. Notify prescriber immediately if patient develops whole-body rash, pruritus, dyspnea, wheezing, hypotension, tachycardia, or diaphoresis, and be prepared to provide supportive care, as needed and ordered.

PATIENT TEACHING
- Tell patient that insulin aspart protamine suspension and insulin aspart injection needs to be resuspended immediately before use. To resuspend, tell patient to roll the vial, cartridge, or prefilled pen syringe between the palms of his hands 10 times. In addition, if the patient is using the prefilled cartridge or pen syringe form, tell him he must then turn the cartridge or syringe upside down so the glass ball moves from one end of the delivery system to the other, and keep turning it at least 10 times to ensure solution becomes uniformly white and cloudy. If needed, instruct patient to repeat rolling and turning procedure until the insulin solution is uniformly white and cloudy.
- Teach patient how to measure insulin dosage and use a standard insulin syringe, the NovoLog Mix 70/30 FlexPen, or Pen-Fill cartridge compatible delivery device prescribed. Inform pa-

tient that drug comes mixed as a 70% insulin aspart protamine suspension and 30% insulin aspart injection solution and shouldn't be mixed with any other insulin.

- Instruct patient how to administer insulin subcutaneously. Review anatomical sites for injection (abdomen [best site for absorption], thigh, upper arm) and stress importance of rotating injection sites within selected area. Alert patient that the rate of insulin absorption and consequently its onset of action can be affected by exercise and by changing the injection site. Urge patient to follow guidelines provided by the prescriber.
- Caution patient only to use insulin aspart protamine suspension and insulin aspart injection if it appears uniformly cloudy after resuspension and not to use after its expiration date.
- Tell patient to keep spare insulin vials, cartridges, or pens in the refrigerator. Remind him that unrefrigerated vials must be used within 28 days of removing from the refrigerator and unrefrigerated prefilled cartridges and pens must be used within 14 days. Tell patient to keep the prefilled cartridge or pen currently in use at room temperature but as cool as possible.
- Caution patient to protect unrefrigerated insulin from direct heat and light.
- Instruct patient to measure insulin dosage carefully and inject it within 15 minutes of eating breakfast and dinner.
- Stress importance of following a regular meal plan and exercise program, monitoring his blood glucose level regularly, and testing glycosylated hemoglobin periodically.
- Explain signs and symptoms and proper management of hypoglycemia and hyperglycemia. Tell patient to notify prescriber episodes are frequent, severe, or difficult to bring under control.
- Stress importance of keeping follow-up appointments to determine effectiveness of prescribed insulin therapy and monitor for diabetes complications.
- Tell female patients to alert the prescriber if they become pregnant or intend to become pregnant because their insulin dosage will need to be adjusted.
- Advise patient to notify prescriber about changes in physical activity or meal plan because insulin dosage will need adjustment.
- Tell patient to notify prescriber about illness, emotional disturbance, or other stress because insulin may need to be adjusted.
- Advise patient to obtain and wear medical identification indicating that he takes insulin.
- Encourage family members to learn signs and symptoms of hypoglycemia and how to administer glucagon in an emergency.

70% insulin isophane (human) suspension and 30% insulin (human) injection
Humulin 70/30, Novolin 70/30

50% insulin isophane (human) suspension and 50% insulin (human) injection
Humulin 50/50

Class and Category
Chemical: Human insulin analogue (human insulin isophane suspension, human insulin injection)
Therapeutic: Antidiabetic (human insulin isophane suspension, human insulin injection)
Pregnancy category: B

Indications and Dosages
▶ *To control hyperglycemia in patients with diabetes mellitus*
SUBCUTANEOUS INJECTION
Adults. Dosage highly individualized based on patient's metabolic needs, eating habits, and other lifestyle variables. Injected b.i.d. 30 to 60 minutes before a meal.
DOSAGE ADJUSTMENT Dosage reduced in patients with renal impairment and possibly those with hepatic impairment

---

Mechanism of Action
Human insulin isophane suspension and human insulin injection bind to insulin receptors in muscle and other tissues (except the brain), causing rapid intracellular transport of glucose and amino acids, promoting anabolism, and inhibiting protein catabolism. In the liver, insulin promotes uptake and storage of glucose as glycogen, inhibits gluconeogenesis, and promotes conversion of excess glucose into fat. These actions lower the blood glucose level.

Contraindications
Episodes of hypoglycemia, diabetic ketoacidosis, hyperosmolar hyperglycemia, hypersensitivity to human insulin or its components

Interactions
DRUGS
human insulin isophane suspension and human insulin injection
anabolic steroids, baclofen, beta blockers, clonidine, corticosteroids, dana-

zol, diuretics, estrogens, hormonal contraceptives, isoniazid, lithium salts, phenothiazines, some lipid-lowering drugs (such as niacin), somatropin, sympathomimetics, thyroid hormone: Possibly increased risk of hyperglycemia

ACE inhibitors, androgens, beta blockers, clonidine, disopyramide, fibrates, fluoxetine, inhibitors of pancreatic function (such as octreotide), lithium salts, MAO inhibitors, oral antidiabetics, propoxyphene, salicylates, sulfa antibiotics: Increased risk of hypoglycemia

beta blockers, clonidine, guanethidine, reserpine: Possibly mask symptoms of hypoglycemia

pentamidine: Possibly hypoglycemia, sometimes followed by hyperglycemia

ACTIVITIES

alcohol use: Possibly increased or decreased blood glucose–lowering effect of insulin

Adverse Reactions

CNS: Headache, hypreflexia, sensory disturbance
CV: Chest pain, hypotension, tachycardia
EENT: Sinusitis
ENDO: Hypoglycemia, insulin resistance
GI: Abdominal pain, diarrhea, nausea
GU: UTI
RESP: Dyspnea, wheezing
SKIN: Diaphoresis, injection site reaction, such as redness, swelling, or pruritus; lipodystrophy; whole-body pruritus or rash
Other: Anaphylaxis, hypokalemia, weight gain

Nursing Considerations

- Inject human insulin isophane suspension and human insulin injection subcutaneously, never intravenously. Rotate injection site within selected anatomical area.
- **WARNING** Monitor patient closely for hypoglycemia, the most common adverse effect of insulin therapy. Evidence may include sudden fatigue or weakness, irritability, shakiness, trouble concentrating, diaphoresis, headache, or change in mental status that may progress to coma, seizure, or neurologic impairment if treatment is delayed. Know that early warning symptoms may be different or less pronounced under certain conditions, such as long-term diabetes, presence of diabetic neuropathy, or use of beta blockers. More intensified diabetes control also increases risk of hypoglycemia.
- If hypoglycemia is suspected, obtain blood glucose level to con-

firm, and treat according to severity.

- For mild hypoglycemia, give 10 to 15 grams of a fast acting carbohydrate, such as 4 ounces of orange juice, 6 ounces of regular soda, 6 to 8 ounces of skim or 1% milk, 2 large lumps or teaspoons of sugar, 5 to 7 Lifesavers, or 2 to 5 glucose tablets. Wait 15 minutes; then retest patient's blood glucose level. If it's still low, treat again. If the patient's next meal or snack is more than 30 minutes away, also provide a follow-up snack. Determine the cause of hypoglycemia to prevent future episodes, if possible, and notify prescriber to determine next insulin dose.

- For severe hypoglycemia, expect to administer subcutaneous or intramuscular glucagon or concentrated intravenous glucose, as ordered. If glucagon is given, remember to keep patient's head turned to the side and elevated because vomiting may occur. If patient doesn't respond within 5 to 20 minutes, repeat glucagon injection. Once patient is awake enough to swallow, provide clear liquids, such as regular non-cola soda, followed by a substantial snack, such as a roll with peanut butter or half of a cheese sandwich. Determine cause of hypoglycemia to prevent future episodes, if possible, and notify prescriber to determine next insulin dose.

- Monitor patient's blood glucose and glycosylated hemoglobin levels, as ordered to determine insulin dosage needs.

- Inspect patient's injection site regularly for signs of adverse reactions such as localized redness, swelling, pruritus, or lipodystrophy.

- Monitor patient's serum potassium level because hypokalemia may occur with insulin use, especially in patients with autonomic neuropathy, patients who are fasting (always check with prescriber before giving insulin to a patient who is fasting), or patients who are using potassium-lowering drugs or taking drugs known to alter serum potassium level.

- **WARNING** Monitor patient closely for hypersensitivity reactions, which may be life-threatening. Notify prescriber immediately if patient develops whole-body rash, pruritus, dyspnea, wheezing, hypotension, tachycardia, or diaphoresis, and be prepared to provide supportive care, as needed and ordered.

PATIENT TEACHING

- Tell patient that human insulin isophane suspension and human insulin injection needs to be resuspended immediately before use. To resuspend, tell patient to roll the vial, cartridge or prefilled pen syringe between the palms of his hands 10 times. In addition, if the patient is using the prefilled cartridge or pen syringe form, tell him he must then turn the cartridge or syringe upside down so that the glass ball moves from one end of the delivery system to the other and keep turning it for at least 10 times to ensure solution becomes uniformly white and cloudy. If necessary, instruct patient to repeat rolling and turning procedure until the insulin solution is uniformly white and cloudy.

- Teach patient how to measure insulin dosage and use a standard insulin syringe, pen, or cartridge compatible delivery device prescribed. Inform patient that drug comes mixed as a 70% human insulin isophane suspension and 30% human insulin injection solution or as 50% human insulin isophane suspension and 50% human insulin injection solution and shouldn't be mixed with any other insulin.

- Instruct patient how to administer insulin subcutaneously. Review anatomical sites for insulin injection (abdomen [best site for absorption], thigh, upper arm) and stress the importance of rotating injection sites within the selected area. Alert patient that the rate of insulin absorption and consequently its onset of action can be affected by exercise and changing the injection area; urge patient to follow guidelines provided by the prescriber.

- Caution patient to use human insulin isophane suspension and human insulin injection only if it appears uniformly cloudy after resuspension and not to use after its expiration date.

- Tell patient to keep spare insulin vials, cartridges, or pens in the refrigerator. Remind him that unrefrigerated vials must be used within 28 days of removing from the refrigerator or it must be discarded and unrefrigerated prefilled cartridges and pens must be used within 10 days or be discarded. Tell patient to keep the prefilled cartridge or pen currently in use at room temperature but as cool as possible.

- Caution patient to protect unrefrigerated insulin from direct heat and light.

- Instruct patient to measure insulin dosage carefully and inject it 30 to 60 minutes before a meal.

- Stress importance of following a regular meal plan and exercise program and of monitoring his blood glucose level regularly and glcosylated hemoglobin periodically.

- Explain signs and symptoms and proper management of hypoglycemia and hyperglycemia. Tell patient to notify prescriber if hypoglycemic episodes are frequent, severe, or difficult to bring under control.

- Stress importance of having follow-up appointments to determine effectiveness of prescribed insulin therapy and check for diabetes complications.
- Tell female patients to alert the prescriber if they become pregnant or intend to become pregnant because their insulin dosage will need to be adjusted.
- Advise patient to notify prescriber about changes in physical activity or usual meal plan because insulin dosage will need adjustment.
- Tell patient to notify prescriber if an illness, emotional disturbance, or other stress occurs because insulin dosage may need to be adjusted.
- Advise patient to obtain and wear medical alert identification showing that the patient takes insulin.
- Encourage family members to learn about the signs and symptoms of hypoglycemia and how to administer glucagon in an emergency.

75% insulin lispro protamine suspension and 25% insulin lispro injection
Humalog Mix 75/25
50% insulin lispro protamine suspension and 50% insulin lispro injection
Humalog Mix 50/50

Class and Category
Chemical: Human insulin analogue (insulin lispro protamine suspension, insulin lispro injection)
Therapeutic: Antidiabetic (insulin lispro protamine suspension, insulin lispro injection)
Pregnancy category: B

Indications and Dosages
▶ *To control hyperglycemia in patients with diabetes mellitus*
SUBCUTANEOUS INJECTION
Adults. Highly individualized dosage based on patient's metabolic needs, eating habits, and other lifestyle variables injected within 15 minutes before selected meals daily.
DOSAGE ADJUSTMENT Dosage reduced in patients with renal impairment and possibly those with hepatic impairment

Mechanism of Action

Insulin lispro protamine suspension and insulin lispro injection bind to insulin receptors located in muscle and other tissues (except brain), which causes rapid intracellular transport of glucose and amino acids, promotes anabolism, and inhibits protein catabolism. In the liver, insulin promotes the uptake and storage of glucose in the form of glycogen, inhibits gluconeogenesis, and promotes conversion of excess glucose into fat. All of these actions contribute to lowering blood glucose levels.

Contraindications

During episodes of hypoglycemia, diabetic coma, diabetic ketoacidosis, hyperosmolar hyperglycemic state, hypersensitivity to insulin lispro or any of its components

Interactions

DRUGS

insulin lispro protamine suspension and insulin lispro injection

anabolic steroids, baclofen, beta blockers, clonidine, corticosteroids, danazol, diuretics, estrogens, hormonal contraceptives, isoniazid, lithium salts, phenothiazines, certain lipid-lowering drugs (such as niacin), somatropin, sympathomimetic agents, thyroid hormone: Increased hyperglycemic activity

ACE inhibitors, androgens, angiotensin II receptor blockers, beta blockers, clonidine, disopyramide, fibrates, fluoxetine, inhibitors of pancreatic function (such as octreotide), lithium salts, MAO inhibitors, oral antidiabetics, propoxyphene, salicylates, sulfa antibiotics: Increased risk of hypoglycemia

beta blockers, clonidine, guanethidine, reserpine: Possibly masked symptoms of hypoglycemia

pentamidine: Possibly hypoglycemia, sometimes followed by hyperglycemia

ACTIVITIES

insulin lispro protamine suspension and insulin lispro injection

alcohol use: Possibly increased or decreased blood glucose–lowering effects of insulin

Adverse Reactions

CNS: Headache, hyperflexia, sensory disturbance
CV: Chest pain, hypotension, tachycardia
EENT: Sinusitis

ENDO: Hypoglycemia, insulin resistance
GI: Abdominal pain, diarrhea, nausea
GU: UTI
RESP: Dyspnea, wheezing
SKIN: Diaphoresis, injection site reaction, such as redness, swelling, or pruritus; lipodystrophy; whole-body pruritus or rash
Other: Anaphylaxis, hypokalemia, weight gain

Nursing Considerations

- Be aware that insulin lispro protamine suspension and insulin lispro injection has a more rapid onset of action and a shorter duration of action than regular human insulin, requiring that it be given within 15 minutes before a meal.
- Inject insulin lispro protamine suspension and insulin lispro injection subcutaneously, never intravenously. Rotate injection site within selected anatomical site.
- Be aware that 1 unit of insulin lispro protamine suspension and insulin lispro injection has the same glucose-lowering effect as 1 unit of regular human insulin, but that its effect is more rapid and of shorter duration.
- **WARNING** Monitor patient closely for hypoglycemia, the most common adverse effect of insulin therapy. Evidence may include sudden fatigue or weakness, irritability, shakiness, trouble concentrating, diaphoresis, headache, or change in mental status that may progress to coma, seizure, or neurologic impairment if treatment is delayed. Know that early warning symptoms may be different or less pronounced under certain conditions, such as long-term diabetes, presence of diabetic neuropathy, or use of beta blockers. More intensified diabetes control also increases risk of hypoglycemia.
- If hypoglycemia is suspected, obtain blood glucose level to confirm, and treat according to severity.
- For mild hypoglycemia, give 10 to 15 grams of a fast-acting carbohydrate, such as 4 ounces of orange juice, 6 ounces of regular soda, 6 to 8 ounces of skim or 1% milk, 2 large lumps or teaspoons of sugar, 5 to 7 Lifesavers, or 2 to 5 glucose tablets. Wait 15 minutes; then retest patient's blood glucose. If blood glucose level is still low, treat again. If the patient's next meal or snack is more than 30 minutes away, also provide a follow-up snack. Determine cause of hypoglycemia to prevent future episodes, if possible, and notify prescriber to determine next insulin dose.
- For severe hypoglycemia, expect to give subcutaneous or intra-

muscular glucagon or concentrated intravenous glucose, as ordered. If glucagon is administered, remember to keep patient's head turned to the side and elevated because vomiting may occur. If patient doesn't respond within 5 to 20 minutes, repeat glucagon injection. Once the patient is awake enough to swallow, provide clear liquids, such as regular non-cola soda followed by a substantial snack, such as a roll with peanut butter or half of a cheese sandwich. Determine cause of hypoglycemia to prevent future episodes, if possible, and notify the prescriber to determine next insulin dose.

- Monitor patient's blood glucose and glycosylated hemoglobin levels, as ordered, to determine insulin dosage needs.
- Inspect the patient's injection site regularly for adverse reactions, such as localized redness, swelling or pruritus or lipodystrophy.
- Monitor patient's serum potassium level because hypokalemia may occur with insulin use, especially in patients with autonomic neuropathy, patients who are fasting (always check with prescriber before administering insulin in a patient who is fasting), or patients who are using potassium-lowering drugs or taking drugs known to alter the serum potassium level.
- **WARNING** Monitor patient closely for hypersensitivity reactions, which may be life-threatening. Notify prescriber immediately if patient develops whole-body rash, pruritus, dyspnea, wheezing, hypotension, tachycardia, or diaphoresis, and be prepared to provide supportive care, as needed and ordered.

PATIENT TEACHING

- Tell patient how to measure insulin dosage using a standard insulin syringe or the Humalog Mix 75/25 pen. Inform patient that drug comes mixed as a 75% insulin lispro protamine suspension and 25% insulin lispro injection solution and shouldn't be mixed with any other insulin.
- Instruct patient how to administer insulin subcutaneously. Review anatomical sites for insulin injection (abdomen being the best site for absorption) and stress importance of rotating injection sites within selected area. Alert patient that the rate of insulin absorption and consequently its onset of action can be affected by changes in injeciton site or exercise, and urge patient to adhere to guidelines provided by the prescriber.
- Caution patient to use insulin lispro protamine suspension and insulin lispro injection only if it appears uniformly cloudy after mixing and not to use after its expiration date.

- Tell patient to keep spare insulin vials or pens in the refrigerator. Remind him that unrefrigerated vials must be used within 28 days of removing from the refrigerator and unrefrigerated pens must be used within 10 days.
- Caution patient to protect unrefrigerated insulin from direct heat and light and to keep at a cool room temperature.
- Instruct patient to measure insulin dosage carefully and inject within 15 minutes before eating a meal.
- Stress importance of adhering to a regular meal plan and exercise program and of monitoring his blood glucose level regularly testing his glycosylated hemoglobin level periodically.
- Explain the signs and symptoms and proper management of hypoglycemia and hyperglycemia. Tell patient to notify prescriber if episodes are freuquent, severe, or difficult to control.
- Stress importance of adhering to follow-up appointments to determine effectiveness of prescribed insulin therapy and monitor for diabetes complications.
- Tell female patients to alert prescriber if they become pregnant or intend to become pregnant because their insulin dosage will need to be adjusted.
- Advise patient to notify prescriber about changes in their physical activity or usual meal plan because insulin dosage will need to be adjusted.
- Tell patient to notify prescriber if an illness, emotional disturbance, or other stress occurs because insulin dosage may need to be adjusted.
- Advise patient to obtain and wear medical alert identification showing that the patient takes insulin.
- Encourage family members to learn signs and symptoms of hypoglycemia and how to administer glucagon in an emergency.

levothyroxine sodium (T₄) and liothyronine sodium (T₃) (liotrix)

Thyrolar ¼, Thyrolar ½, Thyrolar 1, Thyrolar 2, Thyrolar 3

Class and Category

Chemical: Thyroid hormones (levothyroxine, liothyronine)
Therapeutic: Thyroid hormone replacement (levothyroxine, liothyronine)
Pregnancy category: A

Indications and Dosages

▶ *To treat hypothyroidism without myxedema*

TABLETS

Adults. *Initial:* 25 mcg levothyroxine and 6.25 mcg liothyronine (one tablet of Thyrolar ½) daily, increased every 2 to 3 wk by 12.5 mcg levothyroxine and 3.1 mcg liothyronine until therapeutic effects occur. *Maintenance:* 50 mcg levothyroxine and 12.5 mcg liothyronine (one tablet of Thyrolar 1) to 100 mcg levothyroxine and 25 mcg liothyronine (one tablet of Thyrolar 2) daily.

▶ *To treat long-standing myxedema or hypothyroidism in patients with cardiovascular disease*

TABLETS

Adults. *Initial:* 12.5 mcg levothyroxine and 3.1 mcg liothyronine (one tablet of Thyrolar ¼) daily, increased every 2 to 3 wk by 12.5 mcg levothyroxine and 3.1 mcg liothyronine until therapeutic effects occur. *Maintenance:* 50 mcg levothyroxine and 12.5 mcg liothyronine (one tablet of Thyrolar 1) to 100 mcg levothyroxine and 25 mcg liothyronine (one tablet of Thyrolar 2) daily.

DOSAGE ADJUSTMENT For elderly patients, initial dose usually reduced to 25% to 50% of adult dose; dosage then doubled every 6 to 8 wk until therapeutic effects occur.

▶ *To treat congenital hypothyroidism in children*

TABLETS

Children age 12 and over. 75 mcg levothyroxine and 18.75 mcg liothyronine (one tablet of Thyrolar 1 and one tablet of Thyrolar ½) daily.

Children ages 6 to 12. 50 mcg levothyroxine and 12.5 mcg liothyronine (one tablet of Thyrolar 1) daily to 75 mcg levothyroxine and 18.75 mcg liothyronine (one tablet of Thyrolar 1 and one tablet of Thyrolar ½) daily.

Children ages 1 to 6. 37.5 mcg levothyroxine and 9.35 mcg liothyronine (one tablet of Thyrolar ½ and one tablet of Thyrolar ¼) daily to 50 mcg levothyroxine and 12.5 mcg liothyronine (one tablet of Thyrolar 1) daily.

Children ages 6 months to 12 months. 25 mcg levothyroxine and 6.25 mcg liothyronine (one tablet of Thyrolar ½) daily to 37.5 mcg levothyroxine and 9.35 mcg liothyronine (one tablet of Thyrolar ½ and one tablet of Thyrolar ¼) daily.

Newborn infants to age 6 months. 12.5 mcg levothyroxine and 3.1 mcg liothyronine (one tablet of Thyrolar ¼) daily to 25 mcg levothyroxine and 6.25 mcg liothyronine (one tablet of Thyrolar ½) daily.

Mechanism of Action

Both levothyroxine and liothyronine are thyroid hormones and replace endogenous thyroid hormone, which may exert physiologic effects by controlling DNA transcription and protein synthesis. These hormones have all of the following actions of endogenous thyroid hormone. The combination drug:

* increases energy expenditure
* accelerates the rate of cellular oxidation, which stimulates growth, maturation, and metabolism of body tissues
* aids in myelination of nerves and development of synaptic processes in the nervous system
* enhances carbohydrate and protein metabolism, increasing gluconeogenesis and protein synthesis.

Contraindications

Hypersensitivity to levothyroxine, liothyronine, or their components; uncorrected adrenal insufficiency; untreated thyrotoxicosis

Interactions

DRUGS

levothyroxine and liothyronine

adrenocorticoids: Possibly need to adjust adrenocorticoid dosage as thyroid status changes

cholestyramine, colestipol: Decreased absorption of levothyroxine and liothyronine

digoxin: Possibly need to adjust digoxin dosage as thyroid status changes

estrogen: Reduced binding of levothyroxine and liothyronine to protein, possibly requiring increased thyroid hormone dosage

insulin, oral antidiabetics: Possibly need to adjust insulin or oral antidiabetic dosage as thyroid status changes

ketamine: Possibly hypertension and tachycardia

maprotiline: Increased risk of arrhythmias

oral anticoagulants: Altered anticoagulant activity, possibly need to adjust anticoagulant dosage

sympathomimetics: Increased effects of either drug; risk of coronary insufficiency in patients with coronary artery disease

Adverse Reactions

CNS: Anxiety, asthenia, depression, fatigue, headache, insomnia, sluggish feeling, tremor

CV: Arrhythmias, chest pain, hypertension, palpitations, tachycardia

EENT: Keratoconjunctivitis sicca

ENDO: Hyperthyroidism (with overdose), hypothyroidism, increase or decrease in TSH
GI: Nausea
MS: Arthralgia, myalgia
SKIN: Alopecia (transient), dry skin, hyperhidrosis, pruritus, rash, urticaria
Other: Allergic reactions, increased weight

Nursing Considerations
- Administer levothyroxine and liothyronine as a single daily dose before breakfast.
- Expect patient to undergo periodic thyroid function tests during levothyroxine and liothyronine therapy.
- Monitor PT of patient on anticoagulants; she may need a dosage adjustment.
- Check blood glucose level often in diabetic patient. Antidiabetic dosage may need adjustment as hormone replacement occurs.

PATIENT TEACHING
- Inform patient that levothyroxine and liothyronine combination is usually taken for life. Caution her not to stop drug or change dosage unless instructed by prescriber.
- Instruct patient to take drug before breakfast because evening doses may cause insomnia.
- Advise patient to store tablets in refrigerator in a tightly sealed, light-resistant container.
- Instruct patient to report signs of hyperthyroidism, such as chest pain, excessive sweating, heat intolerance, insomnia, palpitations, and weight loss.
- Advise diabetic patient to monitor blood glucose level often because antidiabetic drug dosage may need to be adjusted.
- Inform patient that transient hair loss may occur during first few months of therapy.
- Inform patient of need for periodic thyroid hormone blood tests to monitor drug effectiveness.

norethindrone acetate and ethinyl estradiol
Femhrt

Class and Category
Chemical: Progesterone derivative (norethindrone), estrogen steroid hormone derivative (ethinyl estradiol)

Therapeutic: Antiosteoporotic, ovarian hormone replacement (norethindrone, ethinyl estradiol)
Pregnancy category: X

Indications and Dosages

▶ *To treat moderate to severe vasomotor symptoms of menopause; to prevent osteoporosis from estrogen deficiency in postmenopausal women with an intact uterus*

TABLETS

Adult women. *Initial:* 0.5 mg norethindrone and 2.5 mcg ethinyl estradiol (1 tablet) daily, increased, as needed, to 1 mg norethindrone and 5 mcg ethinyl estradiol (1 tablet of appropriate strength) daily.

Mechanism of Action

Norethindrone is a progestin. Progestins prolong some of the positive effects of estrogens on HDL cholesterol. Norethindrone diffuses freely into target cells of the female reproductive tract, mammary glands, hypothalamus, and pituitary gland and binds to the progesterone cell receptor. It converts a proliferative endometrium into a secretory one in women with adequate estrogen replacement, reducing endometrial growth and the risk of endometrial cancer compared with women who have an intact uterus and take unopposed estrogens. Norethindrone also decreases nuclear estradiol receptors and suppresses epithelial DNA synthesis in endometrial tissues.

Ethinyl estradiol is an estrogen that increases DNA and RNA synthesis in the cells of female reproductive organs, pituitary gland, hypothalamus, and other target organs. In the hypothalamus, estrogens decrease the release of gonadotropin-releasing hormone, which reduces pituitary release of follicle-stimulating hormone and luteinizing hormone. In women, these hormones are required for normal GU and other essential body functions. At the cellular level, estrogens increase cervical secretions, cause endometrial cell proliferation, and improve uterine tone. Estrogen replacement helps maintain GU function and reduces vasomotor symptoms when estrogen production declines from menopause, surgical removal of ovaries, or other estrogen deficiency. Estrogen replacement also helps prevent osteoporosis by inhibiting bone resorption.

Contraindications

Active deep vein thrombosis, pulmonary embolism, or history of these conditions; endometrial hyperplasia; hepatic disorders; hypersensitivity to ethinyl estradiol, norethindrone, or their components; jaundice; known or suspected breast cancer or history of breast cancer from estrogen use; known or suspected estrogen-dependent cancer; new or recent (within past year) MI or stroke; pregnancy; undiagnosed abnormal genital bleeding; vaginal disorders

Interactions
DRUGS
norethindrone and ethinyl estradiol
aminocaproic acid: Possibly an increase in hypercoagulability caused by aminocaproic acid
barbiturates, carbamazepine, hydantoins, rifabutin, rifampin: Possibly reduced activity of estradiol and norethindrone
bromocriptine: Possibly decreased bromocriptine effects
calcium: Possibly increased calcium absorption
corticosteroids: Increased therapeutic and toxic effects of corticosteroids
cyclosporine: Increased risk of hepatotoxicity and nephrotoxicity
hepatotoxic drugs (such as isoniazid): Increased risk of hepatitis and hepatotoxicity
didanosine, lamivudine, zalcitabine: Possibly pancreatitis
oral antidiabetics: Decreased therapeutic effects of these drugs
somatrem, somatropin: Possibly accelerated epiphyseal maturation
warfarin: Altered anticoagulant effect
ethinyl estradiol
thyroid hormones: Decreased effectiveness of thyroid hormones
vitamin C: Decreased metabolism and possibly increased adverse effects of ethinyl estradiol
FOODS
norethindrone and ethinyl estradiol
grapefruit juice: Decreased metabolism and possibly increased adverse effects of ethinyl estradiol
ACTIVITIES
norethindrone and ethinyl estradiol
smoking: Increased risk of pulmonary embolism, thrombophlebitis, stroke, and transient ischemic attack

Adverse Reactions
CNS: Chorea, dementia, depression, dizziness, exacerbation of epilepsy, headache, insomnia, irritability, migraine headache, mood disturbances, nervousness, porphyria, stroke
CV: Deep and superficial venous thrombosis, hypertension, increased triglycerides, MI, peripheral edema, pulmonary embolism,

thromboembolism, thrombophlebitis

EENT: Diplopia, intolerance of contact lenses, retinal vascular thrombosis, sinusitis, vision changes or loss

ENDO: Breast enlargement, pain, tenderness, or tumors; endometrial hyperplasia; galactorrhea; hyperglycemia; nipple discharge

GI: Abdominal cramps or pain, aggravation of hepatic porphyria, anorexia, bloating, constipation, diarrhea, elevated liver function test results, enlargement of hepatic hemangiomas, flatulence, gallbladder obstruction, hepatitis, increased appetite, nausea, pancreatitis, vomiting

GU: Amenorrhea, breakthrough bleeding, cervical erosion, clear vaginal discharge, dysmenorrhea, endometrial or ovarian tumors, increased libido, increased size of uterine leiomyomata, leukorrhea, prolonged or heavy menstrual bleeding, urinary tract infection, vaginitis including vaginal candidiasis

MS: Arthralgias, back or extremity pain, leg cramps

RESP: Bronchitis, exacerbation of asthma, upper respiratory infection

SKIN: Alopecia, application site irritation, chloasma, erythema multiforme or nodosum, hirsutism, jaundice, melasma, pruritus, purpura, rash, urticaria

Other: Anaphylaxis, angioedema, flulike syndrome, folic acid deficiency, hypercalcemia (with bone metastases), hypocalcemia, hyperkalemia, hyponatremia, weight gain or loss, worsening of systemic lupus erythematosus

Nursing Considerations

- Use norethindrone and ethinyl estradiol cautiously in women with asthma, diabetes mellitus, epilepsy, migraine headaches, porphyria, systemic lupus erythematosus, and hepatic hemangiomas because ethinyl estradiol can worsen these conditions.
- Verify that patient has an intact uterus before starting drug. If not, she doesn't need a product that contains a progestin such as norethindrone.
- **WARNING** Assess patient for contact lens intolerance or changes in vision or acuity because estrogens such as ethinyl estradiol can cause keratoconus. Be prepared to stop drug immediately, as prescribed, if patient has sudden partial or complete loss of vision or sudden onset of diplopia or migraine.
- Monitor PT in patients taking warfarin for loss of anticoagulant effect because ethinyl estradiol can increase clotting factors VII, VIII, IX, and X and promote platelet aggregation.
- Watch for elevated liver function test results because norethin-

drone and ethinyl estradiol may worsen such conditions as acute intermittent or variegate hepatic porphyria.

- Closely monitor patient's blood pressure. Some patients may have a substantial increase in blood pressure as an indiosyncratic reaction to estrogens such as ethinyl estradiol. Monitor patients who already have hypertension for increases in blood pressure because estrogens may cause fluid retention. Also monitor patients with asthma, heart disease, migraines, renal disease, or seizure disorder for worsening of these conditions.
- Check serum triglyceride level routinely because, in patients with hypertriglyceridemia, estrogen may increase the level enough to cause pancreatitis and other complications.
- Monitor blood glucose level often in patients wiht diabetes mellitus because estrogens such as ethinyl estradiol may decrease insulin sensitivity and alter glucose tolerance.
- **WARNING** Expect to stop ethinyl estradiol and norethindrone in any woman who develops evidence of dementia, cardiovascular disease, such as MI, pulmonary embolism, stroke, or venous thrombosis.
- Be aware that ethinyl estradiol and norethindrone may worsen mood disorders, including depression. Monitor patient for depression, mood changes, anxiety, fatigue, dizziness, or insomnia.
- **WARNING** Be aware that patients with breast cancer and bone metastasis may develop severe hypercalcemia because estrogens influence calcium and phosphorus metabolism. Watch for toxic effects of increased calcium absorption in patients predisposed to hypercalcemia or nephrolithiasis.
- Assess skin for melasma (tan or brown patches), which may develop on forehead, cheeks, temples, and upper lip. These patches may persist after combination drug is stopped.
- Monitor thyroid function test results in patients with hypothyroidism because long-term use of ethinyl estradiol may decrease effectiveness of thyroid therapy.
- Expect to stop norethindrone and ethinyl estradiol therapy several weeks before patient undergoes major surgery, as prescribed, because prolonged immobilization poses a risk of thromboembolism.

PATIENT TEACHING

- Before therapy starts, inform patient about risks of taking norethindrone and ethinyl estradiol, such as increased risk of cardiovascular disease, breast or endometrial cancer, dementia, gallbladder disease, and vision abnormalities.
- Urge patient to notify prescriber immediately about vaginal

bleeding or any other abnormal signs and symptoms during norethindrone and ethinyl estradiol therapy.
- Caution patient to avoid smoking while using an estrogen-progestin product like norethindrone and ethinyl estradiol.
- Stress importance of keeping follow-up visits every 3 to 6 months to determine effectiveness of drug at relieving menopausal symptoms and osteoporosis as well as having scheduled diagnostic tests to detect adverse reactions.
- Emphasize importance of good dental hygiene and regular dental checkups because an elevated progestin (norethindrone) blood level increases growth of normal oral flora, which may lead to gum tenderness, bleeding, or swelling.

norgestimate and ethinyl estradiol
Ortho-Cyclen, Ortho Tri-Cyclen

Class and Category
Chemical: Progesterone steroid hormone derivative (norgestimate), estrogenic steroid hormone derivative (ethinyl estradiol)
Therapeutic: Ovarian hormone replacement (norgestimate, ethinyl estradiol)
Pregnancy category: X

Indications and Dosages
▶ *To treat moderate acne vulgaris in patients who desire contraception having achieved menarche and who also are unresponsive to topical anti-acne medication*
TABLETS
Women age 15 and over. 0.180 mg, 0.215 mg, or 0.250 mg norgestimate and 0.035 mg ethinyl estradiol (1 active tablet) daily for 21 days starting first day of monthly menstruation followed by 1 inactive tablet daily for 7 days; cycle repeated every 28 days. Or, 0.180 mg, 0.215 mg, or 0.250 mg norgestimate and 0.035 mg ethinyl estradiol (1 active tablet) daily for 21 days starting the first Sunday after monthly menstruation begins, followed by 1 inactive tablet daily for 7 days; cycle repeated every 28 days.

Contraindications
Active deep vein thrombosis, pulmonary embolism, or history of these conditions; cerebral vascular or coronary artery disease; hepatic disorders including cholestatic jaundice in previous pregnancy or prior oral contraceptive pill use; hypersensitivity to norgestimate, ethinyl estradiol, or their components; known or

suspected breast cancer or history of breast cancer from estrogen use; known or suspected estrogen-dependent cancer; migraine with focal aura; new or recent (within past year) stroke or MI; pregnancy; undiagnosed abnormal genital bleeding

---

Mechanism of Action

Norgestimate as a progestin inhibits secretion of gonadotropins from the anterior pituitary to prevent ovulation and follicular maturation. It also thickens cervical secretions making it more difficult for sperm to enter the uterus and produces changes in the endometial lining of the uterus making it more unlikely for implantation to occur. These combined actions interfere with the normal mechanisms of reproduction to prevent pregnancy.

Ethinyl estradiol increases the rate of DNA and RNA synthesis in the cells of female reproductive organs, pituitary gland, hypothalamus, and other target organs. In the hypothalamus, estrogens reduce the release of gonadotropin-releasing hormone, which decreases pituitary release of follicle-stimulating hormone and luteinizing hormone, needed for ovulation and follicular maturation to occur. At the cellular level, estrogens also increase cervical secretions. These combined actions interfere with the normal mechanisms of reproduction to prevent pregnancy.

The combined effect of norgestimate and ethinyl estradiol may increase sex hormone binding globulin and decrease free testosterone, which in turn results in a decreased severity of facial acne.

Interactions

DRUGS

norgestimate and ethinyl estradiol

ampicillin, barbiturates, carbamazepine, griseofulvin, phenylbutazone, phenytoin, rifabutin, rifampin, St. John's Wort, tetracyclines, topiramate: Possibly reduced effectiveness of norgestimate and ethinyl estradiol; increased risk of breakthrough bleeding and menstrual irregularities

ethinyl estradiol

corticosteroids: Increased therapeutic and toxic effects of corticosteroids

cyclosporine: Increased risk of hepatotoxicity and nephrotoxicity

hepatotoxic drugs (such as isoniazid): Increased risk of hepatitis and hepatotoxicity

oral antidiabetics: Decreased therapeutic effects of these drugs

warfarin: Decreased anticoagulant effect

FOODS

ethinyl estradiol

grapefruit juice: Decreased metabolism and possibly increased adverse effects of ethinyl estradiol

ACTIVITIES

ethinyl estradiol

smoking: Increased risk of pulmonary embolism, stroke, thrombophlebitis, and transient ischemic attack

Adverse Reactions

CNS: Chorea, dementia, depression, dizziness, exacerbation of epilepsy, headache, irritability, migraine headache, mood disturbances, nervousness, porphyria, stroke

CV: Hypertension, increased triglycerides, MI, peripheral edema, pulmonary embolism, thromboembolism, thrombophlebitis

EENT: Diplopia, intolerance of contact lenses, retinal vascular thrombosis, sinusitis, vision changes or loss

ENDO: Breast enlargement, pain, tenderness, or tumors; endometrial hyperplasia, galactorrhea; gynecomastia; hyperglycemia; nipple discharge

GI: Abdominal cramps or pain, aggravation of porphyria, anorexia, bloating, constipation, diarrhea, elevated liver function test results, enlargement of hepatic hemangiomas, flatulence, gallbladder obstruction, hepatitis, increased appetite, nausea, pancreatitis, vomiting

GU: Amenorrhea, breakthrough bleeding, cervical erosion, clear vaginal discharge, dysmenorrhea, endometiral or ovarian tumors, increased libido, increased size of uterine leiomyomata, leukorrhea, prolonged or heavy menstrual bleeding, urinary tract infection, vaginitis including vaginal candidiasis

MS: Arthralgias, back or extremity pain, leg cramps

RESP: Bronchitis, exacerbation of asthma, upper respiratory infection

SKIN: Alopecia, application site irritation, chloasma, erythema multiforme or nodosum, hirsutism, jaundice, melasma, pruritus, purpura, rash, urticaria

Other: Anaphylaxis, angioedema, flulike syndrome, folic acid deficiency, hypercalcemia (with bone metastases), hypocalcemia, hyperkalemia, hyponatremia, weight gain or loss

Nursing Considerations

• Use norgestimate and ethinyl estradiol cautiously in women with asthma, diabetes mellitus, epilepsy, migraines, porphyria, systemic lupus erythematosus, and hepatic hemangiomas because ethinyl estradiol can worsen these conditions.

- **WARNING** Assess patient for possible contact lens intolerance or changes in vision or visual acuity because estrogens can cause keratoconus. Be prepared to stop drug immediately, as prescribed, if patient has sudden partial or complete loss of vision or sudden onset of diplopia or migraine.
- Monitor PT for loss of anticoagulant effect in patients taking warfarin because ethinyl estradiol increases production of clotting factors VII, VIII, IX, and X and promotes platelet aggregation.
- Watch for elevated liver function test results because progestins and estrogens may worsen such conditions as acute intermittent and variegate hepatic porphyria.
- Closely monitor patient's blood pressure. Some patients may have a substantial increase in blood pressure as an indiosyncratic reaction to ethinyl estradiol. Monitor patients who already have hypertension for increases in blood pressure because estrogens like ethinyl estradiol may cause fluid retention. Also monitor patients with asthma, heart disease, migraines, renal disease, or seizure disorder for worsening of these conditions.
- Monitor blood glucose level often in patients with diabetes mellitus because ethinyl estradiol may decrease insulin sensitivity and alter glucose tolerance.
- Expect to stop norgestimate and ethinyl estradiol therapy in any woman who develops dementia or signs or symptoms of cardiovascular disease, such as stroke, MI, pulmonary embolism, or venous thrombosis.
- Be aware that norgestimate and ethinyl estradiol may worsen mood disorders, including depression. Monitor patient for depression, mood changes, anxiety, fatigue, dizziness, or insomnia.
- **WARNING** Be aware that patients with breast cancer and bone metastasis may develop severe hypercalcemia because estrogens such as ethinyl estradiol influence calcium and phosphorus metabolism. Watch for toxic effects of increased calcium absorption in patients predisposed to hypercalcemia or nephrolithiasis.
- Assess skin for melasma (tan or brown patches), which may develop on forehead, cheeks, temples, and upper lip. These patches may persist after drug is stopped.
- Monitor thyroid function test results in patients with hypothyroidism because long-term use of the ethinyl estradiol may decrease effectiveness of thyroid therapy.

- Expect to stop norgestimate and ethinyl estradiol therapy several weeks before patient undergoes major surgery, as prescribed, because prolonged immobilization poses a risk of thromboembolism.

PATIENT TEACHING

- Before therapy starts, inform patient of risks involved in taking norgestimate and ethinyl estradiol, such as increased risk of cardiovascular disease, breast or endometrial cancer, dementia, gallbladder disease, and vision abnormalities.
- Alert patient to notify prescriber immediately if vaginal bleeding or any other abnormal signs and symptoms occur while using norgestimate and ethinyl estradiol.
- Advise patient to avoid smoking while taking this drug.
- Stress importance of compliancy with follow up visits.
- Emphasize importance of good dental hygiene and regular dental checkups because an elevated progestin blood level increases the growth of normal oral flora, which may lead to gum tenderness, bleeding, or swelling.

pioglitazone hydrochloride and glimepiride
Duetact

Class and Category
Chemical: Thiazolidinedione (pioglitazone); sulfonylurea (glimepiride)
Therapeutic: Antidiabetic
Pregnancy category: C

Indications and Dosages
▶ *To improve glucose control in patients with type 2 diabetes mellitus who are inadequately controlled by monotherapy with pioglitazone or a sulfonylurea other than glimepiride or by combination therapy with pioglitazone and a sulfonylurea other than glimepiride*
TABLETS
Adults. *Initial:* 30 mg pioglitazone and 2 mg glimepiride once daily; increased if needed.
▶ *To improve glucose control in patients with type 2 diabetes mellitus who are inadequately controlled with glimepiride therapy alone*
TABLETS
Adults. *Initial:* 30 mg pioglitazone and 2 or 4 mg glimepiride once daily; increased if needed.

DOSAGE ADJUSTMENT For elderly, debilitated, or malnourished patients or patients with renal or hepatic insufficiency, initial dosage 30 mg pioglitazone and 1 mg glymepiride, increased slowly. Maximum is 1 tablet of pioglitazone and glimepiride daily regardless of tablet strength.

Mechanism of Action

Pioglitazone decreases insulin resistance by enhancing the sensitivity of insulin-dependent tissues, such as adipose tissue, skeletal muscle, and the liver, and it reduces glucose output from the liver. It activates peroxisome proliferator-activated receptor-gamma (PPARg) receptors, which modulate transcription of insulin-responsive genes involved in glucose control and lipid metabolism. In this way, pioglitazone reduces hyperglycemia, hyperinsulinemia, and hypertriglyceridemia in patients with type 2 diabetes mellitus and insulin resistance. Efficacy depends on the presence of endogenous insulin.

Glimepiride stimulates release of insulin from beta cells in the pancreas. The drug also increases peripheral tissue sensitivity to insulin, either by enhancing insulin binding to cellular receptors or by increasing the number of insulin receptors.

Contraindications

Diabetes complicated by pregnancy; diabetic coma; hypersensitivity to pioglitazone, glimepiride, sulfonylureas, or their components; ketoacidosis; New York Heart Association (NYHA) Class III or IV heart failure; severe hepatic dysfunction; type 1 diabetes mellitus, breast-feeding

Interactions
DRUGS
pioglitazone hydrochloride
fluconazole, itraconazole, ketoconazole, miconazole: Possibly decreased metabolism of pioglitazone
gemfibrozil, rifampin: Possibly altered glucose control
oral contraceptives: Possibly decreased contraceptive effectiveness
glimepiride
ACE inhibitors, anabolic steroids, androgens, azole antifungals, bromocriptine, chloramphenicol, disopyramide, fibric acid derivatives, guanethidine, H_2-receptor antagonists, insulin, magnesium salts, MAO inhibitors, methyldopa, octreotide, oral anticoagulants, oxyphenbutazone, phenylbutazone, probenecid, quinidine, salicylates, sulfonamides, tetracycline, theophylline, tricyclic antidepressants, urinary acidifiers: Increased risk of hypoglycemia

asparaginase, calcium channel blockers, cholestyramine, clonidine, cortico-steroids, danazol, diazoxide, estrogen, glucagon, hydantoins, isoniazid, lithium, morphine, nicotinic acid, oral contraceptives, phenothiazines, rifabutin, rifampin, sympathomimetics, thiazide diuretics, thyroid drugs, urinary alkalinizers: Increased risk of hyperglycemia

beta blockers: Possibly hyperglycemia or masking of hypoglycemia signs

digoxin: Incrased risk of digitalis toxicity

pentamidine: Initially hypoglycemia, then hyperglycemia if beta cell damage occurs

ACTIVITIES

Alcohol use: Altered blood glucose control (usually causing hypoglycemia)

Adverse Reactions

CNS: Abnormal gait, anxiety, asthenia, chills, confusion, depression, dizziness, fatigue, headache, hypertonia, hypoesthesia, insomnia, irritability, malaise, migraine, nervousness, paresthesia, somnolence, syncope, tremor, vertigo

CV: Arrhythmias, congestive heart failure, edema, hypertension, palpitations, sinus tachycardia, vasculitis

EENT: Blurred vision, conjunctivitis, decreased visual acuity, eye pain, macular edema, pharyngitis, retinal hemorrhage, rhinitis, sinusitis, taste perversion, tinnitus, tooth disorders

ENDO: Hypoglycemia

GI: Abdominal pain, anorexia, constipation, diarrhea, elevated liver function test results, epigastric discomfort or fullness, flatulence, heartburn, hunger, nausea, proctocolitis, trace blood in stool, vomiting

GU: Darkened urine, decreased libido, dysuria, polyuria, UTI

HEME: Agranulocytosis, aplastic anemia, eosinophilia, hemolytic anemia, hepatic porphyria, hyperbilirubinemia, leukopenia, pancytopenia, thrombocytopenia

MS: Arthralgia, extremity pain, fractures, leg cramps, myalgia

RESP: Dyspnea, upper respiratory tract infection

SKIN: Allergic reactions, diaphoresis, eczema, erythema multiforme, exfoliative dermatitis, flushing, jaundice, lichenoid reactions, maculopapular or morbilliform rash, photosensitivity, pruritus, urticaria

Other: Disulfiram-like reaction, weight gain

Nursing Considerations

• Be aware that pioglitazone and glimepiride combination isn't recommended for patients with symptomatic heart failure.

- Monitor patient closely for hypoglycemia for 1 to 2 weeks after pioglitazone and glimerpiride therapy starts, especially if patient was taking a sulfonylurea with longer half-life, such as chlorpropamide, because of risk of overlapping drug effects. Also expect a higher risk of hypoglycemia if patient is malnourished, debititated, or has renal, hepatic, pituitary, or adrenal insufficiency.
- Evaluate liver function test results before therapy begins, every 2 months for first year, and annually thereafter, as ordered, because pioglitazone is extensively metabolized by the liver. Expect to stop drug if jaundice develops or ALT values exceed 2½ times normal.
- **WARNING** Monitor patient for evidence of heart failure, such as shortness of breath, rapid weight gain, or edema because pioglitazone can cause fluid retention that may lead to or worsen heart failure. Notify prescriber immediately about any decline in the patient's cardiac status, and expect to discontinue drug, as ordered.
- Be aware that dosage adjustments should be based upon the patient's glycosylated hemoglobin (HbA1C) value rather than fasting blood glucose level alone unless glycemic control declines because HbA1C is a better indicator of long-term glycmeic control.
- Expect to switch patient to insulin, as prescribed, during physical stress, such as infection, surgery, or trauma.

PATIENT TEACHING
- Instruct patient to take drug just before the first meal of the day. Caution him not to skip the meal after taking drug.
- Urge patient not to skip doses or increase dosage without consulting prescriber.
- Tell patient to report signs of hypoglycemia, such as anxiety, confusion, dizziness, excessive sweating, headache, and nausea, or signs of fluid retention, such as shortness of breath, swelling, or sudden weight gain.
- **WARNING** Urge patient to report vision changes promptly and expect to have an eye examination by an ophthalmologist regardless of when the last examination occurred.
- Urge patient to carry hard candy or other simple sugars to treat mild hypoglycemia.
- Advise patient to consult prescriber before taking any OTC drug.
- Teach patient to monitor his blood glucose.

- Teach patient about exercise, diet, signs of hyperglycemia and hypoglycemia, hygiene, foot care, and ways to avoid infection.
- Instruct patient to notify prescriber if he has darkened urine, trouble controlling blood glucose level, easy bruising, fever, rash, sore throat, or unusual bleeding.
- If photosensitivity occurs, instruct patient to avoid direct sunlight and use sunscreen.
- Inform female patient who uses oral contraceptives that drug decreases their effectiveness; suggest another method of contraception while taking pioglitazone.
- Also inform female patient that she may be at risk for fractures during pioglitazone therapy, and urge her to take safety precautions to prevent falls and other injuries.

pioglitazone hydrochloride and metformin hydrochloride

Actoplus Met

Class and Category

Chemical: Thiazolidinedione (pioglitazone), biguanide (metformin)
Therapeutic: Antidiabetic (pioglitazone, metformin)
Pregnancy category: C

Indications and Dosages

▶ *To reduce blood glucose level in patients with type 2 diabetes mellitus who have responded well to pioglitazone initially but need additional glycemic control*

TABLETS

Adults. *Initial:* 15 mg pioglitazone and 500 mg metformin (1 tablet) b.i.d. or 15 mg pioglitazone and 850 mg metformin (1 tablet) daily, gradually adjusted as needed.

▶ *To reduce blood glucose level in patients who haven't achieved adequate glycemic control with metformin alone*

TABLETS

Adults. *Initial:* 15 mg pioglitazone and 500 mg metformin (1 tablet) or 15 mg pioglitazone and 850 mg metformin (1 tablet) daily or b.i.d., gradually adjusted as needed.

▶ *To reduce blood glucose level in patients who already take pioglitazone and metformin separately*

TABLETS

Adults. *Initial:* 15 mg pioglitazone and 500 mg metformin (1 tablet) or 15 mg pioglitazone and 850 mg metformin (1 tablet) daily or b.i.d. depending on dose of pioglitazone and metformin already being taken.

Mechanism of Action

Pioglitazone decreases insulin resistance by enhancing the sensitivity of insulin-dependent tissues, such as adipose tissue, skeletal muscle, and the liver, and reduces glucose output from the liver. Pioglitazone activates peroxisome proliferator-activated receptor-gamma (PRARy) receptors, which modulate transcription of insulin-responsive genes involved in glucose control and lipid metabolism. In this way, pioglitazone reduces hyperglycemia, hyperinsulinemia, and hypertriglyceridemia in patients with type 2 diabetes mellitus and insulin resistance. However to work effectively, pioglitazone depends on the presence of endogenous insulin.

Metformin may promote storage of excess glucose as glycogen in the liver, which reduces glucose production. Metformin also may improve glucose use by skeletal muscle and adipose tissue by increasing glucose transport across cell membranes. It also may increase the number of insulin receptors on cell membranes and make them more sensitive to insulin. In addition, metformin modestly decreases blood triglyceride and total cholesterol levels.

Contraindications

Hypersensitivity to pioglitazone, metformin, or their components; impaired renal function; metabolic acidosis, including diabetic ketoacidosis; severe hepatic dysfunction; type 1 diabetes mellitus; use of iodinated contrast media within preceding 48 hours

Interactions

DRUGS

pioglitazone

hormonal contraceptives: Possibly decreased contraceptive effectiveness

insulin, oral antidiabetics: Increased risk of hypoglycemia

ketoconazole: Possibly decreased metabolism of pioglitazone

metformin

calcium channel blockers, corticosteroids, estrogens, hormonal contraceptives, isoniazid, nicotinic acid, phenothiazines, phenytoin, sympathomimetics, thiazide and other diuretics, thyroid drugs: Possibly hyperglycemia

cationic drugs (such as amiloride, cimetidine, digoxin, morphine, procainamide, quinidine, quinine, ranitidine, triamterene, trimethoprim, vancomycin), nifedipine: Increased metformin level

clofibrate, MAO inhibitors, probenecid, propranolol, rifabutin, rifampin, salicylates, sulfonamides, sulfonylureas: Increased risk of hypoglycemia
furosemide: Possibly increased blood metformin level and decreased blood furosemide level

FOODS

metformin
all foods: Possibly delayed metformin absorption

ACTIVITIES

metformin
alcohol use: Increased risk of hypoglycemia and lactate formation

Adverse Reactions

CNS: Dizziness, headache
CV: Congestive heart failure, edema
EENT: Metallic taste, pharyngitis, sinusitis, tooth disorders
ENDO: Hyperglycemia, hypoglycemia
GI: Abdominal distention, anorexia, constipation, diarrhea, elevated liver transaminase levels, flatulence, indigestion, nausea, vomiting
GU: Urinary tract infection
HEME: Aplastic anemia, decreased hemoglobin and hematocrit, megaloblastic anemia, thrombocytopenia
MS: Myalgia
RESP: Upper respiratory tract infection
SKIN: Photosensitivity, rash
Other: Decreased vitamin B_{12} levels, lactic acidosis, weight gain or loss

Nursing Considerations

- Be aware that pioglitazone and metformin therapy isn't recommended for patients with New York Heart Association Class III or IV status.
- Use drug cautiously in patients with edema because it may occur opr worsen as an adverse reaction to pioglitazone.
- Give pioglitazone and metformin tablets with meals to reduce the risk of adverse GI reactions.
- Expect prescriber to alter dosage if patient has a condition that decreases or delays gastric emptying, such as diarrhea, gastroparesis, GI obstruction, ileus, or vomiting.
- Withhold drug, as ordered, if patient becomes dehydrated because dehydration increases the risk of lactic acidosis.
- Be aware that iodinated contrast media used in radiographic studies increase the risk of renal failure and lactic acidosis dur-

ing pioglitazone and metformin therapy. Expect to withhold drug for 48 hours before and after testing.

- Be prepared to monitor liver function test results before therapy begins, every 2 months during the first year, and annually thereafter, as ordered, because drug is extensively metabolized in the liver. Be prepared to stop drug if patient develops jaundice or if ALT values are greater than 2½ times normal.
- Assess BUN and serum creatinine level, as appropriate, before and during long-term therapy in those at increased risk for lactic acidosis because of the metformin component of drug.
- **WARNING** Monitor patient for signs and symptoms of heart failure—such as shortness of breath, rapid weight gain, or edema—because pioglitazone can cause fluid retention that may lead to or worsen heart failure. Notify prescriber immediately about any deterioration in the patient's cardiac status, and expect to stop the drug, as ordered.
- Watch for signs and symptoms of hypoglycemia, especially if patient also takes another antidiabetic drug.
- Monitor fasting blood glucose level, as ordered, to evaluate effectiveness of therapy. Assess patient for hyperglycemia and the need for insulin during times of increased stress, such as infection or surgery.
- Monitor glycosylated hemoglobin level to assess long-term effectiveness of drug therapy.
- Be aware that patients with inadequate vitamin B_{12} or calcium intake or absorption may develop abnormal vitamin B_{12} levels. Vitamin B_{12} level should be measured every 2 to 3 years, as ordered.
- Expect to withhold drug temporarily, as ordered, before surgical procedures, except for minor procedures that don't need restricted intake of food and fluids. Don't resume drug until patient's oral intake has resumed and renal function is normal.

PATIENT TEACHING
- Stress the need for patient to continue exercise program, diet control, and weight management during pioglitazone and metformin therapy.
- Instruct patient to take drug with breakfast if taking drug once a day, or at breakfast and dinner if taking drug twice a day.
- Direct patient to take drug exactly as prescribed and not to change the dosage or frequency unless instructed.
- Advise patient to notify prescriber immediately if he has shortness of breath, fluid retention, or sudden weight gain because drug may need to be stopped.

- Teach patient how to measure his blood glucose level and recognize hyperglycemia and hypoglycemia. Urge him to notify prescriber about abnormal blood glucose level.
- Caution patient to avoid alcohol, which can increase the risk of hypoglycemia.
- Instruct patient to watch for early evidence of lactic acidosis, including drowsiness, hyperventilation, malaise, and muscle pain, and notify prescriber if such signs develop.
- Instruct patient to keep appointments for liver function tests, as ordered, typically every 2 months during first year of therapy and annually thereafter.
- Inform female patient who uses oral contraceptives that drug decreases their effectiveness; suggest another method of contraception while taking pioglitazone and metformin.
- Warn women of childbearing age who are premenopausal and having periods of anovulation that drug may induce ovulation. Advise using adequate contraception while taking drug.

repaglinide and metformin hydrochloride
PrandiMet

Class and Category
Chemical: Meglitinide (repaglinide), dimethylbiguanide (metformin)
Therapeutic: Antidiabetic (repaglinide, metformin)
Pregnancy category: C

Indications and Dosages
▶ *To reduce blood glucose level in patients with type 2 diabetes mellitus who aren't adequately controlled with metformin alone*
TABLETS
Adults. *Initial:* 1 mg repaglinide and 500 mg metformin (1 tablet) twice daily within 15 minutes of a meal and then increased as needed. *Maximum:* 4 mg repaglinide and 1,000 mg metformin (two 2/500-mg tablets) per meal or 10 mg repaglinide and 2,500 mg metformin (five 2/500-mg tablets) daily.
▶ *To reduce blood glucose level in patients with type 2 diabetes mellitus who aren't adequately controlled with repaglinide alone*
TABLETS
Adults. *Initial:* 1 or 2 mg repaglinide and 500 mg metformin (1 tablet) twice daily within 15 minutes of a meal and then in-

creased as needed. *Maximum:* 4 mg repaglinide and 1,000 mg metformin (two 2/500-mg tablets) per meal or 10 mg repaglinide and 2,500 mg metformin (five 2/500-mg tablets) daily.

▶ *To reduce blood glucose level in patients with type 2 diabetes mellitus who have been receiving repaglinide and metformin separately*

TABLETS

Adults. *Initial:* Dosage similar to but not exceeding patient's current doses, then adjusted to maximum daily dose needed to achieve targeted glycemic control. *Maximum:* 4 mg repaglinide and 1,000 mg metformin (two 2/500-mg tablets) per meal or 10 mg repaglinide and 2,500 mg metformin (five 2/500-mg tablets) daily.

Mechanism of Action

Repaglinide stimulates release of insulin from functioning pancreatic beta cells. In patients with type 2 diabetes mellitus, a shortage of these cells decreases blood insulin levels and causes glucose intolerance. By interacting with the adenosine triphosphatase (ATP)-potassium channel on the beta cell membrane, repaglinide prevents potassium from leaving the cell. This causes the beta cell to depolarize, and the cell membrane's calcium moves into the cell and insulin moves out. The extent of insulin release is glucose dependent; the lower the glucose level, the less insulin is secreted from the cell.

Metformin may promote storage of excess glucose as glycogen in the liver, which reduces glucose production. Metformin also may improve glucose use by skeletal muscle and adipose tissue by increasing glucose transport across cell membranes. This drug also may increase the number of insulin receptors on cell membranes and make them more sensitive to insulin. In addition, metformin modestly decreases blood triglyceride and total cholesterol levels.

Contraindications

Concurrent therapy with both gemfibrozil and itraconazole; hypersensitivity to metformin, repaglinide, or their components; metabolic acidosis (acute or chronic) including diabetic ketoacidosis; renal or severe hepatic impairment; type 1 diabetes mellitus; use of iodinated contrast media within 48 hours

Interactions

DRUGS

repaglinide and metformin

calcium channel blockers, corticosteroids, estrogens, isoniazid, oral contraceptives, phenothiazines, phenytoin, sympathomimetics, thiazide and other diuretics, thyroid drugs: Possibly hyperglycemia

MAO inhibitors, probenecid, salicylates, sulfonamides: Increased risk of hypoglycemia

repaglinide

barbiturates, carbamazepine, rifampin, troglitazone: Possibly increased repaglinide metabolism

beta blockers, chloramphenicol, clarithromycin, NSAIDs, oral anticoagulants: Enhanced hypoglycemic effects

erythromycin, itraconazole, ketoconazole, miconazole: Possibly inhibited repaglinide metabolism

gemfibrozil, trimethoprim: Increased blood repaglinide level resulting in increased and prolonged blood glucose–lowering effects

niacin: Possibly loss of glucose control

NPH insulin: Possibly increased risk of angina

trimethoprim: Increased plasma repaglinide level

metformin

cationic drugs (such as amiloride, cimetidine, digoxin, morphine, procainamide, quinidine, quinine, ranitidine, triamterene, trimethoprim, vancomycin), nifedipine: Increased blood metformin level

clofibrate, propranolol, rifabutin, rifampin, sulfonylureas: Increased risk of hypoglycemia

nicotinic acid: Possibly hyperglycemia

FOODS

metformin

all foods: Possibly delayed metformin absorption

ACTIVITIES

metform

alcohol use: Increased risk of hypoglycemia and lactate formation

Adverse Reactions

CNS: Headache

CV: Angina, myocardial ischemia

EENT: Metallic taste, rhinitis, sinusitis

ENDO: Hypoglycemia

GI: Abdominal distention, anorexia, constipation, diarrhea, elevated liver enzyme levels, flatulence, hepatitis, indigestion, nausea, pancreatitis, vomiting

HEME: Aplastic anemia, hemolytic anemia, leukopenia, megaloblastic anemia, thrombocytopenia

MS: Arthralgia, back pain

RESP: Bronchitis, upper respiratory tract infection

SKIN: Alopecia, photosenstivity, rash, Stevens-Johnson syndrome

Other: Anaphylaxis, decreased vitamin B_{12} level, lactic acidosis, weight loss

Nursing Considerations

- Administer repaglinide and metformin tablets 15 minutes before a meal.
- Monitor patient's blood glucose level to evaluate drug effectiveness. Expect to check Hb_{A1c} level every 3 months, as ordered, to assess patient's long-term control of blood glucose level.
- Assess BUN and serum creatinine levels, as appropriate, before and during long-term therapy in those at increased risk for lactic acidosis.
- Monitor patient's hepatic function, as ordered, because impaired hepatic function may significantly reduce the liver's ability to clear lactate, predisposing the patient to lactic acidosis.
- Monitor patient's hematologic status yearly, as ordered, because drug may cause abnormalities.
- During times of increased stress, such as from infection, surgery, or trauma, monitor blood glucose level often and assess need for additional insulin.
- **WARNING** Withhold drug, as ordered, if patient becomes dehydrated or develops hypoxemia or sepsis because these conditions increase the risk of lactic acidosis. Monitor patient for evidence of lactic acidosis, such as malaise, myalgia, respiratory distress, increasing somnolence, and nonspecific abdominal distress. Expect to institute general supportive measures as prescribed and prepare patient for hemodialysis to correct acidosis and remove accumulated metformin.
- Be aware that iodinated contrast media used in radiographic studies increases the risk of renal failure and lactic acidosis during repaglinide and metformin therapy. Expect to withhold the drug for 48 hours before and after testing.
- Repaglinide shouldn't be used with NPH insulin because doing so may increase the risk of angina.
- Expect to discontinue repgalinide and metformin, as ordered, if patient develops shock, acute congestive heart failure, acute myocardial infarction, or other conditions in which hypoxemia has been linked to lactic acidiosis.

PATIENT TEACHING
- Instruct patient to take repaglinide and metformin tablets within 15 minutes before meals.
- Direct patient to take drug exactly as prescribed and not to change the dosage or frequency unless instructed.
- Stress the importance of following prescribed diet, exercising regularly, controlling weight, and checking blood glucose level.

- Teach patient how to measure blood glucose level and recognize hyperglycemia and hypoglycemia. Urge him to notify prescriber of abnormal blood glucose level. Tell him to carry candy or other simple carbohydrates with him to treat mild episodes of hypoglycemia.
- Caution patient to avoid alcohol, which can increase the risk of hypoglycemia.
- Instruct patient to watch for early signs of lactic acidosis, including drowsiness, hyperventilation, malaise, and muscle pain, and to notify prescriber if such signs develop.
- Advise patient to expect laboratory monitoring of glycosylated hemoglobin level every 3 months until blood glucose is controlled.
- Urge patient to increase his intake of calcium and vitamin B_{12}.

risedronate sodium and calcium carbonate

Actonel with Calcium

Class and Category

Chemical: Pyridinyl bisphosphonate (risedronate), elemental cation (calcium)
Therapeutic: Bone resorption inhibitor (risedronate, calcium)
Pregnancy category: C

Indications and Dosages

▶ *To prevent or treat osteoporosis in postmenopausal women*
TABLETS
Adult women. 35 mg risedronate (1 tablet) every wk on day 1 of 7-day treatment cycle followed by 1,250 mg calcium (1 tablet) daily on days 2 through 7 of 7-day treatment cycle.

Mechanism of Action

Risedronate inhibits osteoclasts at the cellular level. Normally, osteoclasts adhere to the bone surface; risedronate prevents them from doing so. This reduces the rate at which osteoclasts are resorbed by bone.

Calcium suppresses PTH secretion. Increased PTH levels contribute to age-related bone loss, especially at cortical sites, while increased bone turnover is an independent risk factor for fractures. With suppression of PTH secretion, bone turnover decreases.

Contraindications

Hypercalcemia; hypersensitivity to risedronate, calcium, or their components; hypocalcemia; inability to stand or sit uupright for at least 30 minutes; renal calculi; severe renal impairment (creatinine clearance less than 30 ml/min)

Interactions

DRUGS

risedronate

aspirin, NSAIDs: Increased risk of GI irritation

calcium-containing preparations, including antacids: Impaired absorption of risedronate

calcium

bisphosphonates: Decreased absorption of the bisphosphonate

fluoroquinolones: Possibly decreased absorption of the fluoroquinolone

glucocorticoids (systemic): Decreased absorption of calcium

iron: Possibly decreased absorption of iron

levothyroxine: Decreased levothyroxine absorption and increased serum thyrotropin levels

tetracyclines: Possibly decreased absorption of tetracycline

thiazide diuretics: Reduced urinary excretion of calcium, possibly leading to adverse effects

vitamin D, vitamin D analgues (such as calcitriol, doxercalciferol, and paricalcitol): Possibly increased absorption of calcium

FOODS

risedronate

all foods: Decreased risedronate bioavailability

calcium

caffeine, high-fiber food: Possibly decreased calcium absorption

ACTIVITIES

calcium

alcohol use (excessive), smoking: Possibly decreased calcium absorption

Adverse Reactions

CNS: Anxiety, asthenia, depression, dizziness, headache, hypertonia, insomnia, neuralgia, paresthesia, weakness, vertigo

CV: Angina, chest pain, hypertension, hypotension, peripheral edema

EENT: Amblyopia, cataract, conjunctivitis, dry eyes or mouth, eye inflammation, otitis media, pharyngitis, rhinitis, sinusitis, tinnitus

ENDO: Hypercalcemia

GI: Abdominal pain, bloating, colitis, constipation, diarrhea, dysphagia, eructation, esophagitis, esophageal or gastric ulcer, flatulence, gastritis, heartburn, nausea
GU: UTI
HEME: Anemia
MS: Arthralgia; back, bone, or neck pain; bursitis; joint disorder; leg cramps; myasthenia; myalgia; osteonecrosis of the jaw; retrosternal pain
RESP: Bronchitis,dyspnea, pneumonia
SKIN: Bullous skin reactions, ecchymosis, pruritus, rash, skin carcinoma
Other: Angioedema, flulike symptoms

Nursing Considerations

- Use risedronate and calcium cautiously in patients who have a history of kidney stones or hypercalciuria. Be prepared to monitor these patient's urinary calcium excretion regularly, as ordered.
- Check to determine if patient has had a dental examination before starting risedronate and calcium therapy, especially if patient has cancer; is receiving chemotherapy, head or neck radiation, or corticosteroids; or has poor oral hygiene. The risk of developing osteonecrosis is higher in these patients, and invasive dental procedures during risedronate and calcium therapy can exacerbate osteonecrosis.
- Be aware that bisphosphonates like risedronate may interfere with bone-imaging agents.
- Monitor patient's serum calcium levels and bone density scans regularly, as ordered to determine effectiveness of risedronate and calcium therapy.

PATIENT TEACHING

- Instruct patient to take risedronate with a full glass of water at least 30 minutes before she takes her first food or beverage (except water) of the day and not to lie down for 30 minutes. Instruct patient to take calcium tablets with food to improve absorption.
- Tell patient that if she misses taking her weekly risedronate tablet, to take it the morning after she remembers it and to return to taking 1 tablet of risedronate once a week, as originally scheduled on her chosen day. Stress that she should not take 2 risedronate tablets on the same day.
- Advise patient to avoid taking calcium within 2 hours of taking another oral drug because of risk of interaction.

- Caution patient to consult prescriber before taking OTC drugs because of risk of interactions.
- Tell patient to avoid excessive use of tobacco and excessive consumption of alcoholic beverages, caffeine-containing products and high-fiber foods because these substances may decrease calcium absorption.
- Instruct patient on proper oral hygiene and need to notify prescriber before having any invasive dental procedure performed.
- Tell patient to notify prescriber if she develops difficulty or pain with swallowing, retrosternal pain, or severe persistent or worsening heartburn.

rosiglitazone maleate and glimepiride
Avandaryl

Class and Category
Chemical: Thiazolidinedione (rosiglitazone), sulfonylurea (glimepiride)
Therapeutic: Antidiabetic drug
Pregnancy category: C

Indications and Dosages
▶ *To reduce blood glucose level in patients with type 2 diabetes mellitus whose level is inadequately controlled by rosiglitazone or glimepiride alone*
TABLETS
Adults. *Initial:* 4 mg rosiglitazone and 1 mg glimepiride or 4 mg rosiglitazone and 2 mg glimepiride once daily with first meal of the day. Increased as needed after 1 to 2 wk if glimepiride dosage isn't sufficient or after 8 to 12 wk if rosiglitazone dosage isn't sufficient. *Maximum:* 8 mg rosiglitazone and 4 mg glimepiride.

Mechanism of Action
Rosiglitazone and glimepiride each improve glucose control. Rosiglitazone increases tissue sensitivity to insulin. A peroxisome proliferator-activated receptor agonist, it regulates transcription of insulin-responsive genes in key target tissues, such as adipose tissue, skeletal muscle, and liver. Enhanced insulin sensitivity lowers blood glucose level.

Glimepiride stimulates insulin release from beta cells in the pancreas and increases peripheral tissue sensitivity to insulin, either by improving insulin binding to cellular receptors or by increasing the number of insulin receptors.

Contraindications

Active liver disease; diabetic coma; liver enzyme levels more than 2.5 times the upper limit of normal; hypersensitivity to rosiglitazone, glimepiride, sulfonylureas, or their components; ketoacidosis; metabolic acidosis (acute or chronic); New York Heart Association (NYHA) class III or IV heart failure; pregnancy; serum creatinine level of 1.5 mg/dl (men) or 1.4 mg/dl (women) or more; type 1 diabetes mellitus

Interactions

DRUGS

rosiglitazone maleate and glimepiride
rifampin: Increased risk of hyperglycemia
rosiglitazone maleate
CYP2C8 inducers: Possibly decreased effects of rosiglitazone
CYP2C8 inhibitors: Possibly increased effects of rosiglitazone

ACTIVITIES

rosiglitazone maleate and glimepiride
alcohol use: Altered blood glucose control

FOODS

glimepiride
ACE inhibitors, anabolic steroids, androgens, azole antifungals, bromocriptine, chloramphenicol, disopyramide, fibric acid derivatives, guanethidine, H2-receptor antagonists, insulin, magnesium salts, MAO inhibitors, methyldopa, octreotide, oral anticoagulants, oxyphenbutazone, phenylbutazone, probenecid, quinidine, salicylates, sulfonamides, tetracycline, theophylline, tricyclic antidepressants, urine acidifiers: Increased risk of hypoglycemia
asparaginase, calcium channel blockers, cholestyramine, clonidine, corticosteroids, danazol, diazoxide, estrogen, glucagons, hydantoins, isoniazid, lithium, morphine, nicotinic acid, oral contraceptives, phenothiazines, rifabutin, sympathomimetics, thiazide diuretics, thyroid drugs, urine alkalinizers: Increased risk of hyperglycemia
beta blockers: Possibly hyperglycemia or masking of hypoglycemia signs
digoxin: Increased risk of digitalis toxicity
pentamidine: Initially hypoglycemia and then hyperglycemia if beta cell damage occurs

Adverse Reactions

CNS: Abnormal gait, anxiety, asthenia, chills, depression, dizziness, fatigue, headache, hypertonia, hypoesthesia, insomnia, malaise, migraine headache, nervousness, paresthesia, somnolence, syncope, tremor, vertigo

CV: Arrhythmias, congestive heart failure, edema, hypertension, vasculitis

EENT: Blurred vision, conjunctivitis, decreased visual acuity, eye pain, macular edema, pharyngitis, retinal hemorrhage, rhinitis, sinusitis, taste perversion, tinnitus

ENDO: Hyperglycemia, hypoglycemia

GI: Anorexia, constipation, diarrhea, elevated liver enzyme levels, epigastric discomfort or fullness, flatulence, heartburn, hepatotoxicity, hunger, nausea, proctocolitis, trace blood in stool, vomiting

GU: Darkened urine, decreased libido, dysuria, polyuria

HEME: Agranulocytosis, anemia, aplastic anemia, eosinophilia, hemolytic anemia, hepatic porphyria, leukopenia, pancytopenia

MS: Arthralgia, back pain, fractures, leg cramps, myalgia

RESP: Dyspnea, upper respiratory tract infection

SKIN: Allergic skin reactions, diaphoresis, eczema, erythema multiforme, exfoliative dermatitis, flushing, jaundice, lichenoid reactions, maculopapular or morbilliform rash, photosensitivity, pruritus, urticaria

Other: Anaphylaxis, angioedema, disulfiram-like reaction, weight gain

Nursing Considerations

- Be aware that rosiglitazone and glimepiride combination isn't recommended for patients with symptomatic heart failure.
- Give rosiglitazone and glimerpiride cautiously to patients with edema or mild hepatic impairment because of possible adverse reactions.
- Evaulate patient's liver function before starting drug and periodically during therapy, as ordered. Notify prescriber about abnormalities, such as nausea, vomiting, abdominal pain, fatigue, anorexia, and dark urine. Drug may need to be stopped.
- **WARNING** Monitor patient for evidence of heart failure—such as shortness of breath, rapid weight gain, or edema—because rosiglitazone may cause fluid retention that could cause or worsen heart failure. Notify prescriber immediately if patient's cardiac status declines, and expect to stop drug.
- Monitor fasting glucose and glycosylated hemoglobin (Hb_{A1c}) levels periodically, as ordered, to evaluate effectiveness of treatment.
- Be aware that drug is effective only if patient has endogenous insulin. Expect to switch patient to insulin therapy during periods of physical stress, such as infection, surgery, and trauma.
- **WARNING** Monitor patient closely for hypoglycemia, espe-

cially if patient is malnourished or debilitated or has renal, hepatic, pituitary, or adrenal insufficiency.

PATIENT TEACHING

- Instruct patient to take rosigliazone and glimepiride with the first meal of the day.
- Urge patient not to skip doses or increase dosage without consulting prescriber. If a dose is missed, warn patient not to double the next dose.
- Stress the need to follow an exercise program and a diet control program during rosiglitazone therapy.
- Advise patient to notify prescriber immediately about shortness of breath, fluid retention, or sudden weight gain because drug may need to be discontinued.
- Educate patient about signs and symptoms of hypoglycemia, such as anxiety, confusion, dizziness, excessive sweating, headache, and nausea; urge her to notify prescriber if they are severe or persistent.
- Encourage patient to carry candy or other simple sugars to treat mild hypoglycemia.
- Instruct patient to have liver function tests, as prescribed, about every 2 months for first year of therapy and then annually.
- Inform premenopausal, anovulatory patient that rosiglitazone may induce ovulation, increasing risk of pregnancy.
- Advise women to take precautions against falling because rosiglitazone increases risk of fractures.
- Urge patient to wear or carry identification indicating that she has diabetes.
- If photosensitivity is a problem, instruct patient to avoid direct sunlight and to wear sunscreen.

rosiglitazone maleate and metformin hydrochloride

Avandamet

Class and Category

Chemical: Thiazolidinedione (rosiglitazone), dimethylbiguanide (metformin)
Therapeutic: Antidiabetic
Pregnancy category: C

Indications and Dosages

▶ *As adjunct to diet and exercise in patients with type 2 diabetes mellitus when treatment with both rosiglitazone and metformin is considered necessary*

TABLETS

Adults. *Initial:* 2 mg rosiglitazone and 500 mg metformin (1 tablet) once daily; for patient with Hb_{A1c} greater than 11%, 2 mg rosiglitazone and 500 mg metformin (1 tablet) b.i.d. Increased as needed in increments of 2 mg rosiglitazone and 500 mg metformin daily in divided doses every 4 weeks. *Maximum:* 8 mg rosiglitazone and 2,000 mg metformin daily in divided doses.

▶ *To reduce blood glucose level as initial therapy in patients with type 2 diabetes mellitus who aren't adequately controlled with rosiglitazone alone*

TABLETS

Adults. *Initial:* 2 mg rosiglitazone and 500 mg metformin (1 tablet) b.i.d if patient was taking 4 mg daily of rosiglitazone monotherapy; 4 mg rosiglitazone and 500 mg metformin (1 tablet) b.i.d. if 8 mg daily of rosiglitazone monotherapy. Increased as needed after 1 to 2 wk if metformin dosage isn't sufficient or 8 to 12 wk if rosiglitazone dosage isn't sufficient. *Maximum:* 8 mg rosiglitazone and 2,000 mg metformin daily in divided doses.

▶ *To reduce blood glucose level as initial therapy in patients with type 2 diabetes mellitus who aren't adequately controlled with metformin alone*

TABLETS

Adults. *Initial:* 2 mg rosiglitazone and 500 mg metformin (1 tablet) b.i.d. if patient was taking 1,000 mg daily of metformin monotherapy; individualized if patient was taking 1,000 to 2,000 mg daily of metformin monotherapy. Or, 2 mg rosiglitazone and 1,000 mg metformin (2 tablets each containing 1 mg rosiglitazone and 500 mg metformin or 1 tablet containing 2 mg rosiglitazone and 1,000 mg metformin) b.i.d. if patient was taking 2,000 mg daily of metformin monotherapy. Dosage increased, as needed, after 1 to 2 wk if metformin dosage isn't sufficient or after 8 to 12 wk if rosiglitazone dosage isn't sufficient. *Maximum:* 8 mg rosiglitazone and 2,000 mg metformin daily in divided doses.

DOSAGE ADJUSTMENT If patient has been taking rosiglitazone and metformin as separate tablets, usual starting dose of combination drug is that of rosiglitazone and metformin already being taken individually.

Mechanism of Action

Rosiglitazone and metformin each improve glucose control. Rosiglitazone increases tissue sensitivity to insulin. A peroxisome proliferator-activated receptor agonist, it regulates transcription of insulin-responsive genes in key target tissues, such as adipose tissue, skeletal muscle, and liver. Enhanced insulin sensitivity lowers blood glucose level.

Metformin may promote storage of excess glucose as glycogen in the liver, thus reducing glucose production. It also may improve glucose use by skeletal muscle and adipose tissue by facilitating glucose transport across cell membranes. Metformin also may increase the number of insulin receptors on cell membranes and make them more sensitive to insulin.

Contraindications

Diabetic coma; hypersensitivity to metformin, rosiglitazone, or their components; ketoacidosis; metabolic acidosis (acute or chronic); New York Heart Association (NYHA) class III or IV heart failure; renal disease or dysfunction (serum creatinine level of 1.5 mg/dl or more in men or 1.4 mg/dl or more in women); type 1 diabetes mellitus

Interactions

DRUGS

rosiglitazone

CYP 2C8 inducers (such as rifampin): Possibly decreased effects of rosiglitazone

CYP 2C8 inhibitors (such as gemfibrozil): Possibly increased effects of rosiglitazone

metformin

cimetidine: Increased blood metformin level; possibly increased risk of hypoglycemia

furosemide: Increased blood metformin level and decreased blood furosemide level

nifedipine: Enhanced metformin absorption

FOODS

metformin

all foods: Delayed and reduced metformin absorption

ACTIVITIES

metformin

alcohol use: Altered blood glucose control (usually causing hyperglycemia) and possibly potentiated metformin effect on lactate metabolism

Adverse Reactions

CNS: Dizziness, fatigue, headache
CV: Angina, edema, heart failure, MI, pulmonary edema
EENT: Blurred vision, decreased visual acuity, macular edema, nasopharyngitis, sinusitis
ENDO: Hyperglycemia, hypoglycemia
GI: Abdominal pain, constipation, diarrhea, dyspepsia, elevated liver enzymes, hepatotoxicity, nausea, vomiting
HEME: Anemia
MS: Arthralgia, back pain, fracture (women)
RESP: Cough, dyspnea, pleural effusion, upper respiratory tract infection
SKIN: Pruritus, rash, Stevens-Johnson syndrome, urticaria
Other: Anaphylaxis, angioedema, lactic acidosis, viral infection, weight gain

Nursing Considerations

- Be aware that rosiglitazone and metformin therapy isn't recommended for patients with symptomatic heart failure.
- **WARNING** Monitor renal function, as ordered, before starting rosiglitazone and metformin and at least annually thereafter because significant renal impairment can result in tissue hypoperfusion and hypoxemia, leading to lactic acidosis.
- Evaluate patient's liver function before starting drug and periodically throughout therapy, as ordered. Notify prescriber about abnormalities, such as nausea, vomiting, abdominal pain, fatigue, anorexia, and dark urine. Drug may need to be stopped.
- **WARNING** Expect to stop drug for 48 hours before and after radiographic tests involving I.V. iodinated contrast media because of an increased risk of renal failure and lactic acidosis.
- **WARNING** Monitor malnourished or debilitated patients and those with renal, hepatic, pituitary, or adrenal insufficiency because they have an increased risk of hypoglycemia.
- Expect to check vitamin B_{12} blood level at least every 2 to 3 years in patients with inadequate vitamin B_{12} or calcium intake or absorption because prolonged drug use may impair vitamin B_{12} absorption.
- Monitor fasting blood glucose level to determine patient's response to drug. Expect to check glycosylated hemoglobin (HbA_{1c}) level every 3 to 6 months, as ordered, to evaluate long-term blood glucose control.
- Monitor blood glucose level often to detect hyperglycemia and assess the need for supplemental insulin during circumstances

of increased stress, such as infection, surgery, and trauma.
- Arrange for instruction about diabetes and consultation with a dietitian or certified diabetes educator, if possible.
- Monitor patient for evidence of heart failure, such as difficulty breathing, fatigue, abnormal heart sounds, and edema. Notify prescriber if such evidence occurs, and expect to stop drug.

PATIENT TEACHING
- Instruct patient to take drug with morning and evening meals. Caution her not to skip the meal after taking the drug.
- Inform patient that drug is used with diet and exercise therapy and is not a substitute for these additional measures.
- Advise patient not to skip doses, stop drug, or take OTC drugs without consulting prescriber because of risk of hyperglycemia.
- Inform patient that the most common adverse effects are minor and typically occur during first few weeks of therapy.
- Teach patient how to monitor blood glucose level and when to report changes.
- Advise patient to expect laboratory monitoring of HbA_{1c} level every 3 months until blood glucose level is controlled.
- Instruct patient to report signs of hypoglycemia: anxiety, confusion, dizziness, excessive sweating, headache, and nausea.
- Advise patient to carry identification indicating that she has diabetes.
- Advise patient to avoid alcohol because it increases the risk of hypoglycemia.
- Inform women of childbearing age that rosiglitazone may induce ovulation in some premenopausal, anovulatory women, increasing the risk of pregnancy if sexually active. Advise patient to use adequate contraception.
- Instruct female patient of childbearing age to report suspected or confirmed pregnancy to prescriber because she may need to stop rosiglitazone and metformin therapy and switch to insulin therapy, as prescribed, during pregnancy.
- Advise women to guard against falling because drug increases risk of fractures.

sitagliptin and metformin hydrochloride
Janumet

Class and Category
Chemical: Beta amino acid derivative (sitagliptin), dimethyl-biguanide (metformin)

Therapeutic: Antidiabetic
Pregnancy category: B

Indications and Dosages

▶ *To improve glucose control in patients with type 2 diabetes who are inadequately controlled with metformin alone*

TABLETS

Adults. *Initial:* 50 mg sitagliptin b.i.d. along with the dose of metformin already being taken. *Maximum:* 100 mg sitagliptin and 2,000 mg metformin daily.

▶ *To improve glucose control in patients with type 2 diabetes who are inadequately controlled with sitagliptin alone*

TABLETS

Adults. *Initial:* 50 mg sitagliptin and 500 mg metformin b.i.d., increased to 50 mg sitagliptin and 100 mg metformin b.i.d., as needed. *Maximum:* 100 mg sitagliptin and 2,000 mg metformin daily.

Mechanism of Action

Sitagliptin inhibits the dipeptidyl peptidase-4 enzyme to slow inactivation of incretin hormones. These hormones are released by the intestine throughout the day but increase in response to a meal. When blood glucose level is normal or increased, incretin hormones increase insulin synthesis and release from pancreatic beta cells. One type of incretin hormone, glucagon-like peptide (GLP-1) also lowers glucagon secretion from pancreatic alpha cells which reduces hepatic glucose production.

Metformin may promote storage of excess glucose as glycogen in the liver, which reduces glucose production. Drug also may improve glucose use by skeletal muscle and adipose tissue by increasing glucose transport across cell membranes. It also may increase the number of insulin receptors on cell membranes and make them more sensitive to insulin.

These combined actions decrease blood glucose level in type 2 diabetes.

Contraindications

Hepatic or renal dysfunction; hypersensitivity to sitagliptin, metformin, or their components; metabolic acidosis, including diabetic ketoacidosis; use of iodinated contrast media within 48 hours

Interactions

DRUGS

sitagliptin

digoxin: Slightly increased plasma digoxin level

metformin hydrochloride

calcium channel blockers, corticosteroids, estrogens, isoniazid, nicotinic acid, oral contraceptives, phenothiazines, phenytoin, sympathomimetics, thiazide and other diuretics, thyroid drugs: Possibly hyperglycemia
cationic drugs (such as amiloride, cimetidine, digoxin, morphine, procainamide, quinidine, quinine, ranitidine, triamterene, trimethoprim, vancomycin), nifedipine: Increased blood metformin level
clofibrate, MAO inhibitors, probenecid, propranolol, rifabutin, rifampin, salicylates, sulfonamides, sulfonylureas: Increased risk of hypoglycemia

Adverse Reactions

CNS: Asthenia, headache
EENT: Metallic taste, nasopharyngitis
ENDO: Hypoglycemia
GI: Abdominal distention or pain, anorexia, constipation, diarrhea, flatulence, indigestion, nausea, vomiting
HEME: Aplastic anemia, megaloblastic anemia, thromboyctopenia
SKIN: Photosensitivity, rash, Stevens-Johnson syndrome, urticaria
Other: Anaphylaxis, angioedema, decreased vitamin B_{12} level, lactic acidosis, weight loss

Nursing Considerations

• Administer sitagliptin and metformin tablets with food, which decreases and slightly delays absorption, thus reducing the risk of adverse GI reactions.

• Assess patient's renal function before starting sitagliptin and metformin, as ordered, and regularly thereafter; impaired renal function increases risk of lactic acidosis.

• Monitor patient's hepatic function, as ordered, because impaired hepatic function may significantly reduce the liver's ability to clear lactate, predisposing the patient to lactic acidosis.

• Monitor patient's hematologic status annually, as ordered, to detect adverse effects.

• Monitor blood glucose level to evaluate drug effectiveness. Watch for hyperglycemia and the need for insulin during increased stress, such as infection and surgery.

• Withhold drug, as ordered, if patient becomes dehydrated or develops hypoxemia or sepsis because these conditions increase the risk of lactic acidosis.

• Be aware that iodinated contrast media used in radiographic studies increases the risk of renal failure and lactic acidosis during therapy. Expect to withhold drug before and after testing.

- Monitor patient's serum vitamin B_{12} level, as ordered, because metformin may cause it to drop below normal. Although anemia is rare, a vitamin B_{12} supplement may be needed or drug may need to be discontinued.

PATIENT TEACHING

- Instruct patient to take tablets with breakfast and dinner.
- Direct patient to take drug exactly as prescribed and not to change the dosage or frequency unless instructed.
- Stress the importance of following prescribed diet, exercising regularly, controlling weight, and checking blood glucose level.
- Teach patient how to measure his blood glucose level and recognize signs of hyperglycemia and hypoglycemia. Urge him to tell prescriber about abnormal blood glucose levels.
- Caution patient to avoid consuming alcohol because doing so can increase the risk of hypoglycemia.
- Instruct patient to watch for early signs and symptoms of lactic acidosis, including drowsiness, hyperventilation, malaise, and muscle pain, and to notify prescriber if they develop.
- Advise patient to expect laboratory monitoring of glycosylated hemoglobin level every 3 months until blood glucose level is controlled.
- Instruct patient to notify prescriber immediately if he has trouble breathing or develops hives, rash, or swelling.

testosterone cypionate and estradiol cypionate
Depo-Testadiol
testosterone enanthate and estradiol valerate
Valertest No. 1

Class and Category
Chemical: Androgen (testosterone), estrogen (estradiol)
Therapeutic: Hormone replacement (testosterone, estradiol)
Pregnancy category: X

Indications and Dosages
▶ *To treat moderate to severe vasomotor symptoms of menopause*
I.M. INJECTION (DEPO-TESTADIOL)
Adult women. 50 mg testosterone and 2 mg estradiol (1 ml) every 4 wk

I.M. INJECTION (VALERTEST NO. 1)
Adult women. 90 mg testosterone and 4 mg estradiol (1 ml) every 4 wk

Mechanism of Action

Testosterone esters such as cypionate and enanthate first undergo hydrolysis of the ester to the active form, free testosterone, in the liver. Free testosterone is further converted into two of the major active metabolites, DHT and estradiol. Thus, testosterone can produce estrogenic effects as a result of its conversion to estradiol to help maintain GU function and reduce vasomotor symptoms when estrogen production declines from menopause, surgical removal of the ovaries, or other estrogen deficiency.

Estradiol increases DNA and RNA synthesis in the cells of female reproductive organs, pituitary gland, hypothalamus, and other target organs. In the hypothalamus, estrogens decrease release of gonadotropin-releasing hormone, which reduces pituitary release of follicle-stimulating hormone and luteinizing hormone. In women, these hormones are required for normal GU and other essential body functions. At the cellular level, estrogens increase cervical secretions, cause endometrial cell proliferation, and improve uterine tone. Estrogen replacement helps maintain GU function and reduces vasomotor symptoms when estrogen production declines as a result of menopause, surgical removal of ovaries, or other estrogen deficiency.

Contraindications

Active thrombophlebitis or thromboembolic disorders; breast-feeding; hypersensitivity to testosterone, estradiol, or their components; known or suspected breast cancer (except in select patients being treated for metastatic disease); known or suspected estrogen-dependent cancer; pregnancy; severe liver damage; undiagnosed abnormal genital bleeding

Interactions

DRUGS

testosterone and estradiol

corticosteroids: Increased therapeutic and toxic effects of corticosteroids

hepatotoxic drugs (such as isoniazid): Increased risk of hepatitis and hepatotoxicity

oral antidiabetics: Decreased or increased therapeutic effects of these drugs with risk of hyperglycemia or hypoglycemia

warfarin: Altered anticoagulant effect

testosterone
cyclosporine: Possibly increased risk of nephrotoxicity
estradiol, estrogens: Enhanced estrogenic effects
propranolol: Increased clearance of propranolol
estradiol
barbiturates, carbamazepine, hydantoins, rifabutin, rifampin: Possibly reduced activity of estradiol
FOODS
estradiol
grapefruit juice: Decreased metabolism and possibly increased adverse effects of estradiol
ACTIVITIES
testosterone and estradiol
smoking: Increased risk of pulmonary embolism, stroke, thrombophlebitis, and transient ischemic attack

Adverse Reactions

CNS: Chorea, dementia, depression, dizziness, headache, migraine headache, stroke
CV: Elevated cholesterol and triglyceride levels, MI, peripheral edema, pulmonary embolism, thromboembolism, thrombophlebitis
EENT: Diplopia, intolerance of contact lenses, steepening of corneal curvature, vision changes or loss
ENDO: Breast enlargement, pain, tenderness or tumors; gynecomastia; hypercalcemia, hyperglycemia, hypoglycemia, virilization
GI: Abnormal cramps or pain, aggravation of hepatic porphyria , anorexia, constipation, diarrhea, elevated liver function test results, gallbladder obstruction, hepatitis, increased appetite, jaundice, nausea, pancreatitis, vomiting
GU: Alteration in amount of cervical secretions, amenorrhea, breakthrough bleeding, cervical erosion, clear vaginal discharge, dysmenorrhea, increased libido, increased size of uterine leiomyomata, prolonged or heavy menstrual bleeding, vaginal candidiasis
SKIN: Acne, alopecia, chloasma, erythema multiforme or nodosum, hemorrhagic eruption, hirsutism, jaundice, melasma, oily skin, purpura, rash, seborrhea, urticaria
Other: Anaphylaxis, folic acid deficiency, hypercalcemia (in metastatic bone disease), local injection site irritation, weight gain or loss

Nursing Considerations

• For I.M. injection of testosterone and estradiol, before withdrawing drug from vial, warm and shake vial to redissolve any crystals that may have formed during storage at temperatures lower than recommended.

- Give testosterone and estradiol only by I.M. injection.
- **WARNING** Be aware that patients with breast cancer and bone metastasis may develop severe hypercalcemia because estradiol influences calcium and phosphorus metabolism. Watch for toxic effects of increased calcium absorption in patients predisposed to hypercalcemia or nephrolithiasis.
- **WARNING** Assess patient for possible contact lens intolerance or changes in vision or visual acuity because estrogens such as estradiol can cause keratoconus. Be prepared to stop drug immediately, as prescribed, if patient has sudden partial or complete loss of vision or sudden diplopia or migraine.
- Monitor PT for change in anticoagulant effect in patients receiving warfarin because estradiol increases production of clotting factors VII, VIII, IX, and X and promotes platelet aggregation.
- Watch for elevated liver function test results because testosterone and estradiol may worsen such conditions as acute intermittent or variegate hepatic porphyria.
- Closely monitor patient's blood pressure. Some patients may have a substantial increase in blood pressure as an indiosyncratic reaction to estrogens. Monitor patients who already have hypertension for increased blood pressure because estrogens may cause fluid retention. Also monitor patients with asthma, heart disease, migraines, renal disease, or seizure disorder for worsening of these conditions.
- Watch for peripheral edema or mild weight gain because estradiol can cause sodium and fluid retention.
- Monitor blood glucose level often in patients who have diabetes mellitus because estradiol may decrease insulin sensitivity and alter glucose tolerance.
- **WARNING** Expect to stop testosterone and estradiol therapy in any woman who develops signs or symptoms of cardiovascular disease, such as stroke, MI, pulmonary embolism, or venous thrombosis.
- Be aware that estrogens such as estradiol may worsen mood disorders, including depression. Monitor patient for depression, mood changes, anxiety, fatigue, dizziness, or insomnia.
- Assess skin for melasma (tan or brown patches), which may develop on forehead, cheeks, temples, and upper lip. These patches may persist after drug is stopped.
- Monitor thyroid function test results in patients with hypothy-

roidism because long-term use of estradiol may decrease effectiveness of thyroid therapy.

- Expect to stop testosterone and estradiol therapy several weeks before patient undergoes major surgery, as prescribed, because prolonged immobilization poses a risk of thromboembolism.

PATIENT TEACHING

- Before therapy starts, inform patient of risks involved in testosterone and estradiol therapy, such as increased risk of cardiovascular disease, breast or endometrial cancer, dementia, gallbladder disease, and vision abnormalities.
- Inform patient receiving testosterone and estradiol that she should have an annual physical examination, including a pelvic examination, to screen for adverse effects such as cervical dysplasia.
- Inform patient that a cyclic combination regimen of testosterone and estradiol may cause monthly withdrawal bleeding; tell her to notify prescriber if this occurs.
- Instruct patient to notify prescriber about masculine changes, such as a deepening of the voice or facial hair growth.
- Also tell patient to notify prescriber of any unusual signs and symptoms because combination drug can cause serious adverse effects.
- Advise patient taking testosterone and estradiol not to smoke because smoking increases the risk of deep vein thrombosis, heart attack, and other thromboemolic disorders.

Eye and Ear Drugs

bacitracin zinc and polymyxin B sulfate

AK-Poly Bac Ophthalmic, Polysporin

Class and Category

Chemical: Bacillus subtilis derivative (bacitracin), bacillus polymyxa derivative (polymyxin B)
Therapeutic: Antibiotics (bacitracin, polymyxin B)
Pregnancy category: C

Indications and Dosages

▶ *To treat superficial ocular infections of the conjunctiva or cornea caused by gram-negative bacilli, including virtually all strains of* Pseudomonas aeruginosa *and* Haemophilus influenzae *and most gram-positive bacilli and cocci, including hemolytic streptococci*

OPHTHALMIC OINTMENT

Adults. Applied as a thin ribbon into conjunctival sac every 3 to 4 hr for 7 to 10 days, depending on severity of infection.

Mechanism of Action

Bacitracin interferes with bacterial cell wall synthesis by binding with iso-prenyl pyrophosphate (a lipid-carrying molecule that transports substances out of bacterial cells to help build new cell walls), forming an unusable complex in bacterial cells. This weakens the bacterial cell wall and causes lysis and death. Bacitracin is considered a bacteriostatic and bactericidal drug.

Polymyxin B binds to cell membrane phospholipids in gram-negative bacteria, increasing the permeability of the cell membrane. Polymyxin B also acts as a cationic detergent altering the osmotic barrier of the membrane and causing essential intracellular metabolites to leak out. Both actions lead to bacterial cell death.

Contraindications

Hypersensitivity to bacitracin, polymyxin B or their components

Adverse Reactions
EENT: Delayed corneal healing, secondary ocular infection

Nursing Considerations
- Monitor patient for evidence of secondary ocular infection, such as signs and symptoms not alleviated within 7 to 10 days. If infection continues after bacitracin and polymyxin B therapy, expect to obtain culture and sensitivity samples, as ordered, and administer additional antibiotic therapy as indicated.

PATIENT TEACHING
- Stress importance of using bacitracin and polymyxin B ophthalmic ointment exactly as prescribed, even if feeling better.
- Instruct patient or caregiver how to use ophthalmic ointment.
- Remind patients and caregivers to wash their hands before and after using drug.
- Caution patient or caregiver not to touch tube to eye or to share drug to avoid contaminatubg drug or spreading infection.
- Tell patient to notify prescriber if symptoms do not improve or become worse by the end of the prescribed therapy time.

brimonidine tartrate 0.2% and timolol maleate 0.5%
Combigan

Class and Category
Chemical: Alpha$_2$ adrenergic receptor agonist (brimonidine), nonselective beta-adrenergic receptor inhibitor (timolol)
Therapeutic: Ocular antihypertensive
Pregnancy category: C

Indications and Dosages
▶ *To reduce elevated intraocular pressure (IOP) in patients with glaucoma or ocular hypertension who have not responded well to other therapies*
OPHTHALMIC SOLUTION
Adults. 1 drop instilled twice daily about 12 hours apart in affected eye or eyes.

Contraindications
Bronchial asthma; cardiogenic shock; hypersensitivity to brimonidine, timolol or their components; overt cardiac failure; second- or third-degree atrioventricular block; severe chronic obstructive pulmonary disease; sinus bradycardia

Mechanism of Action

Brimonidine activates alpha receptors in the eye to decrease vasoconstriction. This action reduces aqueous humor production and increases uveoscleral outflow, which lowers intraocular pressure.

Timolol reduces aqueous humor secretion by blocking beta1 and beta2 receptors in the ciliary processes of the eye. It also slightly increases the outflow of aqueous humor. These combined actions lower intraocular pressure.

Interactions

DRUGS

brimonidine

antihypertensives, digitalis: Possibly reduced pulse rate and blood pressure

CNS depressants: Possibly additive or potentiating effect

MAO inhibitors: Increased adverse reactions, such as hypotension

tricyclic antidepressants: Possibly blunted therapeutic effect of brimonidine in lowering intraocular pressure

timolol

beta blockers (oral): Possibly additive beta blocker effect

calcium antagonists: Possibly increased risk of atrioventricular conduction disturbances, left ventricular failure, and hypotension

calcium antagonists, digitalis: Possibly additive effects in prolonging atrioventricular conduction time

catecholamine-depleting agents, such as reserpine: Possibly additive effects and development of hypotension or marked bradycardia

clonidine: Increased risk of rebound hypertension when clonididne is discontinued

epinephrine (injectable): Possibly unresponsive therapeutic effect to epinephrine use in treatment of anaphylaxis

quinidine, selective serotonin reuptake inhibitors: Possibly decreased heart rate and depression

ACTIVITIES

brimonidine

alcohol use: Possibly additive or potentiating effect

Adverse Reactions

CNS: Asthenia, behavioral changes, cerebral ischemia, change in level of consciousness, depression, dizziness, diminished concentration, emotional lability, fatigue, headache, hypothermia, hypotonia, insomnia, nightmares, paresthesia, psychic disturbances, somnolence, stroke, syncope, vertigo, weakness

CV: Angina, arrhythmias, bradycardia, cardiac arrest and failure, chest pain, claudication, edema, heart block, hypertension, hypotension, palpitations, pulmonary edema, Raynaud's phenomenon, tachycardia, worsening of arterial insufficiency

EENT: Abnormal taste; allergic conjunctivitis; blepharitis; blurred vision; cataract; choroidal detachment following filtration surgery; conjunctival edema, folliculosis, hemorrhage, and hyperemia; conjunctivitis; corneal erosion; cystoid macular edema; decreased corneal sensitivity and visual acuity; diplopia; eye discharge, dryness, irritation, pain, and pruritus; eyelid edema, erythema, and pruritus; foreign body sensation; iritis; keratitis; keratoconjunctivitis sicca; laryngospasm; miosis; nasal dryness; ocular burning or stinging; oral dryness; pharyngitis; photophobia; pseudopemphigoid; ptosis; rhinitis; sinus infection; sinusitis; superficial punctate keratitis; tearing; tinnitus; visual disturbances; visual field defect; vitreous detachment and floaters

ENDO: Hyperglycemia, hypoglycemia, masked symptoms of hypoglycemia in patients with diabetes

GI: Dyspepsia, gastric pain, hepatomegaly, ischemic colitis, mesenteric arterial thrombosis, nausea, vomiting

GU: Decreased libido, difficulty urinating, impotence, Peyronie's disease, retroperitoneal fibrosis

HEME: Agranulocytosis, nonthrombocytopenic purpura, thrombocytopenic purpura

MS: Arthralgia, cold hands and feet

RESP: Apnea, bronchitis, bronchospasms, cough, crackles, diaphoresis, dyspnea, respiratory distress or failure

SKIN: Alopecia, increased pigmentation, irritation, pruritus, rash, urticaria, worsening of psoriasis

Other: Anaphylaxis, angioedema, flulike symptoms, hypersensitivity reaction, systemic lupus erythematosus, weight loss, worsening of myasthenia gravis

Nursing Considerations

- Administer brimonidine and timolol cautiously in patients with diabetes mellitus or hyperthyroidism because timolol may mask evidence of acute hypoglycemia and thyrotoxicosis.
- Monitor patient closely for systemic adverse reactions because the drug may be absorbed systemically and may cause severe reactions. If patient develops a systemic adverse reaction, withhold drug and notify prescriber. Be especially alert for serious respiratory reactions (including asthma), cardiac failure, and vascular insufficiency.

- **WARNING** Be aware that patients with a history of atopy or severe anaphylactic reactions may not respond to doses of epinephrine usually given for anaphylaxis.
- Inspect patient for adverse ocular reactions. Reactions such as conjunctivitis and lid reactions suggest an allergic response. If they occur, notify prescriber and expect drug to be discontinued.
- Monitor patients with myasthenia gravis closely because timolol may potentiate muscle weakness. Notify prescriber immediately.

PATIENT TEACHING

- Teach patient how to instill brimonidine and timolol eye drops, and remind patient to use drug exactly as prescribed.
- Instruct patient not to touch the bottle tip to his eyelids or any other surface and not to share the drug with anyone else to avoid contaminating drug and spreading eye infection.
- Advise patient to withhold brimonidine and timolol and notify prescriber if serious or unusual reactions occur or if he has indications of a localized allergic response such as conjunctivitis or eyelid abnormalities.
- If patient uses other topical eye drugs, tell him to space them at least 5 minutes apart.
- If patient has ocular surgery or develop a new ocular problem such as trauma or infection, tell him to cinslut with prescriber about continued use of drug.
- If patient wears soft contact lenses, tell him to remove them before using drug and to wait 15 minutes before reinserting them.
- Caution patient to avoid alcohol and hazardous activities during brimonidine and timolol therapy because drug can cause dizziness, decreased mental alertness, and fatigue.

chloroxylenol, pramoxine hydrochloride, and hydrocortisone

Cortane B Cortic, Cortic-ND, Oti-med, Otomar-HC, Tri-Otic

Class and Category

Chemical: Dimethylbenzene (chloroxylenol), morpholine derivative (pramoxine), glucocorticoid (hydrocortisone)
Therapeutic: Topical antiseptic, germicide and antifungal (chloroxylenol), local anesthetic (pramoxine), anti-inflammatory (hydrocortisone)
Pregnancy category: C

Indications and Dosages

▶ *To treat superficial infections of external auditory canal caused by sensitive gram-positive and gram-negative bacteria, such as* Streptococcus pneumoniae *and* Haemophilus influenzae

EARDROPS

Adults. Wick saturated with drug and inserted into ear canal followed by instillation of several drops as often as needed to keep wick moistened for 24 hr. Wick removed at end of 24 hr, followed by instillation of 5 drops, t.i.d. or q.i.d. Or, drops instilled without use of wick t.i.d. or q.i.d.

Children. Wick saturated with drug and inserted into ear canal followed by instillation of several drops as often as needed to keep wick moistened for 24 hr. Wick removed at end of 24 hr, followed by instillation of 3 drops, t.i.d. or q.i.d. Or, drops instilled without use of wick t.i.d. or q.i.d.

▶ *To prevent superficial infection of the external auditory canal in an unaffected ear when infection is present in the other ear*

EARDROPS

Adults. 5 drops instilled t.i.d.

Mechanism of Action

Chloroxylenol destroys bacterial microorganisms by breaking down the bacterial cell wall. This results in cell death.

Hydrocortisone binds to intracellular glucocorticoid receptors in the ear and suppresses the inflammatory and immune responses by:

- inhibiting neutrophil and monocyte accumulation at the inflammation site and suppressing their phagocytic and bactericidal activity
- stabilizing lysosomal membranes
- suppressing the antigen response of macrophages and helper T cells
- inhibiting the synthesis of cellular mediators of the inflammatory response, such as cytokines, interleukins, and prostaglandins.

Pramoxine provides temporary relief from auricular itching and pain by stabilizing the neuronal membrane of nerve endings with which it comes into contact.

Contraindications

Hypersensitivity to chloroxylenol, hydrocortisone, other steroids, pramoxine, or their components; ophthalmic use; perforated eardrums; presence of varicella or vaccinia infections

Adverse Reactions

EENT: Ear canal burning, dryness, irritation or pruritus

ENDO: Systemic hypercorticoidism (with prolonged use)
SKIN: Acneform eruptions, folliculitis, hypertrichosis, hypopigmentation

Nursing Considerations

• Before inserting wick into ear canal, carefully remove all cerumen and debris.
• Monitor patient closely for signs and symptoms of systemic hypercorticoidism if drug is given over prolonged period of time because hydrocortisone may be absorbed enough to increase glucocorticoid blood levels.
• Inspect ear canal for evidence of irritation or allergic response. If present, stop drug and notify prescriber.

PATIENT TEACHING

• Instruct patient or caregiver to use chloroxylenol, pramoxine, and hydrocortisone eardrops exactly as prescribed.
• Teach the patient or caregiver how to use the eardrops, if necessary.
• Tell patient to stop using drug and notify prescriber if allergic response or local irritation occurs.

ciprofloxacin hydrochloride 0.3% and dexamethasone 0.1%

Ciprodex

Class and Category

Chemical: Fluoroquinolone derivative (ciprofloxacin), glucocoritcoid (dexamethasone)
Therapeutic: Antibiotic (ciprofloxacin), anti-inflammatory (dexamethasone)
Pregnancy category: C

Indications and Dosages

▶ *To treat acute otitis media caused by* Staphylococcus aureus, Streptococcus pneumoniae, Haemophilus influenzae, Moraxella catarrhalis, *or* Pseudomonas aeruginosa
SUSPENSION

Children age 6 months and over with tympanostomy tube or tubes. 4 drops in affected ear or ears b.i.d. for 7 days.
▶ *To treat acute otitis externa caused by* S. aureus *or* P. aeruginosa
SUSPENSION

Adults and children age 6 months and over. 4 drops instilled into affected ear or ears b.i.d. for 7 days.

Mechanism of Action

Ciprofloxacin inhibits the enzyme DNA gyrase, which is responsible for the unwinding and supercoiling of bacterial DNA before it replicates. By inhibiting this enzyme, ciprofloxacin causes bacterial cells to die.

Dexamethasone binds to intracellular glucocorticoid receptors in external and media ear tissue and suppresses the inflammatory and immune responses by:

- inhibiting neutrophil and monocyte accumulation at the inflammation site and suppressing their phagocytic and bactericidal activity
- stabilizing lysosomal membranes
- suppressing the antigen response of macrophages and helper T cells
- inhibiting the synthesis of cellular mediators of the inflammatory response, such as cytokines, interleukins, and prostaglandins.

Contraindications

Hypersensitivity to ciprofloxacin, other quinolone antibiotics, dexamethasone, other corticosteroids, or their components; viral infection of external ear canal such as herpes simplex or varicella

Adverse Reactions

CNS: Irritability
EENT: Decreased hearing; ear congestion, discomfort, erythema, pain, precipitate, or pruritus; taste perversion; secondary ear infection
SKIN: Rash

Nursing Considerations

- Don't instill ciprofloxacin and dexamethasone otic suspension into eye or inject parenterally.
- If patient develops a rash, stop drug and notify prescriber.
- If there's no improvement in 1 week, obtain culture and sensitivity samples, as ordered, to rule out possibility of secondary infection, particularly fungal infection.

PATIENT TEACHING

- Instruct patient or caregiver to use ciprofloxacin and dexamethasone eardrops exactly as prescribed, for length of time prescribed, even if feeling better.
- Show patient or caregiver how to use eardrops, if needed. Tell him to lie down with the affected ear upward before instilling the drops. After instillation, tell him to stay in this position for 30 to 60 seconds so the drops can penetrate into the ear.

- Tell patient to shake suspension well before using and to warm bottle by holding it in his hands for 1 or 2 minutes to avoid dizziness that may occur with the instillation of a cold solution into the ear canal.
- Tell patient to protect bottle from light.
- Tell patient to stop using drug and notify prescriber if a rash occurs.
- Advise patient to contact prescriber if signs and symptoms worsen or do not improve in 7 days.

ciprofloxacin hydrochloride and hydrocortisone
Cipro HC Otic

Class and Category
Chemical: Fluoroquinolone derivative (ciprofloxacin), glucocoritcoid (hydrocortisone)
Therapeutic: Antibiotic (ciprofloxacin), anti-inflammatory (hydrocortisone)
Pregnancy category: C

Indications and Dosages
▶ *To treat otitis externa caused by* Pseudomonas aeruginosa, Staphylococcus aureus, *or* Proteus mirabilis
SUSPENSION
Adults and children age 1 and over. 3 drops instilled into affected ear b.i.d. for 7 days.

Mechanism of Action
Ciprofloxacin inhibits the enzyme DNA gyrase, which is responsible for the unwinding and supercoiling of bacterial DNA before it replicates. By inhibiting this enzyme, ciprofloxacin causes bacterial cells to die.

Hydrocortisone binds to intracellular glucocorticoid receptors in external ear tissue and suppresses the inflammatory and immune responses by:
- inhibiting neutrophil and monocyte accumulation at the inflammation site and suppressing their phagocytic and bactericidal activity
- stabilizing lysosomal membranes
- suppressing the antigen response of macrophages and helper T cells
- inhibiting the synthesis of cellular mediators of the inflammatory response, such as cytokines, interleukins, and prostaglandins.

Contraindications
Hypersensitivity to ciprofloxacin, other quinolone antibiotics, hydrocortisone, other corticosteroids, or their components; perforated tympanic; viral infection of external ear canal, such as herpes simplex or varicella

Adverse Reactions
CNS: Headache including migraine, hyperesthesia, paresthesia
EENT: Secondary fungal ear infection
RESP: Cough
SKIN: Alopecia, fungal dermatitis, pruritus, rash, urticaria

Nursing Considerations
- Don't instill ciprofloxacin and hydrocortisone otic suspension into eye or inject it parenterally.
- Stop drug and notify prescriber about evidence of hypersensitivity (rash, pruritus, urticaria), because systemic quinolones can cause anaphylaxis; ensure immediate emergency treatment.
- If there's no improvement in 1 week, obtain culture and sensitivity samples, as ordered, to rule out possibility of secondary infection, particularly fungal infection.

PATIENT TEACHING
- Instruct patient or caregiver to use eardrops exactly as prescribed, for length of time prescribed, even if feeling better.
- Show patient or caregiver how to instill eardrops, if needed. Tell him to lie down with the affected ear upward before instilling the drops. After instillation, tell him to stay in this position for 30 to 60 seconds so the drops can penetrate into the ear.
- Tell patient to shake suspension well before using and to warm bottle by holding it in his hands for 1 or 2 minutes to avoid possible dizziness from instilling a cold solution into the ear.
- Tell patient to protect bottle from light.
- Tell patient to stop using drug and notify prescriber if allergic response or local irritation occurs.
- Advise patient to contact prescriber if signs and symptoms worsen or do not improve in 7 days.

colistin sulfate, neomycin sulfate, thonzonium bromide, hydrocortisone acetate
Coly-Mycin S, Cortisporin-TC

Class and Category

Chemical: Polypeptide (colistin), aminoglucoside (neomycin), unclassified (thonzonium), glucocorticoid (hydrocortisone)
Therapeutic: Antibiotics (colistin, neomycin), surface activator (thonzonium), anti-inflammatory (hydrocortisone)
Pregnancy category: C

Indications and Dosages

▶ *To treat superficial bacterial infections of the external auditory canal or mastoidectomy and fenestration cavities caused by* Enterobacter aerogenes, Escherichia coli, Klebsiella pneumoniae, Pseudomonas aeruginosa, *or* Staphylococcus aureus

OTIC SUSPENSION

Adults. 5 drops instilled into the affected ear or ears t.i.d. or q.i.d. for 10 days. Or, cotton wick inserted into ear canal and then saturated with solution followed by repeat saturation every 4 hr with cotton wick replaced every 24 hr for 10 days.
Children. 4 drops instilled into the affected ear or ears t.i.d. or q.i.d. for 10 days. Or, cotton wick inserted into ear canal and then saturated with solution followed by repeat saturation every 4 hr with cotton wick replaced every 24 hr for 10 days.

Mechanism of Action

Colistin penetrates and disrupts bacterial cell membranes, killing the cells.

Neomycin competes with messenger RNA to bind with a receptor protein on the 30S ribosomal subunit of DNA in bacterial cells. This action causes abnormal, nonfunctioning proteins to form, which kills the cells.

Thonzonium is a surface-active agent that promotes tissue contact among other drugs in the mix. It does this by dispersing and penetrating cellular debris and exudate.

Hydrocortisone binds to intracellular glucocorticoid receptors in the ear and suppresses inflammatory and immune responses by:

- inhibiting neutrophil and monocyte accumulation at the inflammation site and suppressing their phagocytic and bactericidal activity
- stabilizing lysosomal membranes
- suppressing the antigen response of macrophages and helper T cells
- inhibiting the synthesis of cellular mediators of the inflammatory response, such as cytokines, interleukins, and prostaglandins.

These actions inhibit the edema, fibrin deposition, capillary dilation, leukocyte migration, capillary proliferation, fibroblast proliferation, deposition of collagen, and scar formation associated with inflammation.

Contraindications

Hypersensitivity to colistin, neomycin, thonzonium, hydrocortisone, or their components; presence of or suspected external auditory canal viral infection caused by herpes simplex virus or varicella zoster virus

Adverse Reactions

EENT: Ear canal edema, erythema, irritation or pruritus; hearing loss, ototoxicity
GU: Nephrotoxicity
SKIN: Rash

Nursing Considerations

- Use colistin, neomycin, thonzonium, and hydrocortisone cautiously in patients with perforated tympanic membrane.
- Don't administer otic suspension into the eye or inject it parenterally.
- Stop drug and notify prescriber if patient develops a rash or localized reactions, such as ear canal edema, erythema, irritation, or pruritus.
- Monitor patient's hearing. If hearing loss develops, stop drug immediately and notify prescriber.
- If there's no improvement in 1 week, obtain culture and sensitivity samples, as ordered, to rule out possibility of secondary infection, particularly fungal infection.

PATIENT TEACHING

- Instruct patient or caregiver to administer the eardrops exactly as prescribed, for the length of time prescribed, even if the patient feels better.
- Tell patient or caregiver to clean external auditory canal and dry with sterile cotton applicator before instilling drops.
- Tell patient to shake suspension well before using and to warm bottle by holding it in his hands for 1 or 2 minutes to avoid dizziness that may occur with the instillation of a cold solution.
- Show patient or caregiver how to administer eardrops, if necessary. Tell patient to lie down with the affected ear upward before instilling the drops. After instillation, tell him to keep this position for 5 minutes so the drops can penetrate into the ear.
- Caution patient not to touch tip of dropper to ear, fingers, or other surfaces to avoid contamination.
- Tell patient to stop using drug and notify prescriber if allergic response or local irritation occurs.
- Advise patient to contact prescriber if signs and symptoms worsen or do not improve in 7 days.

cyclopentolate hydrochloride 0.2% and phenylephrine 1%
Cyclomydril

Class and Category
Chemical: Tertiary amine (cyclopentolate), sympathomimetic amine (phenylephrine)
Therapeutic: Mydriatic and cycloplegic (cyclopentolate), vasoconstrictor (phenylephrine)
Pregnancy category: C

Indications and Dosages
▶ *To produce mydriasis and cycloplegia before diagnostic ophthalmic procedures are performed*
SOLUTION
Adults and children age 1 and over. 1 drop instilled in each eye, repeated every 5 to 10 minutes, as needed. *Maximum:* 3 drops per eye.

Mechanism of Action
Cyclopentolate blocks the action of acetylcholine, which causes relaxation of the cholinergically innervated sphincter muscle of the iris. Cyclopentolate also blocks cholinergic stimulation of the accommodative ciliary muscle of the lens, resulting in dilation of the pupil and paralysis of accommodation.

Phenylephrine stimulates alpha-adrenergic receptors and inhibits activity of the intracellular enzyme adenyl cyclase, which then inhibits production of cAMP. The inhibition of cAMP causes constriction of the arterioles. Phenylephrine also acts directly on the adrenergic receptors in the eye producing contraction of the dilator muscles.

Contraindications
Angle-closure glaucoma; hypersensitivity to cyclopentolate, phenylephrine or their components; severe coronary artery disease or hypertension; use within 14 days of MAO inhibitor therapy; ventricular tachycardia

Interactions
DRUGS
phenylephrine
MAO inhibitors: Increased and prolonged cardiac stimulation, increased vasopressor effect, increased risk of severe cardiovascular and cerebrovascular effects, hyperpyrexia, vomiting

Adverse Reactions

CNS: Confusion, dizziness, excitation, headache, insomnia, nervousness, paresthesia, psychotic reactions (children), restlessness, tremor, weakness

CV: Angina, bradycardia, hypertension, hypotension, palpitations, peripheral vasoconstriction that may lead to necrosis or gangrene, tachycardia, ventricular arrhythmias

EENT: Blocked lacrimal drainage system, blurred vision, dry mouth, increased intraocular pressure, superficial punctate epithelial ocular lesions, transient ocular burning, ocular erythema or irritation

GI: Constipation, nausea, vomiting

GU: Urinary hesitancy or retention

RESP: Dyspnea

SKIN: Photophobia

Other: Allergic reaction

Nursing Considerations

- Use cautiously in elderly patients and those predisposed to increased intraocular pressure. Prepare these patients to have a tonometric examination, as ordered, and an estimation of the depth of the angle of the posterior chamber before instillation of cyclopentolate and phenylephrine drops.
- After administering eyedrops, compress lacrimal sac for several minutes to minimize systemic absorption.
- Be aware that patients with heavily pigmented irises may need a higher dosage to obtain same effect.
- Monitor patient closely for systemic adverse reactions from absorption. Notify prescriber if present and be prepared to provide supportive treatment, as ordered, until drug has worn off (typically 24 hours but may persist for several days).
- Monitor children, patients with Down syndrome, and the elderly who are more susceptible to adverse reactions, especially psychotic reactions and excitation that often occur within 30 to 45 minutes following administration of drug.
- Observe patient for signs and symptoms of an allergic response such as persistent irritation and diffuse redness of eyes that occurs within minutes of administering drug.

PATIENT TEACHING

- Warn patient that cyclopentolate and phenylephrine may cause a transient burning sensation when instilled.
- Caution patient to avoid hazardous activities until the effects of the drug have worn off.

dorzolamide hydrochloride and timolol maleate
Cosopt

Class and Category
Chemical: Carbonic anhydrase inhibitor (dorzolamide), beta blocker (timolol)
Therapeutic: Ocular Antihypertensives (dorzolamide, timolol)
Pregnancy category: C

Indications and Dosages
▶ *To reduce elevated intraocular pressure in patients with open-angle glaucoma or ocular hypertension who have not responded well to beta blocker alone*
OPHTHALMIC SOLUTION
Adults and children age 2 and over. 1 drop instilled into affected eye or eyes b.i.d.

Mechanism of Action
Dorzolamide inhibits human carbonic anhydrase II. When carbonic anhydrase II is inhibited in the ciliary processes of the eye, aqueous humor secretion is decreased because the formation of bicarbonate ions is slowed reducing sodium and fluid transport. This results in lowered intraocular pressure.

Timolol reduces acqueous humor secretion by blocking $beta_1$ and $beta_2$ receptors in the ciliary processes of the eye. It also slightly increases the outflow of aqueous humor. These combined actions lowers intraocular pressure.

Contraindications
Bronchial asthma including history; cardiogenic shock; hypersensitivity to dorzolamide, timolol, or their components; overt cardiac failure; second or third degree atrioventricular block; severe chronic obstructive pulmonary disease; sinus bradycardia

Interactions
DRUGS
dorzolamide
carbonic anhydrase inhibitors: Possibly additive effects
salicylate (high-dose): Increased risk of salicylate toxicity
timolol
beta blockers (oral): Possibly additive beta blocker effect
calcium antagonists: Possibly increased risk of atrioventricular conduction disturbances, left ventricular failure, and hypotension

catecholamine-depleting agents, such as reserpine: Possibly additive effects and development of hypotension or marked bradycardia
clonidine: Increased risk of rebound hypertension when clonidine is discontinued
CYP2D6 inhibitors such as quinidine and SSRIs: Decreased heart rate or depression
digitalis and calcium antagonists: Possibly additive effects in prolonging atrioventricular conduction time
epinephrine (injectable): Possibly unresponsive therapeutic effect to epinephrine use in treatment of anaphylaxis
quinidine: Possibly decreased heart rate

Adverse Reactions

CNS: Asthenia, cerebral ischemia, dizziness, headache, insomnia, nightmares, psychic disturbances, somnolence, syncope
CV: Arrhythmia, bradycardia, cardiac failure, chest pain, claudication, edema, heart block, hypertension, hypotension, MI, palpitation, pulmonary edema, Raynaud's phenomenon, stroke, worsening of angina
EENT: Blepharitis; blurred or cloudy vision; bitter, sour, or unusual taste; conjunctival discharge, edema, hyperemia, infection, or pain; corneal erosion or staining; cortical lens opacity; decreased corneal sensitivity; diplopia; dry eyes; eyelid edema, erythema, exudates, pain, or scales; foreign body sensation; glaucomatous cupping; lens nucleus coloration or opacity; macular edema; ocular burning, discharge, pain, pruritus, stinging, or tearing; pharyngitis; post-subcapsular cataract; ptosis; sinusitis; superficial punctate keratitis; tinnitus; visual field defect; vitreous detachment
GI: Abdominal pain, anorexia, dyspepsia, nausea
ENDO: Hypoglycemia (in diabetics)
GU: Decreased libido, impotence, Peyronie's disease, UTI
MS: Back pain
RESP: Bronchitis, bronchospasm, cough, respiratory failure, upper respiratory tract infection
SKIN: Alopecia, pruritus, rash, urticaria, worsening of psoriasis
Other: Anaphylaxis, angioedema, flulike symptoms, systemic lupus erythematosus

Nursing Considerations

• Avoid giving dorzolamide and timolol to patients with severe renal impairment because drug is excreted mainly by the kidneys and its effects on such patients are unknown.

- Administer dorzolamide and timolol cautiously in patients with diabetes mellitus or hyperthyroidism because timolol, a beta blocker, may mask signs and symptoms of acute hypoglycemia and thyrotoxicosis. Also administer cautiously in patients with hepatic dysfunction because adverse effects of this drug aren't known in this patient population.
- Monitor patient closely for systemic adverse reactions because even though drug is administered topically, it's absorbed systemically and can cause severe reactions. If patient develops a systemic adverse reaction, withhold drug and notify prescriber
- Monitor patient closely for adverse reactions associated with sulfonamide use because dorzolamide is a sulfonamide. Although these reactions haven't occurred with dorzolamide and timolol, the possibility exists for serious reactions, such as Stevens-Johnson syndrome, toxic epidermal necrolysis, fulminant hepatic necrosis, agranulocytosis, aplastic anemia, and other blood dyscrasias. If these types of adverse reactions occur during therapy with dorzolamide and timolol, withhold drug and notify prescriber.
- Also monitor the patient closely for adverse reactions associated with beta blocker use because timolol is a beta blocker. Although these reactions haven't occurred with dorzolamide and timolol, the possibility exists. For example, beta-adrenergic blockade may precipitate heart failure or increase muscle weakness in patients with myasthenia gravis. If these types of adverse reactions occur during therpy with dorzolamide and timolol, withhold drug and notify prescriber.
- Inspect patient for ocular adverse reactions. If reactions such as conjunctivitis and lid reactions occur suggesting the presence of an allergic response, notify prescriber and expect dorzolamide and timolol to be discontinued.

PATIENT TEACHING
- Instruct patient to use dorzolamide and timolol solution exactly as prescribed.
- Show patient how to open the bottle for the first time by unscrewing the cap as indicated by the arrows on the top of the cap. Warn him that if cap is pulled directly up and away from the bottle, the dispenser will not work properly.
- Teach patient how to use eyedrops, if necessary.
- Instruct patient not to touch the bottle tip to his eyelids or any other surface and not to share the drug with anyone else to avoid contaminating drug and spreading eye infection.

- If patient wears soft contact lenses, tell him to remove them before instilling drug and to wait 15 minutes before reinserting them.
- Tell patient that if other topical eye drugs are used, he should space them at least 10 minutes apart.
- Advise patient to withhold dorzolamide and timolol and notify prescriber if serious or unusual reactions occur or if indications of a localized allergic response such as conjunctivitis or eyelid abnormalities appear while using the drug.
- Caution patient that if trauma or infection occurs in a treated eye, he should contact prescriber for advice on continuing therapy with dorzolamide and timolol.

fluorescein sodium 0.25% and benoxinate hydrochloride 0.4%

Flurate, Fluress

Class and Category

Chemical: Water-soluble dibasic acid xanthine dye (fluorescein), diethylamino ethyl amino butoxybenzoate (benoxinate)
Therapeutic: Disclosing agent (fluorescein), local anesthetic (benoxinate)
Pregnancy category: NR

Indications and Dosages

▶ *To prevent eye pain and identify corneal scratches or tears during ophthalmic procedures such as tonometry, gonioscopy, removal of corneal foreign bodies, and other short corneal or conjunctival procedures*

OPHTHALMIC SOLUTION

Adults. 1 or 2 drops instilled into affected eye or eyes as a one-time instillation before surgery.

▶ *To provide deep ophthalmic anesthesia*

OPTHTHALMIC SOLUTION

Adults. 2 drops instilled into affected eye or eyes at 90-second intervals for three instillations.

Contraindications

Hypersensitivity to fluorescein, benoxinate, or any of their components

Adverse Reactions

EENT: Acute, diffuse epithelial keratitis; corneal filaments; gray, ground, glass corneal appearance; iritis with descemetitis; sloughing of necrotic epithelium; temporary burning, conjunctival redness, or stinging

SKIN: Contact allergic dermatitis with drying and fissuring of fingertips

---

Mechanism of Action

Fluorescein reveals defects in the corneal epithelium because any break in the normally intact epithelium will allow the dye to penetrate, causing a green color at the site. Intact corneal epithelium resists fluorescein penetration and doesn't change color. Precorneal tear film will appear yellow or orange. If epithelial loss is extensive, topical fluorescein penetrates into the aqueous humor and can be seen biomicroscopically as a green flare.

Benoxinate stabilizes the neuronal membrane so the neuron is less permeable to ions. This prevents the initiation and transmission of nerve impulses, thereby preventing the perception of eye pain.

Nursing Considerations

- Use cautiously in patients with allergies, cardiac disease, or hyperthyroidism because they're at increased risk for adverse reactions to fluorescein and benoxinate.
- Monitor patient closely after instillation of fluorescein and benoxinate drops for adverse systemic effects because, although rare, toxicity causing central nervous system stimulation followed by depression may occur.
- Protect treated eyes from irritating chemicals and foreign bodies until effects of anesthesia have worn off.

PATIENT TEACHING

- Warn patient that instillation of fluorescein and benoxinate eyedrops may cause a transient burning or stinging.
- Caution patient not to touch or rub affected eye or eyes until the effects of anesthesia is gone.

fluorescein sodium 0.25% and proparacaine hydrochloride 0.5%

Fluoracaine

Class and Category

Chemical: Water-soluble dibasic acid xanthine dye (fluorescein), diethylamino ethyl ester (proparacaine)

Therapeutic: Disclosing agent (fluorescein), local anesthetic (proparacaine)
Pregnancy category: NR

Indications and Dosages

▶ *To prevent or relieve eye pain and identify corneal scratches or tears during ophthalmic procedures such as tonometry, gonioscopy, removal of corneal foreign bodies, and other short corneal or conjunctival procedures*

OPHTHALMIC SOLUTION

Adults. 1 or 2 drops instilled in affected eye or eyes as a one-time instillation before surgery.

▶ *To provide deep ophthalmic anesthesia*

OPTHTHALMIC SOLUTION

Adults. 1 drop instilled in affected eye or eyes every 5 to 10 minutes for 5 to 7 doses.

Mechanism of Action

Fluorescein reveals defects in the corneal epithelium because any break in the normally intact corneal epithelium will allow the dye to penetrate, causing a green color at the site. Intact corneal epithelium resists fluorescein penetration and doesn't change color. Precorneal tear film will appear yellow or orange. If epithelial loss is extensive, topical fluorescein penetrates into the aqueous humor and can be seen biomicroscopically as a green flare.

Proparacaine stabilizes the neuronal membrane so the neuron is less permeable to ions. This prevents the initiation and transmission of nerve impulses, thereby preventing the perception of eye pain.

Contraindications

Hypersensitivity to fluorescein, proparacaine, or their components

Adverse Reactions

EENT: Acute, diffuse epithelial keratitis; corneal filaments; gray, ground, glass corneal appearance; iritis with descemetitis; sloughing of necrotic epithelium; temporary burning, conjunctival redness, or stinging

SKIN: Contact allergic dermatitis with drying and fissuring of fingertips

Nursing Considerations

• Use cautiously in patients with allergies, cardiac disease, or hyperthyroidism because they're at increased risk for adverse reactions to fluorescein and proparacaine.

- Monitor patient closely for adverse systemic effects after instillation of fluorescein and proparacaine drops because, although rare, toxicity causing CNS stimulation followed by depression may occur.
- Apply an eye patch, as ordered, following instillation of fluoresceine and proparacaine eyedrops, and protect treated eye from irritating chemicals and foreign bodies until effects of anesthesia have worn off.

PATIENT TEACHING

- Warn patient that fluorescein and proparacaine eyedrops may cause burning or stinging several hours after instillation.
- Caution patient not to touch or rub his eye and to leave the eye patch on, if present, until the effects of anesthesia is gone.

fluorometholone 0.1% and sulfacetamide sodium 10%
FML-S

Class and Category
Chemical: Fluorinated glucocorticoid (fluorometholone), sulfonamide (sulfacetamide sodium)
Therapeutic: Anti-inflammatory (fluorometholone), antibiotic (sulfacetamide sodium)
Pregnancy category: C

Indications and Dosages
▶ *To treat inflammatory ocular conditions of the palpebral and bulbar conjunctiva, cornea, and anterior segment of the globe; chronic anterior uveitis and corneal injury from chemical, radiation, or thermal burns or penetration of foreign bodies when superficial ocular infection is present (or risk is high) caused by* Enterobacter *species,* Escherichia coli, Klebsiella species, Staphylococcus aureus, Streptococcus pneumoniae, *and* Streptococcus viridans *group*
OPHTHALMIC SUSPENSION
Adults. 1 drop instilled into conjunctival sac q.i.d.

Incompatibilities
Silver preparations are incompatible with sulfonamide preparations such as sulfacetamide

Contraindications
Fungal diseases affecting ocular structures; hypersensitivity to fluorometholone, other corticosteroids, sulfacetamide sodium,

other sulfonamides, or their components; mycobacterial infection of the eye; viral diseases of the cornea and conjunctiva, including epithelial herpes simplex keratitis, vaccinia, and varicella

---

Mechanism of Action
Fluorometholone binds to intracellular glucocorticoid receptors in the eye and suppresses inflammatory and immune responses by:
- inhibiting neutrophil and monocyte accumulation at the inflammation site and suppressing their phagocytic and bactericidal activity
- stabilizing lysosomal membranes
- suppressing the antigen response of macrophages and helper T cells
- inhibiting the synthesis of cellular mediators of the inflammatory response, such as cytokines, interleukins, and prostaglandins.

These actions inhibit the edema, fibrin deposition, capillary dilation, leukocyte migration, capillary proliferation, fibroblast proliferation, deposition of collagen and scar formation associated with inflammation.

Sulfacetamide sodium interferes with utilization of para-aminobenzoic acid (PABA) thus inhibiting biosynthesis of folic acid, which is essential for growth of susceptible organisms.

Interactions
DRUGS
fluorometholone
corticosteroids: Increased risk of cross-sensitivity
sulfacetamide sodium
local anesthetics: Possibly antagonized effects of sulfacetamide
sulfonamides: Increased risk of cross-sensitivity

Adverse Reactions
EENT: Acute anterior uveitis; conjunctivitis; conjunctival hyperemia, corneal ulcers or secondary fungal infections; elevated intraocular pressure; eye irritation; glaucoma; keratitis; loss of accommodation; mydriasis; optic nerve damage; perforation of the globe; posterior subcapsular cataract formation; ptosis; secondary ocular bacterial infections
ENDO: Systemic hypercorticoidism (with prolonged use)
GI: Fulminant hepatic necrosis
HEME: Agranulocytosis, aplastic anemia, blood dyscrasias
SKIN: Stevens-Johnson syndrome, toxic epidermal necrolysis
Other: Allergic reactions, delayed wound healing

Nursing Considerations

- Use fluorometholone and sulfacetamide sodium with great caution in the patient with a history of herpes simplex because use of an ocular steroid preparation such as fluorometholone may exacerbate the severity of many ocular viral infections.
- Use cautiously in patients with glaucoma because fluorometholone increase intraocular pressure. Be prepared to check intraocular pressure often in patients with glaucoma or routinely if drug is used for 10 days or longer in patients without glaucoma.
- Obtain eyelid culture and sensitivity tests as ordered before giving first dose, if infection is already present. Expect to begin drug therapy before test results are known.
- Be aware that the use of topical corticosteroids like fluorometholone in the presence of thin corneal or scleral tissue may lead to perforation.
- Assess patient's vision, and inspect eyes for abnormalities because prolonged use of ophthalmic corticosteroids may cause glaucoma, damage to the optic nerve, defects in visual acuity and fields of vision, and posterior subcapsular cataract formation. Prolonged use also increases risk of secondary ocular infections.
- Question patient about eye discomfort because fluorometholone may mask signs and symptoms of acute purulent eye infections.
- **WARNING** Don't inject fluorometholone and sulfacetamide sodium suspension into the eye.
- Monitor patient for serious adverse reactions including allergic response. If suspected, notify prescriber, withhold fluorometholone and sulfacetamide sodium, and be prepared to administer appropriate supportive treatment.
- If patient has persistent corneal ulceration and has used fluorometholone and sulfacetamide sodium suspension long-term, obtain fungal cultures because fungal corneal infections are particularly likely with long-term local corticosteroid use.

PATIENT TEACHING

- Instruct patient to use fluorometholone and sulfacetamide sodium suspension exactly as prescribed.
- Teach patient how to use eyedrops, if necessary.
- Tell patient to shake the bottle well before using.
- Caution patient to discard the suspension if it appears dark brown and obtain a new suspension.

- Advise patient to discontinue using fluorometholone and sulfacetamide sodium and notify prescriber if signs and symptoms such as ocular pain or inflammation do not improve after two days or becomes worse.
- Instruct patient to take care not to touch the bottle tip to eyelids or any other surface to avoid contamination.
- Inform patient that no one else should use the drug because infection may be spread in this manner.

neomycin sulfate, polymyxin B sulfate, and bacitracin zinc

AK-Spore, Neocidin, Neosporin Ointment, Neotal, Ocu-Spor-B, Ocusporin, Ocutricin, Spectro-Sporin, Triple Antibiotic

Class and Category

Chemical: Aminoglucoside (neomycin), bacillus polymyxa derivative (polymyxin B), bacillus subtilis derivative (bacitracin)
Therapeutic: Antibiotics (neomycin, polymyxin B, bacitracin
Pregnancy category: C

Indications and Dosages

▶ *To treat superficial bacterial infections of the external eye and surrounding area, such as conjunctivitis, keratitis, keratoconjunctivitis, blepharitis, or blepharoconjunctivitis caused by* Enterobacter *species,* Escherichia coli, Haemophilus influenzae, Klebsiella species, Neisseria *species,* Pseudomonas aeruginosa, Staphylococcus aureus, *and streptococci, including* Streptococcus pneumoniae

OPHTHALMIC OINTMENT

Adults. Thin ribbon (about ½ inch) applied into conjunctival sac of affected eye or eyes every 3 or 4 hr for 7 to 10 days

Contraindications

Hypersensitivity to neomycin, polymyxin B, bacitracin, or their components

Adverse Reactions

EENT: Conjunctival or eyelid edema, erythema, or pruritus; delayed eye wound healing; elevation of intraocular pressure; glaucoma; local eye irritation, optic nerve damage; posterior subcapsular cataract formation; secondary eye infection
GU: Nephrotoxicity
SKIN: Pruritus, rash, urticaria
Other: Allergic reactions, anaphylaxis

Mechanism of Action

Neomycin competes with messenger RNA to bind with a receptor protein on the 30S ribosomal subunit of DNA in bacterial cells. This action causes abnormal, nonfunctioning proteins to form, which kills the cells.

Polymyxin B binds to cell membrane phospholipids in gram-negative bacteria, increasing cell membrane permeability. Polymyxin B also acts as a cationic detergent, altering the osmotic barrier of the membrane and causing essential intracellular metabolites to leak. Both actions lead to cell death.

Bacitracin interferes with bacterial cell wall synthesis by binding with isoprenyl pyrophosphate (a lipid-carrying molecule that transports substances out of bacterial cells to help build new cell walls), forming an unusable complex in bacterial cells. This weakens cell walls and causes cell lysis and death. Bacitracin is bacteriostatic and bactericidal.

Nursing Considerations

- Obtain eyelid culture and sensitivity tests as ordered before giving first dose, if infection is already present. Expect to begin drug therapy before test results are known.
- Monitor patient for signs of hypersensitivity such as conjunctiva and eyelid edema, erythema, or prurituis and notify prescriber, if present, and expect to discontinue drug. Be aware that failure to heal may also be a sensitization reaction.
- Monitor patient for development of secondary ocular infections because overgrowth of nonsusceptible organisms, including fungi, may occur.
- Notify prescriber if patient's eye discomfort or inflammation does not improve or purulent discharge becomes worse.

PATIENT TEACHING

- Instruct patient to use neomycin, polymyxin B, and bacitracin ointment exactly as prescribed, even when feeling better.
- Teach patient how to self-administer eye ointment, if appropriate.
- Advise patient to stop using neomycin, polymyxin B, and bacitracin and notify prescriber if ocular pain and inflammation don't improve, if they become worse, or if an allergic reaction occurs.
- Instruct patient to take care not to touch the tube tip to eyelids or any other surface to avoid contamination.
- Inform patient that no one else should use the drug because infection may be spread in this manner.

neomycin sulfate, polymyxin B sulfate, bacitracin zinc, and hydrocortisone

AK-Spore HC, Cortisporin

Class and Category

Chemical: Aminoglucoside (neomycin), bacillus polymyxa derivative (polymyxin B), bacillus subtilis derivative (bacitracin), synthetic glucocorticoid (hydrocortisone)

Therapeutic: Antibiotics (neomycin, polymyxin B, bacitracin), antiinflammatory (hydrocortisone)

Pregnancy category: C

Indications and Dosages

▶ *To treat inflammatory ocular conditions of the palpebral and bulbar conjunctiva, cornea, and anterior segment of the globe; chronic anterior uveitis and corneal injury from chemical, radiation, or thermal burns or penetration of foreign bodies when superficial ocular infection is present (or risk is high) caused by* Enterobacter *species,* Escherichia coli, Haemophilus influenzae, Klebsiella *species,* Neisseria *species,* Pseudomonas aeruginosa, Staphylococcus aureus, *and streptococci, including* Streptococcus pneumoniae

OPHTHALMIC OINTMENT

Adults. Thin ribbon (about ½ inch) applied into conjunctival sac of affected eye or eyes every 3 or 4 hr.

Contraindications

Fungal diseases affecting ocular structures; hypersensitivity to neomycin, polymyxin B, bacitracin, hydrocortisone, other corticosteroids, or their components; mycobacterial infection of the eye; viral diseases of the cornea and conjunctiva, including epithelial herpes simplex keratitis, vaccinia, and varicella

Adverse Reactions

EENT: Conjunctival or eyelid edema, erythema, or pruritus; delayed eye wound healing; elevation of intraocular pressure; glaucoma; local eye irritation; optic nerve damage; posterior subcapsular cataract formation; secondary eye infection

GU: Nephrotoxicity

SKIN: Pruritus, rash, urticaria

Other: Allergic reactions, anaphylaxis

Mechanism of Action

Neomycin competes with messenger RNA to bind with a receptor protein on the 30S ribosomal subunit of DNA in bacterial cells. This action causes abnormal, nonfunctioning proteins to form, which kills the cells.

Polymyxin B binds to cell membrane phospholipids in gram-negative bacteria, increasing cell membrane permeability. Polymyxin B also acts as a cationic detergent, altering the osmotic barrier of the membrane and causing essential intracellular metabolites to leak. Both actions lead to cell death.

Bacitracin interferes with bacterial cell wall synthesis by binding with isoprenyl pyrophosphate (a lipid-carrying molecule that transports substances out of bacterial cells to help build new cell walls), forming an unusable complex in bacterial cells. This weakens cell walls and causes lysis and death. Bacitracin is bacteriostatic and bactericidal.

Hydrocortisone binds to intracellular glucocorticoid receptors in the eye and suppresses inflammatory and immune responses by:

- inhibiting neutrophil and monocyte accumulation at the inflammation site and suppressing their phagocytic and bactericidal activity
- stabilizing lysosomal membranes
- suppressing the antigen response of macrophages and helper T cells
- inhibiting the synthesis of cellular mediators of the inflammatory response, such as cytokines, interleukins, and prostaglandins.

These actions inhibit the edema, fibrin deposition, capillary dilation, leukocyte migration, capillary proliferation, fibroblast proliferation, deposition of collagen and scar formation associated with inflammation.

Nursing Considerations

- Use neomycin, polymyxin B, bacitracin, and hydrocortisone with great caution if patient has a history of herpes simplex because ocular steroids such as hydrocortisone may worsen the severity of many ocular viral infections.
- Use cautiously in patients with glaucoma because hydrocortisone may increase intraocular pressure. Be prepared to check intraocular pressure often in patients with glaucoma or routinely if drug is used for 10 days or longer in patients without glaucoma.
- Obtain eyelid culture and sensitivity tests as ordered before giving first dose, if infection is already present. Expect to begin drug therapy before test results are known.

- Be aware that the use of topical corticosteroids like hydrocortisone in the presence of thin corneal or scleral tissue may lead to perforation.
- Assess patient's vision and inspect eyes for abnormalities because prolonged use of ophthalmic corticosteroids may cause glaucoma, with damage to the optic nerve, defects in visual acuity and fields of vision, and forkation of posterior subcapsular cataracts. Prolonged use also increases risk of secondary ocular infections.
- Notify prescriber if patient's eye discomfort or inflammation does not improve within 48 hours or worsens.
- Question patient regarding the presence of eye discomfort because hydrocortisone may mask signs and symptoms of acute purulent infections.
- **WARNING** Do not inject neomycin, polymyxin B, bacitracin, and hydrocortisone solution into the eye or introduce it directly into the anterior chamber of the eye.
- If patient has persistent corneal ulceration and has used suspension long-term, obtain fungal cultures. Fungal corneal infections are particularly likely with long-term local corticosteroid use.

PATIENT TEACHING
- Instruct patient to administer neomycin, polymyxin B, bacitracin, and hydrocortisone ointment exactly as prescribed, even when feeling better.
- Teach patient how to use eye ointment, if appropriate.
- Advise patient to stop using neomycin, polymyxin B, bacitracin, and hydrocortisone and notify prescriber if ocular pain or inflammation don't improve within 48 hours, become worse, or patient has an allergic reaction.
- Instruct patient to take care not to touch the tube tip to eyelids or any other surface to avoid contamination.
- Inform patient that no one else should use the drug because infection may be spread in this manner.

neomycin sulfate, polymyxin B sulfate, and dexamethasone sodium phosphate
AK-Trol, Dexacine, Maxitrol

Class and Category
Chemical: Aminoglucoside (neomycin), bacillus polymyxa derivative (polymyxin B), synthetic glucocorticoid (dexamethasone)

Therapeutic: Antibiotics (neomycin, polymyxin B), anti-inflammatory (dexamethasone)
Pregnancy category: C

Indications and Dosages

▶ *To treat inflammatory ocular conditions of the palpebral and bulbar conjunctiva, cornea, and anterior segment of the globe; chronic anterior uveitis and corneal injury from chemical, radiation, or thermal burns or penetration of foreign bodies when superficial ocular infection is present (or risk is high) caused by* Enterobacter *species,* Escherichia coli, Haemophilus influenzae, Klebsiella *species,* Neisseria *species,* Pseudomonas aeruginosa, *and* Staphylococcus aureus

OPHTHALMIC SUSPENSION

Adults. If severe, 1 or 2 drops instilled into conjuctival sac of affected eyes hourly and then tapered to discontinuation as infection and inflammation subsides. If mild, 1 or 2 drops instilled into conjunctival sac of affected eyes 4 to 6 times daily and then tapered to discontinuation as infection and inflammation subsides.

OPTHALMIC OINTMENT

Adults. Applied as a thin ribbon (about ½ inch) into conjunctival sac t.i.d. or q.i.d.

Mechanism of Action

Neomycin competes with messenger RNA to bind with a receptor protein on the 30S ribosomal subunit of DNA in bacterial cells. This action causes abnormal, nonfunctioning proteins to form, which kills the cells.

Polymyxin B binds to cell membrane phospholipids in gram-negative bacteria, increasing the permeability of the cell membranes. Polymyxin B also acts as a cationic detergent, altering the osmotic barrier of the membrane and causing essential intracellular metabolites to leak. Both actions lead to cell death.

Dexamethasone binds to intracellular glucocorticoid receptors in the eye and suppresses inflammatory and immune responses by:

• inhibiting neutrophil and monocyte accumulation at the inflammation site and suppressing their phagocytic and bactericidal activity
• stabilizing lysosomal membranes
• suppressing the antigen response of macrophages and helper T cells
• inhibiting the synthesis of cellular mediators of the inflammatory response, such as cytokines, interleukins, and prostaglandins.

These actions inhibit the edema, fibrin deposition, capillary dilation, leukocyte migration, capillary proliferation, fibroblast proliferation, deposition of collagen and scar formation associated with inflammation.

Contraindications

Fungal diseases affecting ocular structures; hypersensitivity to neomycin, polymyxin B, dexamethasone, other corticosteroids, or their components; mycobacterial infection of the eye; viral diseases of the cornea and conjunctiva, including epithelial herpes simplex keratitis, vaccinia, and varicella

Adverse Reactions

EENT: Delayed eye wound healing, elevation of intraocular pressure, glaucoma, optic nerve damage, posterior subcapsular cataract formation, secondary eye infection
SKIN: Pruritus, rash, urticaria
Other: Allergic reactions

Nursing Considerations

- Use neomycin, polymyxin B, and dexamethasone with great caution in the patient with a history of herpes simplex because use of an ocular steroid preparation such as dexamethasone may exacerbate the severity of many ocular viral infections.
- Use cautiously in patients with glaucoma because dexamethasone may increase intraocular pressure. Be prepared to check intraocular pressure often in patients with glaucoma or routinely if drug is used for 10 days or longer in patients without glaucoma.
- Obtain eyelid culture and sensitivity tests as ordered before giving first dose, if infection is already present. Expect to begin drug therapy before test results are known.
- Be aware that topical corticosteroids such as dexamethasone may lead to perforation if the patient has thin corneal or scleral tissue.
- Assess patient's vision and inspect eyes for abnormalities as prolonged use of ophthalmic corticosteroids may cause glaucoma, damage to the optic nerve, defects in visual acuity and fields of vision, and posterior subcapsular cataract formation. Prolonged use also increases risk of secondary ocular infections.
- Notify prescriber if patient's eye discomfort or inflammation worsens.
- Question patient about eye discomfort because dexamethasone may mask signs and symptoms of acute purulent eye infections.
- **WARNING** Don't inject neomycin, polymyxin B, and dexamethasone solution into the eye.
- If patient has persistent corneal ulceration and has used neomycin, polymyxin B, and dexamethasone suspension longterm, obtain fungal cultures because fungal corneal infections are particularly likely with long-term local corticosteroid use.

PATIENT TEACHING
• Instruct patient to use neomycin, polymyxin B and dexamethasone solution exactly as prescribed.
• If needed, teach patient how to use eyedrops or ointment.
• To use suspension form, tell patient to shake the container first.
• Advise patient to discontinue using neomycin, polymyxin B, and dexamethasone and notify prescriber if signs and symptoms such as ocular pain or inflammation do not improve after 2 days or becomes worse or if an allergic reaction occurs.
• Instruct patient to take care not to touch the bottle tip or tube tip to eyelids or any other surface to avoid contamination.
• Inform patient that no one else should use the drug because infection may be spread in this manner.

neomycin, polymyxin B sulfate, and gramicidin

Neosporin Solution

Class and Category

Chemical: Aminoglucoside (neomycin), bacillus polymyxa derivative (polymyxin B), and bacillus brevis derivative (gramicidin)
Therapeutic: Antibiotics (neomycin, polymyxin B, gramicidin)
Pregnancy category: C

Indications and Dosages

▶ *To treat superficial infections of the external eye and surrounding area, such as conjunctivitis, keratitis, keratoconjunctivitis, blepharitis, and blepharoconjunctivitis caused by susceptible bacteria*
OPHTHALMIC SOLUTION
Adults. For severe infections, 2 drops in affected eye or eyes every 1 hr initially. With positive response, taper to every 2 to 4 hr for total of 7 to 10 days. For mild to moderate infection, 1 or 2 drops in affected eye or eyes every 2 to 4 hr for 7 to 10 days.

Contraindications

Hypersensitivity to neomycin, polymyxin B, gramicidin, or their components

Adverse Reactions

EENT: Conjunctival or eyelid edema, erythema, or pruritus; delayed healing; local eye irritation; secondary eye infection
SKIN: Rash
Other: Anaphylaxis

Mechanism of Action

Neomycin competes with messenger RNA to bind with a receptor protein on the 30S ribosomal subunit of DNA in bacterial cells. This action causes abnormal, nonfunctioning proteins to form, which kills the cells.

Polymyxin B binds to cell membrane phospholipids in gram-negative bacteria, increasing cell membrane permeability. Polymyxin B also acts as a cationic detergent, altering the osmotic barrier of the membrane and causing essential intracellular metabolites to leak. Both actions lead to cell death.

Gramicidin increases bacterial cell membrane permeability to inorganic cations by forming a network of channels through the normal lipid bilayer of the membrane. This results in the death of susceptible gram-positive bacteria.

Nursing Considerations

- **WARNING** Be aware that neomycin, polymyxin B, and gramicidin should never be introduced into the anterior chamber of the eye or injected subconjunctivally.
- Monitor patient for evidence of allergic reaction, such as rash, localized conjunctival or eyelid edema, erythema, or pruritus. If present, withhold drug and notify prescriber.
- Know that if an allergic reaction occurs, patient may also be allergic to gentamicin, kanamycin, paromomycin, and streptomycin because of cross-sensitivity.
- Monitor patient for evidence of secondary ocular infection such as signs and symptoms not alleviated within 7 to 10 days. If infection is not eradicated at completion of neomycin, polymyxin B, and gramicidin therapy, expect to obtain culture and sensitivity samples, as ordered, and administer additional antibiotic therapy as indicated.

PATIENT TEACHING

- Stress importance of administering neomycin, polymyxin B, and gramicidin ophthalmic solution exactly as prescribed, even when feeling better.
- Instruct patient or caregiver how to use eyedrops, if necessary.
- Remind patients and caregivers to wash their hands before and after administering drug.
- Caution patient or caregiver not to touch eye with tip of dropper or to share the drug with anyone else because of risk of contamination or spread of infection.
- Tell patient to notify prescriber if symptoms do not improve or become worse by the end of the prescribed therapy time.

neomycin sulfate, polymyxin B sulfate, and hydrocortisone

Antibiotic Ear Suspension, Octicair, Pediotic

Class and Category

Chemical: Aminoglucoside (neomycin), bacillus polymyxa derivative (polymyxin B),synthetic glucocorticoid (hydrocortisone)
Therapeutic: Antibiotics (neomycin, polymyxin B), anti-inflammatory (hydrocortisone)
Pregnancy category: C

Indications and Dosages

▶ *To treat inflammatory ocular conditions of the palpebral and bulbar conjunctiva, cornea, and anterior segment of the globe; chronic anterior uveitis and corneal injury from chemical, radiation, or thermal burns or penetration of foreign bodies when superficial ocular infection is present (or risk is high) from bacteria caused by* Enterobacter *species,* Escherichia coli, Haemophilus influenzae, Klebsiella species, Neisseria *species,* Pseudomonas aeruginosa, *and* Staphylococcus aureus

OPHTHALMIC SUSPENSION

Adults. 1 or 2 drops instilled into the affected eye or eyes every 3 or 4 hr.

▶ *To treat superficial bacterial infections of the external auditory canal or mastoidectomy and fenestration cavities caused by* Enterobacter *species,* Escherichia coli, Haemophilus influenzae, Klebsiella *species,* Neisseria *species,* Pseudomonas aeruginosa, *and* Staphylococcus aureus

OTIC SOLUTION

Adults. 4 drops instilled into the affected ear or ears t.i.d. or q.i.d. for 10 days. Or, cotton wick inserted into ear canal and then saturated with solution followed by repeat saturation every 4 hr, with cotton wick replaced every 24 hr for 10 days.
Children age 2 and over. 3 drops instilled into the affected ear or ears t.i.d. or q.i.d. for 10 days. Or, cotton wick inserted into ear canal and then saturated with solution followed by repeat saturation every 4 hr, with cotton wick replaced every 24 hr for 10 days.

Contraindications

Fungal diseases affecting ocular or auricular structures; hypersensitivity to neomycin, polymyxin B, hydrocortisone, other corticosteroids, or their components; mycobacterial infection of the eye or ear; viral diseases of the cornea, conjunctiva and ear, including epithelial herpes simplex keratitis, vaccinia, and varicella

---

Mechanism of Action

Neomycin competes with messenger RNA to bind with a receptor protein on the 30S ribosomal subunit of DNA in bacterial cells. This action causes abnormal, nonfunctioning proteins to form, which kills the cells.

Polymyxin B binds to cell membrane phospholipids in gram-negative bacteria, increasing cell membrane permeability. Polymyxin B also acts as a cationic detergent, altering the osmotic barrier of the membrane and causing essential intracellular metabolites to leak. Both actions lead to cell death.

Hydrocortisone binds to intracellular glucocorticoid receptors in the eye and ear and suppresses inflammatory and immune responses by:

- inhibiting neutrophil and monocyte accumulation at the inflammation site and suppressing their phagocytic and bactericidal activity
- stabilizing lysosomal membranes
- suppressing the antigen response of macrophages and helper T cells
- inhibiting the synthesis of cellular mediators of the inflammatory response, such as cytokines, interleukins, and prostaglandins.

These actions inhibit the edema, fibrin deposition, capillary dilation, leukocyte migration, capillary proliferation, fibroblast proliferation, deposition of collagen and scar formation associated with inflammation.

Adverse Reactions

EENT: Burning or stinging in ear (if drug has gained access to middle ear); conjunctival, eyelid or ear canal edema, erythema, or pruritus; delayed eye or ear wound healing; elevation of intraocular pressure; glaucoma; hearing loss; optic nerve damage; ototoxicity; posterior subcapsular cataract formation; secondary eye infection

GU: Nephrotoxicity

SKIN: Pruritus, rash, urticaria

Other: Allergic reactions

Nursing Considerations

- Use neomycin, polymyxin B, and hydrocortisone with great caution in patients with a history of herpes simplex because ocular or otic steroids such as hydrocortisone may worsen the severity of many ocular or otic viral infections.
- Use cautiously in patients with glaucoma because hydrocortisone may increase intraocular pressure. Monitor intraocular

pressure often in patients with glaucoma and routinely if drug is used for 10 days or longer in patients without glaucoma.
- If infection is already present, obtain eyelid or ear culture and sensitivity tests as ordered before giving first dose. Expect to begin drug therapy before test results are known.
- Be aware that topical corticosteroids like hydrocortisone may lead to perforation if patient has thin corneal or scleral tissue.
- Assess patient's vision and inspect eyes for abnormalities because prolonged use of ophthalmic corticosteroids may cause glaucoma, damage to the optic nerve, defects in visual acuity and fields of vision, and posterior subcapsular cataract formation. Prolonged use also increases the risk of secondary ocular or otic infections.
- Notify prescriber if patient's discomfort or inflammation worsens.
- Question patient about eye or ear discomfort because hydrocortisone may mask evidence of acute purulent infections.
- **WARNING** Don't inject neomycin, polymyxin B, and hydrocortisone solution into the eye.
- If patient has persistent corneal ulceration and has used neomycin, polymyxin B, and hydrocortisone suspension long-term, obtain fungal cultures because fungal corneal infections are particularly likely with long-term local corticosteroid use.

PATIENT TEACHING
- Instruct patient to use neomycin, polymyxin B, and hydrocortisone solution exactly as prescribed, even when feeling better.
- Teach patient how to use eyedrops or eardrops, if appropriate.
- Instruct patient prescribed suspension form of drug to shake container well before administering.
- Advise patient to discontinue using neomycin, polymyxin B, and hydrocortisone and notify prescriber if signs and symptoms such as ocular or ear pain or inflammation do not improve or becomes worse or if an allergic reaction occurs.
- Instruct patient to take care not to touch the bottle tip to eyelids or ear or any other surface to avoid contamination.
- Inform patient that no one else should use the drug because infection may be spread in this manner.

neomycin sulfate, polymyxin B sulfate, and prednisolone
Poly-Pred Liquifilm

Class and Category
Chemical: Aminoglucoside (neomycin), bacillus polymyxa derivative (polymyxin B), glucocorticoid (prednisolone)
Therapeutic: Antibiotics (neomycin, polymyxin B), anti-inflammatory (prednisolone)
Pregnancy category: C

Indications and Dosages
▶ *To treat inflammatory ocular conditions of the palpebral and bulbar conjunctiva, cornea, and anterior segment of the globe; chronic anterior uveitis and corneal injury from chemical, radiation, or thermal burns or penetration of foreign bodies when superficial ocular infection is present (or risk is high) caused by* Enterobacter *species,* Escherichia coli, Haemophilus influenzae, Klebsiella *species,* Neisseria *species,* Pseudomonas aeruginosa, *and* Staphylococcus aureus

OPHTHALMIC SUSPENSION

Adults. For severe eye infection, 1 or 2 drops in affected eye or eyes every 30 minutes, decreasing in frequency as infection is controlled. For mild to moderate eye infection, 1 or 2 drops instilled into affected eye or eyes every 3 to 4 hr. For eyelid infection, 1 or 2 drops instilled in the eye; then have patient close the eye, and rub excess on lid and lid margins every 3 to 4 hr.

Mechanism of Action
Neomycin competes with messenger RNA to bind with a receptor protein on the 30S ribosomal subunit of DNA in bacterial cells. This action causes abnormal, nonfunctioning proteins to form, which kills the cells.

Polymyxin B binds to cell membrane phospholipids in gram-negative bacteria, increasing cell membrane permeability. Polymyxin B also acts as a cationic detergent, altering the osmotic barrier of the membrane and causing essential intracellular metabolites to leak. Both actions lead to cell death.

Prednisolone binds to intracellular glucocorticoid receptors in the eye and suppresses inflammatory and immune responses by:
- inhibiting neutrophil and monocyte accumulation at the inflammation site and suppressing their phagocytic and bactericidal activity
- stabilizing lysosomal membranes
- suppressing the antigen response of macrophages and helper T cells
- inhibiting the synthesis of cellular mediators of the inflammatory response, such as cytokines, interleukins, and prostaglandins.

These actions inhibit the edema, fibrin deposition, capillary dilation, leukocyte migration, capillary proliferation, fibroblast proliferation, deposition of collagen and scar formation associated with inflammation.

Contraindications

Fungal diseases affecting ocular structures; hypersensitivity to neomycin, polymyxin B, prednisolone, other corticosteroids, or their components; mycobacterial infection of the eye; uncomplicated removal of a corneal foreign body; viral diseases of the cornea and conjunctiva, including epithelial herpes simplex keratitis, vaccinia, and varicella

Adverse Reactions

EENT: Conjunctival or eyelid edema, erythema, or pruritus; delayed eye wound healing; elevation of intraocular pressure; glaucoma; optic nerve damage; posterior subcapsular cataract formation; secondary eye infection
SKIN: Pruritus, rash, urticaria
Other: Allergic reactions

Nursing Considerations

- Use neomycin, polymyxin B, and prednisolone with great caution if patient has a history of herpes simplex because ocular steroids such as prednisolone may worsen the severity of many ocular viral infections.
- Use cautiously in patients with glaucoma because prednisolone may increase intraocular pressure. Be prepared to check intraocular pressure often in patients with glaucoma and routinely when therapy lasts 10 days in patients without glaucoma.
- Obtain eyelid culture and sensitivity tests as ordered before giving first dose, if infection is already present. Expect to begin drug therapy before test results are known.
- Be aware that topical corticosteroids such as prednisolone may lead to perforation if patient has thin corneal or scleral tissue.
- Assess patient's vision and inspect eyes for abnormalities as prolonged use of ophthalmic corticosteroids may cause glaucoma, damage to the optic nerve, defects in visual acuity and fields of vision, and posterior subcapsular cataract formation. Prolonged use also increases risk of secondary ocular infections.
- Notify prescriber if patient's eye discomfort or inflammation does not improve within 48 hours or worsens.
- Question patient about eye discomfort because prednisolone may mask signs and symptoms of acute purulent infections.
- **WARNING** Do not inject neomycin, polymyxin B, and prednisolone subconjunctivally nor should the drug be introduced directly into the anterior chamber of the eye.
- If patient has persistent corneal ulceration and has used neomycin, polymyxin B, and prednisolone suspension long-

term, obtain fungal cultures because fungal corneal infections are particularly likely with long-term local corticosteroid use.

PATIENT TEACHING

- Instruct patient to use neomycin, polymyxin B, and prednisolone suspension exactly as prescribed, even when feeling better.
- Teach patient how to use eyedrops, if appropriate.
- Tell patient to shake suspension well before using drops.
- Advise patient to discontinue using neomycin, polymyxin B, and prednisolone and notify prescriber if signs and symptoms such as ocular pain or inflammation do not improve within 48 hours, becomes worse or an allergic reaction occurs.
- Instruct patient to take care not to touch the eyedropper to eyelids or any other surface to avoid contamination.
- Inform patient that no one else should use the drug because infection may be spread in this manner.

oxytetracycline hydrochloride and polymyxin B sulfate

Terramycin with Polymyxin B Sulfate Ophthalmic Ointment

Class and Category

Chemical: Tetracycline derived from *Streptomyces rimosus* (oxytetracycline), *Bacillus polymyxa* derivative (polymyxin B)
Therapeutic: Antibiotics (oxytetracycline, polymyxin B)
Pregnancy category: C

Indications and Dosages

▶ *To treat superficial ocular infection involving the conjunctiva or cornea caused by susceptible strains of staphylococci, streptococci, pneumococci,* Hemophilus influenzae, Pseudomonas aeruginosa, *Koch-Weeks bacillus, or* Proteus

OPHTHALMIC OINTMENT

Adults. Applied as a thin ribbon (about ½ inch) into conjunctival sac b.i.d. to q.i.d.

Contraindications

Hypersensitivity to oxytetracycline, polymyxin B, or their components

Adverse Reactions

EENT: Erythema, pruritus, rash, or swelling of eye and surrounding area; secondary eye infection

Mechanism of Action

Oxytetracycline binds with ribosomal subunits of susceptible bacteria and alters the cytoplasmic membrane, inhibiting bacterial protein synthesis and rendering the organism ineffective.

Polymyxin B binds to cell membrane phospholipids in gram-negative bacteria, increasing cell membrane permeability. Polymyxin B also acts as a cationic detergent, altering the osmotic barrier of the membrane and causing essential intracellular metabolites to leak. Both actions lead to cell death.

Nursing Considerations

- Assess patient for adverse reactions. If signs and symptoms of an allergic response such as local rash or pruritus occur, withhold drug and notify prescriber.
- Monitor patient for evidence of secondary ocular infection. If infection remains when oxytetracycline and polymyxin B therapy ends, expect to obtain culture and sensitivity samples, as ordered, and give additional antibiotic therapy as indicated.

PATIENT TEACHING

- Stress importance of instilling oxytetracycline and polymyxin B ophthalmic ointment exactly as prescribed, even when eye(s) is feeling better.
- Instruct patient or caregiver how to use ophthalmic ointment.
- Remind patients and caregivers to wash their hands before and after administering drug.
- Caution patient or caregiver not to touch eye with tip of tube or to share the drug with anyone else because of risk of contamination or spread of infection.
- Tell patient to notify prescriber if symptoms do not improve or become worse by the end of the prescribed therapy time.

phenylephrine hydrochloride 0.25%, antipyrine 5%, and benzocaine 5%

Tympagesic

Class and Category

Chemical: Sympathomimetic amine (phenylephrine), pyrazolone derivative (antipyrine), ethyl aminobenzoate (benzocaine)
Therapeutic: Vasoconstrictor and decongestant (phenylephrine), analgesic (antipyrine) and local anesethetic (benzocaine)

Pregnancy category: C

Indications and Dosages

▶ *To relieve ear pain in treatment of painful ear conditions, such as acute otitis media*

OTIC SOLUTION

Adults. External ear canal filled with solution followed by insertion of cotton pledget moistened with otic solution. Pledget moistened every 2 to 4 hr, as needed, until pain is relieved

---

Mechanism of Action

Phenylephrine stimulates alpha-adrenergic receptors and inhibits the activity of the intracellular enzyme adenyl cyclase, which then inhibits production of cAMP. Inhibition of cAMP causes arteriole constriction, which decreases blood flow and mucosal edema. Phenylephrine also enhances the effects of anesthetics such as benzocaine by decreasing their rate of absorption and prolonging their duration of action.

Antipyrine blocks conduction of nerve impulses to the brain, thereby disrupting impulse transmission and preventing the perception of ear pain.

Benzocaine blocking nerve conduction, first in autonomic and then in sensory and finally in motor nerve fibers. Its effect appears to stem from decreased permeability of nerve cell membranes to sodium ions or competition with calcium ions for membrane binding sites.

Contraindications

Hypersensitivity to phenylephrine, antipyrine, benzocaine, or their components; perforated tympanic membrane; presence of ear discharge

Interactions

DRUGS

phenylephrine

beta blockers, MAO inhibitors: Enhanced sympathomimetic effects

benzocaine

sulfonamides: Reduced sulfonamide effectiveness

Adverse Reactions

CNS: Anxiety, chills, dizziness, headache, nervousness, restlessness, weakness

EENT: Ear canal irritation, redness, or swelling; tinnitus

GI: Nausea, vomiting

HEME: Agranulocytosis

SKIN: Contact dermatitis, erythema, pallor, pruritus, rash, urticaria, vesiculation with oozing

Nursing Considerations

- Use cautiously in elderly patients and those with hypertension, increased intraocular pressure, diabetes mellitus, ischemic heart disease, hyperthyroidism, or prostatic hypertrophy because of the vasoconstrictive properties of phenylephrine.
- Monitor patient closely for systemic adverse reactions, although they're rare because absorption from the eardrum or external ear canal is minimal. If irritation or an allergic response occurs, such as rash, pruritus, or urticaria, withhold drug and notify prescriber.
- Be aware that drug contains a sulfite that can cause serious to life-threatening allergic-type reactions, including anaphylaxis, in susceptible patients such as those with asthma.
- Withhold drug and notify prescriber about nausea, vomiting, and CNS stimulation. These rare symptoms may signal high levels of antipyrine and benzocaine.

PATIENT TEACHING

- Instruct patient or caregiver to use phenylephrine, antipyrine, and benzocaine eardrops exactly as prescribed.
- Show patient or caregiver how to administer eardrops, if necessary, telling him to use the dropped to fill the ear canal with the drug and then insert a cotton pledget saturated with the drug into the ear canal until the next application. Remind him to replace the dropper into the bottle without rinsing it.
- Tell patient to stop using drug and notify prescriber if allergic response or local irritation occurs.
- Tell patient to stop drug when ear pain has stopped. If pain persists, tell patient to notify prescriber; drug is for short-term use.

prednisolone acetate and gentamicin sulfate

Pred-G, Pred G Liquilfilm, Pred-G S.O.P.

Class and Category

Chemical: Glucocorticoid (prednisolone), aminoglycoside derived from *Micromonospora purpurea* (gentamicin)
Therapeutic: Anti-inflammatory (prednisolone), antibiotic (gentamicin)

Pregnancy category: C

Indications and Dosages

▶ *To treat inflammatory ocular conditions of the palpebral and bulbar conjunctiva, cornea, and anterior segment of the globe; chronic anterior uveitis and corneal injury from chemical, radiation, or thermal burns or penetration of foreign bodies when superficial ocular infection is present (or risk is high) caused by* Enterobacter aerogenes, Escherichia coli, Hemophilus influenzae, Klebsiella pneumoniae, Neisseria gonorrhoeae, Pseudomonas aeruginosa, Serratia marcescens, Staphylococcus aureus, Streptococcus pneumoniae, *or* Streptococcus pyogenes

OINTMENT

Adults. A small ribbon (about ½ inch) applied into the conjunctival sac once daily to t.i.d.

SUSPENSION

Adults. If severe infection, 1 drop instilled into conjunctival sac of affected eye or eyes every 1 hr and then tapered to b.i.d. to q.i.d. with positive response. If mild to moderate infection, 1 drop instilled into conjunctival sac b.i.d. to q.i.d.

Mechanism of Action

Prednisolone binds to intracellular glucocorticoid receptors in the eye and suppresses inflammatory and immune responses by:

- inhibiting neutrophil and monocyte accumulation at the inflammation site and suppressing their phagocytic and bactericidal activity
- stabilizing lysosomal membranes
- suppressing the antigen response of macrophages and helper T cells
- inhibiting the synthesis of cellular mediators of the inflammatory response, such as cytokines, interleukins, and prostaglandins.

These actions inhibit the edema, fibrin deposition, capillary dilation, leukocyte migration, capillary proliferation, fibroblast proliferation, deposition of collagen, and scar formation associated with inflammation.

Gentamicin binds to negatively charged sites on the outer cell membrane of bacteria, thereby disrupting the membrane's integrity. Gentamicin also binds to bacterial ribosomal subunits and inhibits protein synthesis. Both actions lead to cell death.

Contraindications

Fungal diseases affecting ocular structures; hypersensitivity to gentamicin, prednisolone, other corticosteroids, or their components; mycobacterial infection of the eye; viral diseases of the cornea and conjunctiva, including epithelial herpes simplex keratitis, vaccinia, and varicella

Adverse Reactions

EENT: Conjunctival or eyelid edema, erythema, or pruritus; delayed eye wound healing; elevation of intraocular pressure; glaucoma; local eye burning, irritation, or stinging; optic nerve damage; posterior subcapsular cataract formation; secondary eye infection; superficial punctate keratitis

Nursing Considerations

- Use prednisolone and gentamicin with great caution in patients with a history of herpes simplex because ocular steroids such as prednisolone may worsen the severity of ocular viral infections.
- Use cautiously in patients with glaucoma because prednisolone may increase intraocular pressure. Be prepared to monitor intraocular pressure often in patients with glaucoma or routinely if therapy lasts 10 days or more in patients without glaucoma.
- If infection is already present, obtain eyelid culture and sensitivity tests, as ordered, before giving first dose. Expect to start drug therapy before test results are known.
- Be aware that topical corticosteroids such as prednisolone may lead to perforation if patient has thin corneal or scleral tissue.
- Assess patient's vision and inspect eyes for abnormalities as prolonged use of ophthalmic corticosteroids may cause glaucoma, damage to the optic nerve, defects in visual acuity and fields of vision, and posterior subcapsular cataract formation. Prolonged use also increases risk of secondary ocular infections.
- Notify prescriber if patient's eye discomfort or inflammation doesn't improve within 48 hours or it worsens.
- Question patient about eye discomfort because prednisolone may mask signs and symptoms of acute purulent infections.
- **WARNING** Do not inject prednisolone and gentamicin suspension subconjunctivally nor should the drug be introduced directly into the anterior chamber of the eye.
- If patient has persistent corneal ulceration and has used prednisolone and gentamicin solution long-term, obtain fungal cultures because fungal corneal infections are particularly likely with long-term local corticosteroid use.

PATIENT TEACHING

- Instruct patient to use prednisolone and gentamicin suspension or ointment exactly as prescribed, even when feeling better.
- Teach patient how to use eyedrops or ointment, if appropriate.

- Tell patient to shake suspension well before using eyedrops.
- Advise patient to stop using prednisolone and gentamicin and to notify prescriber if ocular pain or inflammation don't improve within 48 hours, they become worse, or patient has an allergic reaction.
- Instruct patient to take care not to touch the eyedropper or tube tip to eyelids or any other surface to avoid contamination.
- Inform patient that no one else should use the drug because infection may be spread in this manner.

prednisolone acetate and sulfacetamide sodium

Blephamide, Cetapred, Isopto, Metimyd, Sulster, Vasocidin

Class and Category

Chemical: Glucocorticoid (prednisolone), sulfonamide (sulfacetamide sodium)

Therapeutic: Anti-inflammatory (prednisolone), antibiotic (sulfacetamide sodium)

Pregnancy category: C

Indications and Dosages

▶ *To treat inflammatory ocular conditions of the palpebral and bulbar conjunctiva, cornea, and anterior segment of the globe; chronic anterior uveitis and corneal injury from chemical, radiation, or thermal burns or penetration of foreign bodies when superficial ocular infection is present (or risk is high) caused by* Enterobacter *species,* Escherichia coli, Haemophilus influenzae, Klebsiella *species,* Staphylococcus aureus, Streptococcus pneumoniae, *and* Streptococcus viridans *group*

OPHTHALMIC SUSPENSION

Adults. 2 drops instilled into conjunctival sac every 4 hr while awake and at bedtime.

Incompatibilities

Silver preparations are incompatible with sulfacetamide preparations

Contraindications

Fungal diseases affecting ocular structures; hypersensitivity to prednisolone, other corticosteroids, sulfacetamide sodium, other sulfonamides, or their components; mycobacterial infection of the eye; viral diseases of the cornea and conjunctiva, including epithelial herpes simplex keratitis, vaccinia, and varicella

Mechanism of Action

Prednisolone binds to intracellular glucocorticoid receptors in the eye and suppresses inflammatory and immune responses by:

- inhibiting neutrophil and monocyte accumulation at the inflammation site and suppressing their phagocytic and bactericidal activity
- stabilizing lysosomal membranes
- suppressing the antigen response of macrophages and helper T cells
- inhibiting the synthesis of cellular mediators of the inflammatory response, such as cytokines, interleukins, and prostaglandins.

These actions inhibit the edema, fibrin deposition, capillary dilation, leukocyte migration, capillary proliferation, fibroblast proliferation, deposition of collagen, and scar formation associated with inflammation.

Sulfacetamide sodium hinders bacterial cell growth by restricting the synthesis of folic acid required for growth through competition with para-aminobenzoic acid (PABA).

Interactions

DRUGS

prednisolone

corticosteroids: Increased risk of cross-sensitivity

sulfacetamide sodium

local anesthetics: Possibly antagonized effects of sulfacetamide sodium

sulfonamides: Increased risk of cross-sensitivity

Adverse Reactions

EENT: Acute anterior uvetitis, conjunctivitis, conjunctival hyperemia, corneal ulcers or secondary fungal infections, elevated intraocular pressure, eye irritation, glaucoma, keratitis, loss of accommodation, mydriasis, optic nerve damage, perforation of the globe of the eye, posterior subcapsular cataract formation, ptosis, secondary ocular bacterial infections

ENDO: Systemic hypercorticoidism

GI: Fulminant hepatic necrosis

HEME: Agranulocytosis, aplastic anemia, blood dyscrasias

SKIN: Stevens-Johnson syndrome, toxic epidermal necrolysis

Other: Allergic reactions, delayed wound healing

Nursing Considerations

- Use prednisolone and sulfacetamide sodium with great caution in patients with a history of herpes simplex because ocular steroids may worsen many ocular viral infections.

- Use cautiously in patients with glaucoma because prednisolone may increase intraocular pressure. Be prepared to monitor intraocular pressure often in patients with glaucoma or routinely if therapy lasts 10 days or longer in patients without glaucoma.
- Also use cautiously in African-Americans, who have a greater risk of acute anterior uveitis than other populations.
- If infection is already present, obtain eyelid culture and sensitivity tests as ordered before giving first dose. Expect to start drug therapy before test results are known.
- Be aware that topical corticosteroids such as prednisolone may lead to perforation if patient has thin corneal or scleral tissue.
- Assess patient's vision and inspect eyes for abnormalities as prolonged use of ophthalmic corticosteroids may cause glaucoma, with damage to the optic nerve, defects in visual acuity, and fields of vision and in posterior subcapsular cataract formation. Prolonged use also increases risk of secondary ocular infections.
- Notify prescriber if patient's eye pain or inflammation worsens.
- Question patient about eye discomfort because prednisolone may mask signs and symptoms of acute purulent eye infections.
- **WARNING** Don't inject prednisolone and sulfacetamide sodium suspension into the eye.
- Monitor patient for serious adverse reactions, including allergic response. If suspected, notify prescriber, withhold prednisolone and sulfacetamide sodium, and be prepared to administer appropriate supportive treatment.
- If patient has persistent corneal ulceration and has used prednisolone and sulfacetamide suspension long-term, obtain fungal cultures because fungal corneal infections are particularly likely with long-term local corticosteroid use.

PATIENT TEACHING
- Instruct patient to use prednisolone and sulfacetamide sodium suspension exactly as prescribed even when feeling better.
- Teach patient how to administer eyedrops, if necessary.
- Tell patient to shake the bottle well before using.
- Caution patient to discard the suspension if it appears dark brown and obtain a new suspension.
- Advise patient to stop using prednisolone and sulfacetamide sodium and notify prescriber if ocular pain or inflammation don't improve or they worsen after 2 days.
- Instruct patient to take care not to touch the bottle tip to eyelids or any other surface to avoid contamination.
- Inform patient that no one else should use the drug because infection may be spread in this manner.

scopolamine hydrobromide 0.3% and phenylephrine 10%
Murocoll-2

Class and Category
Chemical: Naturally occurring tertiary amine (scopolamine), sympathomimetic amine (phenylephrine)
Therapeutic: Mydriatic and cycloplegic (scopolamine), mydriatic (phenylephrine)
Pregnancy category: NR

Indications and Dosages
▶ *To produce mydriasis for diagnostic eye exam*
SOLUTION
Adults. 1 or 2 drops instilled into each eye, repeated in 5 minutes if needed.
▶ *To break posterior synechiae in iritis*
SOLUTION
Adults. 1 or 2 drops instilled into affected eye or eyes t.i.d. to q.i.d. postoperatively.

Mechanism of Action
Scopolamine blocks the action of acetylcholine, which relaxes the cholinergically innervated sphincter muscle of the iris. The drug also blocks cholinergic stimulation of the accommodative ciliary muscle of the lens, resulting in dilation of the pupil and paralysis of accommodation.

Phenylephrine acts on adrenergic receptors in the eye, contracting the dilator muscle of the pupil and constricting the arterioles of the conjunctiva.

Contraindications
Angle-closure glaucoma; hypersensitivity to scopolamine, phenylephrine, sulfites or their components; severe coronary artery disease or hypertension; use within 14 days of MAO inhibitor therapy; ventricular tachycardia

Interactions
DRUGS
phenylephrine
MAO inhibitors: Increased and prolonged cardiac stimulation, increased vasopressor effect, increased risk of severe cardiovascular and cerebrovascular effects, hyperpyrexia, and vomiting

Adverse Reactions

CNS: Amnesia, confusion, dizziness, excitation, hallucinations, headache, insomnia, nervousness, paresthesia, psychotic reactions, restlessness, somnolence, tremor, weakness

CV: Angina, bradycardia, hypertension, hypotension, palpitations, peripheral vasoconstriction that may lead to necrosis or gangrene, tachycardia, ventricular arrhythmias

EENT: Blocked lacrimal drainage system; blurred vision; dry mouth; follicular conjunctivitis; increased intraocular pressure; ocular vascular congestion, edema, erythema, irritation or exudates

GI: Constipation, nausea, vomiting

GU: Urinary hesitancy, incontinence or retention

MS: Spastic extremities

RESP: Dyspnea

SKIN: Photophobia

Other: Allergic reaction, anaphylaxis

Nursing Considerations

- Use cautiously in elderly patients and those predisposed to increased intraocular pressure. Prepare them for estimation of the the angle depth of their anterior chamber before instillation.
- Monitor patient closely for adverse systemic reactions. If they occur, notify prescriber and expect to give supportive treatment until drug has worn off—which may take several days.
- Monitor elderly patients and those with Down syndrome. They're more susceptible to adverse reactions, especially excitation and psychosis, often within 30 to 45 minutes after use.
- **WARNING** Drug contains a bisulfite that may cause severe allergic-type reactions, especially in patients with asthma. Monitor these patients closely for anaphylaxis, and withhold drug and be prepared to provide supportive care, if indicated.
- Watch for evidence of allergic response, such as persistent irritation and diffuse eye redness minutes of administering drug.

PATIENT TEACHING

- Instruct patient or caregiver how to administer eyedrops.
- Advise patient or caregiver to press a finger on the lacrimal sac for 1 to 2 minutes after administration.
- Stress importance of using eyedrops exactly as prescribed.
- Caution patient to avoid hazardous activities until CNS effects of the drug are known.
- Tell patient to stop drug and tell prescriber about allergic reaction.
- Instruct patient to take care not to touch the eyedropper to eyelids or any other surface to avoid contamination.

tobramycin and dexamethasone
TobraDex

Class and Category
Chemical: Aminoglycoside (tobramycin), synthetic glucocorticoid (dexamethasone)
Therapeutic: Antibiotic (tobramycin), anti-inflammatory (dexamethasone)
Pregnancy category: C

Indications and Dosages
▶ *To treat inflammatory ocular conditions of the palpebral and bulbar conjunctiva, cornea, and anterior segment of the globe; chronic anterior uveitis and corneal injury from chemical, radiation, or thermal burns or penetration of foreign bodies when superficial ocular infection is present (or risk is high) caused by* Acinetobacter calcoaceticus, Enterobacter aerogenes, Escherichia coli, Haemophilus influenzae, Haemophilus aegyptius, Klebsiella pneumoniae, Moraxella lacunata, Morganella morganii, *most* Proteus vulgaris *strains,* Proteus mirabilis, Pseudomonas aeruginosa, Staphylococcus aureus, Staphylococcus epidermidis, Streptococcus pneumoniae, *some* Streptococcus *group A beta-hemolytic and nonhemolytic species, or some* Neisseria *species*

OPHTHALMIC SUSPENSION

Adults and children age 2 and over. *Initial:* 1 or 2 drops instilled into conjunctival sac every 2 hr for 24 to 48 hr, followed by 1 or 2 drops instilled into conjunctival sac every 4 to 6 hr. Or, 1 or 2 drops instilled into conjunctival sac every 4 to 6 hr.

OPHTHALMIC OINTMENT

Adults and children age 2 and over. Applied as a thin ribbon (about ½ inch) into conjunctival sac t.i.d. or q.i.d.

Contraindications
Fungal diseases affecting ocular structures; hypersensitivity to tobramycin, other aminoglycosides, dexamethasone, other corticosteroids, or their components; mycobacterial infection of the eye; viral diseases of the cornea and conjunctiva, including epithelial herpes simplex keratitis, vaccinia, and varicella

Interactions
DRUGS
tobramycin
aminoglycosides: Increased risk of cross-sensitivity
dexamethasone
corticosteroids: Increased risk of cross-sensitivity

Mechanism of Action

Tobramycin inhibits bacterial protein synthesis by binding irreversibly to one of two aminoglycoside-binding sites on the 30S ribosomal subunit, resulting in bacteriostatic effects. Bactericidal effects may stem from accumulation of tobramycin in cells, so intracellular drug level exceeds the extracellular level.

Dexamethasone binds to intracellular glucocorticoid receptors in the eye and suppresses inflammatory and immune responses by:

- inhibiting neutrophil and monocyte accumulation at the inflammation site and suppressing their phagocytic and bactericidal activity
- stabilizing lysosomal membranes
- suppressing the antigen response of macrophages and helper T cells
- inhibiting the synthesis of cellular mediators of the inflammatory response, such as cytokines, interleukins, and prostaglandins.

These actions inhibit the edema, fibrin deposition, capillary dilation, leukocyte migration, capillary proliferation, fibroblast proliferation, deposition of collagen and scar formation associated with inflammation.

Adverse Reactions

EENT: Conjunctival erythema, delayed eye wound healing, elevation of intraocular pressure, eyelid itching and swelling, glaucoma, optic nerve damage, posterior subcapsular cataract formation, secondary eye infection
SKIN: Pruritus, rash, urticaria
Other: Allergic reactions

Nursing Considerations

- Use tobramycin and dexamethasone with great caution if patient has a history of herpes simplex because ocular steroids may worsen the severity of many ocular viral infections.
- Use cautiously in patients with glaucoma because dexamethasone may increase intraocular pressure. Check intraocular pressure often in patients with glaucoma or routinely if drug is used for 10 days or longer in patients without glaucoma.
- Obtain eyelid culture and sensitivity tests as ordered before giving first dose, if infection is already present. Expect to begin drug therapy before test results are known.
- Be aware that topical corticosteroids such as dexamethasone may lead to perforation if patient has thin corneal or scleral tissue.
- Assess patient's vision and inspect eyes for abnormalities as prolonged use of ophthalmic corticosteroids may cause glaucoma, damage to the optic nerve, defects in visual acuity and fields of

vision and posterior subcapsular cataract formation. Prolonged use also increases risk of secondary ocular infections.

- Tell prescriber if patient's discomfort or inflammation worsens.
- Question patient about eye discomfort because dexamethasone may mask signs and symptoms of acute purulent eye infections.
- **WARNING** Don't inject suspension into the eye.
- Monitor patient for serious eye adverse reactions including allergic response. If suspected, notify prescriber, withhold tobramycin and dexamethasone, and be prepared to administer appropriate supportive treatment.
- If patient has persistent corneal ulceration and has used tobramycin and dexamethasone suspension long-term, obtain fungal cultures because fungal corneal infections are particularly likely with long-term local corticosteroid use.

PATIENT TEACHING
- Instruct patient to use drug exactly as prescribed.
- Teach patient how to use eyedrops or ointment, if necessary.
- Tell patient to shake suspension well before using.
- Advise patient to stop drug and notify prescriber if signs and symptoms such as ocular pain or inflammation do not improve after 2 days or becomes worse or if an allergic reaction occurs.
- Instruct patient to take care not to touch the bottle or tube tip to eyelids or any other surface to avoid contamination.
- Inform patient that no one else should use the drug because infection may be spread in this manner.

trimethoprim sulfate and polymyxin B sulfate

Polytrim

Class and Category

Chemical: Dihydrofolic acid analogue (trimethorprim), bacillus polymyxa derivative (polymyxin B)
Therapeutic: Antibiotics (trimethorprim, polymyxin B)
Pregnancy category: C

Indications and Dosages

▶ *To treat mild to moderate superficial ocular bacterial infections including acute bacterial conjunctivitis and blepharoconjunctivitis caused by susceptible strains of* Staphylococcus aureus, Staphylococcus epidermidis, Streptococcus pneumoniae, Streptococcus viridans, Haemophilus influenzae, *and* Pseudomonas aeruginosa

OPHTHALMIC SOLUTION
Adults and children age 2 months and over. 1 drop instilled into affected eye or eyes every 3 hr while awake for 7 to 10 days. *Maximum:* 6 drops per eye daily.

Mechanism of Action
Trimethorprim inhibits formation of tetrahydrofolic acid, the metabolically active form of folic acid, in susceptible bacteria. This action depletes folate, an essential component of bacterial development, thereby disrupting production of bacterial nucleic acid and protein.

Polymyxin B binds to cell membrane phospholipids in gram-negative bacteria, increasing cell membrane permeability. Polymyxin B also acts as a cationic detergent, altering the osmotic barrier of the membrane and causing essential intracellular metabolites to leak. Both actions lead to cell death.

Contraindications
Hypersensitivity to trimethorprim, polymyxin B, or their components

Adverse Reactions
EENT: Circumocular rash surrounding eye; eyelid or local burning, edema, itching, increased redness and stinging; secondary eye infection; tearing

Nursing Considerations
- Be aware that trimethorprim and polymyxin B shouldn't be used to prevent or treat ophthalmic neonatorium.
- **WARNING** Don't inject drug solution into the eye.
- Monitor patient for sensitivity reaction, such as rash. If present, notify prescriber and expect drug to be stopped.
- Monitor patient for evidence of secondary eye infection, such as discharge or continued signs and symptoms. Notify prescriber, and expect to obtain culture and sensitivity samples, as ordered.

PATIENT TEACHING
- Instruct patient to use trimethorprim and polymyxin B solution exactly as prescribed even when feeling better.
- Teach patient how to administer eyedrops, if necessary.
- Advise patient to stop using drug and to notify prescriber if redness, irritation, swelling, or pain persists or increases.
- Instruct patient to take care not to touch the bottle tip to eyelids or any other surface to avoid contamination.
- Inform patient that no one else should use the drug because infection may be spread in this manner.

Gastrointestinal Drugs

bismuth subsalicylate, metronidazole, and tetracycline hydrochloride
Helidac Therapy
bismuth subcitrate potassium, metronidazole, and tetracycline hydrochloride
Pylera

Class and Category
Chemical: 2-hydroxybenzoic acid bismuth salt and salicylic acid (bismuth subsalicylate), synthetic nitroimidazole derivative (metronidazole), chlortetracycline derivative (tetracycline)
Therapeutic: Antibiotic (bismuth, metronidazole, tetracycline)
Pregnancy category: D

Indications and Dosages
▶ *To eradicate* Helicobacter pylori *infection in patients with duodenal ulcer, to be given with an* H_2 *antagonist approved to treat acute duodenal ulcer*

CHEWABLE TABLETS (BISMUTH SUBSALICYLATE), TABLETS (METRONIDAZOLE), CAPSULES (TETRACYCLINE)

Adults. 525 mg bismuth subsalicyate (2 chewable tablets), 250 mg metronidazole (1 tablet), and 500 mg tetracycline (1 capsule) q.i.d. for 14 days.

▶ *To eradicate* H. pylori *infection in patients with active duodenal ulcer or a history of duodenal ulcer within past 5 years, to be given with omeprazole*

CAPSULES (BISMUTH SUBCITRATE POTASSIUM, METRONIDAZOLE, AND TETRACYCLINE)

Adults. 420 mg bismuth subcitrate potassium, 375 mg metronidazole, and 375 mg tetracycline (3 capsules) after breakfast, lunch, dinner, and at bedtime for 10 days.

Mechanism of Action

Bismuth subsalicylate is almost completely hydrolyzed in the GI tract to bismuth and salicylic acid. It disrupts the integrity of *Helicobacter pylori* cells and prevents their adhesion to the gastric epithelium. It also kills *H. pylori* by inhibiting its urease, phospholipase, and proteolytic activity.

Metronidazole is un-ionized at physiologic pH and is readily taken up by *H. pylori* cells. Once inside the cells, metronidazole is reduced to unidentified polar products that lack the nitro group; they disrupt bacterial DNA and inhibit nucleic acid synthesis to cause cell death.

Tetracycline exerts a bacteriostatic effect against *H. pylori* by passing through the bacterial lipid bilayer, where it binds reversibly to 30S ribosomal subunits. Bound tetracycline blocks the binding of aminoacyl transfer RNA to messenger RNA, thus inhibiting bacterial protein synthesis.

Contraindications

Breast-feeding; children; hepatic or renal impairment; hypersensitivity to bismuth subsalicylate, bismuth citrate, aspirin, other salicylates, metronidazole, other nitromidazole derivatives, tetracycline, other tetracyclines, or their components; pregnancy

Interactions

DRUGS

bismuth subsalicylate, metronidazole, and tetracycline
aspirin, anticogulants: Increased risk for bleeding

bismuth subsalicylate
insulin, oral antidiabetics: Increased risk of hypoglycemia
probenecid, sulfinpyrazone: Decreased effectiveness of these drugs

metronidazole
cimetidine: Possibly prolonged metronidazole half-life and decreased plasma clearance
disulfiram: Increased risk of psychotic reactions
lithium: Increased serum lithium level and toxicity
phenobarbital, phenytoin: Reduced metronidazole plasma level and possibly impaired phenytoin clearance

tetracycline
aluminum-, calcium-, or magnesium-containing antacids; iron supplements (oral); magnesium-containing laxatives; magnesium salicylate; multivitamins (containing manganese or zinc salts); sodium bicarbonate: Possibly impaired absorption of tetracycline and formation of nonabsorbable complexes
cholestyramine, colestipol: Possibly impaired tetracycline absorption

digoxin: Possibly increased blood digoxin level
methoxyflurane: Possibly nephrotoxicity
oral contraceptives (containing estrogen): Possibly reduced contraceptive reliability
penicillins: Possibly decreased bactericidal effect of penicillins
FOODS
tetracycline
dairy products, other foods: Possibly impaired tetracycline absorption
ACTIVITIES
metronidazole
alcohol use: Possibly increased incidence of abdominal cramps, nausea, vomiting, headache, and flushing

Adverse Reactions

CNS: Asthenia, cerebral ischemia, depression, dizziness, headache, insomnia, malaise, nervousness, paresthesia, peripheral neuropathy, seizures, somnolence, syncope, weakness
CV: Chest pain, hypertension, MI
EENT: Conjunctivitis, discolored tongue, dry mouth, enamel hypoplasia, glossitis, metallic taste, oral candidiasis, rhinitis, sinusitis, stomatitis, taste perversion
GI: Abdominal pain, anal discomfort, anorexia, constipation, diarrhea, duodenal ulcer, dyspepsia, dysphagia, elevated liver enzymes, flatulence, GI hemorrhage, hepatotoxicity, intestinal obstruction, melena, nausea, rectal candidiasis or hemorrhage, vomiting
GU: Incontinence, UTI, vaginal candidiasis
HEME: Mild leukopenia
MS: Arthritis, musculoskeletal pain, rheumatoid arthritis, tendonitis
RESP: Upper respiratory infection
SKIN: Acne, ecchymosis, photosensitivity, pruritus, rash
Other: Flulike syndrome, neoplasms

Nursing Considerations

• Use cautiously in patients with CNS disease; those with blood dyscrasia or a history of it; and elderly patients who may have asymptomatic renal and hepatic dysfunction.
• Be aware that bismuth subsalicylate, metronidazole, and tetracycline is packaged in 14 blister cards, each containing the following daily dose: eight chewable 262.4-mg bismuth subsalicylate tablets, four 250-mg metronidazole tablets, and four 500-mg tetracycline capsules. Be aware that each Pylera capsule

contains 140 mg bismuth subcitrate, 125 mg metronidazole, and 125 mg tetracycline.

- Know that bismuth subsalicylate and bismuth subcitrate are used in these combinations for their antimicrobial effects and not for relief of upset stomach.
- Monitor anticoagulant therapy closely because triple therapy may interact with anticoagulants.
- Monitor diabetic patients receiving insulin or oral antidiabetic agents for hypoglycemia.
- Monitor patient for signs of central nervous system effects such as seizures and peripheral neuropathy. If present, contact prescriber and expect to discontinue triple therapy.
- Be aware that if candidiasis infection occurs, it will require treatment with a candicidal agent.

PATIENT TEACHING

- Instruct patient to take the prescribed triple therapy exactly as prescribed for the length of time prescribed.
- Tell patient to chew and then swallow bismuth subsalicylate pink tablets and then swallow the metronidazole white tablet and tetracycline white capsule whole with a full glass of water.
- Tell patient prescribed bismuth subcitrate, metronidazole, and tetracycline triple therapy to swallow the three capsules of each dose with a full glass of water.
- Instruct patient to avoid antacids; preparations containing iron, zinc, or sodium bicarbonate; and milk or dairy products while taking triple therapy.
- If patient misses a dose, caution against doubling the next dose. Instead, tell him to make up the missed dose by continuing the normal dose schedule until the drug is gone. If he misses more than four doses, instruct patient to notify prescriber.
- Caution patient to avoid alcohol during drug therapy and for at least 1 day after taking all doses.
- Tell patient that bismuth subsalicylate and bismuth subcitrate may cause a transient and harmless darkening of the tongue and stool.
- Instruct patient to report blood in his stool or any other troublesome or serious adverse effect, such as a yeast infection.
- Warn patient to avoid sun exposure as much as possible and to use sunscreen when out of doors.
- Tell women using oral contraceptives to use an additional or different form of contraception throughout bismuth, metronidazole, and tetracycline triple therapy.

chlordiazepoxide hydrochloride and clidinium bromide

Clindex, Clinoxide, Clipoxide, Librax, Lidox, Lidoxide, Zebrax

Class, Category, and Schedule

Chemical: Benzodiazepine (chlordiazepoxide), synthetic quaternary ammonium derivative (clidinium)
Therapeutic: Sedative (chlordiazepoxide), anticholinergic (clidinium)
Pregnancy category: NR
Controlled substance schedule: IV

Indications and Dosages

▶ *As adjunct therapy in the treatment of peptic ulcer; to treat irritable bowel syndrome and acute enterocolitis*

CAPSULE

Adults. 5 to 10 mg clordiazepoxide and 2.5 to 5 mg clidinium (1 to 2 capsules) daily up to q.i.d. 30 to 60 minutes before meals or food intake

---

Mechanism of Action

Chlordiazepoxide may potentiate the effects of gamma-aminobutyric acid (GABA) and other inhibitory neurotransmitters by binding to specific benzodiazepine receptors in the limbic and cortical areas of the CNS. By binding to these receptors, chlordiazepoxide increases GABA's inhibitory effects and blocks cortical and limbic arousal, which helps relax and slow the digestive system.

Clidinium inhibits acetylcholine's muscarinic actions at postganglionic parasympathetic receptor sites, including smooth muscles, secretory glands, and the CNS. These actions relax smooth muscles, including those in the GI tract, and diminish GI and biliary tract secretions to reduce gastric acid formation.

Contraindications

Angle-closure glaucoma; benign bladder neck obstruction; hypersensitivity to chlordiazepoxide, clidinium, or their components; ileus, intestinal atony (elderly or debilitated patients), intestinal obstruction, myasthenia gravis; myocardial ischemia; ocular adhesions between lens and iris; prostatic hypertrophy; renal disease; severe ulcerative colitis; tachycardia; toxic megacolon; unstable cardiovascular status in acute hemorrhage

Interactions

DRUGS

chlordiazepoxide and clidinium

antidiarrheal drugs containing attapulgitel or kaolin: Decreased blood levels of chlordiazepoxide and clidinium

CNS depressants: Increased clidinium and CNS effects

ketoconazole: Decreased blood level of ketoconazole

oral potassium chloride: Increased risk of causing or worsening gastric or intestinal ulceration

chlordiazepoxide

antacids: Altered rate of chlordiazepoxide absorption

cimetidine, disulfiram, fluoxetine, hormonal contraceptives, isoniazid, ketoconazole, metoprolol, propoxyphene, propranolol, valproic acid: Increased blood chlordiazepoxide level

digoxin: Increased blood digoxin level and risk of digitalis toxicity

levodopa: Decreased efficacy of levodopa's antiparkinsonian effects

neuromuscular blockers: Potentiated, counteracted, or diminished effects of neuromuscular blockers

phenytoin: Possibly increased phenytoin toxicity

probenecid: Shortened onset of action or prolonged effect of chlordiazepoxide

rifampin: Decreased chlordiazepoxide effect

theophyllines: Antagonized sedative effects of chlordiazepoxide

clidinium

amantadine: Increased risk of clidinium adverse effects

atenolol: Increased atenolol effects

other anticholinergics: Possibly increased adverse effects

phenothiazines: Decreased antipsychotic effectiveness

tricyclic antidepressants: Increased clidinium adverse effects

ACTIVITIES

chlordiazepoxide and clidinium

alcohol use: Increased CNS effects

Adverse Reactions

CNS: Ataxia, confusion, depression, dizziness, drowsiness, excitement, fever, headache, insomnia, irritability, memory loss, nervousness, weakness

CV: Bradycardia, hypotension, palpitations, tachycardia

EENT: Blurred vision, cycloplegia, dry mouth, increased intraocular pressure, loss of taste, mydriasis, nasal congestion, pharyngitis, photophobia

GI: Bloating, constipation, dysphagia, heartburn, hepatic dysfunction, jaundice, ileus, nausea, vomiting

GU: Impotence, urinary hesitancy, urine retention
HEME: Agranulocytosis
RESP: Dyspnea, shortness of breath
SKIN: Decreased sweating, flushing, rash, urticaria

Nursing Considerations

- Use chlordiazepoxide and clindinium cautiously in patients with heart failure, arrhythmias, hypertension, autonomic neuropathy, hyperthyroidism, allergies, asthma, debilitating chronic lung disease, renal or hepatic impairment, or porphyria.
- **WARNING** Be aware that prolonged use of therapeutic doses can lead to dependence.
- Monitor liver function test results during therapy.
- If patient has a history of psychiatric disorders, monitor for paradoxical reactions, such as excitement, stimulation, and acute rage, during first 2 weeks of therapy.
- **WARNING** Monitor for excitement, agitation, drowsiness, and confusion in elderly patients because they're more sensitive to clindinium's effects. If these reactions occur, notify prescriber and expect to decrease dosage.
- Take safety precautions to protect patient from falling.

PATIENT TEACHING

- Instruct patient to take drug 30 to 60 minutes before meals.
- Tell patient to take chlordiazepoxide and clindinium exactly as prescribed and not to alter dosage or dosing frequency without consulting prescriber first.
- Alert patient that chlordiazepoxide and clindinium may become habit forming, causing mental or physical dependence. Stress importance of not abruptly stopping chlordiazepoxide and clindinium therapy because withdrawal symptoms, such as vomiting, diaphoresis, and dizziness may occur.
- Caution patient to avoid hazardous activities until drug's CNS effects are known.
- Instruct patient to avoid alcohol and other CNS depressants during chlordiazepoxide and clindinium therapy.
- Advise patient to avoid using antacids during chlordiazepoxide and clindinium therapy.
- Instruct patient to report adverse effects of chlordiazepoxide and clindinium, such as constipation, vision changes, sore throat, trouble urinating, and palpitations.
- Tell patient to avoid taking chlordiazepoxide and clindinium within an hour of antidiarrheal drugs because chlordiazepoxide and clindinium will be less effective.

- Alert patient that drug will make him sweat less, which may cause his body temperature to increase, especially during exercise, hot weather, or hot baths or saunas. Advise using extra care not to become overheated as heat stroke could occur.
- Advise patient to use sugarless candy or gum, melt bits of ice in his mouth, or use a saliva substitute if his mouth, nose, or throat feels dry. If mouth dryness continues for more than 2 weeks, tell patient to contact prescriber because continued dryness may increase his risk for dental disease, which can include tooth decay, gum disease, and fungus infections.

diphenoxylate hydrochloride and atropine sulfate

Lofene, Logen, Lomocot, Lomotil, Lonox, Vi-Atro

Class, Category, and Schedule

Chemical: Belladonna alkaloid, tertiary amine (atropine), phenylpiperidine derivative opioid (diphenoxylate)
Therapeutic: Antidiarrheal
Pregnancy category: C
Controlled substance schedule: V

Indications and Dosages

▶ *To treat acute and chronic diarrhea*

ORAL SOLUTION, TABLETS

Adults and adolescents. *Initial:* 5 mg of diphenoxylate and 0.05 mg of atropine t.i.d. or q.i.d. *Maintenance:* 5 mg of diphenoxylate and 0.05 mg of atropine daily, p.r.n. *Maximum:* 20 mg of diphenoxylate daily.

DOSAGE ADJUSTMENT Dosage reduced as soon as symptoms are controlled. Expect prescriber to consider alternative treatment if no improvement occurs after 10 days at maximum dosage. Dosage also reduced in elderly or very ill patients and in those with respiratory problems.

Mechanism of Action

Diphenoxylate directly affects circular smooth muscles of the GI tract, reducing intestinal motility.

Subtherapeutic doses of atropine are added to diphenoxylate to reduce its potential for abuse.

Contraindications
Diarrhea caused by pseudomembranous enterocolitis or entero-toxin-producing bacteria; hypersensitivity to atropine, diphenoxy-late, or their components; obstructive jaundice; ulcerative colitis

Interactions
DRUGS
anticholinergics: Possibly enhanced effects of atropine
barbiturates, tranquilizers, and other habit-forming CNS depressants: Potentiated CNS depression; possibly increased risk of drug dependence
MAO inhibitors: Possibly hypertensive crisis
naltrexone: Withdrawal symptoms if patient is physically dependent on diphenoxylate
opioid analgesics: Increased risk of severe constipation; additive CNS depression
ACTIVITIES
alcohol use: Possibly potentiated CNS depression

Adverse Reactions
CNS: Confusion, depression, dizziness, drowsiness, euphoria, fever, headache, hyperthermia, lethargy, malaise, paresthesia, restlessness, sedation
CV: Tachycardia
EENT: Gingival hyperplasia
GI: Abdominal cramps or pain, anorexia, ileus, nausea, pancreatitis, toxic megacolon, vomiting
GU: Urine retention
RESP: Respiratory depression
SKIN: Dry skin and mucous membranes, flushing, pruritus, urticaria
Other: Anaphylaxis, physical and psychological dependence

Nursing Considerations
- **WARNING** Use diphenoxylate-atropine combination with extreme caution in patients with abnormal hepatic or renal function because drug can cause hepatic coma. Monitor liver function test results as appropriate during long-term therapy.
- **WARNING** Monitor for respiratory depression, especially in elderly or very ill patients and in those with respiratory problems; expect to give lower doses as prescribed.
- If severe fluid or electrolyte imbalance develops, expect to withhold diphenoxylate and atropine as ordered until imbalance is corrected. Drug-induced ileus or toxic megacolon may cause

fluid retention in the intestine, aggravating dehydration and electrolyte imbalance.
- Closely monitor patient with ulcerative colitis because drug has caused toxic megacolon. Notify prescriber immediately about unexpected adverse reactions, especially abdominal distention and hypoactive or absent bowel sounds.
- During long-term therapy, assess for tolerance to drug's antidiarrheal effects.

PATIENT TEACHING
- Caution patient not to exceed the prescribed dosage because of the risk of adverse reactions, including drug dependence.
- Stress the importance of keeping drug away from children because overdose can cause permanent brain damage in them.
- Instruct patient to take drug with food if GI distress occurs.
- Advise patient to avoid hazardous activities until drug's CNS effects are known.
- Urge patient to avoid alcohol and CNS depressants because of additive effects.
- Instruct patient to notify prescriber if diarrhea isn't improved or controlled within 48 hours or if a fever develops.

lansoprazole, amoxicillin, and clarithromycin

Prevpac

Class and Category

Chemical: Substituted benzimidazole (lansoprazole), aminopenicillin (amoxicillin), macrolide derivative (clarithromycin)
Therapeutic: Antisecretory, antiulcer (lansoprazole), antiobiotics (amoxicillin, clarithromycin)
Pregnancy category: C

Indications and Dosages

▶ *To reduce the risk of duodenal ulcer recurrence by eradicating the presence of* Helicobacter pylori *in the stomach*

E.R. CAPSULES (LANSOPRAZOLE), CAPSULES (AMOXICILLIN), TABLETS (CLARITHROMYCIN)

Adults. 30 mg lansoprazole, 1 gram amoxicillin, and 500 mg clarithromycin (one 30-mg capsule lansoprazole, two 500-mg capsules amoxicillin, and one 500-mg tablet clarithromycin) b.i.d. morning and evening for 10 to 14 days.

DOSAGE ADJUSTMENT For patients with renal impairment

(creatinine clearance less than normal but greater than 30 ml/min), hepatic impairment, or both, clarithromycin dosage may need to be reduced or dosing interval increased.

Mechanism of Action

Lansoprazole binds to and inactivates the hydrogen-potassium-adenosine triphosphate enzyme system (also called the proton pump) in gastric parietal cells. This action blocks the final step of gastric acid production.

Amoxicillin kills bacteria by binding to and inactivating penicillin-binding proteins on the inner membrane of bacterial cell walls. Penicillin-binding proteins play a role in bacterial cell wall synthesis and cell division. By binding to these proteins, the drug weakens bacterial cell walls and causes lysis.

Clarithromycin inhibits RNA-dependent protein synthesis in many types of aerobic, anaerobic, gram-positive, and gram-negative bacteria. By binding with the 50S ribosomal subunit of the bacterial 70S ribosome, clarithromycin causes bacterial cells to die.

Contraindications

Concurrent therapy with astemizole, cisapride, dihydroergotamine, ergotamine, pimozide, or terfenadine; hypersensitivity to lansoprazole, amoxicillin, other penicillins, clarithromycin, erythromycin, other macrolides, or their components

Interactions

DRUGS

lansoprazole

ampicillin, atazanavir, digoxin, iron salts, ketoconazole, other drugs that depend on low gastric pH for bioavailability: Inhibited absorption of these drugs

fluvoxamine: Elevated plasma lansoprozole level

sucralfate: Delayed lansoprazole absorption

theophylline: Slightly decreased blood theophylline level

warfarin: Possibly increased risk of bleeding

amoxicillin

allopurinol: Possibly increased incidence of rash

chloramphenicol, macrolides, sulfonamides, tetracyclines: Reduced bactericidal effect of amoxicillin

methotrexate: Increased risk of methotrexate toxicity

oral contraceptives with estrogen: Possibly reduced contraceptive effectiveness

probenecid: Increased amoxicillin effects

clarithromycin

astemizole, disopyramide, quinidine: Possibly prolonged QT interval or torsades de pointes

carbamazepine, other drugs metabolized by cytochrome P450 enzyme system: Increased blood levels of these drugs

cisapride, disopyramide, pimozide, quinidine, terfenadine: Increased risk of arrhythmias

digoxin: Increased serum digoxin level

dihydroergotamine, ergotamine: Risk of acute ergot toxicity

lovastatin, simvastatin: Risk of rhabdomyolysis

oral anticoagulants: Potentiated anticoagulant effects

rifabutin, rifampin: Decreased blood clarithromycin level by more than 50%

sildenafil: Possibly prolonged blood sildenafil level

theophylline: Increased blood theophylline level

triazolam: Possibly increased CNS effects

zidovudine: Decreased blood zidovudine level

FOODS

lansoprazole

all food: Possibly reduced absorption of lansoprazole

Adverse Reactions

CNS: Agitation, anxiety, behavior changes, confusion, dizziness, fatigue, headache, insomnia, reversible hyperactivity, seizures, somnolence, vertigo

CV: QT-interval prolongation, torsades de pointes, vasculitis, ventricular arrhythmias

EENT: Altered taste, glossitis, hearing loss, oral moniliasis, stomatitis, tongue discoloration

ENDO: Hypoglycemia

GI: Abdominal pain, anorexia, constipation, diarrhea, elevated liver enzymes, hepatitis, hepatotoxicity, jaundice, increased appetite, indigestion, nausea, pancreatitis, pseudomembranous colitis, vomiting

GU: Elevated BUN level, interstitial nephritis, urine retention

HEME: Agranulocytosis, aplastic and hemolytic anemia, eosinophilia, granulocytosis, leukopenia, neutropenia, pancytopenia, thrombocytopenia, thrombocytopenic purpura

MS: Arthralgia, myositis

SKIN: Acute generalized exanthematous pustulosis, erythema multiforme, erythematous maculopapular rash, exfoliative dermatitis, Stevens-Johnson syndrome, toxic epidermal necrolysis, pruritus, rash, urticaria

Other: Allerigc reaction, anaphylaxis, serum sickness–like reactions, superinfection

Nursing Considerations

- Use lansoprazole, amoxicillin, and clarithromycin cautiously in patients with renal impairment because of clarithromycin and in patients with infectious mononucleosis or who are breast-feeding because of amoxicillin.
- Administer lansoprazole, amoxicillin, and clarithromycin 30 minutes before breakfast and dinner.
- WARNING If allergic reaction occurs, stop lansoprazole, amoxicillin, and clarithromycin immediately and start emergency care as indicated and ordered. It may include epinephrine, oxygen, intravenous steroids, and airway management.
- Monitor patient closely for diarrhea, which may be caused by antibiotic-induced pseudomembranous colitis. If diarrhea occurs, notify prescriber and expect to withhold drug therapy and administer treatment for diarrhea, as ordered.

PATIENT TEACHING

- Instruct patient to take lansoprazole, amoxicillin, and clarithromycin exactly as prescribed even when feeling better.
- Tell patient to swallow each capsule and tablet whole.
- Let patient know he may take antacids with lansoprazole, amoxicillin, and clarithromycin therapy.
- Advise patient to report diarrhea, severe headache, severe nausea, rash, itching, or worsening of symptoms immediately.

omeprazole and sodium bicarbonate
Zegerid

Class and Category

Chemical: Substituted benzimidazole (omeprazole), electrolyte (sodium bicarbonate)
Therapeutic: Antiulcer, proton pump inhibitor (omeprazole), antacid (sodium bicarbonate)
Pregnancy category: C

Indications and Dosages

▶ *To treat gastroesophageal reflux disease (GERD) with erosive esophagitis diagnosed by endoscopy*
CAPSULES, ORAL SUSPENSION
Adults. 20 mg omeprazole and 1,100 mg sodium bicarbonate (1 capsule) or 20 mg omeprazole and 1,680 mg sodium bicarbon-

ate (1 packet) once daily for 4 to 8 weeks. *Maintenance of healing:* 20 mg omeprazole and 1,100 mg sodium bicarbonate (1 capsule) or 20 mg omeprazole and 1,680 mg sodium bicarbonate (1 packet) once daily for up to 12 months total (including 4- to 8-week treatment period).

▶ *To provide short-term treatment of active duodenal ulcer*
CAPSULES, ORAL SUSPENSION
Adults. 20 mg omeprazole and 1,100 mg sodium bicarbonate (1 capsule) or 20 mg omeprazole and 1,680 mg sodium bicarbonate (1 packet) once daily for 4 to 8 weeks.

▶ *To provide short-term treatment of active benign gastric ulcer*
CAPSULES, ORAL SUSPENSION
Adults. 40 mg omeprazole and 1,100 mg sodium bicarbonate (1 capsule) or 40 mg omeprazole and 1,680 mg sodium bicarbonate (1 packet) once daily for 4 to 8 weeks.

▶ *To treat heartburn and other symptoms of GERD without evidence of esophageal erosion*
CAPSULES, ORAL SUSPENSION
Adults. 20 mg omeprazole and 1,100 mg sodium bicarbonate (1 capsule) or 20 mg omeprazole and 1,680 mg sodium bicarbonate (1 packet) once daily for up to 4 weeks.

▶ *To reduce risk of upper GI bleeding in critically ill patients*
ORAL SUSPENSION
Adults. *Initial:* 40 mg omeprazole and 1,680 mg sodium bicarbonate (1 packet) followed by 40 mg omeprazole and 1,680 mg sodium bicarbonate (1 packet) 6 to 8 hours later and then 40 mg omeprazole and 1,680 mg sodium bicarbonate (1 packet) once daily for 14 days.

Mechanism of Action

Omeprazole interferes with gastric acid secretion by inhibiting the hydrogen-potassium-adenosine triphosphatase ($H+K+$-ATPase) enzyme system, or proton pump, in gastric parietal cells. Normally, the proton pump uses energy from ATP hydrolysis to drive hydrogen ($H+$) and chloride ($Cl-$) out of parietal cells and into the stomach lumen in exchange for potassium ($K+$), which leaves the stomach lumen and enters parietal cells. After this exchange, $H+$ and $Cl-$ combine in the stomach to form hydrochloric acid (HCl). Omeprazole irreversibly blocks exchange of intracellular $H+$ and extracellular $K+$. By keeping $H+$ from the stomach lumen, it prevents more HCl from forming.

Sodium bicarbonate relieves hyperacidity by neutralizing or buffering existing stomach acid, thereby increasing the pH of stomach contents.

Contraindications

Hypersensitivity to omeprazole, other proton pump inhibitors, or their components

Interactions

DRUGS

omeprazole and sodium bicarbonate

digoxin: Increased digoxin bioavailability; possibly digitalis toxicity
iron supplements or preparation, ketoconazole: Decreased absorption of these drugs
sucralfate: Decreased omeprazole absorption; interference with binding of sucralfate to gastric mucosa

omeprazole

alprazolam, astemizole, carbamazepine, cisapride, cyclosporine, diazepam, diltiazem, erythromycin, felodipine, lidocaine, lovastatin, midazolam, quinidine, simvastatin, terfenadine, triazolam, verapamil, voriconazole: Decreased clearance and increased blood levels of these drugs
ampicillin, itraconazole, vitamin B_{12}: Impaired absorption of these drugs
atazanavir: Decreased plasma atazanavir level
cilostazol: Increased blood cilostazol level
clarithromycin: Increased blood levels of clarithromycin and omeprazole
levobupivacaine: Increased risk of levobupivacaine toxicity
methotrexate: Possibly delayed methotrexate elimination
nifedipine: Decreased nifedipine clearance; increased risk of hypotension
phenytoin: Decreased phenytoin clearance; increased risk of phenytoin toxicity
tacrolimus: Possibly increased tacrolimus levels
warfarin: Possibly increased risk of abnormal bleeding

sodium bicarbonate

amphetamines, quinidine: Decreased urinary excretion of these drugs, possibly resulting in toxicity
anticholinergics: Decreased anticholinergic absorption and effectiveness
calcium-containing products: Increased risk of milk-alkali syndrome
chlorpropamide, lithium, salicylates, tetracyclines: Increased renal excretion and decreased absorption of these drugs
ciprofloxacin, norfloxacin, ofloxacin: Decreased solubility of these drugs, leading to crystalluria and nephrotoxicity
citrates: Increased risk of systemic alkalosis; increased risk of cal-

cium calculus formation and hypernatremia in patients with history of uric acid calculi

enteric-coated drugs: Increased risk of gastric or duodenal irritation from rapid removal of eneric coating

ephedrine: Increased ephedrine half-life and duration of action

H₂-receptor antagonists: Decreased absorption of these drugs

mecamylamine: Decreased excretion and prolonged effect of mecamylamine

methenamine: Decreased methenamine effectiveness

mexiletine: Possibly mexiletine toxicity

potassium supplements: Decreased serum potassium level

urinary acidifiers (ammonium chloride, ascorbic acid, potassium and sodium phosphates): Counteracted effects of urinary acidifiers

FOODS

sodium bicarbonate

dairy products: Increased risk of milk-alkali syndrome with prolonged use of sodium bicarbonate

Adverse Reactions

CNS: Agitation, asthenia, dizziness, drowsiness, fatigue, fever, headache, hepatic encephalopathy, psychic disturbances, seizures, somnolence, thirst

CV: Angina, atrial fibrillation, bradycardia, fluid overload, hypertension, hypotension, peripheral edema, supraventricular tachycardia, tachycardia, ventricular tachycardia, weak pulse

EENT: Anterior ischemic optic neuropathy, dry mouth, optic atrophy or neuritis, optic neuropathy, oral candidiasis, stomatitis

ENDO: Hyperglycemia, hypoglycemia

GI: Abdominal cramps or pain, acid regurgitation, constipation, diarrhea, dyspepsia, elevated liver enzyme levels, flatulence, gastric hypomotility, hepatitis, hepatic failure, liver necrosis, nausea, pancreatitis, vomiting

GU: Interstitial nephritis, UTI

HEME: Agranulocytosis, anemia, hemolytic anemia, leukopenia, leukocytosis, neutropenia, pancytopenia, thrombocytopenia

MS: Back pain, muscle spasms, myalgia, tetany

RESP: Acute respiratory distress syndrome, cough, pneumonia, pneumothorax, respiratory failure, upper respiratory tract infection

SKIN: Erythema multiforme, photosensitivity, pruritus, rash, Stevens-Johnson syndrome, toxic epidermal necrolysis, urticaria

Other: Anaphylaxis, angioedema, candidal infection, electrolyte imbalance, metabolic alkalosis, milk-alkali syndrome, sepsis

Nursing Considerations

- Use caution when giving omeprazole and sodium bicarbonate to patients with hypocalcemia or metabolic alkalosis.
- Be aware that both the 20-mg and 40-mg capsules and oral suspension packets contain the same amount of sodium bicarbonate. Therefore, two packets or capsules containing 20 mg of the drug should not be substituted for one packet or capsule containing 40 mg of the drug.
- Give drug on an empty stomach at least 1 hour before a meal. If patient is receiving continuous tube feedings, the enteral feeding should be suspended about 3 hours before to 1 hour after administration of the oral drug suspension.
- Administer capsule form with only water. Don't open the capsule and sprinkle its contents onto food.
- Prepare suspension form of drug by emptying packet contents into a small cup containing 1 to 2 tablespoons of water. Stir well and have patient drink immediately. Refill cup with water and have patient drink again.
- When giving drug through a nasogastric or orogastric tube, mix packet contents with about 20 ml of water. Stir well, and give immediately. After giving drug, flush tube with 20 ml of water.
- Monitor sodium intake of patient taking omeprazole and sodium bicarbonate because each capsule contains 304 mg and each packet contains 460 mg of sodium.
- If patient receiving long-term omeprazole and sodium bicarbonate therapy is consuming a diet that includes calcium or milk, monitor her for milk-alkali syndrome, characterized by anorexia, confusion, headache, hypercalcemia, metabolic acidosis, nausea, renal insufficiency, and vomiting.

PATIENT TEACHING

- Instruct patient to take drug on an empty stomach at least 1 hour before a meal, preferably breakfast.
- Tell patient to swallow capsule whole with only water. Stress importance of not opening capsule. If patient has been prescribed the powder form for oral suspension, tell her to empty packet contents into a small cup containing 1 to 2 tablespoons of only water. She should then stir the mixture well and drink immediately. Lastly, she should refill the cup with water and drink all the water.
- Encourage patient to inform all prescribers that she takes omeprazole and sodium bicarbonate because of the risk of drug interactions.

phenobarbital, hyoscyamine sulfate (or hydrobromide), atropine sulfate, and scopolamine hydrobromide

Barophen, Donnamor, Donnapine, Donnatal, Donnatal Extentabs, Hyosophen, Kinesed, Spasmophen, Spasquid, Susano

Class and Category

Chemical: Barbiturate (phenobarbital), tertiary amine (hyoscyamine, atropine, scopolamine)
Therapeutic: Sedative-hypnotic (phenobarbital), anticholinergic (hyoscyamine, atropine, scopolamine)
Pregnancy category: C

Indications and Dosages

▶ *As adjunct to treat irritable bowel syndrome, acute enterocolitis, and duodenal ulcer*

CAPSULE, TABLET

Adults and adolescents. 16 to 32 mg phenobarbital, 0.104 to 0.208 mg hyoscyamine, 0.0194 to 0.0388 mg atropine, and 0.0065 to 0.0125 mg scopolamine (1 or 2 capsules or tablets) b.i.d. to q.i.d.

CHEWABLE TABLETS

Adults and adolescents. 16 to 32 mg phenobarbital, 0.12 to 0.24 mg hyoscyamine, 0.12 to 0.24 mg atropine, and 0.007 to 0.014 mg scopolamine (1 or 2 tablets) b.i.d. to q.i.d.

E.R. TABLETS

Adults and adolescents. 48.6 mg phenobarbital, 0.3111 mg hyoscyamine, 0.0582 mg atropine, and 0.0195 mg scopolamine (1 tablet) every 8 to 12 hr.

ELIXIR

Adults and adolescents. 16 to 32 mg phenobarbital, 0.104 to 0.208 mg hyoscyamine, 0.0194 to 0.0388 mg atropine, and 0.0065 to 0.0125 mg scopolamine (5 or 10 ml) b.i.d. to q.i.d.

Contraindications

Acute intermittent porphyria; glaucoma; hiatal hernia associated with reflux esophagitis; hypersensitivity to phenobarbital, other barbiturates, hyoscyamine, atropine, scopolamine or their components; idiosyncratic reaction of phenobarbital-induced excitement or restlessness; intestinal atony in elderly or debilitated patients; myasthenia gravis; paralytic ileus; obstructive uropathy or GI disorders; severe ulcerative colitis; toxic megacolon; unstable cardiovascular status in acute hemorrhage

Mechanism of Action

Phenobarbital inhibits ascending conduction in the reticular formation, which produces drowsiness, hypnosis, and sedation. Phenobarbital also decreases the spread of seizure activity in the cortex, thalamus, and limbic system.

Belladonna alkaloids (hyoscyamine, atropine, scopolamine) inhibit acetylcholine's muscarinic actions at postganglionic parasympathetic receptor sites, including smooth muscles, secretory glands, and CNS. These actions relax smooth muscles and diminish GI, GU, and biliary tract secretions.

Interactions

DRUGS

phenobarbital

acetaminophen: Decreased acetaminophen effectiveness with long-term phenobarbital therapy

amphetamines: Delayed intestinal absorption of phenobarbital

anesthetics (halogenated hydrocarbon): Possibly hepatotoxicity

anticonvulsants (hydantoin): Unpredictable effects anticonvulsant metabolism

anticonvulsants (succinimide), including carbamazepine: Decreased blood levels and elimination half-lives of these drugs

calcium channel blockers: Possibly excessive hypotension

carbonic anhydrase inhibitors: Enhanced osteopenia induced by phenobarbital

chloramphenicol, corticosteroids, cyclosporine, dacarbazine, digoxin, metronidazole, quinidine: Decreased effectiveness of these drugs from enhanced metabolism

CNS depressants: Additive CNS depression

cyclophosphamide: Possibly reduced half-life and increased leukopenic activity of cyclophosphamide

disopyramide: Possibly ineffectiveness of disopyramide

doxycycline, fenoprofen: Shortened half-life of these drugs

griseofulvin: Possibly decreased absorption and effectiveness of griseofulvin

guanadrel, guanethidine: Possibly increased orthostatic hypotension

haloperidol: Decreased seizure threshold, decreased blood haloperidol level

ketamine (high doses): Increased risk of hypotension and respiratory depression

leucovorin: Interference with phenobarbital's anticonsulsant effect

levothyroxine, oral contraceptives, phenylbutazone, tricyclic antidepressants: Decreased effectiveness of these drugs

loxapine, phenothiazines, thioxanthenes: Decreased seizure threshold
MAO inhibitors: Prolonged phenobarbital effects and possibly altered pattern of seizure activity
maprotiline: Increased CNS depression, decreased seizure threshold at high doses, and decreased phenobarbital effectiveness
methoxyflurane: Possibly hepatotoxicity and nephrotoxicity
methylphenidate: Increased risk of phenobarbital toxicity
mexiletine: Decreased blood mexiletine level
oral anticoagulants: Decreased anticoagulant activity and increased risk of bleeding when phenobarbital is discontinued
pituitary hormones (posterior): Increased risk of arrhythmias and coronary insufficiency
primidone: Altered pattern of seizures and increased CNS effects of both drugs
valproate, valproic acid: Decreased phenobarbital metabolism and increased risk of barbiturate toxicity
vitamin D: Decreased phenobarbital effectiveness
xanthines: Increased xanthine metabolism and antagonized hypnotic effect of phenobarbital
belladonna alkaloids
amantadine: Increased adverse anticholinergic effects
atenolol, digoxin: Possibly increased therapeutic and adverse effects of these drugs
phenothiazines: Possibly decreased phenothiazine effectiveness and increased adverse effects of belladonna alkaloids
tricyclic antidepressants: Possibly increased adverse anticholinergic effects
ACTIVITIES
phenobarbital
alcohol use: Additive CNS depression

Adverse Reactions

CNS: Anxiety, CNS stimulation (with high doses), confusion, depression, dizziness, drowsiness, headache, insomnia, irritability, lethargy, mood changes, nervousness, paradoxical stimulation, sedation, vertigo, weakness
CV: Bradycardia, hypotension, palpitations, tachycardia
EENT: Altered taste, blurred vision, cycloplegia, dry mouth, increased intraocular pressure, miosis, mydriasis, nasal congestion, photophobia, ptosis
ENDO: Suppression of lactation
GI: Bloating, constipation, diarrhea, dysphagia, heartburn, ileus, nausea, vomiting

GU: Decreased libido, impotence, urinary hesitancy, urine retention

MS: Arthralgia, bone tenderness, musculoskeletal pain

RESP: Bronchospasm, respiratory depression

SKIN: Decreased sweating, dermatitis, flushing, photosensitivity, rash, urticaria, xerostomia

Other: Anaphylaxis, physical and psychological dependence

Nursing Considerations

- Be aware that drug shouldn't be given during third trimester of pregnancy because repeated use of phenobarbital can cause dependence in neonate. Drug also shouldn't be given to breast-feeding women because it may cause CNS depression in infants.

- Use drug cautiously in patients with allergies, arrhythmias, asthma, autonomic neuropathy, coronary artery disease, debilitating chronic lung disease, heart failure, hepatic or renal dysfunction, hypertension, hyperthyroidism, tachycardia, and prostatic hypertrophy because of adverse effects of drug.

- Monitor patient's respiratory status before each dose because drug can cause respiratory depression, especially in patient with bronchopneumonia, pulmonary disease, respiratory tract infection, or status asthmaticus.

- Monitor patient for diarrhea, which may be an early sign of incomplete intestinal obstruction, especially in patients with ileostomy or colostomy. If present, withhold drug and notify prescriber.

- **WARNING** Monitor elderly patients for excitement, agitation, drowsiness, and confusion, even with small doses. Elderly patients are more sensitive to the effects of the combination drug and are more likely to develop these adverse reactions. If they develop, notify prescriber because dosage may need to be decreased.

- Anticipate that phenobarbital may worsen major depression, suicidal tendencies, or other mental disorders.

- Monitor patient receiving anticoagulant therapy because phenobarbital may necessitate larger doses of the anticoagulant for optimal effect. When drug is stopped, the anticoagulant dose may have to be decreased.

- Take safety precautions to protect patient from injury from falling.

- If patient has received drug for a prolonged period, expect to taper dosage slowly to prevent withdrawal symptoms when drug is discontinued because of phenobarbital.

PATIENT TEACHING
- Tell patient to take drug exactly as prescribed and not to increased dosage or dosing frequency without consulting prescriber because drug may become habit forming.
- Instruct patient to take elixir form undiluted or to mix it with water, milk, or fruit juice and to use a calibrated device to ensure accurate dosage.
- Tell patient to notify prescriber if she has persistent or severe diarrhea, constipation, or difficulty urinating.
- Caution patient to avoid driving and similar activities until the effects of the drug is known.
- **WARNING** Urge patient to avoid extremely hot or humid conditions because heatstroke may occur.
- Urge patient to avoid alcohol during therapy.
- Caution patient on prolonged therapy not to stop drug abruptly because withdrawal symptoms may result from stopping phenobarbital.
- Alert female patient to notify prescriber about suspected, known, or intended pregnancy. Advise against breast-feeding during therapy.

polyethylene glycol, sodium sulfate, sodium chloride, and potassium chloride

MoviPrep

Class and Category

Chemical: Polymer of ethylene oxide (polyethylene glycol), electrolyte minerals (sodium sulfate, sodium chloride, potassium chloride)

Therapeutic: Colon cleanser (polyethylene glycol, sodium sulfate, sodium chloride, potassium chloride)

Pregnancy category: C

Indications and Dosages

▶ *To cleanse the colon in preparation for colonoscopy*

ORAL SOLUTION

Adults. *For split-dose regimen:* 1 liter (100 grams polyethylene glycol, 7.5 grams sodium sulfate, 2.64 grams sodium chloride, 1.015 grams potassium chloride) split into 8 ounces of solution every 15 minutes until 1 liter is consumed followed by 0.5 liters of clear fluid the evening before the colonoscopy. Then, on the morning of the colonoscopy, 1 liter (100 grams polyethylene glycol, 7.5 grams sodium sulfate, 2.64 grams sodium chloride, 1.015 grams potassium chloride) split into 8 ounces of solution every 15 minutes until 1 liter is consumed followed by 0.5 liters of clear fluid at least 1 hr before colonoscopy. *For evening-only regimen:* 1 liter (100 grams polyethylene glycol, 7.5 grams sodium sulfate, 2.64 grams sodium chloride, 1.015 grams potassium chloride) split into 8 ounces of solution every 15 minutes until 1 liter is consumed starting about 6 PM the night before the colonoscopy, followed in 1.5 hours with another 1 liter (100 grams polyethylene glycol, 7.5 grams sodium sulfate, 2.64 grams sodium chloride, 1.015 grams potassium chloride) split into 8 ounces of solution every 15 minutes until 1 liter is consumed followed by 1 liter of clear liquids of additional fluid during the evening before the colonoscopy.

Mechanism of Action
Collectively, polyethylene glycol, sodium sulfate, sodium chloride, and potassium chloride produce an osmotic action in the intestines that causes large amounts of water to be drawn into the colon. This action stimulates the colon to evacuate its contents. The end result is a purgative effect.

Contraindications
Hypersensitivity to polyethylene glycol, sodium sulfate, sodium chloride, or potassium chloride, or their components

Interactions
DRUGS

polyethylene glycol, sodium sulfate, sodium chloride, or potassium chloride
all oral drugs: Decreased absorption of oral drugs if given within 1 hour of start of colon-cleansing preparation

Adverse Reactions
CNS: Dizziness, headache, malaise, rigors, seizures, sleep disturbance, thirst
CV: Asystole, chest tightness
EENT: Throat tightness
GI: Abdominal distention or pain, anal discomfort, dyspepsia, esophageal perforation, GI bleeding, hunger, nausea
RESP: Acute pulmonary edema, dyspnea
SKIN: Rash, urticaria

Other: Anaphylaxis, angioedema of lip and face, hyperphosphatemia, hypokalemia, thirst

Nursing Considerations

- Use polyethylene glycol, sodium sulfate, sodium chloride, and potassium chloride with extreme caution in a patient with significant GI dysfunction, such as severe ulcerative colitis, gastric retention, or toxic colitis.
- Expect additional testing for a patient with suspected GI obstruction or perforation to determine if the drug can be given safely.
- Use cautiously in patients taking drugs that increase the risk of electrolyte abnormalities, such as diuretics and ACE inhibitors. Also use cautiously in patients with hyponatremia. Expect to obtain a baseline and post-procedure measures of electrolyte status, as ordered, when using this combination as a bowel cleanser.
- Use polyethylene glycol, sodium sulfate, sodium chloride, and potassium chloride cautiously in patients with glucose-6-phosphate dehydrogenase deficiency, especially if patient also has an active infection, a history of hemolysis, or concurrent drug therapy known to precipitate hemolytic reactions because it contains sodium ascorbate and ascorbic acid.
- Monitor patient for seizure activity because, although rare, generalized tonic-clonic seizures may occur in patients with no history of seizures when polyethylene glycol is used.
- Assess patient's tolerance of the drug throughout administration, especially if patient has an impaired gag reflex or is prone to regurgitate or aspirate.
- Expect to withhold or slow delivery of the drug until symptoms subside, as ordered, in patients who complain of severe bloating, abdominal distention, or abdominal pain.

PATIENT TEACHING

- Instruct patient to take polyethylene glycol, sodium sulfate, sodium chloride, and potassium chloride exactly as prescribed and not to add ingredients, such as flavoring, to it.
- Advise patient to maintain adequate hydration throughout drug administration as well as after the colonoscopy.
- Tell him he may have clear soup or plain yogurt for dinner the night before the procedure but no solid foods from about 1 hour before starting the colonoscopy preparation until after the procedure is over. Urge him to continue drinking clear fluids during the preparation time.

- Alert patient that the first bowel movement may occur within 1 hour of starting the drug therapy and that he should stay close to the toilet throughout administration.
- Instruct patient to stop drinking solution until symptoms subside or to drink each portion at longer intervals if he has severe abdominal discomfort or distention.
- Tell patient to stop drug administration and seek emergency care if he has a seizure.

sodium phenylacetate 10% and sodium benzoate 10%

Ammonul, Ucephan

Class and Category

Chemical: Naturally occurring peptide fraction (sodium phenylacetate), salt of benzoic acid (sodium benzoate)

Therapeutic: Antihyperammonemic (sodium phenylacetate, sodium benzoate)

Pregnancy category: C

Indications and Dosages

▶ *As adjunct to treat acute hyperammonemia and associated encephalopathy in patients with enzyme deficiencies in the urea cycle*

I.V. INFUSION (AMMONUL)

Adults and children weighing more than 20 kg (44 lb). *Initial:* 5,500 mg sodium phenylacetate and 5,500 mg sodium benzoate (55 ml)/m^2 infused over 90 to 120 minutes as a loading dose. *Maintenance:* Following loading dose, 5,500 mg sodium phenylacetate and 5,500 mg sodium benzoate (55 ml)/m^2 infused over 24 hours daily until plasma ammonia level has returned to normal or patient can tolerate oral nutrition and oral medication. Loading and maintenance doses given with arginine hydrochloride 10%.

Children weighing 20 kg or less. *Initial:* 250 mg sodium phenylacetate and 250 mg sodium benzoate (2.5 ml)/kg infused over 90 to 120 minutes as a loading dose. *Maintenance:* Following loading dose, 250 mg sodium phenylacetate and 250 mg sodium benzoate (2.5 ml)/kg infused over 24 hours daily until plasma ammonia level has returned to normal or patient can tolerate oral nutrition and oral medication. Loading and maintenance doses given with arginine hydrochloride 10%.

▶ *To prevent or treat hyperammonemia in patients with urea cycle enzymopathy (UCE) from carbamylphosphate synthetase, ornithine transcarbamylase, or arginosuccinate synthetase deficiency.*

ORAL SOLUTION (UCEPHAN)

Adults and children. 250 mg sodium phenylacetate and 250 mg sodium benzoate (2.5 ml)/kg daily divided into three to six doses. *Maximum:* 10 grams sodium phenylacetate and 10 grams sodium benzoate (100 ml) daily.

Mechanism of Action

Sodium phenylacetate conjugates with glutamine in the liver and kidneys to form phenylacetylglutamine, via acetylation. Phenylacetylglutamine is excreted by the kidneys through glomerular filtration and tubular secretion. The nitrogen content of phenylacetylglutamine per mole is identical to that of urea, so it can serve as an alternative to urea for excretion of waste nitrogen.

Benzoate undergoes acetylation and then conjugates with glycine to form hippuric acid, which is rapidly excreted by the kidneys through glomerular filtration and tubular secretion. One mole of hippuric acid contains one mole of waste nitrogen, which serves as an alternative to urea for excretion of waste nitrogen.

Since both sodium phenylacetate and sodium benzoate are metabolically active compounds that can serve as alternatives to urea for excretion of waste nitrogen, they can significantly reduce waste nitrogen levels in patients with deficiencies of urea cycle enzymes. This action decreases ammonia levels in the body and the risk of glutamine-induced neurotoxicity.

Contraindications

Hypersensitivity to sodium phenylacetate, sodium benzoate, or their components

Interactions

DRUGS

sodium phenylacetate and sodium benzoate

pencillin, valproic acid: Possibly decreased effectiveness of sodium phenylacetate and sodium benzoate

probenecid: Possibly decreased excretion of sodium phenylacetate and sodium benzoate

Adverse Reactions

CNS: Acute psychosis, aggression, agitation, asthenia, ataxia, cerebral edema, coma, confusion, fever, hallucinations, increased intracranial pressure, mental impairment, paralysis, subdural hematoma, seizures, stroke, tremor, tetany

CV: Atrial rupture, cardiac arrest or failure, cardiogenic shock, cardiomopathy, chest pain, edema, hypertension, hypotension, pericardial effusion, phlebothrombosis, thrombosis

EENT: Blindness

ENDO: Hyperglycemia, hypoglycemia

GI: Cholestasis, diarrhea, GI hemorrhage, hepatic artery stenosis, hepatic failure, jaundice, nausea, vomiting

GU: Anuria, renal failure, urine retention, UTI

HEME: Anemia, coagulopathy, disseminated intravascular coagulation, hemorrhage, pancytopenia, thrombocytopenia

RESP: Acute respiratory distress syndrome, dyspnea, hypercapnia, hyperventilation, pneumothorax, pulmonary edema or hemorrhage, respiratory acidosis or alkalosis, respiratory distress or failure, tachypnea

SKIN: Alopecia, flushing, generalized or maculo-papular rash, pruritus, urticaria

Other: Dehydration, hyperammonemia, hyperkalemia, hypernatremia, hypocalcemia, hypokalemia, infusion site infection, metabolic acidosis or alkalosis, sepsis, septic shock

Nursing Considerations

- Administer sodium phenylacetate and sodium benzoate cautiously to patients with hepatic or renal insufficiency because drug is metabolized in the liver and excreted by the kidneys.
- Dosage for intravenous sodium phenylacetate and sodium benzoate is determined by weight for children weighing 20 kg (44 lb) or less and body surface area for adults and for children weighing more than 20 kg.
- Dilute intravenous form of sodium phenylacetate and sodium benzoate with sterile dextrose injection, 10% ($D_{10}W$) following manufacturer guidelines to obtain a dilution that is greater than 25 ml/kg before administration. During the admixture process, when injecting the intravenous form of the drug into the $D_{10}W$ bag, use a Millex Durapore GV 33 mm sterile syringe filter to prevent any particulate matter that might be present in the drug from entering the final mixture.
- **WARNING** Administer intravenous sodium phenylacetate and sodium benzoate only through a central line because burns may occur if drug is infused through a peripheral line. Monitor infusion closely for any evidence of infiltration because infiltration into perivenous tissues may cause skin ne-

crosis. If infiltration occurs, change infusion site, monitor infiltrated site closely, aspirate residual drug from catheter, elevate affected arm, and apply cold packs intermittently, as ordered.

- Intravenous arginine must be given with intravenous sodium phenylacetate and sodium benzoate for acute treatment of hyperammonia caused by carbamyl phosphate synthetase, omithine transcarbamylase, arginosuccinate synthetase, or argininosuccinate lyase deficiency. It may be mixed in the same solution as sodium phenylacetate and sodium benzoate and given together.

- Other than arginine, don't mix any other drug in the same intravenous solution with sodium phenylacetate and sodium benzoate.

- Before starting intravenous sodium phenylacetate and sodium benzoate therapy, stop giving analogous drugs, such as oral sodium phenylbutyrate or an oral sodium phenylbutyrate and sodium benzoate combination, as ordered. Start or resume oral therapy with sodium phenylacetate alone or sodium phenylacetate and sodium benzoate together, as ordered, when ammonia level has returned to normal and intravenous delivery is no longer needed.

- Dilute each oral dose of sodium phenylacetate and sodium benzoate in 4 to 8 ounces of infant formula or milk, and administer with meals.

- Avoid letting drug contact skin or clothing when diluting or administering because drug has a lingering odor.

- Prepare patient for hemodialysis in cases of hyperammonemic coma or life-threatening ammonia levels. Expect hemodialysis to be repeated until patient's plasma ammonia level is near normal.

- Provide supportive care during therapy, with supplemental caloric intake and restriction of dietary protein, as ordered.

- **WARNING** Monitor patient closely for edema because drug has a high sodium content. If patient develops congestive heart failure or severe renal failure, notify prescriber and expect to stop sodium phenylacetate and sodium benzoate and provide supportive care, as ordered.

- If patient has nausea or vomiting during intravenous delivery, notify prescriber and, if ordered, give an antiemetic during the infusion.

- Monitor patient's neurologic status and response to treatment closely.

- Monitor patient's electrolyte and plasma ammonia levels, as ordered.

PATIENT TEACHING

- Instruct patient or caregiver to mix each oral dose of sodium phenylacetate and sodium benzoate with 4 to 8 ounces of infant formula or milk and to take with meals.
- Caution patient or caregiver not to mix oral drug with other liquids.
- Tell patient to avoid letting drug contact his skin or clothing because drug has a lingering odor.
- Advise patient to report any adverse effects during and after administration of sodium phenylacetate and sodium benzoate because they may become severe quickly.
- Tell patient prescribed the intravenous form of the drug that it will need to be given as a continuous infusion through a central line.
- Explain hemodialysis to the patient who must undergo this procedure.

sodium phosphate monobasic monohydrate and sodium phosphate dibasic anhydrous

Visicol

Class and Category

Chemical: Electrolyte minerals (sodium phosphate monobasic monohydrate, sodium phosphate dibasic anhydrous)
Therapeutic: Colon cleanser (sodium phosphate monobasic monohydrate, sodium phosphate dibasic anhydrous)
Pregnancy category: C

Indications and Dosages

▶ *To cleanse the colon before colonoscopy*

TABLETS

Adults. 3.306 grams sodium phosphate monobasic monohydrate and 1.194 grams sodium phosphate dibasic anhydrous (3 tablets) with 8 oz of water every 15 minutes until 18 tablets have been ingested, followed by 2.204 grams sodium phosphate monobasic monohydrate and 0.797 grams sodium phosphate dibasic anhydrous (2 tablets) with 8 oz of water for a total dose of 30 grams of sodium phosphate monobasic monohydrate and sodium phosphate dibasic anhydrous (20 tablets) the evening before the colonoscopy. Then, starting 3 to 5 hours before the colonoscopy, 3.306 grams sodium phosphate monobasic monohydrate and 1.194 grams sodium phosphate dibasic anhydrous (3 tablets) with 8 oz of water every 15 minutes until 18 tablets have been ingested followed by 2.204 grams sodium phosphate monobasic monohydrate and 0.797 grams sodium phosphate dibasic anhydrous (2 tablets) with 8 oz of water for a total of 30 grams (20 tablets).

Mechanism of Action
Both sodium phosphate monobasic monohydrate and sodium phosphate dibasic anhydrous produce an osmotic action in the colon through sodium accumulating in the colon, which causes large amounts of water to be drawn into the colon. The result is a purgative effect.

Contraindications
Acute phosphate nephropathy, hypersensitivity to sodium phosphate salts or their components

Interactions
DRUGS
sodium phosphate monobasic monohydrate and sodium phosphate dibasic anhydrous
all drugs during administration of sodium phosphate salts: Lack of absorption

Adverse Reactions
CNS: Paresthesia of the lips, seizures
CV: Arrhythmias
EENT: Tongue edema
GI: Abdominal bloating and pain, mucosal bleeding, nausea, vomiting
GU: Acute phosphate nephropathy, acute renal failure
SKIN: Paresthesia of the lips, pruritus, rash, urticaria
Other: Hyperphosphatemia, hypophosphatemia, hypocalcemia, hypokalemia

Nursing Considerations
• Use sodium phosphate salts cautiously in patients with severe renal insufficiency, congestive heart failure, ascites, unstable angina, acute bowel obstruction, bowel perforation, irritable bowel disorder, toxic megacolon, gastric retention, ileus,

pseudo-obstruction of the bowel, severe chronic constipation, acute colitis, gastric bypass surgery, gastric stapling surgery, gastric hypomotility syndrome, recent cardiac surgery, or therapy with drugs that affect renal perfusion or function, such as diuretics, ACE inhibitors, angiotensin receptor blockers, and possibly NSAIDs because of the increased risk of serious adverse effects.

• Be prepared to obtain a baseline and then post-colonoscopy evaluation of the patient's serum phosphate, calcium, potassium, sodium, creatinine, and BUN levels, as ordered, especially in patients at risk for serious adverse effects, such as those with a history of renal insufficiency; those who might be prone to acute phosphate nephropathy; those with electrolyte disorders, seizures, arrhythmias, cardiomyopathy, a prolonged QT interval, or a recent history of MI; and those who develop vomiting or signs of dehydration with drug administration.

• Correct any electrolyte imbalance, as ordered, before giving sodium phosphate salts.

• Because of the phosphate content of sodium phosphate monobasic monohydrate and sodium phosphate dibasic anhydrous, monitor patient closely for fluid and electrolyte abnormalities and cardiac arrhythmias, especially if patient has renal insufficiency, bowel perforation, or previous misuse or overdose of this drug.

• Institute seizure precautions in patients who have a history of seizures and patients at increased risk of seizures, such as those taking drugs that lower the seizure threshold (such as tricyclic antidepressants), those withdrawing from alcohol or benzodiazepines, and those with hyponatremia.

• Expect to obtain a pre-dose and post-colonoscopy ECG, as ordered, in patients at high risk for serious cardiac arrhythmias such as patients with cardiomyopathy, prolonged QT interval, history of uncontrolled arrhythmias, or a recent history of myocardial infarction.

PATIENT TEACHING

• Instruct patient to take sodium phosphate salts exactly as prescribed and to drink 8 ounces of clear liquids with every 3-tablet dose and final 2-tablet dose for each of the two regimens for a total of 3.6 quarts of fluids.

• Caution patient to avoid taking additional laxatives or purgatives, especially sodium phosphate–based products to prepare for colonoscopy.

- Stress the need to stop taking the drug and contact the prescriber immediately if vomiting or other serious adverse reactions develop, such as hives, rash, or a sudden change in sense of well-being.
- Alert patient that blood tests and an ECG may be needed before and after drug administration.

Genitourinary Drugs

belladonna and opium

B & O Suppositories, B & O Supprettes No. 15A,
B & O Supprettes No. 16A

Class, Category, and Schedule

Chemical: Naturally occurring belladonna leaf herb (belladonna),
naturally occurring dried milky exudate of the Papaver som-
niferum Linne or its variety album De Candolle plant (opium)
Therapeutic: Geniturinary analgesic
Pregnancy category: C
Controlled substance schedule: II

Indications and Dosages

▶ *To relieve moderate to severe pain from ureteral spasm following GU
surgery that is unresponsive to nonopioid analgesics*
SUPPOSITORY
Adults. 16.2 mg belladonna and 30 mg opium (1 suppository) or
16.2 mg belladonna and 60 mg opium (1 suppository) daily or
b.i.d.

Mechanism of Action

Belladonna leaf contains several alkaloids, mainly L-hyoscyamine (which
probably racemizes to atropine during extraction) and scopolamine. Atropine
dominates belladonna's effect, inhibiting acetylcholine's muscarinic action at
the neuroeffector junctions of smooth muscles of the urinary bladder. It decreases urinary tract motility and smooth muscle contractions, thereby relieving ureteral spasms and pain.

Opium contains several opioid alkaloids, including morphine. Morphine
dominates the effect of opium binding with and activating opioid receptors
(primarily mu receptors) in the brain and spinal cord to produce analgesia
and euphoria.

Contraindications

Acute alcoholism, angle-closure glaucoma; asthma; GI obstructive disease (alchalasia, pyloric obstruction, pyloroduodenal stenosis); hepatic disease; hypersensitivity to belladonna, atropine, opium, morphine, or their components; ileus; intestinal atony; labor (with premature delivery); myasthenia gravis; myocardial ischemia; obstructive uropathy; renal disease; respiratory depression, severe ulcerative colitis; tachycardia; toxic megacolon; unstable cardiovascular status in acute hemorrhage; upper airway obstruction

Interactions

DRUGS

belladonna and opium

anticholinergics: Increased risk of severe constipation leading to ileus, urine retention

antihistamines: Possibly excessive anticholinergic activity

belladonna

amantadine, antidyskinetics, meperidine, muscle relaxants, phenothiazines, tricyclic antidepressants and other drugs with anticholinergic properties including antiarrhythmics (disopyramide, procainamide, quinidine), buclizine, meclizine: Increased anticholinergic effect

antimyasthenics: Reduced intestinal motility

cyclopropane: Increased risk of ventricular arrhythmias

metoclopramide: Decreased effect on GI motility

opioid analgesics: Increased risk of ileus, severe constipation, and urine retention

potassium chloride, especially wax-matrix forms: Possibly GI ulcers

opium

amitriptyline, clomipramine, nortriptyline: Increased CNS and respiratory depression

anticholinergics: Possibly severe constipation leading to ileus, urine retention

antidiarrheals such as loperamide and paregoric: CNS depression, possibly severe constipation

antihistamines, chloral hydrate, glutethimide, MAO inhibitors, methocarbamol: Increased CNS and respiratory depressant effects of opium

antihypertensives, hypotension-producing drugs: Increased hypotension, risk of orthostatic hypotension

buprenorphine: Decreased therapeutic effects of morphine, increased respiratory depression, possibly withdrawal symptoms

cimetidine: Increased analgesic and CNS and respiratory depressant effects of opium

CNS depressants: Possibly coma, hypotension, respiratory depression, severe sedation

diuretics: Decreased diuretic efficacy

metoclopramide: Possibly antagonized metoclopramide effect on GI motility

mixed agonist-antagonist analgesics: Possibly withdrawal symptoms

naloxone: Antagonized analgesic and CNS and respiratory depressant effects of opium (morphine), possibly withdrawal symptoms

naltrexone: Possibly induction or worsening of withdrawal symptoms if opium given within 7 to 10 days before naltrexone

neuromuscular blockers: Increased or prolonged respiratory depression

opioid analgesics: Increased CNS and respiratory depression, increased hypotension

ACTIVITIES

opium

alcohol use: Increased CNS and respiratory depression, increased hypotension

Adverse Reactions

CNS: Agitation, amnesia, anxiety, ataxia, Babinski's or Chaddock's reflex, behavioral changes, coma, confusion, decreased concentration, decreased tendon reflexes, delirium, delusions, depression, dizziness, drowsiness, euphoria, fever, hallucinations, headache, hyperreflexia, insomnia, lethargy, light-headedness, malaise, mania, nervousness, paranoia, psychosis, restlessness, sedation, seizures, somnolence, stupor, syncope, tremor, vertigo, weakness

CV: Arrhythmias, bradycardia, cardiac arrest, cardiac dilation, chest pain, hypertension, hypotension, orthostatic hypotension, left ventricular failure, MI, palpitations, shock, tachycardia, weak or impalpable peripheral pulses

EENT: Acute angle-closure glaucoma, altered taste, blepharitis, blindness, blurred vision, conjunctivitis, cyclophoria, cycloplegia, decreased visual acuity or accommodation, diplopia, dry mouth, eye irritation, eyelid crusting, heterophoria, increased intraocular pressure, keratoconjunctivitis, lacrimation, laryngitis, laryngeal edema or laryngospasm (allergic), miosis, mydriasis, nasal congestion, nystagmus, oral lesions, photophobia, pupils poorly reactive to light, rhinitis, strabismus, tongue chewing

GI: Abdominal cramps or distention, abdominal pain, anorexia, biliary tract spasm, bloating, constipation, decreased bowel sounds, delayed gastric emptying, diarrhea, dysphagia, elevated liver function test results, gastroesophageal reflux, heartburn, hiccups, ileus and toxic megacolon in patients with inflammatory bowel disease, intestinal obstruction, indigestion, nausea, vomiting

GU: Bladder distention, decreased ejaculate potency, decreased libido, difficult ejaculation, enuresis, impotence, prolonged labor, urinary hesitancy, urinary urgency, urine retention

HEME: Anemia, leukopenia, thrombocytopenia

MS: Arthralgia, dysarthria, hypertonia, muscle twitching

RESP: Apnea, asthma exacerbation, atelectasis, bradypnea, bronchospasm, depressed cough reflex, dyspnea, hypoventilation, inspiratory stridor, pulmonary edema, respiratory depression or arrest, shallow breathing, subcostal recession, tachypnea, wheezing

SKIN: Cold skin, cyanosis, decreased sweating, dermatitis, diaphoresis, flushing, pallor, pruritus, rash, urticaria

Other: Allergic reaction, anaphylaxis, dehydration, facial edema, physical and psychological dependence, polydipsia, sensations of warmth, withdrawal symptoms

Nursing Considerations
- Before therapy begins, assess patient's current drug use, including all prescription and OTC drugs.
- If rectal suppository is too soft to insert, chill it in refrigerator for 30 minutes or run wrapped suppository under cold water.
- **WARNING** Monitor patient's respiratory and cardiovascular status carefully and frequently during belladonna and opium therapy. Be alert for changes in vital signs that could signal presence of arrhythmias, respiratory depression, and hypotension.
- Evaluate patient for therapeutic response, including report of decreased pain and body movements that suggest pain relief.
- Watch for excessive or persistent sedation; if patient is on higher dosage of opium, it may need to be lowered.
- Be aware that belladonna and opium may cause physical and psychological dependence; watch carefully for drug tolerance and withdrawal symptoms, such as body aches, diaphoresis, diarrhea, fever, piloerection, rhinorrhea, sneezing, and yawning.
- Be aware that opium may have a prolonged duration and cumulative effect in patients with impaired hepatic or renal function. Monitor patient carefully.
- Assess bowel and bladder elimination. Notify prescriber if diarrhea, constipation, urinary hesitancy, or urine retention develop.

PATIENT TEACHING
- Instruct patient to take belladonna and opium exactly as prescribed and not to change dosage without consulting prescriber.
- Tell patient to moisten rectal suppository before inserting it.
- Urge patient to avoid alcohol and other CNS depressants during belladonna and opium therapy.
- Advise patient to avoid hazardous activities while taking belladonna and opium until the CNS effects are known.
- Teach patient to change position slowly to minimize effects of orthostatic hypotension.
- Instruct patient to notify prescriber about worsening or breakthrough pain.
- Inform patient that belladonna and opium may be habit-forming. Urge him to notify prescriber if he experiences anxiety, decreased appetite, excessive tearing, irritability, muscle aches or twitching, rapid heart rate, or yawning.
- Advise patient to notify prescriber if he has persistent or severe diarrhea, constipation, or difficulty urinating.

citric acid monohydrate, potassium citrate monohydrate, and sodium citrate dihydrate

Tricitrates

Class and Category
Chemical: Base (citric acid), potassium derivative of base (potassium citrate), sodium derivative of base (sodium citrate)
Therapeutic: Urinary alkalinizers (citric acid, potassium citrate, sodium citrate)
Pregnancy category: NR

Indications and Dosages
▶ *To provide long-term maintenance of alkaline urine when managing chronic metabolic acidosis caused by such conditions as chronic renal insufficiency or renal tubular acidosis*
SOLUTION
Adults. 1,002 to 2,004 mg citric acid, 1,650 to 3,300 mg potassium citrate, and 1,500 to 3,000 mg sodium citrate (15 to 30 ml) q.i.d. after meals and at bedtime.
Children. 334 to 1,002 mg citric acid, 550 to 1,650 mg potassium citrate, and 500 to 1,500 mg sodium citrate (5 to 15 ml) q.i.d. after meals and at bedtime.

> ## Mechanism of Action
> Citrate acid, potassium citrate, and sodium citrate are oxidized in the body to form bicarbonate, a buffer, which increases urinary pH as it is readily excreted in urine.

Contraindications
Azotemia, hyperkalemia, hypernatremia, oliguria, severe myocardial damage or renal impairment, untreated Addison's disease, use with sodium restricted diets

Adverse Reactions
GI: Laxative effect, nausea, vomiting
Other: Hyperkalemia, hypernatremia, metabolic alkalosis

Nursing Considerations
- Use with extreme caution in patients who need to limit intake of sodium and potassium and in patients with heart failure, hypertension, renal dysfunction, peripheral or pulmonary edema, or toxemia of pregnancy.
- Use cautiously in patients with low urine output.
- Monitor patient's serum electrolyte and acid-base status, as ordered, because electrolyte imbalance or metabolic alkalosis may occur, especially in patients with renal impairment.

PATIENT TEACHING
- Instruct patient to take citric acid, potassium citrate, and sodium citrate exactly as prescribed because excessive amounts can cause tetany or depress heart function.
- Instruct patient to store drug solution in a tight container and protect from extreme heat or cold.
- Tell patient to take drug after meals and at bedtime to minimize the laxative effect of the drug.
- Reassure patient that the drug is pleasant tasting.

neomycin sulfate and polymyxin B sulfate irrigant
Neosporin G.U. Irrigant

Class and Category
Chemical: Aminoglycoside (neomycin), polypeptide (polymyxin B sulfate)

Therapeutic: Antibiotic
Pregnancy category: D

Indications and Dosages

▶ *To prevent bacteriuria and gram-negative rod septicemia associated with the use of indwelling catheters*

IRRIGANT

Adults. 1-ml ampule diluted in 1,000 ml of isotonic saline solution, continuously irrigating the urinary bladder over 24 hr via a three-way catheter every day for up to 10 days.

Mechanism of Action

Both neomycin and polymyxin B are bactericidal. Neomycin competes with messenger RNA in bacterial cells to bind with a specific receptor protein on the 30S ribosomal subunit of DNA. This action causes abnormal, nonfunctioning proteins to form. A lack of functional proteins causes bacterial cell death.

Polymyxin B binds to cell membrane phospholipids in gram-negative bacteria, increasing the permeability of the cell membrane. It also acts as a cationic detergent, altering the osmotic barrier of the membrane and causing essential intracellular metabolites to leak. These actions results in cell death.

Contraindications

Bladder mucosa or wall tears, bladder surgery involving bladder wall, hypersensitivity to neomycin, other aminoglycosides, polymyxin B or other polymyxins or their components, or history of a serious reaction to neomycin or other aminoglycosides

Interactions

DRUGS

neomycin and polymyxin B

general anesthetics, neuromuscular blockers, skeletal muscle relaxants: Increased or prolonged skeletal muscle relaxation, possibly respiratory paralysis

neomycin

dimenhydrinate: Possibly masked symptoms of neomycin-induced ototoxicity

oral anticoagulants: Possibly potentiated anticoagulant effects

polymyxin B

nephrotoxic and neurotoxic drugs (such as aminoglycosides, amphotericin B, colistin, sodium citrate, streptomycin, tobramycin, and vancomycin): Increased risk of nephrotoxicity and neurotoxicity

Adverse Reactions

EENT: Hearing impairment (only if absorption inadvertently occurs), tinnitus (only if absorption inadvertently occurs)
GU: Irritation of urinary bladder mucosa, renal dysfunction (only if absorption inadvertently occurs)

Nursing Considerations

• Add 1 ampule of neomycin and polymyxin B to a 1,000-ml container of isotonic saline solution using aseptic technique. Use within 48 hours. When ready to use, connect the 1,000-ml container to the inflow lumen of the three-way urinary catheter and begin flow.
• Monitor flow rate of the irrigation solution to deliver 1,000 ml continuously over 24 hours. If the patient's urine output exceeds 2 liters in 24 hours, notify prescriber to determine if rate should be adjusted to deliver 2,000 ml of neomycin and polymyxin B solution over 24 hours.
• Don't interrupt the flow of irrigation solution into the bladder for longer than a few minutes, and only if absolutely necessary because effectiveness to prevent a bladder infection will be compromised with less than continuous irrigation.
• Obtain urine specimens for urinalysis and culture and sensitivity testing routinely throughout neomycin and polymyxin B therapy, as ordered. Notify prescriber of any abnormal findings.
• Be aware that neomycin and polymyxin B usually isn't absorbed systemically as long as the irrigation does not go beyond 10 days.
• Watch closely for neuromuscular blockade, nephrotoxicity, or ototoxicity if patient is receiving high doses or prolonged treatment or patient is elderly, dehydrated, or has impaired renal function.

PATIENT TEACHING
• Advise patient to notify prescriber about hearing loss or ringing in the ears.
• Tell patient to alert prescriber if she suspects or knows she is pregnant because the neomycin portion of the drug can cross the placenta if it is inadvertently absorbed.

potassium acid phosphate and sodium acid phosphate

K-Phos M.F., K Phos No. 2

Class and Category
Chemical: Electrolyte minerals (potassium acid phosphate, sodium acid phosphate)
Therapeutic: Urinary acidifiers (potassium acid phosphate, sodium acid phosphate)
Pregnancy category: C

Indications and Dosages
▶ *To acidify urine and lower urinary calcium concentration*
TABLETS
Adults. 155 mg to 610 mg potassium acid phosphate and 350 mg to 1,400 mg sodium acid phosphate (1 to 2 tablets depending on product used) q.i.d. *Maximum:* 8 tablets daily.

Mechanism of Action
Potassium acid phosphate and sodium acid phosphate increases serum phosphate levels. At the renal distal tubule, hydrogen secretion by the tubular cell in exchange for sodium in the tubular urine converts dibasic phosphate salts to monobasic phosphate salts. This causes large amounts of acid to be excreted without lowering urine pH to a degree that would block hydrogen transport by a high concentration gradient between the tubular cell and luminal fluid. Phosphate salts lower urinary calcium level because an increase in serum phosphorus level causes a decrease in calcium level. This effect may involve increased bone formation, movement of calcium into cells, decreased bone resorption, or decreased calcium absorption.

Contraindications
Hyperkalemia, hyperphosphatemia, infected magnesium ammonium phosphate stones, renal insufficiency less than 30% normal

Interactions
DRUGS
potassium acid phosphate and sodium acid phosphate
potassium supplements: Increased risk of hyperkalemia
salicylates: Reduced excretion of salicylates which may lead to salicylate toxicity
FOODS
potassium acid phosphate and sodium acid phosphate
sodium-rich foods, salt: Increased risk of hypernatremia

Adverse Reactions
CNS: Confusion, dizziness, headache, numbness, seizures, thirst, tingling, tiredness, weakness

CV: Irregular heartbeat, peripheral edema, tachycardia
EENT: Numbness or tingling around lips
GI: Abdominal discomfort, diarrhea, nausea, vomiting
GU: Low urine output
MS: Bone and joint pain, heaviness of legs, muscle cramps, pain or weakness in hands and feet
RESP: Shortness of breath
Other: Weight gain

Nursing Considerations

- Use cautiously in patients with cardiac disease (including heart failure), Addison's disease, acute dehydration, hepatic or renal impairment, extensive tissue breakdown (as with burns), congenital myotonia, hypernatremia, hypertension, toxemia of pregnancy, hypoparathyroidism, acute panceatitis, and rickets.
- Monitor renal function and serum electrolyte test results, as ordered because electrolyte imbalances can result in serious adverse effects.
- Be aware that high serum phosphate levels increase the risk of extra skeletal calcification.

PATIENT TEACHING

- Instruct patient to take potassium acid phosphate and sodium acid phosphate exactly as prescribed.
- Tell patient to take drug with a full glass of water.
- Caution patient to avoid eating excessive amounts of potassium- or sodium-rich foods and to limit salt intake.
- Advise patient to notify prescriber if abdominal pain, nausea, or vomiting occurs.
- Warn patient with kidney stones of the possibility of passing old stones when phosphate therapy is started.
- Instruct patient to avoid antacids that contain aluminum, calcium, or magnesium while taking phosphate drug because they may hinder phosphate absorption.

potassium citrate monohydrate and citric acid monohydrate

Cytra-K, Cytra-K Crystals, Polycitra-K, Polycitra-L Crystals

Class and Category

Chemical: Potassium derivative of base (potassium citrate), base (citric acid)
Therapeutic: Urinary alkalinizes (potassium citrate, citric acid)

Pregnancy category: NR

Indications and Dosages

▶ *To provide long-term maintenance of alkaline urine in the management of chronic metabolic acidosis caused by such conditions as chronic renal insufficiency or renal tubular acidosis*

POWDER FOR MIX (CYTRA-L CRYSTALS, POLYCITRA-K CRYSTALS)

Adults. 3,300 mg potassium citrate monohydrate and 1,002 mg citric acid monohydrate (number of packets varies depending on manufacturer) q.i.d. after meals and at bedtime.

SOLUTION, SYRUP (CYTRA-K, POLYCITRA-K)

Adults. 3,300 to 6,600 mg potassium citrate monohydrate and 1,002 to 2,004 mg citric acid monohydrate (15 to 30 ml) q.i.d. after meals and at betime.

Children. 1,100 to 3,300 mg potassium citrate monohydrate and 334 to 1,002 mg citric acid monohydrate (5 to 15 ml) q.i.d. after meals and at bedtime.

Mechanism of Action

Potassium citrate and citrate acid are oxidized in the body to form bicarbonate, a buffer, which increases urinary pH as it is readily excreted in urine.

Contraindications

Acute dehydration, adynamia episodica hereditaria, anuria, azotemia, heat cramps, hyperkalemia, oliguria, severe myocardial damage or renal impairment, untreated Addison's disease

Adverse Reactions

GI: Laxative effect, nausea, vomiting
Other: Hyperkalemia, metabolic alkalosis

Nursing Considerations

- Use with extreme caution in patients who need to limit intake of potassium.
- Monitor patient's serum electrolytes and acid-base status, as ordered, because hyperkalemia or metabolic alkalosis may occur, especially in patients with renal impairment.

PATIENT TEACHING

- Instruct patient to take potassium citrate and citric acid exactly as prescribed because excessive amounts can cause tetany or depress heart function.
- Instruct patient to mix drug exactly as described on packets and to protect packets from extreme heat or cold.

- Instruct patient prescribed solution form to store in a tight container and protect from extreme heat or cold.
- Tell patient to take drug after meals and at bedtime to minimize the GI effects of the drug.
- Reassure patient that the drug is pleasant tasting.

probenecid and colchicine

ColBenemid, Col-Probenecid, Proben-C

Class and Category

Chemical: Sulfonamide derivative (probenecid), colchicium alkaloid derivative (colchicine)
Therapeutic: Antigout
Pregnancy category: Not rated

Indications and Dosages

▶ *To treat chronic gouty arthritis in patients who experience frequent attacks*

TABLETS

Adults. *Initial:* 500 mg of probenecid and 0.5 mg of colchicine (1 tablet) daily for 1 wk; then increased to maintenance dosage. *Maintenance:* 1 tablet b.i.d.; if not effective or if 24-hr uric acid excretion isn't greater than 700 mg, dosage increased by 1 tablet daily every 4 wk, as needed and prescribed, up to a maximum of 4 tablets daily. If no acute gout attacks occur over next 6 mo and serum uric acid level is within normal limits, dosage decreased, as prescribed, by 1 tablet every 6 mo until lowest effective maintenance dose is reached.

DOSAGE ADJUSTMENT Dosage possibly increased for patients with mild renal dysfunction.

Mechanism of Action

Reduces the frequency of gout attacks through several mechanisms. Probenecid increases urinary excretion of uric acid and reduces serum uric acid level, which may prevent or resolve urate deposits, tophus formation, and joint changes. Eventually, the incidence of acute gout attacks may decrease.

Colchicine helps to stop inflammation, probably by disrupting microtubules in leukocytes. Microtubules contribute to cell structure and movement. When colchicine binds to tubulin (the protein from which microtubules are made), it causes microtubules to fall apart. This, in turn, disrupts cell function and prevents leukocytes from continuing to invade joints and produce inflammation.

Contraindications

Age less than 2 years; blood dyscrasias; hypersensitivity to colchicine, probenecid, or their components; renal calculi (urate)

Interactions

DRUGS

acyclovir: Decreased renal tubular secretion of acyclovir
allopurinol: Additive antihyperuricemic effects
aminosalicylate sodium, cephalosporins, ciprofloxacin, clofibrate, dapsone, ganciclovir, imipenem, methotrexate, nitrofurantoin, norfloxacin, penicillins: Increased and possibly prolonged blood levels of these drugs and increased risk of toxicity
antineoplastics (rapidly cytolytic): Possibly uric acid nephropathy
cyclosporine: Possibly impaired renal function and risk of nephrotoxicity
diazoxide, mecamylamine, pyrazinamide: Increased risk of hyperuricemia; decreased probenecid effectiveness
dyphylline: Increased half-life of dyphylline
erythromycin: Impaired metabolism of colchicine
furosemide: Increased blood furosemide level
heparin: Increased and prolonged anticoagulant effect
indomethacin, ketoprofen, other NSAIDs: Possibly increased adverse effects
lorazepam, oxazepam, temazepam: Increased effects of these drugs and, possibly, excessive sedation
riboflavin: Decreased GI absorption of riboflavin
rifampin, sulfonamides: Increased blood levels of these drugs and, possibly, toxicity
salicylates: Decreased uricosuric effects of probenecid and colchicine
sodium benzoate and sodium phenylacetate: Decreased renal elimination of these drugs
sulfonylureas: Increased sulfonylurea half-life
thiopental: Prolonged thiopental effect
vitamin B_{12} (cyanocobalamin): Reversible decrease in blood vitamin B_{12} level
zidovudine: Increased risk of zidovudine toxicity

ACTIVITIES

alcohol use: Increased risk of hyperuricemia, decreased antigout effects

Adverse Reactions

CNS: Dizziness, fever, headache, peripheral neuritis

EENT: Sore gums

GI: Abdominal pain, anorexia, diarrhea, hepatic necrosis, nausea, vomiting

GU: Hematuria, nephropathy (urate), nephrotic syndrome, renal calculi (urate), renal colic, urinary frequency

HEME: Agranulocytosis, anemia, aplastic anemia, hemolytic anemia, leukopenia

MS: Back or rib pain, gout attacks, muscle weakness

SKIN: Alopecia, dermatitis, flushing, purpura

Other: Anaphylaxis

Nursing Considerations

- Be aware that probenecid and colchicine therapy shouldn't be started until acute gout attack has subsided. If acute gout attack begins during therapy, however, expect to continue therapy.
- Use drug cautiously in patients with peptic ulcer disease.
- Expect to give sodium bicarbonate (3 to 7.5 grams daily) or potassium citrate (7.5 grams daily), as prescribed, to keep urine alkaline and prevent renal calculus formation.
- Monitor CBC, serum uric acid level, and liver and renal function test results during therapy.
- Closely monitor patients receiving intermittent therapy because they're more prone to allergic reactions.
- Monitor blood glucose level often in diabetic patient who takes a sulfonylurea because of the risk of drug interactions.

PATIENT TEACHING

- Advise patient to take probenecid and colchicine with meals to minimize stomach upset.
- Encourage increased fluid intake (up to 3 liters daily, if not contraindicated) to help prevent renal calculus formation.
- Instruct patient to notify prescriber immediately if she has a gouty arthritis flare-up (joint pain, swelling, and redness) or signs of kidney stones, such as flank pain and blood in urine.
- Caution patient against taking salicylates during therapy. Instead, urge her to use acetaminophen for mild pain or fever.

sodium citrate dihydrate and citric acid monohydrate

Bicitra, Cytra-2, Oracit, Shohl's Solution

Class and Category

Chemical: Salt derivative of base (sodium citrate), base (citric acid)

Therapeutic: Urinary alkalinizes (sodium citrate, citric acid)
Pregnancy category: NR

Indications and Dosages

▶ *To provide long-term maintenance of alkaline urine in the management of chronic metabolic acidosis associated with conditions such as chronic renal insufficiency or renal tubular acidosis*

SOLUTION (ORACIT)

Adults. 980 to 2,940 mg sodium citrate dihydrate and 1,280 to 3,840 mg citric acid monohydrate (10 to 30 ml) q.i.d. after meals and at bedtime.

Children. 490 to 1,470 mg sodium citrate dihydrate and 640 to 1,920 mg citric acid monohydrate (5 to 15 ml) q.i.d. after meals and at bedtime.

SOLUTION (BICITRA, CYTRA-2, SHOHL'S SOLUTION)

Adults. 1,000 to 3,000 mg sodium citrate dihydrate and 668 to 2,004 mg citric acid monohydrate (10 to 30 ml) q.i.d. after meals and at bedtime.

Children. 500 to 1,500 mg sodium citrate dihydrate and 334 to 1,002 mg citric acid monohydrate (5 to 15 ml) q.i.d. after meals and at bedtime.

Mechanism of Action

Sodium citrate dihydrate and citrate acid monohydrate are oxidized in the body to form bicarbonate, a buffer, which increases urinary pH as it is readily excreted in urine.

Contraindications

Severe renal impairment, sodium-restricted diet

Adverse Reactions

GI: Laxative effect, nausea, vomiting
Other: Hypernatremia, metabolic alkalosis

Nursing Considerations

• Use sodium citrate dihydrate and citric acid monohydrate with extreme caution in patients with heart failure, hypertension, renal dysfunction, peripheral or pulmonary edema, or toxemia of pregnancy.
• Use with caution in patients with low urine output.
• Monitor patient's serum electrolytes and acid-base status, as ordered, because hypernatremia or metabolic alkalosis may occur, especially in patients with renal impairment.

PATIENT TEACHING

- Instruct patient to take drug exactly as prescribed because excessive amounts can cause tetany or depress heart function.
- Tell patient to take drug after meals and at bedtime to minimize the GI effects of the drug.
- Reassure patient that the drug is pleasant tasting.
- Instruct patient to store drug solution in a tight container and protect from extreme heat or cold.

trimethoprim, sulfamethoxazole, and phenazopyridine hydrochoride

Zotrim

Class and Category

Chemical: Dihydrofolic acid analogue (trimethoprim), sulfonamide derivative (sulfamethoxazole, azo dye (phenazopyridine)
Therapeutic: Antibiotics (trimethoprim, sulfamethoxazole), urinary analgesic (phenazopyridine)
Pregnancy category: C

Indications and Dosages

▶ *To treat urinary tract infections caused by susceptible strains of* Escherichia coli, Enterobacer *or* Klebsiella *species,* Morganella morganii, Proteus mirabilis, *and* Proteus vulgaris
DOUBLE-STRENGTH TABLET (TRIMETHOPRIM AND SULFAMETHOXAZOLE)

Adults. 160 mg trimethoprim and 800 mg sulfamethoxazole (1 tablet) every 12 hr for 10 days.

DOSAGE ADJUSTMENT For patients with creatinine clearance between 15 ml/min and 30 ml/min, dosage decreased by half.

▶ *To relieve pain, burning, urgency, frequency, and other discomforts caused by infection-related irritation of the lower urinary tract mucosa*
TABLET (PHENAZOPYRIDINE)

Adults. 200 mg phenazopyridine (1 tablet) t.i.d. after meals for no longer than 2 days.

Contraindications

Age less than 2 months; breast-feeding; hypersensitivity to trimethoprim, sulfamethoxazole, other sulfonamides, phenazopyridine, or their components; megaloblastic anemia caused by folate deficiency; renal insufficiency (creatinine clearance less than 15 ml/min); term pregnancy

Mechanism of Action

Trimethoprim and sulfamethoxazole block two consecutive steps in the formation of essential nucleic acids and proteins in susceptible organisms. Sulfamethoxazole inhibits synthesis of dihydrofolic acid (a nucleic acid) by completing with para-aminobenzoic acid. Trimethoprim inhibits the action of the enzyme dihydro-folate reductase, thus blocking production of tetrahydrofolic acid. These actions result in bacterial cell death.

Phenazopyridine exerts a topical or local anesthetic effect on the mucosa of the urinary tract as drug is excreted in urine to relieve discomfort associated with urinary tract infection.

Interactions

DRUGS

trimethoprim and sulfamethoxazole

ACE inhibitors: Possibly increased risk of hyperkalemia in elderly patients

cyclosporine: Decreased blood level and therapeutic effectiveness of cyclosporine, increased risk of nephrotoxicity

digoxin: Possibly increased blood digoxin level resulting in increased risk of digoxin toxicity

diuretics: Increased risk of thrombocytopenic purpura in elderly patients

indomethacin: Possibly increased blood trimethoprim and sulfamethoxazole levels

methotrexate: Increased blood methotrexate level and risk of methotrexate toxicity

phenytoin: Possibly decreased hepatic clearance and prolonged half-life of phenytoin

pyrimethamine (dosage greater than 25 mg/wk): Increased risk of megaloblastic anemia

sulfonylureas: Possibly increased hypoglycemic effects of sulfonylureas

tricyclic antidepressants: Decreased effectiveness of tricyclic antidepressant

warfarin: Increased anticoagulant effects

Adverse Reactions

CNS: Anxiety, aseptic meningitis ataxia, chills, depression, fatigue, hallucinations, headache, insomnia, seizures, vertigo
EENT: Glossitis, stomatitis
GI: Abdominal pain, anorexia, diarrhea, hepatitis, indigestion, nausea, pancreatitis, pseudomembranous enterocolitis, vomiting

GU: Crystalluria, reddish orange urine, renal failure, toxic nephrosis

HEME: Agranulocytosis, eosinophilia, hemolytic anemia, leukopenia, methemoglobinemia, neutropenia, thrombocytopenia

RESP: Cough, dyspnea

SKIN: Dermatitis, erythema, photosensitivity, pruritus, rash, Stevens-Johnson syndrome, toxic epidermal necrolysis, urticaria

Other: Anaphylaxis, discoloration of body fluids

Nursing Considerations

- Be aware that blister card contains 20 double-strength trimethoprim and sulfamethoxazole tablets and 6 phenazopyridine tablets.
- Expect to obtain culture and sensitivity test results before starting antibiotic therapy with trimethroprin and sulfamethoxazole.
- Assess patient for evidence of blood dyscrasia, including bleeding, ecchymosis, and joint pain. This is especially important in elderly patients who also take a thiazide diuretic during the 10 days of trimethroprin and sulfamethoxazole therapy.
- Notify prescriber if yellowish skin or sclera develop in patient during 2-day therapy with phenazopyridine because this may indicate drug accumulation from impaired renal excretion. Expect prescriber to discontinue drug.

PATIENT TEACHING

- If GI distress develops, advise patient to take drug with meals.
- Instruct patient not to take phenazopyridine in package for longer than 2 days and to notify prescriber if symptoms persist beyond that time.
- Warn patient that during use of phenazopyridine, his urine will turn orange to red and other body fluids such as tears may become discolored. Explain that this effect is harmless and will resolve when drug is stopped.
- Advise patient not to wear contact lenses while using phenazopyridine because they may become stained from discoloration of tears.
- Instruct patient to notify prescriber immediately if rash, severe diarrhea, or other serious adverse reactions occur.
- To minimize photosensitivity, advise patient to avoid direct sunlight and to use sunscreen.

Respiratory Drugs

acrivastine and pseudoephedrine sulfate

Semprex-D

Class and Category

Chemical: Alkylamine antihistamine (acrivastine), sympatho-mimetic amine (pseudoephedrine)
Therapeutic: Antihistaminic (acrivastine), decongestant (pseudo-ephedrine)
Pregnancy category: B

Indications and Dosages

▶ *To relieve symptoms of seasonal allergic rhinitis*

CAPSULES

Adults and children age 12 and over. 8 mg acrivastine and 60 mg pseudoephedrine (1 capsule) every 4 to 6 hr. *Maximum:* 8 mg acrivastine and 60 mg pseudoephedrine (1 capsule) every 4 to 6 hr daily.

Mechanism of Action

Acrivastine competes with histamine for histamine H_1 receptor sites on effector cells and antagonizes the vasodilator effect of endogenously released histamine. This prevents vascular engorgement, mucosal edema, sneezing, and profuse watery secretion and irritation that normally result from histamine action on peripheral afferent nerve terminals.

Pseudoephedrine acts on alpha$_1$-adrenergic receptors in the mucosa of the respiratory tract to produce vasoconstriction. This process shrinks swollen nasal mucous membranes; reduces tissue hyperemia, edema, and nasal congestion; and increases nasal airway patency. It also may increase drainage of sinus secretions and open obstructed eustachian ostia.

Contraindications

Hypersensitivity or idiosyncractic reactions to acrivastine, other alkylamine antihistamines, pseudoephedrine, other sympathomimetic amines, or their components; severe coronary artery disease or hypertension; use within 14 days of MAO inhibitor therapy

Interactions

DRUGS

acrivastine

barbiturates, CNS depressants, tricyclic antidepressants: Additive effects

pseudoephedrine

antacids: Increased absorption of pseudoephedrine

antihypertensives, diuretics: Possibly decreased antihypertensive effects

beta blockers: Decreased therapeutic effects of both drugs

citrates: Possibly inhibited urinary excretion and prolonged duration of action of pseudoephedrine

CNS stimulants, sympathomimetics: Possibly increased additive CNS stimulation to excessive levels

cocaine (mucosal-local): Possibly increased cardiovascular effects of either drug and CNS stimulation

digoxin, levodopa: Increased risk of cardiac arrhythmias

hydrocarbon inhalation anesthetics: Increased risk of serious arrhythmias

kaolin: Decreased pseudoephedrine absorption

MAO inhibitors: Increased and prolonged cardiac stimulation, increased vasopressor effect, increased risk of severe cardiovascular and cerebrovascular effects, hyperpyrexia, and vomiting

nitrates: Reduced antianginal effects of nitrates

rauwolfia alkaloids: Possibly inhibited pseudoephedrine action

thyroid hormones: Increased cardiovascular effects of both drugs

ACTIVITIES

acrivastine

alcohol use: Additive effects

Adverse Reactions

CNS: Asthenia, dizziness, headache, insomnia, light-headedness, nervousness, restlessness, somnolence, trembling, weakness

CV: Palpitations, tachycardia

EENT: Dry mouth, pharyngitis

ENDO: Dysmenorrhea

GI: Dyspepsia, nausea, vomiting

GU: Dysuria
RESP: Bronchospasm, increased cough
SKIN: Diaphoresis, erythema multiforme, pallor
Other: Anaphylaxis, angioedema

Nursing Considerations

- Use cautiously in patients with diabetes, hypertension, increased intraocular pressure, ischemic heart disease, prostatic hypertrophy, stenosing peptic ulcer, or pyloroduodenal obstruction because of the vasoconstrictive action of pseudoephedrine.
- Monitor elderly patients closely for dizziness, sedation, confusion, hallucinations, convulsions, CNS depression, and hypotension because these patients are more likely to develop such adverse effects.
- Monitor renal function, as ordered, because pseudoephedrine is substantially excreted by the kidneys. Be aware that drug isn't recommended for patients with impaired renal function.
- Evaluate effectiveness of acrivastine and pseudoephedrine in relieving symptoms of seasonal allergic rhinitis, such as sneezing, rhinorrhea, pruritus, lacrimation, and nasal congestion.
- Be aware that patient shouldn't undergo intradermal allergen tests within 4 days of receiving drug because the results may be altered.

PATIENT TEACHING

- Urge patient to avoid alcohol, other antidepressants, and OTC medications containing other antihistamines or sympathomimetics while taking acrivastine and pseudoephedrine.
- Instruct patient to avoid hazardous activities until drug's CNS effects are known.
- Suggest that patient relieve dry mouth with frequent rinsing and use of sugarless gum or hard candy.

azatadine maleate and pseudoephedrine sulfate

Trinalin Repetabs

Class and Category

Chemical: Piperidine derivative (azatadine), sympathomimetic amine (pseudoephedrine)
Therapeutic: Antihistamine (azatadine), decongestant (pseudoephedrine)
Pregnancy category: NR

Indications and Dosages

▶ *To relieve symptoms of upper respiratory mucosal congestion in perennial and allergic rhinitis; to relieve nasal congestion and eustachian tube congestion*

E.R. TABLETS

Adults. 1 mg azatadine and 120 mg pseudoephedrine (1 tablet) b.i.d.

Mechanism of Action

Azatadine competes with histamine for histamine H_1 receptor sites on effector cells and antagonizes the vasodilator effect of endogenously released histamine. This prevents vascular engorgement, mucosal edema and profuse watery secretion, irritation, and sneezing that normally result from histamine action on peripheral afferent nerve terminals in nasal passages.

Pseudoephedrine acts on alpha$_1$-adrenergic receptors in the mucosa of the respiratory tract to produce vasoconstriction. This process shrinks swollen nasal mucous membranes; reduces tissue hyperemia, edema, and nasal congestion; and increases nasal airway patency. It also may increase drainage of sinus secretions and open obstructed eustachian ostia.

Contraindications

Hypersensitivity or idiosyncratic reactions to azatadine, pseudoephedrine or their components; hyperthyroidism; narrow-angle glaucoma; severe coronary artery disease or hypertension; urine retention; use within 14 days of MAO inhibitor therapy

Interactions

DRUGS

azatadine

barbiturates, CNS depressants, tricyclic antidepressants: Additive effects

pseudoephedrine

antacids: Increased pseudoephedrine absoprtion

antihypertensives, diuretics: Possibly decreased antihypertensive effects

beta blockers: Decreased therapeutic effects of both drugs

citrates: Possibly inhibited urinary excretion and prolonged duration of pseudoephedrine action

CNS stimulants, sympathomimetics: Possibly increased additive CNS stimulation to excessive levels

cocaine (mucosal-local): Possibly increased cardiovascular effects of either drug and CNS stimulation

digoxin, levodopa: Increased risk of cardiac arrhythmias

hydrocarbon inhalation anesthetics: Possibly serious arrhythmias
kaolin: Decreased pseudoephedrine absorption
MAO inhibitors: Increased and prolonged cardiac stimulation, increased vasopressor effect, increased risk of severe cardiovascular and cerebrovascular effects, hyperpyrexia, and vomiting
nitrates: Reduced antianginal effects of nitrates
rauwolfia alkaloids: Possibly inhibited action of pseudoephedrine
thyroid hormones: Increased cardiovascular effects of both drugs
ACTIVITIES
azatadine
alcohol use: Additive effects

Adverse Reactions

CNS: Anxiety, CNS stimulation or depression, confusion, disturbed coordination, dizziness, drowsiness, fear, hallucinations, headache, insomnia, light-headedness, mood shifts, nervousness, restlessness, sedation, seizures, sleepiness, tenseness, trembling, weakness
CV: Arrhythmias, hypertension, hypotension, palpitations, tachycardia
EENT: Dry mouth, nose, or throat
GI: Abdominal pain, epigastric distress, nausea, vomiting
GU: Dysuria, urine retention
HEME: Hemolytic anemia, pancytopenia, thrombocytopenia
RESP: Dyspnea, thickened bronchial secretions
SKIN: Diaphoresis, pallor, rash

Nursing Considerations

- Use cautiously in patients with bladder neck obstruction, cardiovascular disease, diabetes, increased intraocular pressure, pyloroduodenal obstruction, prostatic hypertrophy, or stenosing peptic ulcer because of the vasoconstrictive action of pseudoephedrine. Also use cautiously in patients with a history of bronchial asthma because of the atropine-like action of azatadine.
- Monitor elderly patients for dizziness, sedation, confusion, hallucinations, CNS depression, hypotension, and seizures because these patients are more likely to develop such adverse effects.
- Monitor renal function, as ordered, because pseudoephedrine is substantially excreted by the kidneys.
- Regularly evaluate effectiveness of azatadine and pseudoephedrine in relieving upper respiratory congestion.
- Patient shouldn't undergo intradermal allergen tests within 4 days of receiving drug because the results may be altered.

PATIENT TEACHING
- Urge patient to avoid alcohol, other antidepressants and OTC medications containing other antihistamines or sympathomimetics while taking azatadine and pseudoephedrine.
- Instruct patient to avoid hazardous activities until drug's CNS effects are known.
- Suggest that patient relieve dry mouth with frequent rinsing and use of sugarless gum or hard candy.

brompheniramine maleate and pseudoephedrine hydrochloride

AccuHist Pediatric Drops, Andehist, Brofed, Bromadrine TR, Bromfed, Bromfed-PD, Bromfenex, Bromfenex PD, Dimetapp Cold & Allergy, Histex SR, Iofed, Iofed PD, Lodrane, Lodrane 12 D, Lodrane LD, Respahist, Rondec, Rondec Chewables, Touro, UTRAbrom, UTRAbrom PD

dexbrompheniramine maleate and pseudoephedrine sulfate

Dexaphen SA, Disobrom

Class and Category

Chemical: Propylamine derivative (brompheniramine, dexbrompheniramine), sympathomimetic amine (pseudoephedrine)

Therapeutic: Antihistamines (brompheniramine, dexbrompheniramine), decongestant (pseudoephedrine)

Pregnancy category: B

Indications and Dosages

▶ *To relieve persistent runny nose, sneezing, and nasal congestion caused by upper respiratory infections, sinus inflammation, or hay fever*
E.R. CAPSULES

Adults and children age 12 and over. 6 or 12 mg brompheniramine and 60 or 120 mg pseudoephedrine (1 to 2 capsules depending on product used) every 12 hr.

Children ages 6 to 12. 6 mg brompheniramine and 60 mg pseudoephedrine (1 capsule) every 12 hr.

TABLETS, CHEWABLE TABLETS

Adults and children age 12 and over. 4 mg brompheniramine and 60 mg pseudoephedrine (1 tablet) every 4 hr.

Children ages 6 to 12. 2 mg brompheniramine and 30 mg pseudoephedrine (½ tablet) every 4 hr.

E.R. TABLETS
Adults. 6 to 12 mg brompheniramine or dexbrompheniramine and 45 to 120 mg pseudoephedrine (1 or 2 tablets depending on product used) every 12 hr.
ORAL SOLUTION
Adults and children age 12 and over. 8 mg brompheniramine and 60 mg pseudoephedrine (10 ml) every 8 hr. Or, 4 mg brompheniramine and 60 mg pseudoephedrine (5 ml) every 4 to 6 hr.
Children ages 6 to 12. 4 mg brompheniramine and 30 mg pseudoephedrine (5 ml) every 8 hr.
Children ages 2 to 6. 2 mg bromopheniramine and 15 mg pseudoephedrine (2.5 ml) every 8 hr.
SYRUP
Adults and children age 12 and over. 4 mg brompheniramine and 60 mg pseudoephedrine (10 ml) every 4 to 6 hr.
Children ages 6 to 12. 2 mg brompheniramine and 30 mg pseudoephedrine (5 ml) every 4 to 6 hr.
DROPS
Children ages 12 months to 24 months. 1 mg brompheniramine and 15 mg pseudoephedrine (1 ml) q.i.d.
Children ages 6 to 12 months. 0.75 mg brompheniramine and 11.25 mg pseudoephedrine (0.75 ml) q.i.d.
Infants ages 3 months to 6 months. 0.5 mg brompheniramine and 7.5 mg pseudoephedrine (0.5 ml) q.i.d.
Infants ages 1 month to 3 months. 0.25 mg brompheniramine and 3.75 mg pseudoephedrine (0.25 ml) q.i.d.

Mechanism of Action

Brompheniramine and dexbrompheniramine compete with histamine for H_1 receptor sites, thereby antagonizing many histamine effects and reducing allergy signs and symptoms.

Pseudoephedrine acts on $alpha_1$-adrenergic receptors in the mucosa of the respiratory tract to produce vasoconstriction. This process shrinks swollen nasal mucous membranes; reduces tissue hyperemia, edema, and nasal congestion; and increases nasal airway patency. It also may increase drainage of sinus secretions and open obstructed eustachian ostia.

Contraindications

Breast-feeding; hypersensitivity or idiosyncractic reactions to brompheniramine, dexbrompheniramine, pseudoephedrine, or their components; hyperthyroidism; narrow-angle glaucoma; severe coronary artery disease or hypertension; urine retention; use within 14 days of MAO inhibitor therapy

Interactions

DRUGS

brompheniramine, dexbrompheniramine, and pseudoephedrine

MAO inhibitors: Increased and prolonged cardiac stimulation, increased vasopressor effect, increased risk of severe cardiovascular and cerebrovascular effects, hyperpyrexia, and vomiting

brompheniramine and dexbrompheniramine

anticholinergics: Additive anticholinergic effects

CNS depressants: Additive CNS effects

pseudoephedrine

antacids: Increased pseudoephedrine absorption

antihypertensives, diuretics: Possibly decreased antihypertensive effects

beta blockers: Decreased therapeutic effects of both drugs

citrates: Possibly inhibited urinary excretion and prolonged duration of pseudoephedrine action

CNS stimulants, sympathomimetics: Possibly increased additive CNS stimulation to excessive levels

cocaine (mucosal-local): Possibly increased cardiovascular effects of either drug and CNS stimulation

digoxin, levodopa: Increased risk of cardiac arrhythmias

hydrocarbon inhalation anesthetics: Increased risk of serious arrhythmias

kaolin: Decreased pseudoephedrine absorption

nitrates: Reduced antianginal effects of nitrates

rauwolfia alkaloids: Possibly inhibited pseudoephedrine action

thyroid hormones: Increased cardiovascular effects of both drugs

ACTIVITIES

brompheniramine and dexbrompheniramine

alcohol use: Additive CNS effects

Adverse Reactions

CNS: Anxiety, chills, confusion, coordination disturbance, dizziness, drowsiness, excitation (children), fatigue, fear, hallucinations, headache, hysteria, insomnia, irritability, lightheadedness, nervousness, numbness, restlessness, sedation, seizures, tenseness, trembling, vertigo, weakness

CV: Arrhythmias, chest tightness, hypotension, palpitations, tachycardia
EENT: Blurred or double vision; dry mouth, nose, and throat; nasal congestion; tinnitus
ENDO: Early menstruation
GI: Anorexia, constipation, diarrhea, nausea, stomach upset or pain, vomiting
GU: Dysuria, frequent urination, urinary hesitancy, urine retention
HEME: Anemia, unusual bleeding or bruising
RESP: Dyspnea, increased chest congestion, wheezing
SKIN: Diaphoresis, pallor, photosensitivity, rash, urticaria
Other: Anaphylaxis

Nursing Considerations

- Use cautiously in patients with asthma, cardiovascular disease, diabetes, emphysema or other chronic lung disease, hypertension, peptic ulcer, hyperthyroidism, narrow-angle glaucoma, or prostatic hypertrophy.
- Monitor children for excitation and elderly patients for dizziness, sedation, and hypotension; such patients may have an increased risk for these effects.
- Monitor renal function, as ordered, because pseudoephedrine is substantially excreted by the kidneys.
- Regularly evaluate effectiveness of brompheniramine or dexbrompheniramine and pseudoephedrine in reducing upper respiratory symptoms.
- Patient shouldn't undergo intradermal allergen tests within 72 hours of receiving drug because results may be altered.

PATIENT TEACHING

- Instruct patient to use a calibrated measuring device for syrup or oral solution form of brompheniramine and pseudoephedrine to ensure accurate dose.
- Urge patient to avoid alcohol and other antidepressants while taking brompheniramine or dexbrompheniramine and pseudoephedrine.
- Instruct patient to avoid hazardous activities until drug's CNS effects are known.
- Suggest that patient relieve dry mouth with frequent rinsing and use of sugarless gum or hard candy.
- Tell patient to take last dose of the day a few hours before bedtime if brompheniramine or dexbrompheniramine and pseudoephedrine makes him nervous or restless.

budesonide and formoterol fumarate dehydrate

Symbicort

Class and Category

Chemical: Glucocorticoid (budesonide), racemic acid salt (formoterol)

Therapeutic: Antiasthmatic, anti-inflammatory (budesonide), bronchodilator, beta$_2$-adrenergic agonist (formoterol)

Pregnancy category: C

Indications and Dosages

▶ *To provide long-term maintenance treatment of asthma in patients not currently using an inhaled corticosteroid*

ORAL INHALATION

Adults and children age 12 and over. Two inhalations (80 mcg or 160 mcg budesonide and 4.5 mcg formoterol/inhalation) twice daily, morning and evening, depending upon asthma severity.

▶ *To provide long-term maintenance treatment of asthma in patients currently using low to medium doses of inhaled corticosteroid therapy*

ORAL INHALATION

Adults and children age 12 and over. Two inhalations (80 mcg budesonide and 4.5 mcg formoterol/inhalation) twice daily, morning and evening.

▶ *To provide long-term maintenance treatment of asthma in patients currently receiving medium to high doses of inhaled corticosteroid therapy*

ORAL INHALATION

Adults and children age 12 and over. Two inhalations (160 mcg budesonide and 4.5 mcg formoterol/inhalation) twice daily, morning and evening.

▶ *To provide maintenance treatment of airflow obstruction in patients with COPD, including chronic bronchitis and emphysema*

ORAL INHALATION

Adults and children age 12 and over. Two inhalations (160 mcg budesonide and 4.5 mcg formoterol/inhalation) twice daily, morning and evening.

Contraindications

Hypersensitivity to budesonide, formoterol fumarate, or their components; primary treatment of status asthmaticus or other acute episodes of asthma or COPD that require intensive measures

Mechanism of Action

Budesonide inhibits inflammatory cells and mediators, possibly by decreasing their influx into nasal passages or bronchial walls. As a result, nasal or airway inflammation decreases. The drug also inhibits mucus secretion in airways, decreasing the amount and viscosity of sputum.

Formoterol selectively attaches to beta2 receptors on bronchial membranes, stimulating the intracellular enzyme adenyl cyclase to convert adenosine triphosphate to cAMP. The resulting increase in the intracellular cAMP level relaxes bronchial smooth-muscle cells, stabilizes mast cells, and inhibits histamine release.

Interactions

DRUGS

budesonide

clarithromycin, erythromycin, itraconazole, ketoconazole, other CYP3A4 inhibitors: Possibly increased blood budesonide level

formoterol

adrenergics: Possibly increased sympathetic effects of formoterol

beta blockers: Decreased effects of formoterol, possibly severe broncospasm

corticosteroids, non–potassium-sparing diuretics, xanthine derivatives: Possibly increased hypokalemic effect of formoterol

disopyramide, MAO inhibitors, phenothiazines, procainamide, quinidine, tricyclic antidepressants: Possibly prolonged QTc interval, increasing risk of ventricular arrhythmias

Adverse Reactions

CNS: Amnesia, anxiety, asthenia, dizziness, fatigue, fever, headache, insomnia, malaise, tremor

CV: Angina, arrhythmias, chest pain, hypertension, hypotension, palpitations, tachycardia

EENT: Bad taste; cataracts; dry mouth; epistaxis; glaucoma; hoarseness; laryngeal spasm, irritation, or swelling; nasal irritation; oral or pharyngeal candidiasis; pharyngitis; rhinitis and tonsillitis (in children); sinusitis

ENDO: Growth suppression in children, hyperglycemia, suppressed adrenal function

GI: Abdominal pain, diarrhea, dyspepsia, flatulence, gastroenteritis, indigestion, nausea, vomiting

GU: UTI

MS: Arthralgia, back pain, leg cramps, muscle spasms

RESP: Asthma exacerbation, bronchitis, bronchospasm (paradoxical or hypersensitivity induced), cough, dyspnea, increased sputum production, respiratory tract infection
SKIN: Dermatitis, pruritus, purpura, rash, urticaria
Other: Anaphylaxis, angioedema, hypokalemia, metabolic acidosis, viral infection (in children)

Nursing Considerations

- Use budesonide and formoterol cautiously in patients with cardiovascular disorders because formoterol may increase blood pressure, heart rate, and level of excitement. Also use budesonide and formoterol with extreme caution if patient has a tubercular infection; untreated fungal, bacterial, or systemic viral infection; or ocular herpes simplex because budesonide is a corticosteroid.
- Budesonide and formoterol should not be used for quick relief of bronchospasm because of the prolonged onset of action. If patient needs increasing use of rescue inhaler or develops respiratory distress, notify prescriber because patient will need to be reassessed immediately.
- Monitor patient closely for hypersensitivity reactions such as angioedema, bronchospasm, rash, and urticaria after giving drug. Notify prescriber immediately if a reaction occurs, and expect to provide emergency supportive care.
- **WARNING** Asthma-related deaths may increase in asthmatics receiving the long-acting beta$_2$ agonist, salmeterol. Because formoterol is also a long-acting beta$_2$ agonist, monitor patient closely throughout therapy, and notify prescriber immediately of any changes in respiratory status.
- Closely monitor a child's growth pattern; budesonide may stunt growth.
- Be prepared to give varicella zoster immune globulin or pooled I.V. immunoglobulin if patient is exposed to chickenpox. If chickenpox develops, give antiviral as ordered. A patient exposed to measles may need pooled I.M. immunoglobulin.
- Assess effectiveness of budesonide and formoterol regularly.
- Watch closely for paradoxical bronchospasm; if it occurs, stop drug immediately and notify prescriber.
- Monitor patients with a history of cardiovascular disorders, especially coronary insufficiency, arrhythmias, or hypertension. Notify prescriber of any significant increases in pulse rate or blood pressure or worsening of chronic conditions because formoterol may produce cardiovascular reactions, including

angina, arrhythmias, hypertension, hypotension, palpitations, and tachycardia. Drug may need to be discontinued if such reactions occur.

- Monitor patient closely for major adverse reactions because budesonide and formoterol may be absorbed systemically. Although rare, potential effects could include decreased bone mineral density, increased blood glucose level in diabetic patients, decreased serum potassium level, and suppressed adrenal function.

PATIENT TEACHING

- Tell patient to use drug exactly as prescribed and not to exceed recommended dosage.
- Instruct her to rinse her mouth with water after each dose and to spit the water out. Tell her to contact her prescriber if she develops a mouth or throat infection.
- Caution patient not to use budesonide and formoterol as a rescuer inhaler.
- Instruct patient to contact prescriber if symptoms persist or have worsened after 3 weeks. Caution against increasing the dose on her own.
- Instruct patient to notify prescriber immediately if she has palpitations, chest pain, rapid heart rate, tremor, or nervousness while taking drug because dosage may need to be adjusted.
- Caution patient to avoid exposure to chickenpox and measles and, if exposed, to contact prescriber immediately.
- Instruct patient against stopping drug abruptly.
- Advise patient to have regular eye examinations.
- Urge female patient to notify the prescriber if she is or could be pregnant.
- Advise patient with diabetes to monitor her blood glucose level closely.

carbetapentane tannate and chlorpheniramine tannate

Tannic-12, Trionate, Tussi-12, Tussi-12 S, Tussizone-12 RF

Class and Category

Chemical: Cyclopentane carbolic ester (carbetapentane), propylamine derivative (chlorpheniramine)
Therapeutic: Antitussive (carbetapentane) and antihistaminic (chlorpheniramine)

Pregnancy category: C

Indications and Dosages

▶ *To relieve cough in such respiratory tract conditions as the common cold, bronchial asthma, and acute and chronic bronchitis*

TABLETS

Adults. 60 or 120 mg carbetapentane and 5 or 10 mg chlorpheniramine (1 or 2 tablets) every 12 hr.

SUSPENSION

Adults and children age 6 and over. 30 or 60 mg carbetapentante and 4 or 8 mg chlorpheniramine (5 or 10 ml) every 12 hr.

Children ages 2 to 6. 15 or 30 mg carbetapentante and 2 or 4 mg chlorpheniramine (2.5 or 5 ml) every 12 hr.

Mechanism of Action

Carbetapentane has atropine-like and local anesthetic actions that suppresses the cough reflex through selective depression of the medullary cough center in the brain.

Chlorpheniramine competes with histamine for H_1 receptor sites, thereby antagonizing many histamine effects and reducing allergy effects.

Contraindications

Breast-feeding; hypersensitivity to carbetapentane, chlorpheniramine, or their components; use of MAO inhibitors within 14 days

Interactions

DRUGS

carbetapentane and chlorpheniramine (suspension form)

tartrazine (FD & C Yellow No. 5): Possibly induced allergic-type reactions in susceptible people

chlorpheniramine

CNS depressants: Additive CNS effects

MAO inhibitors: Possibly prolonged and intensified anticholinergic effects of chlorpheniramine

phenytoin: Possibly increased serum phenytoin levels and toxicity

ACTIVITIES

chlorpheniramine

alcohol use: Additive CNS effects

Adverse Reactions

CNS: Confusion, dizziness, drowsiness, excitation (children), hallucinations, headache, insomnia, restlessness, sedation

CV: Bradycardia, hypotension, palpitations, tachycardia
EENT: Blurred vision, dry mouth or eyes
GI: Abdominal pain, constipation, nausea, vomiting
GU: Urinary hesitancy, urine retention
HEME: Agranulocytosis, aplastic anemia, thrombocytopenia

Nursing Considerations

• Use cautiously in patients with cardiovascular disease, hypertension, hyperthyroidism, narrow-angle glaucoma, or prostatic hypertrophy.
• Monitor children for excitation and elderly patients for dizziness, sedation, and hypotension; such patients may have an increased risk for these effects.
• Monitor patient's CBC and platelet count, as ordered. Rarely, drug may cause serious adverse reactions, such as agranulocytosis, aplastic anemia, and thrombocytopenia.
• Regularly evaluate effectiveness of carbetapentane and chlorpheniramine in reducing cough and allergy symptoms.
• Be aware that patient shouldn't have intradermal allergen tests within 72 hours of receiving drug because results may be altered.

PATIENT TEACHING

• Instruct patient to use a calibrated measuring device for suspension form of carbetapentane and chlorpheniramine to ensure accurate dose.
• Urge patient to avoid alcohol and other antidepressants while taking carbetapentane and chlorpheniramine.
• Instruct patient to avoid hazardous activities until drug's CNS effects are known.
• Suggest that patient relieve dry mouth with frequent rinsing and use of sugarless gum or hard candy.

carbetapentane tannate, chlorpheniramine tannate, ephedrine tannate, and phenylephrine tannate

Quad Tann, Renatamine Pediatric Suspension, Rynatuss, Rynatuss Pediatric Suspension

Class and Category

Chemical: Cyclopentane carbolic ester (carbetapentane), propylamine derivative (chlorpheniramine), sympathomimetic amines (ephedrine, phenylephrine)
Therapeutic: Antitussive (carbetapentane), antihistaminic (chlor-

peniramine), bronchodilator (ephedrine), decongestant (phenylephrine)

Pregnancy category: C

Indications and Dosages

▶ *To relieve cough in such respiratory tract conditions as the common cold, bronchial asthma, and acute and chronic bronchitis*

TABLETS

Adults. 60 or 120 mg carbetapentane, 5 or 10 mg chlorpheniramine, 10 or 20 mg ephedrine, and 10 or 20 mg phenylephrine (1 or 2 tablets) every 12 hr.

SUSPENSION

Adults and children age 6 and over. 30 or 60 mg carbetapentante, 4 or 8 mg chlorpheniramine, 5 or 10 mg ephedrine, and 5 or 10 mg phenylephrine (5 or 10 ml) every 12 hr.

Children ages 2 to 6. 15 or 30 mg carbetapentante, 2 or 4 mg chlorpheniramine, 2.5 or 5 mg ephedrine and 2.5 or 5 mg phenylephrine (2.5 or 5 ml) every 12 hr.

Mechanism of Action

Carbetapentane has atropine-like and local anesthetic actions that suppress the cough reflex in the medullary cough center in the brain.

Chlorpheniramine competes with histamine for H_1 receptor sites, thereby antagonizing many histamine effects and reducing allergy effects.

Ephedrine stimulates beta-adrenergic receptors in the lungs, relaxing bronchial smooth muscle and relieving bronchospasm. It also stimulates alpha-adrenergic receptors in nasal passages to produce vasoconstriction and a drying effect on nasal mucous membranes.

Phenylephrine stimulates alpha-adrenergic receptors and inhibits the intracellular enzyme adenyl cyclase, which then inhibits production of cAMP. Inhibition of cAMP causes arterial and venous constriction in nasal passages, which decreases blood flow and mucosal edema caused by allergic response.

Contraindications

Breast-feeding; hypersensitivity to carbetapentane, chlorpheniramine, ephedrine, or phenylephrine or their components; use of MAO inhibitors within 14 days

Interactions

DRUGS

carbetapentane, chlorpheniramine, ephedrine, and phenylephrine (suspension form)

tartrazine (FD & C Yellow No. 5): Possibly induced allergic-type reactions in susceptible persons

chlorpheniramine, ephedrine, and phenylephrine

MAO inhibitors: Possibly prolonged and intensified anticholinergic effects

phenytoin: Possibly increased serum phenytoin levels and toxicity

chlorpheniramine and phenylephrine

CNS depressants: Additive CNS effects

ephedrine and phenylephrine

alpha blockers, haloperidol, loxapine, phenothiazines, thioxanthenes: Possibly decreased vasoconstrictor effect of phenylephrine

beta blockers: Decreased therapeutic effects of each drug

ergot alkaloids: Possibly rupture of cerebral blood vessel, increased vasopressor effect, peripheral vascular ischemia, and gangrene (with ergotamine)

hydrocarbon inhalation anesthetics: Increased risk of serious arrhythmias

thyroid hormones: Increased cardiovascular effects of each drug

ephedrine

guanadrel, guanethidine: Possibly decreased hypotensive effects of these agents

guanethidine, methyldopa, reserpine: Reduced pressor response of ephedrine

theophylline: Possibly enhanced toxicity, especially increased nausea, nervousness, and insomnia

tricyclic antidepressants: Possibly increased pressor response

urinary acidifers: May decrease half-life of ephedrine, which may lead to decreased effects

urinary alkalizers: May increase ephadrine half-life and effects

phenylephrine

antihypertenisves, diuretics: Possibly decreased antihypertensive effects

atropine: Possibly enhanced vasopressor effect of phenylephrine

bretylium: Possibly potentiated vaopressor effect and arrhythmias

doxapram: Increased vasopressor effect of both drugs

guanadrel, guanethidine: Increased vasopressor effect of phenylephrine; increased risk of severe hypertension and arrhythmias

mecamylamine, methyldopa: Decreased hypotensive effects of these drugs; increased vasopressor effect of phenylephrine

nitrates: Possibly decreased vasopressor effect of phenylephrine and decreased antianginal effect of nitrates

oxytocin: Possibly severe, persistent hypertension

phenoxybenzamine: Decreased vasoconstrictor effect of phenylephrine; possibly hypotension and tachycardia

theophylline: Possibly enhanced toxicity (including cardiac toxicity)
ACTIVITIES
chlorpheniramine and phenylephrine
alcohol use: Additive CNS effects

Adverse Reactions

CNS: Confusion, dizziness, drowsiness, excitation (children), headache, impaired cognition, insomnia, nervousness, paresthesia, restlessness, sedation, tremor, weakness
CV: Angina, bradycardia, hypertension, hypotension, palpitations, peripheral vasoconstriction that may lead to necrosis or gangrene, tachycardia, ventricular arrhythmias
EENT: Blurred vision, dry eyes or mouth
GI: Abdominal pain, constipation, nausea, vomiting
GU: Urinary hesitancy, urine retention
HEME: Agranulocytosis, aplastic anemia, thrombocytopenia
RESP: Dyspnea

Nursing Considerations

- Use cautiously in patients with cardiovascular disease, diabetes, hypertension, hyperthyroidism, narrow-angle glaucoma, or prostatic hypertrophy.
- Monitor children for excitation and elderly patients for dizziness, sedation, and hypotension; such patients may have an increased risk for these effects.
- Monitor patient's CBC and platelet counts, as ordered, because, although rare, drug may cause serious hematologic adverse reactions such as agranulocytosis, aplastic anemia, and thrombocytopenia.
- Regularly evaluate effectiveness of carbetapentane, chlorpheniramine, ephedrine, and phenylephrine in reducing cough and allergy symptoms.
- Be aware that patient shouldn't have intradermal allergen tests within 72 hours of receiving drug because results may be altered.

PATIENT TEACHING
- Instruct patient to use a calibrated measuring device for suspension form of carbetapentane, chlorpheniramine, ephedrine, and phenylephrine to ensure accurate dose.
- Urge patient to avoid alcohol and other antidepressants while taking drug.
- Instruct patient to avoid hazardous activities until drug's CNS effects are known.
- Suggest that patient relieve dry mouth with frequent rinsing and use of sugarless gum or hard candy.

carbetapentane citrate, phenylephrine hydrochloride, and guaifenesin

Levall

Class and Category

Chemical: Cyclopentane carbolic ester (carbetapentane), sympatho-mimetic amine (phenylephrine), glyceryl guaiacolate (guaifenesin)

Therapeutic: Antitussive (carbetapentane), decongestant (phenyl-ephrine), expectorant (guaifenesin)

Pregnancy category: C

Indications and Dosages

▶ *To provide temporary relief of nonproductive cough and nasal congestion from the common cold, bronchitis, or sinusitis*

ORAL SOLUTION

Adults. 20 mg carbetapentane, 15 mg phenylephrine, and 100 mg guaifenesin (5 ml) every 4 to 6 hr. *Maximum:* 20 ml daily.

Mechanism of Action

Carbetapentane has atropine-like and local anesthetic actions, which suppress the cough reflex in the medullary, cough center in the brain.

Phenylephrine stimulates alpha-adrenergic receptors and inhibits the intracellular enzyme adenyl cyclase, which then inhibits production of cAMP. Inhibition of cAMP causes arterial and venous constriction in nasal passages, which decreases blood flow and mucosal edema caused by allergic response.

Guaifenesin increases fluid and mucus removal from the upper respiratory tract by increasing the volume of secretions and reducing their adhesiveness and surface tension.

Contraindications

Hypersensitivity to bisulfites, carbetapentane, phenylephrine, guaifenesin, or their components; severe coronary artery disease or hypertension; use within 14 days of MAO inhibitor therapy; ventricular tachycardia

Interactions

DRUGS

phenylephrine

alpha blockers, haloperidol, loxapine, phenothiazines, thioxanthenes: Possibly decreased vasoconstrictor effect of phenylephrine

antihypertenisves, diuretics: Possibly decreased antihypertensive effects *atropine:* Possibly enhanced vasopressor effect of phenylephrine

beta blockers: Decreased therapeutic effects of both drugs

bretylium: Possibly potentiated vaopressor effect and arrhythmias

doxapram: Increased vasopressor effect of both drugs

ergot alkaloids: Possibly cerebral blood vessel rupture, increased vasopressor effect, peripheral vascular ischemia, and gangrene (with ergotamine)

guanadrel, guanethidine: Increased vasopressor effect of phenylephrine; increased risk of severe hypertension and arrhythmias

hydrocarbon inhalation anesthetics: Increased risk of serious arrhythmias

MAO inhibitors: Increased and prolonged cardiac stimulation, increased vasopressor effect, increased risk of severe cardiovascular and cerebrovascular effects, hyperpyrexia, and vomiting

maprotiline, tricyclic antidepressants: Increased risk of severe cardiovascular effects (including arrhythmias, hyperpyrexia, severe hypertension)

mecamylamine, methyldopa: Decreased hypotensive effects of these drugs and increased vasopressor effect of phenylephrine

nitrates: Possibly decreased vasopressor effect of phenylephrine and decreased antianginal effect of nitrates

oxytocin: Possibly severe, persistent hypertension

phenoxybenzamine: Decreased vasoconstrictor effect of phenylephrine and possible hypotension and tachycardia

theophylline: Possibly enhanced toxicity (including cardiac toxicity)

thyroid hormones: Increased cardiovascular effects of each drug

Adverse Reactions

CNS: Anxiety, confusion, dizziness, hallucinations, headache, insomnia, nervousness, paresthesia, restlessness, tremor, weakness

CV: Angina, bradycardia, hypertension, hypotension, palpitations, peripheral vasoconstriction that may lead to necrosis or gangrene, tachycardia, ventricular arrhythmia

GI: Nausea, vomiting

GU: Dysuria, urine retention

RESP: Dyspnea

SKIN: Pallor, rash, urticaria

Other: Allergic reaction

Nursing Considerations

- Assess patient for signs and symptoms of angina, arrhythmias, and hypertension because phenylephrine may increase myocardial oxygen demand and the risk of proarrhythmias and blood pressure changes.

- **WARNING** Monitor patient with thyroid disease for increased sensitivity to catecholamines and for possible thyrotoxicity or cardiotoxicity.
- Regularly evaluate effectiveness of carbetapentane, phenylephrine, and guaifenesin in relieving cough and other upper respiratory symptoms. Notify prescriber if symptoms don't improve or if they worsen.

PATIENT TEACHING
- Caution patient to take drug exactly as prescribed and not to increase dosage or frequency without first consulting prescriber.
- Instruct patient to increase fluid intake (unless contraindicated) to help thin secretions.
- Advise patient to avoid hazardous activities until drug's CNS effects are known.

carbetapentane tannate, phenylephrine tannate, and pyrilamine tannate

Tussi-12D, Tussi-12D S

Class and Category

Chemical: Cyclopentane carbolic ester (carbetapentane), sympathomimetic amine (phenylephrine), ethylenediamine antihistamine (pyrilamine)

Therapeutic: Antitussive (carbetapentane), decongestant (phenylephrine), antihistaminic (pyrilamine)

Pregnancy category: C

Indications and Dosages

▶ *To relieve cough and nasal congestion from the common cold, sinusitis, allergic rhinitis, and other upper respiratory tract conditions*

SUSPENSION

Adults. 30 to 60 mg carbetapentane, 5 to 10 mg phenylephrine, and 30 to 60 mg pyrilamine (5 to 10 ml) every 12 hr.

TABLETS

Adults. 60 to 120 mg carbetapentane, 10 to 20 mg phenylephrine, and 40 to 80 mg pyrilamine (1 to 2 tablets) every 12 hr.

Contraindications

Acute MI; angina; breast-feeding; cardiac arrhythmias; coronary artery disease; hypersensitivity to carbetapentane, phenylephrine, pyrilamine or their components; use of MAO inhibitors within 14 days; ventricular tachycardia

Mechanism of Action
Carbetapentane has atropine-like and local anesthetic actions that suppress the cough reflex in the medullary cough center in the brain.

Phenylephrine stimulates alpha-adrenergic receptors and inhibits the intracellular enzyme adenyl cyclase, which then inhibits production of cAMP. Inhibition of cAMP causes arterial and venous constriction in nasal passages, which decreases blood flow and mucosal edema caused by allergic response.

Pyrilamine competes with histamine for H_1 receptor sites, thereby antagonizing many histamine effects to reduce allergy signs and symptoms.

Interactions
DRUGS

phenylephrine and pyrilamine
MAO inhibitors: Possibly prolonged and intensified anticholinergic effects of pyrilamine and overall effects of phenylephrine
carbetapentane
tartrazine (FD & C Yellow No. 5 contained in certain products): Possibly induced allergic-type reactions in susceptible persons
phenylephrine
alpha blockers, haloperidol, loxapine, phenothiazines, thioxanthenes: Possibly decreased vasoconstrictor effect of phenylephrine
antihypertenisves, diuretics: Possibly decreased antihypertensive effects
atropine: Possibly enhanced vasopressor effect of phenylephrine
beta blockers: Decreased therapeutic effects of both drugs
bretylium: Possibly potentiated vaopressor effect and arrhythmias
doxapram: Increased vasopressor effect of both drugs
ergot alkaloids: Possibly cerebral blood vessel rupture, increased vasopressor effect, peripheral vascular ischemia, and gangrene (with ergotamine)
guanadrel, guanethidine: Increased vasopressor effect of phenylephrine, increased risk of severe hypertension and arrhythmias
hydrocarbon inhalation anesthetics: Possibly serious arrhythmias
maprotiline, tricyclic antidepressants: Increased risk of severe cardiovascular effects (including arrhythmias, hyperpyrexia, severe hypertension)
mecamylamine, methyldopa: Decreased hypotensive effects of these drugs, increased vasopressor effect of phenylephrine
nitrates: Possibly decreased vasopressor effect of phenylephrine and decreased antianginal effect of nitrates
oxytocin: Possibly severe, persistent hypertension

phenoxybenzamine: Decreased vasoconstrictor effect of phenylephrine, possibly hypotension and tachycardia
theophylline: Possibly enhanced toxicity (including cardiac toxicity)
thyroid hormones: Increased cardiovascular effects of each drug
chlorpheniramine
CNS depressants: Additive CNS effects
ACTIVITIES
chlorpheniramine
alcohol use: Additive CNS effects

Adverse Reactions
CNS: Confusion, dizziness, drowsiness, hallucinations, headache, insomnia, nervousness, paresthesia, restlessness, sedation, seizures, tremor, weakness
CV: Angina, bradycardia, hypertension, hypotension, palpitations, peripheral vasoconstriction that may lead to necrosis or gangrene, tachycardia, ventricular arrhythmias
EENT: Blurred vision; dry eyes, mouth, and nose
GI: Constipation, nausea, vomiting
GU: Urinary hesitancy, urine retention
RESP: Dyspnea

Nursing Considerations
- Use cautiously in patients with cardiovascular disease, diabetes, hypertension, hyperthyroidism, narrow-angle glaucoma, or prostatic hypertrophy.
- Monitor patients who may be more susceptible to dizziness, sedation, and hypotension, such as the elderly.
- Regularly evaluate effectiveness of carbetapentane, phenylephrine, and pyrilamine in reducing cough and nasal congestion.
- Patient shouldn't have intradermal allergen tests within 72 hours of receiving drug because results may be altered.

PATIENT TEACHING
- Instruct patient to use a calibrated measuring device when using suspension form of carbetapentane, phenylephrine, and pyrilamine to ensure accurate dose.
- Instruct patient to take drug exactly as prescribed and not to increase dosage or frequency without consulting prescriber.
- Urge patient to avoid alcohol and other antidepressants while taking carbetapentane, phenylephrine, and pyrilamine.
- Instruct patient to avoid hazardous activities until drug's CNS effects are known.
- Suggest that patient relieve dry mouth with frequent rinsing and use of sugarless gum or hard candy.

carbinoxamine maleate and pseudoephedrine hydrochloride

Andehist Drops, Cardec-S, Coldec D, CP Oral, Mooredec, Palgic-D, Rinade B.I.D. Tablets, Rondec, Rondec Drops, Rondec-TR

Class and Category

Chemical: Ethanolamine derivative (carbinoxamine), sympathomimetic amine (pseudoephedrine)

Therapeutic: Antihistaminic (carbinoxamine), decongestant (pseudoephedrine)

Pregnancy category: C

Indications and Dosages

▶ *To relieve persistent runny nose, sneezing, and nasal congestion caused by upper respiratory infections, sinus inflammation, hay fever, or the common cold*

E.R. TABLETS

Adults. 6 to 8 mg carbinoxamine and 60 to 120 mg pseudoephedrine (1 tablet) every 12 hr.

TABLETS

Adults. 4 mg carbinoxamine and 120 mg pseudoephedrine (1 tablet) every 12 hr. Or, 4 mg carbinoxamine and 60 mg pseudoephedrine (1 tablet) every 6 hr. Or, 8 mg carbinoxamine and 90 mg pseudoephedrine (1 tablet) every 12 hr.

Children age 6 and over. 4 mg carbinoxamine and 60 mg pseudoephedrine (1 tablet) every 6 hr.

CHEWABLE TABLETS

Adults and children age 12 and over. 4 mg carbinoxamine and 60 mg pseudoephedrine (1 tablet) every 4 hr.

Children ages 6 to 12. 2 mg carbinoxamine and 30 mg pseudoephedrine (½ tablet) every 4 hr.

SYRUP

Adults and children age 6 and over. 4 mg carbinoxamine and 60 mg pseudoephedrine (5 ml) every 6 hr.

Children age 18 months to 6 years. 2 mg carbinoxamine and 30 mg pseudoephedrine (2.5 ml) every 6 hr.

ORAL SOLUTION

Children ages 9 months to 18 months. 2 mg carbinoxamine and 25 mg pseudoephedrine (1 ml) every 6 hr.

Children ages 6 months to 9 months. 1.5 mg carbinoxamine and 18.75 mg pseudoephedrine (0.75 ml) every 6 hr.

Infants ages 3 months to 6 months. 1 mg carbinoxamine and 12.5 mg pseudoephedrine (0.5 ml) every 6 hr.

Infants ages 1 month to 3 months. 0.5 mg carbinoxamine and 6.25 mg pseudoephedrine (0.25 ml) every 6 hr.
DROPS
Children ages 12 months to 24 months. 1 or 2 mg carbinoxamine and 15 mg pseudoephedrine (1 ml) q.i.d.
Children ages 6 months to 12 months. 0.75 or 1.5 mg carbinoxamine and 11.25 mg psuedoephedrine (0.75 ml) q.i.d.
Infants ages 3 months to 6 months. 0.5 or 1 mg carbinoxamine and 7.5 mg pseudoephedrine (0.5 ml) q.i.d.
Infants ages 1 month to 3 months. 0.25 or 0.5 mg carbinoxamine and 3.75 mg pseudoephedrine (0.25 ml) q.i.d.

Mechanism of Action

Carbinoxamine competes with histamine for H$_1$ receptor sites, thereby antagonizing many histamine effects and reducing allergy signs and symptoms.

Pseudoephedrine acts on alpha$_1$-adrenergic receptors in the mucosa of the respiratory tract to produce vasoconstriction. This process shrinks swollen nasal mucous membranes; reduces tissue hyperemia, edema, and nasal congestion; and increases nasal airway patency. It also may increase drainage of sinus secretions and open obstructed eustachian ostia.

Contraindications

Angina; breast-feeding; cardiac arrhythmias; hypersensitivity or idiosyncractic reactions to carbinoxamine, pseudoephedrine, or their components; hyperthyroidism; MI; narrow-angle glaucoma; severe coronary artery disease or hypertension; urine retention; use within 14 days of MAO inhibitor therapy

Interactions
DRUGS
carbinoxamine and pseudoephedrine
MAO inhibitors: Increased and prolonged cardiac stimulation, increased vasopressor effect, increased risk of severe cardiovascular and cerebrovascular effects, hyperpyrexia, and vomiting
carbinoxamine
anticholinergics: Additive anticholinergic effects
CNS depressants: Additive CNS effects
pseudoephedrine
antacids: Increased absorption of pseudoephedrine
antihypertensives, diuretics: Possibly decreased antihypertensive effects

beta blockers: Decreased therapeutic effects of both drugs
citrates: Possibly inhibited urinary pseudoephedrine excretion and prolonged duration of action
CNS stimulants, sympathomimetics: Possibly increased additive CNS stimulation to excessive levels
cocaine (mucosal-local): Possibly increased cardiovascular effects of either drug and CNS stimulation
digoxin, levodopa: Increased risk of cardiac arrhythmias
hydrocarbon inhalation anesthetics: Increased risk of serious arrhythmias
kaolin: Decreased pseudoephedrine absorption
MAO inhibitors: Increased and prolonged cardiac stimulation, increased vasopressor effect, increased risk of severe cardiovascular and cerebrovascular effects, hyperpyrexia, and vomiting
nitrates: Reduced antianginal effects of nitrates
rauwolfia alkaloids: Possibly inhibited pseudoephedrine action
thyroid hormones: Increased cardiovascular effects of both drugs
ACTIVITIES
carbinoxamine
alcohol use: Additive CNS effects

Adverse Reactions

CNS: Anxiety, chills, confusion, coordination disturbance, dizziness, drowsiness, excitation (children), fatigue, fear, hallucinations, headache, hysteria, insomnia, irritability, light-headedness, nervousness, numbness, restlessness, sedation, seizures, tenseness, trembling, vertigo, weakness
CV: Angina, arrhythmias, chest tightness, hypertension, palpitations, tachycardia
EENT: Blurred or double vision; dry eyes, mouth, nose, and throat; nasal congestion; tinnitus
ENDO: Early menstruation
GI: Anorexia, constipation, diarrhea, nausea, stomach upset or pain, vomiting
GU: Dysuria, frequent urination, urinary hesitancy, urine retention
HEME: Anemia, unusual bleeding or bruising
RESP: Dyspnea, increased chest congestion, wheezing
SKIN: Diaphoresis, pallor, photosensitivity, rash, urticaria
Other: Anaphylaxis

Nursing Considerations

• Use carbinoxamine and pseudoephedrine cautiously in patients with asthma, cardiovascular disease, diabetes, emphysema or other chronic lung disease, hypertension, peptic ulcer, hyper-

thyroidism, narrow-angle glaucoma, or prostatic hypertrophy.
- Monitor children for excitation and elderly patients for dizziness, sedation, and hypotension; such patients may have an increased risk for these effects.
- Monitor renal function, as ordered, because pseudoephedrine is substantially excreted by the kidneys.
- Regularly evaluate effectiveness of carbinoxamine and pseudoephedrine in reducing upper respiratory symptoms.
- Be aware that patient shouldn't have intradermal allergen tests within 72 hours of receiving drug because results may be altered.

PATIENT TEACHING
- Instruct patient to use a calibrated measuring device for syrup or oral solution form of carbinoxamine and pseudoephedrine to ensure accurate dose.
- Urge patient to avoid alcohol and other antidepressants while taking carbinoxamine and pseudoephedrine.
- Instruct patient to avoid hazardous activities until drug's CNS effects are known.
- Suggest that patient relieve dry mouth with frequent rinsing and use of sugarless gum or hard candy.
- Tell patient to take last dose of the day a few hours before bedtime if carbinoxamine and pseudoephedrine makes her nervous or restless.

cetirizine hydrochloride and pseudoephedrine hydrochloride
Zyrtec-D 12 Hour

Class and Category
Chemical: H_1 receptor antagonist (cetirizine), sympathomimetic amine (pseudoephedrine)
Therapeutic: Antihistamine (cetirizine), decongestant (pseudoephedrine)
Pregnancy category: C

Indications and Dosages
▶ *To relieve nasal and non-nasal symptoms of seasonal or perennial allergic rhinitis*

E.R. TABLETS
Adults and children age 12 and over. 5 mg cetirizine and 120 mg pseudoephedrine (1 tablet) every 12 hr.

DOSAGE ADJUSTMENT For patients with decreased renal

function (creatinine clearance of 11 to 31 ml/min/1.73 m^2), patients on hemodialysis (creatinine clearance less than 7 ml/min/1.73 m^2), or patients with decreased hepatic function, dosage decreased to 5 mg cetirizine and 120 mg pseudoephedrine (1 tablet) every 24 hr.

Mechanism of Action

Cetirizine competes with histamine for histamine H$_1$ receptor sites on effector cells and antagonizes the vasodilator effect of endogenously released histamine. This prevents the peripheral vascular engorgement, mucosal edema, sneezing, and profuse watery nasal secretion and irritation that normally result from histamine action on peripheral afferent nerve terminals.

Pseudoephedrine acts on alpha$_1$-adrenergic receptors in the mucosa of the respiratory tract to produce vasoconstriction. This process shrinks swollen nasal mucous membranes; reduces tissue hyperemia, edema, and nasal congestion; and increases nasal airway patency. It also may increase drainage of sinus secretions and open obstructed eustachian ostia.

Contraindications

Angina; cardiac arrhythmias; hypersensitivity or idiosyncratic reactions to cetirizine, pseudoephedrine, or their components; hyperthyroidism; narrow-angle glaucoma; severe coronary artery disease or hypertension; urine retention; use within 14 days of MAO inhibitor therapy

Interactions

DRUGS

cetirizine

barbiturates, CNS depressants, tricyclic antidepressants: Additive effects
theophylline: Possibly decreased cetirizine clearance

pseudoephedrine

antacids: Increased pseudoephedrine absorption
antihypertensives, diuretics: Possibly decreased antihypertensive effects
beta blockers: Decreased therapeutic effects of both drugs
citrates: Possibly inhibited urinary pseudoephedrine excretion and prolonged duration of action
CNS stimulant, other sympathomimetics: Possibly increased additive CNS stimulation to excessive levels
cocaine (mucosal-local): Possibly increased cardiovascular effects of either drug and CNS stimulation
digoxin, levodopa: Increased risk of cardiac arrhythmias

hydrocarbon inhalation anesthetics: Possibly serious arrhythmias
kaolin: Decreased pseudoephedrine absorption
MAO inhibitors: Increased and prolonged cardiac stimulation, increased vasopressor effect, increased risk of severe cardiovascular and cerebrovascular effects, hyperpyrexia, vomiting
nitrates: Reduced antianginal effects of nitrates
rauwolfia alkaloids: Possibly inhibited pseudoephedrine action
thyroid hormones: Increased cardiovascular effects of both drugs
ACTIVITIES
cetirizine
alcohol use: Additive effects

Adverse Reactions

CNS: Anxiety, dizziness, drowsiness, excitability, fatigue, fear, hallucinations, headache, insomnia, light-headedness, nervousness, restlessness, seizures, somnolence, trembling, weakness
CV: Angina, arrhythmias, hypertension, palpitations, tachycardia
EENT: Dry mouth, epistaxis, ocular hypertension, pharyngitis, sinusitis
GI: Nausea, vomiting
GU: Dysuria
RESP: Dyspnea
SKIN: Diaphoresis, pallor

Nursing Considerations

- Use cetirizine and pseudoephedrine cautiously in patients with hypertension, diabetes mellitus, ischemic heart disease, increased intraocular pressure, hyperthyroidism, renal impairment, or prostatic hypertrophy because of pseudoephedrine.
- Monitor children for excitation and elderly patients for dizziness, sedation, and hypotension; such patients may have an increased risk for these effects.
- Monitor renal function, as ordered, because pseudoephedrine is substantially excreted by the kidneys.
- Evaluate effectiveness of cetirizine and pseudoephedrine in relieving seasonal or perennial allergic rhinitis.
- Be aware that patient shouldn't have intradermal allergen tests within 4 days of receiving drug because results may be altered.
PATIENT TEACHING
- Urge patient to avoid alcohol, other antidepressants, and OTC medication containing other antihistamines or sympathomimetics while taking cetirizine and pseudoephedrine.
- Instruct patient to avoid hazardous activities until drug's CNS effects are known.

• Suggest that patient relieve dry mouth with frequent rinsing and use of sugarless gum or hard candy.

chlorpheniramine maleate and hydrocodone bitartrate
S-T Forte 2

chlorpheniramine polistirex and hydrocodone polistirex
Tussionex Pennkinetic Suspension

Class, Category, and Schedule
Chemical: Alkylamine (chlorpheniramine), opioid and phenanthrene derivative (hydrocodone)
Therapeutic: Antihistamine (chlorpheniramine), antitussive (hydrocodone),
Pregnancy category: C
Controlled substance schedule: III

Indications and Dosages
▶ *To relieve cough and respiratory symptoms from colds and allergies*
E.R. SUSPENSION
Adults. 8 mg chlorpheniramine and 10 mg hydrocodone (5 ml) every 12 hr. *Maximum:* 16 mg chlorpheniramine and 20 mg hydrocodone every 24 hr.
Children age 6 and over. 4 mg chlorpheniramine and 5 mg hydrocodone (2.5 ml) every 12 hr. *Maximum:* 8 mg chlorpheniramine and 10 mg hydrocodone every 24 hr.
ORAL SOLUTION
Adults and children age 12 and over. 2 mg chlorpheniramine and 2.5 mg hydrocodone (5 ml) every 6 to 8 hr.
Children ages 3 to 12. 1 mg chlorpheniramine and 1.25 mg hydrocodone (2.5 ml) every 6 to 8 hr.

Mechanism of Action
Chlorpheniramine competes with histamine for H_1 receptor sites, thereby antagonizing many histamine effects and reducing allergy signs and symptoms.
  Hydrocodone suppresses cough by acting directly on opiate receptors in the medulla's cough center.

Contraindications
Children under age 6 (E.R. suspension), hypersensitivity to chlor-

pheniramine, hydrocodone, other opioids, or their components; respiratory depression; severe asthma; upper airway obstruction; use of MAO inhibitors within 14 days

Interactions

DRUGS

chlorpheniramine and hydrocodone

anticholinergics, paregoric: Possibly intensified anticholinergic adverse effects, such as paralytic ileus

CNS depressants: Additive CNS effects

MAO inhibitors: Increased and prolonged cardiac stimulation, increased vasopressor effect, increased risk of severe cardiovascular and cerebrovascular effects, hyperpyrexia, and vomiting

chlorpheniramine

phenytoin: Possibly increased serum phenytoin levels and toxicity

hydrocodone

antihypertensives, diuretics: Potentiated hypotensive effects

buprenorphine: Decreased hydrocodone effectiveness

hydroxyzine: Increased hydrocodone analgesic effect; increased CNS depressant and hypotensive effects

metoclopramide: Antagonized effect of metoclopramide on GI motility

naloxone: Antagonized hydrocodone analgesic effect

naltrexone: Precipitated withdrawal symptoms in hydrocodone-dependent patients

neuromuscular blockers: Additive respiratory depressant effects

opioids: Additive CNS and respiratory depressants effects and hypotensive effects

ACTIVITIES

chlorpheniramine and hydrocodone

alcohol use: Additive CNS effects

Adverse Reactions

CNS: Anxiety, confusion, decreased mental and physical performance, depression, dizziness, drowsiness, euphoria, faintness, fear, headache, light-headedness, mood changes, nervousness, restlessness, sedation, seizures, tiredness, weakness

CV: Bradycardia, chest tightness, hypotension, palpitations, tachycardia

EENT: Blurred or double vision, dry mouth, laryngeal edema, laryngospasm

GI: Anorexia, constipation, nausea, paralytic ileus, toxic megacolon, vomiting

GU: Dysuria, frequent urination

RESP: Dyspnea, shortness of breath, slow or irregular breathing, wheezing
Skin: Diaphoresis, facial flushing, pruritus, rash, uriticaria
Other: Angioedema, atelectasis, mental or physical dependence

Nursing Considerations

- Use cautiously in patients with a recent head injury and those with Addison's disease, asthma or other chronic respiratory disease, increased intraocular pressure, hypothyroidism, liver or renal impairment, or prostatic hypertrophy. Also use cautiously in children because of an increased risk of respiratory depression.
- Monitor children for excitation and elderly patients for dizziness, sedation, and hypotension; they have an increased risk.
- Regularly evaluate effectiveness of chlorpheniramine and hyrdocodone in reducing symptoms.
- Monitor patient's respiratory status closely. Expect to give naloxone if respiratory depression occurs and to provide other supportive measures, as indicated and ordered.
- Be aware that patient shouldn't have intradermal allergen tests within 72 hours of receiving drug because results may be altered.

PATIENT TEACHING

- Instruct patient to shake suspension well before measuring dose and to use a calibrated device to ensure accurate dose.
- Urge patient to avoid alcohol and other antidepressants while taking chlorpheniramine and hydrocodone.
- Instruct patient to avoid hazardous activities until drug's CNS effects are known.
- Suggest that patient relieve dry mouth with frequent rinsing and use of sugarless gum or hard candy.
- Tell patient to take last dose of the day a few hours before bedtime if drug makes her nervous or restless.

chlorpheniramine maleate, hydrocodone bitartrate, and phenylephrine hydrochloride

Atuss MS, Chlorgest-HD, Comtussin HC, Cytuss HC, ED-TLC, ED Tuss HC, Endagen-HD, Endal HD, Endal HD Plus, Histinex HC, Histussin HC, Hydrocodone CP, Hydrocodone HD, Hydron CP, Hydro-PC, Hydro-PC II, Iodal HD, Iotussin HC, Maxi-Tuss HC, Poly-Tussin, Unituss HC, Vanex-HD, Z-Cof HC

Class, Category, and Schedule
Chemical: Alkylamine (chlorpheniramine), opioid and phenanthrene derivative (hydrocodone), and sympathomimetic amine (phenylephrine)
Therapeutic: Antihistamine (chlorpheniramine), antitussive (hydrocodone), and decongestant (phenylephrine)
Pregnancy category: C
Controlled substance schedule: III

Indications and Dosages
▶ *To relieve cough and upper respiratory symptoms of colds and allergies*
SYRUP, ORAL SOLUTION
Adults and children age 12 and over. 2 to 4 mg chlorpheniramine, 1.67 mg to 5 mg hydrocodone, and 5 to 10 mg phenylephrine (5 to 10 ml depending on product used) every 4 hr or t.i.d. to q.i.d. Or, 8 mg chlorpheniramine, 3.34 mg hydrocodone, and 10 mg phenylephrine (10 ml) every 6 to 8 hr. *Maximum:* 4 doses daily.
Children age 6 to 12. 2 to 4 mg chlorpheniramine, 1.25 to 2.5 mg hydrocodone, and 5 to 10 mg phenylephrine (2.5 or 5 ml depending on product) every 4 to 8 hr. *Maximum:* 4 doses daily.
Children age 2 to 6. 1 mg chlorpheniramine, 0.625 mg hydrocodone, and 2.5 mg phenylephrine (1.25 ml) every 4 to 6 hr.
DOSAGE ADJUSTMENT For patients with renal impairment, dosage may need to be reduced.

Mechanism of Action
Chlorpheniramine competes with histamine for H_1 receptor sites, thereby antagonizing many histamine effects and reducing allergy signs and symptoms.

Hydrocodone suppresses cough by directly acting on opiate receptors in the medulla's cough center.

Phenylephrine stimulates alpha-adrenergic receptors and inhibits the intracellular enzyme adenyl cyclase, which then inhibits production of cAMP. Inhibition of cAMP causes arterial and venous constriction in nasal passages, which decreases blood flow and mucosal edema caused by allergic response.

Contraindications
Breast-feeding; closed-angle glaucoma; hypersensitivity to chlorpheniramine, hydrocodone, other opioids, phenylephrine, or their components; prostate disease; respiratory depression; severe

asthma; thyroid disease; upper airway obstruction, use of MAO inhibitors within 14 days

Interactions

DRUGS

chlorpheniramine, hydrocodone and phenylephrine

MAO inhibitors: Increased and prolonged cardiac stimulation, increased vasopressor effect, increased risk of severe cardiovascular and cerebrovascular effects, hyperpyrexia, vomiting

chlorpheniramine and hydrocodone

anticholinergics: Possibly intensified anticholinergic adverse effects

CNS depressants: Additive CNS effects

chlorpheniramine

phenytoin: Possibly increased serum phenytoin levels and toxicity

hydrocodone

antihypertensives, diuretics: Potentiated hypotensive effects

buprenorphine: Decreased effectiveness of hydrocodone

hydroxyzine: Increased hydrocodone analgesic effect; increased CNS depressant and hypotensive effects

metoclopramide: Antagonized effect of metoclopramide on GI motility

naloxone: Antagonized hydrocodone analgesic effect

naltrexone: Precipitated withdrawal symptoms in hydrocodone-dependent patients

neuromuscular blockers: Additive respiratory depressant effects

opioids: Additive CNS and respiratory depressants effects and hypotensive effects

phenylephrine

alpha blockers, haloperidol, loxapine, phenothiazines, thioxanthenes: Possibly decreased vasoconstrictor effect of phenylephrine

antihypertenisves, diuretics: Possibly decreased antihypertensive effects

atropine: Possibly enhanced vasopressor effect of phenylephrine

beta blockers: Decreased therapeutic effects of both drugs

bretylium: Possibly potentiated vaopressor effect and arrhythmias

doxapram: Increased vasopressor effect of both drugs

ergot alkaloids: Possibly cerebral blood vessel rupture, increased vasopressor effect, peripheral vascular ischemia, and gangrene (with ergotamine)

guanadrel, guanethidine: Increased vasopressor effect of phenylephrine, increased risk of severe hypertension and arrhythmias

hydrocarbon inhalation anesthetics: Increased risk of serious arrhythmias *maprotiline, tricyclic antidepressants:* Increased risk of severe cardiovascular effects (including arrhythmias, hyperpyrexia, severe hypertension)

mecamylamine, methyldopa: Decreased hypotensive effects of these drugs, increased vasopressor effect of phenylephrine

nitrates: Possibly decreased vasopressor effect of phenylephrine and decreased antianginal effect of nitrates

oxytocin: Possibly severe, persistent hypertension

phenoxybenzamine: Decreased vasoconstrictor effect of phenylephrine, possibly hypotension and tachycardia

theophylline: Possibly increased toxicity (including cardiac toxicity)

thyroid hormones: Increased cardiovascular effects of each drug

ACTIVITIES

chlorpheniramine and hydrocodone
alcohol use: Additive CNS effects

Adverse Reactions

CNS: Anxiety, confusion, decreased mental and physical performance, depression, dizziness, drowsiness, excitation (children), euphoria, faintness, fear, hallucinations, headache, insomnia, irritability, lethargy, light-headedness, mood changes, nervousness, paresthesia, psychosis, restlessness, sedation, seizures, tiredness, tremor, weakness

CV: Angina, bradycardia, chest tightness, hypertension, hypotension, palpitations, peripheral vasoconstriction, tachycardia, ventricular arrhythmias

EENT: Blurred or double vision, dry mouth, laryngeal edema, laryngospasm, mydriasis, ocular hypertension, photophobia

GI: Abdominal pain, anorexia, constipation, nausea, paralytic ileus, toxic megacolon, vomiting

GU: Dysuria, frequent urination, urinary hesitancy, urine retention

RESP: Dyspnea, shortness of breath, slow or irregular breathing, wheezing

Skin: Diaphoresis, facial flushing, pruritus, rash, uriticaria

Other: Angioedema, anaphylaxis, physical or psychological dependence

Nursing Considerations

• Use cautiously in patients with a recent head injury and those with Addison's disease, asthma or other chronic respiratory disease, increased intraocular pressure, hypothyroidism, or liver or renal impairment.

- Monitor children for excitation and elderly patients for dizziness, sedation, and hypotension; such patients may have an increased risk for these effects.
- Regularly evaluate effectiveness of chlorpheniramine, hydrocodone, and phenylephrine in reducing cough and upper respiratory symptoms.
- Be aware that patient shouldn't have intradermal allergen tests within 72 hours of receiving drug because results may be altered.

PATIENT TEACHING

- Instruct patient to use a calibrated measuring device to ensure accurate dose of chlorpheniramine, hydrocodone, and phenylephrine.
- Urge patient to avoid alcohol and other antidepressants while taking chlorpheniramine, hydrocodone, and phenylephrine.
- Instruct patient to avoid hazardous activities until drug's CNS effects are known.
- Suggest that patient relieve dry mouth with frequent rinsing and use of sugarless gum or hard candy.
- Tell patient to take last dose of the day a few hours before bedtime if chlorpheniramine, hydrocodone, and phenylephrine makes him nervous or restless.

chlorpheniramine maleate, hydrocodone bitartrate, and pseudoephedrine hydrochloride

Histinex PV, Hydron PSC, Hydro-Tussin HC, Hyphed, Pancof-HC, P-V Tussin, Tussend

Class, Category, and Schedule

Chemical: Alkylamine (chlorpheniramine), opioid and phenanthrene derivative (hydrocodone), sympathomimetic amine (pseudoephedrine)
Therapeutic: Antihistamine (chlorpheniramine), antitussive (hydrocodone), decongestant (pseudoephedrine)
Pregnancy category: C
Controlled substance schedule: III

Indications and Dosages

▶ *To relieve cough and upper respiratory symptoms of colds and allergies*

ORAL SOLUTION, SYRUP

Adults and children age 12 and over. 2 to 4 mg chlorpheni-

ramine, 3 to 6 mg hydrocodone, and 15 to 60 mg pseudoephedrine (5 to 10 ml depending on product) every 4 to 6 hr. Or,
doses may be given t.i.d or q.i.d. *Maximum:* 4 doses daily.
Children ages 6 to 12. 2 mg chlorpheniramine, 2.5 mg hydrocodone, and 30 mg pseudoephedrine (5 ml) every 4 to 6 hr. *Maximum:* 4 doses daily.
Children ages 2 to 6. 1 mg chlorpheniramine, 1.25 mg hydrocodone, and 15 mg pseudoephedrine (2.5 ml) every 4 to 6 hr.
Maximum: 4 doses daily.
TABLETS
Adults. 4 mg chlorpheniramine, 5 mg hydrocodone, and 60 mg
pseudoephedrine (1 tablet) every 6 hr.

Mechanism of Action

Chlorpheniramine competes with histamine for H_1 receptor sites, thereby antagonizing many histamine effects and reducing allergy signs and symptoms.
   Hydrocodone suppresses cough by directly acting on opiate receptors in
the medulla's cough center.
   Pseudoephedrine acts on $alpha_1$-adrenergic receptors in the mucosa of the
respiratory tract to produce vasoconstriction. This process shrinks swollen
nasal mucous membranes; reduces tissue hyperemia, edema, and nasal congestion; and increases nasal airway patency. It also may increase drainage of
sinus secretions and open obstructed eustachian ostia.

Contraindications
Hypersensitivity or idiosyncractic reactions to chlorpheniramine,
hydrocodone, other opioids, pseuodephedrine, or their components; hyperthyroidism; narrow-angle glaucoma; prostatic hypertrophy; respiratory depression; severe asthma, coronary artery
disease or hypertension; upper airway obstruction, urine retention, use of MAO inhibitors within 14 days

Interactions
DRUGS
chlorpheniramine, hydrocodone, and pseudoephedrine
MAO inhibitors: Increased and prolonged cardiac stimulation, increased vasopressor effect, increased risk of severe cardiovascular
and cerebrovascular effects, hyperpyrexia, and vomiting
chlorpheniramine and hydrocodone
anticholinergics, paregoric: Possibly intensified anticholinergic adverse effects
CNS depressants: Additive CNS effects

chlorpheniramine
phenytoin: Possibly increased serum phenytoin level and toxicity
hydrocodone
antihypertensives, diuretics: Potentiated hypotensive effects
buprenorphine: Decreased hydrocodone effectiveness
hydroxyzine: Increased hydrocodone analgesic effect; increased CNS depressant and hypotensive effects
metoclopramide: Antagonized metoclopramide effect on GI motility
naloxone: Anatagonized hydrocodone analgesic effect
naltrexone: Precipitated withdrawal symptoms in hydrocodone-dependent patients
neuromuscular blockers: Additive respiratory depressant effects
opioids: Additive CNS and respiratory depressants effects and hypotensive effects
pseudoephedrine
antacids: Increased pseudoephedrine absorption
antihypertensives, diuretics: Possibly decreased antihypertensive effects
beta blockers: Decreased therapeutic effects of both drugs
citrates: Possibly inhibited urinary pseudoephedrine excretion and prolonged duration of action
CNS stimulant, other sympathomimetics: Possibly increased additive CNS stimulation to excessive levels
cocaine (mucosal-local): Possibly increased cardiovascular effects of either drug and CNS stimulation
digoxin, levodopa: Increased risk of cardiac arrhythmias
hydrocarbon inhalation anesthetics: Possibly serious arrhythmias
kaolin: Decreased pseudoephedrine absorption
nitrates: Reduced antianginal effects of nitrates
rauwolfia alkaloids: Possibly inhibited pseudoephedrine action
thyroid hormones: Increased cardiovascular effects of both drugs
ACTIVITIES
chlorpheniramine and hydrocodone
alcohol use: Additive CNS effects

Adverse Reactions

CNS: Angina, anxiety, arrhythmia exacerbation, confusion, decreased mental and physical performance, depression, dizziness, drowsiness, excitation (children), euphoria, faintness, fear, headache, insomnia, light-headedness, mood changes, nervousness, restlessness, sedation, seizures, tiredness, trembling, weakness
CV: Bradycardia, chest tightness, hypotension, palpitations, tachycardia

EENT: Blurred or double vision, dry mouth, laryngeal edema, laryngospasm, photophobia

GI: Anorexia, constipation, nausea, paralytic ileus, toxic megacolon, vomiting

GU: Dysuria, frequent urination, urine retention

RESP: Dyspnea, shortness of breath, slow or irregular breathing, wheezing

Skin: Diaphoresis, facial flushing, pallor, pruritus, rash, uriticaria

Other: Angioedema, atelectasis, mental or physical dependence

Nursing Considerations

• Use cautiously in patients with a recent head injury and those with Addison's disease, asthma or other chronic respiratory disease, increased intraocular pressure, or liver or renal impairment.

• Monitor children for excitation and elderly patients for dizziness, sedation, and hypotension; such patients may have an increased risk for these effects.

• Monitor renal function, as ordered, because pseudoephedrine is substantially excreted by the kidneys.

• Regularly evaluate effectiveness of chlorpheniramine, hydrocodone, and pseudoephedrine in reducing symptoms.

• Be aware that patient shouldn't have intradermal allergen tests within 72 hours of receiving drug because it may alter results.

PATIENT TEACHING

• Instruct patient to use a calibrated measuring device to ensure accurate dose.

• Urge patient to avoid alcohol and other antidepressants while taking chlorpheniramine, hydrocodone, and pseudoephedrine.

• Instruct patient to avoid hazardous activities until drug's CNS effects are known.

• Suggest that patient relieve dry mouth with frequent rinsing and use of sugarless gum or hard candy.

• Tell patient to take last dose of the day a few hours before bedtime if chlorpheniramine, hydrocodone, and pseudoephedrine makes her nervous or restless.

chlorpheniramine maleate, hydrocodone bitartrate, pseudoephedrine hydrochloride, and guaifenesin

Ztuss Expectorant

Class, Category, and Schedule

Chemical: Alkylamine (chlorpheniramine), opioid and phenan-threne derivative (hydrocodone), sympathomimetic amine (pseudoephedrine), glyceryl guaiacolate (guaifenesin)
Therapeutic: Antihistamine (chlorpheniramine), antitussive (hydrocodone), decongestant (pseudoephedrine), expectorant (guaifenesin)
Pregnancy category: C
Controlled substance schedule: III

Indications and Dosages

▶ *To relieve cough and upper respiratory symptoms of colds and allergies*

ORAL SOLUTION

Adults. 4 mg chlorpheniramine, 5 mg hydrocodone, 30 mg pseudoephedrine, and 200 mg guaifenesin (10 ml) every 4 to 6 hr.

Mechanism of Action

Chlorpheniramine competes with histamine for H_1 receptor sites, thereby antagonizing many histamine effects and reducing allergy signs and symptoms.

Hydrocodone suppresses cough by directly acting on opiate receptors in the medulla's cough center.

Pseudoephedrine acts on $alpha_1$-adrenergic receptors in the mucosa of the respiratory tract to produce vasoconstriction. This process shrinks swollen nasal mucous membranes; reduces tissue hyperemia, edema, and nasal congestion; and increases nasal airway patency. It also may increase drainage of sinus secretions and open obstructed eustachian ostia.

Guaifenesin increases fluid and mucus removal from upper respiratory tract by increasing secretion volume and reducing adhesiveness and surface tension.

Contraindications

Hypersensitivity or idiosyncratic reactions to chlorpheniramine, hydrocodone, other opioids, pseudodephedrine, guaifenesin, or their components; hyperthyroidism; narrow-angle glaucoma; prostatic hypertrophy; respiratory depression; severe asthma, coronary artery disease or hypertension; upper airway obstruction, urine retention, use of MAO inhibitors within 14 days

Interactions

DRUGS

chlorpheniramine, hydrocodone, and pseudoephedrine

MAO inhibitors: Increased and prolonged cardiac stimulation, increased vasopressor effect, increased risk of severe cardiovascular and cerebrovascular effects, hyperpyrexia, and vomiting

chlorpheniramine and hydrocodone

anticholinergics, paregoric: Possibly intensified adverse anticholinergic effects

CNS depressants: Additive CNS effects

chlorpheniramine

phenytoin: Possibly increased serum phenytoin level and toxicity

hydrocodone

antihypertensives, diuretics: Potentiated hypotensive effects

buprenorphine: Decreased hydrocodone effectiveness

hydroxyzine: Increased hydrocodone analgesic effect; increased CNS depressant and hypotensive effects

metoclopramide: Antagonized effect of metoclopramide on GI motility

naloxone: Anatagonized hydrocodone analgesic effect

naltrexone: Precipitated withdrawal symptoms in hydrocodone-dependent patients

neuromuscular blockers: Additive respiratory depressant effects

opioids: Additive CNS and respiratory depressants effects and hypotensive effects

pseudoephedrine

antacids: Increased pseudoephedrine absorption

antihypertensives, diuretics: Possibly decreased antihypertensive effects

beta blockers: Decreased therapeutic effects of both drugs

citrates: Possibly inhibited urinary excretion and prolonged duration of pseudoephedrine action

CNS stimulant, other sympathomimetics: Possibly increased additive CNS stimulation to excessive levels

cocaine (mucosal-local): Possibly increased cardiovascular effects of either drug and CNS stimulation

digoxin, levodopa: Increased risk of cardiac arrhythmias

hydrocarbon inhalation anesthetics: Increased risk of serious arrhythmias

kaolin: Decreased pseudoephedrine absorption

nitrates: Reduced antianginal effects of nitrates

rauwolfia alkaloids: Possibly inhibited pseudoephedrine action

thyroid hormones: Increased cardiovascular effects of both drugs

ACTIVITIES

chlorpheniramine and hydrocodone

alcohol use: Additive CNS effects

Adverse Reactions

CNS: Anxiety, confusion, decreased mental and physical performance, depression, dizziness, drowsiness, euphoria, faintness, fear, headache, insomnia, light-headedness, mood changes, nervousness, restlessness, sedation, seizures, tiredness, trembling, weakness

CV: Angina, arrhythmia exacerbation, bradycardia, chest tightness, hypotension, palpitations, tachycardia

EENT: Blurred or double vision, dry mouth, laryngeal edema, laryngospasm, photophobia

GI: Anorexia, constipation, nausea, paralytic ileus, toxic megacolon, vomiting

GU: Dysuria, frequent urination, urine retention

RESP: Dyspnea, shortness of breath, slow or irregular breathing, wheezing

Skin: Diaphoresis, facial flushing, pallor, pruritus, rash, uriticaria

Other: Angioedema, atelectasis, mental or physical dependence

Nursing Considerations

- Use chlorpheniramine, hydrocodone, pseudoephedrine, and guaifenesin cautiously in patients with recent head injury, Addison's disease, asthma or other chronic respiratory disease, increased intraocular pressure, or liver or renal impairment.
- Monitor patients who may be more susceptible to dizziness, sedation, and hypotension, such as the elderly.
- Monitor renal function, as ordered, because pseudoephedrine is substantially excreted by the kidneys.
- Regularly evaluate effectiveness of drug in reducing symptoms.
- Patient shouldn't have intradermal allergen tests within 72 hours of receiving drug because results may be altered.

PATIENT TEACHING

- Instruct patient to use a calibrated measuring device to ensure accurate dose.
- Urge patient to avoid alcohol and other antidepressants while taking chlorpheniramine, hydrocodone, pseudoephedrine, and guaifenesin.
- Instruct patient to avoid hazardous activities until drug's CNS effects are known.
- Suggest that patient relieve dry mouth with frequent rinsing and use of sugarless gum or hard candy.
- Tell patient to take last dose of the day a few hours before bedtime if chlorpheniramine, hydrocodone, pseudoephedrine, and guaifenesin makes him nervous or restless.

chlorpheniramine maleate and pseudoephedrine hydrochloride

Amerifed, Anaplex, Atrohist Pediatric, Biohist-LA, Chlordrine S.R., Chlorfed-A, Chlor-Trimeton Allergy Decongestant, Codimal LA, Colfed-A, Deconamine, Deconamine SR, Deconomed SR, Dura-Tap PD, Histade, Histex, Kronofed-A, Kronofed-A Jr., ND Clear, ND Clear T.D., Novafed A, Pseudo-Chlor, Rescon, Rescon-ED, Rescon-JR, Rinade B.I.D. Capsules, Ryna, Sudafed Cold & Allergy, Time-Hist

chlorpheniramine tannate and pseudoephedrine tannate

C-PHED, CP-TANNIC, Tanafed

Class and Category

Chemical: Alkylamine (chlorpheniramine), sympathomimetic amine (pseudoephedrine)
Therapeutic: Antihistamine (chlorpheniramine), decongestant (pseudoephedrine)
Pregnancy category: C

Indications and Dosages

▶ *To relieve persistent runny nose, sneezing, and nasal congestion caused by upper respiratory infections, sinus inflammation, or hay fever; to relieve sinus pressure and drain sinuses*

SYRUP

Adults and children age 12 and over. 2 to 4 mg chlorpheniramine and 30 to 60 mg pseudoephedrine (5 to 10 ml) every 6 to 8 hr.

Children ages 6 to 12. 1 to 2 mg chlorpheniramine and 15 to 30 mg pseudoephedrine (2.5 to 5 ml) every 6 to 8 hr.

Children ages 2 to 6. 1 mg chlorpheniramine and 15 mg pseudoephedrine (2.5 ml) every 6 to 8 hr.

ORAL SOLUTION

Adults. 4 mg chlorpheniramine and 60 mg pseudoephedrine (10 ml) every 4 to 6 hr. Alternatively, 4 mg chlorpheniramine and 80 mg pseudoephedrine (5 ml) every 8 hr.

SUSPENSION (TANNATE)

Adults and children age 12 and over. 9 to 18 mg chlorpheniramine and 150 to 300 mg pseudoephedrine (10 to 20 ml) every 12 hr.

Children ages 6 to 12. 4.5 to 9 mg chlorpheniramine and 75 to 150 mg pseudoephedrine (5 to 10 ml) every 12 hr.

Children ages 2 to 6. 2.25 to 4.5 mg chlorpheniramine and 37.5 to 75 mg pseudoephedrine (2.5 to 5 ml) every 12 hr.
TABLETS
Adults. 4 mg chlorpheniramine and 60 mg pseudoephedrine (1 tablet) every 4 to 8 hr. *Maximum:* 4 doses daily.
E.R. TABLETS
Adults. 6 to 12 mg chlorpheniramine and 60 to 120 mg pseudo-ephedrine (½ to 1 tablet depending on product) every 12 hr.
E.R. CAPSULES
Adults and children age 12 and over. 4 to 8 mg chlorphen-iramine and 60 to 120 mg pseudoephedrine (1 or 2 capsules de-pending on product) every 12 hr.
Children ages 6 to 12. 4 mg chlorpheniramine and 60 mg pseu-doephedrine (1 capsule) every 12 hr.

Mechanism of Action

Chlorpheniramine competes with histamine for H_1 receptor sites, thereby an-tagonizing many histamine effects and reducing allergy signs and symptoms.

Pseudoephedrine acts on $alpha_1$-adrenergic receptors in the mucosa of the respiratory tract to produce vasoconstriction. This process shrinks swollen nasal mucous membranes; reduces tissue hyperemia, edema, and nasal con-gestion; and increases nasal airway patency. It also may increase drainage of sinus secretions and open obstructed eustachian ostia.

Contraindications

Breast-feeding; hypersensitivity or idiosyncractic reactions to chlorpheniramine, pseudoephedrine, or their components; hyper-thyroidism; narrow-angle glaucoma; severe coronary artery dis-ease or hypertension; urine retention; use within 14 days of MAO inhibitor therapy

Interactions

DRUGS

chlorpheniramine and pseudoephedrine
MAO inhibitors: Increased and prolonged cardiac stimulation, in-creased vasopressor effect, increased risk of severe cardiovascular and cerebrovascular effects, hyperpyrexia, and vomiting
chlorpheniramine
anticholinergics: Additive anticholinergic effects
CNS depressants: Additive CNS effects
phenytoin: Possibly increased serum phenytoin levels and toxicity

pseudoephedrine

antacids: Increased pseudoephedrine absorption

antihypertensives, diuretics: Possibly decreased antihypertensive effects

beta blockers: Decreased therapeutic effects of both drugs

citrates: Possibly inhibited urinary excretion and prolonged duration of pseudoephedrine action

CNS stimulant, other sympathomimetics: Possibly increased additive CNS stimulation to excessive levels

cocaine (mucosal-local): Possibly increased cardiovascular effects of either drug and CNS stimulation

digoxin, levodopa: Increased risk of cardiac arrhythmias

hydrocarbon inhalation anesthetics: Possibly serious arrhythmias

kaolin: Decreased pseudoephedrine absorption

nitrates: Reduced antianginal effects of nitrates

rauwolfia alkaloids: Possibly inhibited pseudoephedrine action

thyroid hormones: Increased cardiovascular effects of both drugs

ACTIVITIES

chlorpheniramine

alcohol use: Additive CNS effects

Adverse Reactions

CNS: Anxiety, chills, confusion, coordination disturbance, dizziness, drowsiness, excitation (children), fatigue, fear, hallucinations, headache, hysteria, insomnia, irritability, light-headedness, nervousness, numbness, restlessness, sedation, seizures, tenseness, trembling, vertigo, weakness

CV: Arrhythmias, chest tightness, hypotension, palpitations, tachycardia

EENT: Blurred or double vision; dry mouth, nose, and throat; nasal congestion, tinnitus

ENDO: Early menstruation

GI: Anorexia, constipation, diarrhea, nausea, stomach upset or pain, vomiting

GU: Dysuria, frequent urination, urinary hesitancy or retention

HEME: Anemia, unusual bleeding or bruising

RESP: Dyspnea, increased chest congestion, wheezing

SKIN: Diaphoresis, pallor, photosensitivity, rash, urticaria

Other: Anaphylaxis

Nursing Considerations

- Use chlorpheniramine and pseudoephedrine cautiously in patients with asthma, cardiovascular disease, diabetes, emphysema or other chronic lung disease, hypertension, peptic ulcer, nar-

row-angle glaucoma, or prostatic hypertrophy.
- Monitor children for excitation and elderly patients for dizziness, sedation, and hypotension; such patients may have an increased risk for these effects.
- Monitor renal function, as ordered, because pseudoephedrine is substantially excreted by the kidneys.
- Regularly evaluate effectiveness of chlorpheniramine and pseudoephedrine in reducing upper respiratory symptoms regularly.
- Be aware that patient shouldn't have intradermal allergen tests within 72 hours of receiving drug because results may be altered.

PATIENT TEACHING
- Instruct patient to use a calibrated measuring device when using syrup form of chlorpheniramine and pseudoephedrine to ensure accurate dose.
- Urge patient to avoid alcohol and other antidepressants while taking chlorpheniramine and pseudoephedrine.
- Instruct patient to avoid hazardous activities until drug's CNS effects are known.
- Suggest that patient relieve dry mouth with frequent rinsing and use of sugarless gum or hard candy.
- Tell patient to take last dose of the day a few hours before bedtime if chlorpheniramine and pseudoephedrine makes her nervous or restless.

chlorpheniramine maleate, pseudoephedrine hydrochloride, and methscopolamine nitrate

CPM 8/PSE 90/MSC 2.5, Durahist, Mescolor, Pannaz, Rescon-MX, Xiral

Class and Category

Chemical: Alkylamine (chlorpheniramine), sympathomimetic amine (pseudoephedrine), hyoscine methobromide (methscopolamine)

Therapeutic: Antihistamine (chlorpheniramine), decongestant (pseudoephedrine), anticholingeric (methscopolamine)

Pregnancy category: C

Indications and Dosages

▶ *To relieve persistent runny nose, sneezing, and nasal congestion caused by upper respiratory infections, sinus inflammation, or hay fever; to relieve sinus pressure and drain sinuses*

E.R. TABLETS

Adults. 8 mg chlorpheniramine, 120 mg pseudoephedrine, and 2.5 mg methscopolamine (1 tablet) every 12 hr. *Maximum:* 16 mg chlorpheniramine, 240 mg pseudoephedrine, and 5 mg methscopolamine in 24 hr.

Children ages 6 to 12. 4 mg chlorpheniramine, 60 mg pseudoephedrine, and 1.25 mg methscopolamine (½ tablet) every 12 hr. *Maximum:* 8 mg chlorpheniramine, 120 mg pseudoephedrine, and 2.5 mg methscopolamine in 24 hr.

Mechanism of Action

Chlorpheniramine competes with histamine for H_1 receptor sites, thereby antagonizing many histamine effects and reducing allergy signs and symptoms.

Pseudoephedrine acts on $alpha_1$-adrenergic receptors in the mucosa of the respiratory tract to produce vasoconstriction. This process shrinks swollen nasal mucous membranes; reduces tissue hyperemia, edema, and nasal congestion; and increases nasal airway patency. It also may increase drainage of sinus secretions and open obstructed eustachian ostia.

Methscopolamine competitively inhibits acetylcholine at autonomic postganglionic cholinergic receptors. Because the most sensitive receptors are in salivary, bronchial, and sweat glands, this action reduces secretions from these glands. It also reduces nasal, oropharyngeal, and bronchial secretions and decreases airway resistance by relaxing smooth muscles in the bronchi and bronchioles.

Contraindications

Breast-feeding; cardiac disease such as arrhythmias, congestive heart failure, coronary artery disease, severe hypertension, and mitral stenosis; hemorrhage with hemodynamic instability; hepatic dysfunction; hypersensitivity or idiosyncractic reactions to chlorpheniramine, pseudoephedrine, methscopolamine, or their components; hyperthyroidism; ileus; intestinal atony; myasthenia gravis; narrow-angle glaucoma; obstructive GI or uropathic disease; prostatic hypertrophy; renal impairment; toxic megacolon; ulcerative colitis; urine retention; use within 14 days of MAO inhibitor therapy

Interactions

DRUGS

chlorpheniramine and pseudoephedrine

MAO inhibitors: Increased and prolonged cardiac stimulation, in-

creased vasopressor effect, increased risk of severe cardiovascular and cerebrovascular effects, hyperpyrexia, and vomiting

chlorpheniramine and methscopolamine

anticholinergics: Additive anticholinergic effects

CNS depressants: Additive CNS effects

chlorpheniramine

phenytoin: Possibly increased serum phenytoin level and toxicity

pseudoephedrine

antacids: Increased pseudoephedrine absorption

antihypertensives, diuretics: Possibly decreased antihypertensive effects

beta blockers: Decreased therapeutic effects of both drugs

citrates: Possibly inhibited urinary excretion and prolonged duration of pseudoephedrine action

CNS stimulant, other sympathomimetics: Possibly increased additive CNS stimulation to excessive levels

cocaine (mucosal-local): Possibly increased cardiovascular effects of either drug and CNS stimulation

digoxin, levodopa: Increased risk of cardiac arrhythmias

hydrocarbon inhalation anesthetics: Increased risk of serious arrhythmias

kaolin: Decreased pseudoephedrine absorption

nitrates: Reduced antianginal effects of nitrates

rauwolfia alkaloids: Possibly inhibited action of pseudoephedrine

thyroid hormones: Increased cardiovascular effects of both drugs

methscopolamine

adsorbent antidiarrheals, antacids: Decreased absorption and therapeutic effects of methoscopolamine

antimyasthenics: Possibly reduced intestinal motility

CNS depressants: Possibly potentiated effects of either drug, resulting in additive sedation

haloperidol: Decreased antipsychotic effect of haloperidol

ketoconazole: Decreased ketoconazole absorption

lorazepam (parenteral): Possibly hallucinations, irrational behavior, and sedation

metoclopramide: Possibly antagonized effect of metoclopramide on GI motility

opioid analgesics: Increased risk of severe constipation and ileus

potassium chloride: Possibly increased severity of potassium chloride-induced GI lesions

sildenafil, tadalafil, vardenafil: Possibly increased risk of hypotension

urinary alkalizers (antacids, carbonic anhydrase inhibitors, citrates, so-

dium bicarbonate): Delayed excretion of methscopolamine, possibly leading to increased therapeutic and adverse effects
ACTIVITIES
chlorpheniramine and methscopolamine
alcohol use: Additive CNS effects

Adverse Reactions

CNS: Anxiety, chills, confusion, coordination disturbance, dizziness, drowsiness, euphoria, fatigue, fear, hallucinations, headache, hysteria, insomnia, irritability, light-headedness, memory loss, nervousness, numbness, paradoxical stimulation, restlessness, sedation, seizures, tenseness, trembling, vertigo, weakness
CV: Arrhythmias, chest tightness, hypotension, palpitations, tachycardia
EENT: Blurred or double vision; dry eyes, mouth, nose, and throat; mydriasis; nasal congestion; tinnitus
ENDO: Early menstruation
GI: Anorexia, constipation, diarrhea, dysphagia, nausea, stomach upset or pain, vomiting
GU: Dysuria, frequent urination, urinary hesitancy or retention
HEME: Anemia, unusual bleeding or bruising
RESP: Dyspnea, increased chest congestion, wheezing
SKIN: Decreased sweating, diaphoresis, dry skin, flushing, pallor, photosensitivity, rash, urticaria
Other: Anaphylaxis

Nursing Considerations

- Use chlorpheniramine, pseudoephedrine, and methscopolamine cautiously in patients with asthma, diabetes, emphysema or other chronic lung disease, hypertension, or peptic ulcer.
- Monitor patients who may be more susceptible to dizziness, sedation, and hypotension, such as the elderly.
- Monitor renal function, as ordered, because pseudoephedrine is substantially excreted by the kidneys.
- Regularly evaluate effectiveness of chlorpheniramine, pseudoephedrine, and methscopolamine in reducing upper respiratory symptoms.
- Be aware that patient shouldn't have intradermal allergen tests within 72 hours of receiving drug because results may be altered.
PATIENT TEACHING
- Urge patient to avoid alcohol and other antidepressants during therapy.

- Instruct patient to avoid hazardous activities until drug's CNS effects are known.
- Suggest that patient relieve dry mouth with frequent rinsing and use of sugarless gum or hard candy. Suggest lubricating drops for dry eyes.
- Tell patient to take last dose of the day a few hours before bedtime if chlorpheniramine, pseudoephedrine, and methscopolamine makes him nervous or restless.

chlorpheniramine maleate, pyrilamine maleate, hydrocodone bitartrate, phenylephrine hydrochloride, and pseudoephedrine hydrochloride

Statuss Green

Class, Category, and Schedule

Chemical: Alkylamine (chlorpheniramine), ethylenediamine antihistamine (pyrilamine), opioid and phenanthrene derivative (hydrocodone), sympathomimetic amines (phenylephrine, pseudoephedrine)

Therapeutic: Antihistamines (chlorpheniramine, pyrilamine), antitussive (hydrocodone), decongestants (phenylephrine, pseudoephedrine)

Pregnancy category: C

Controlled substance schedule: III

Indications and Dosages

▶ *To relieve cough and upper respiratory symptoms of colds and allergies*

ORAL SOLUTION

Adults. 4 mg chlorpheniramine, 6.6 mg pyrilamine, 5 mg hydrocodone, 10 mg phenylephrine, and 6.6 mg pseudoephedrine (10 ml) every 4 to 6 hr. *Maximum:* 40 ml daily.

Contraindications

Breast-feeding; hypersensitivity or idiosyncractic reactions to chlorpheniramine, pyrilamine, hydrocodone, other opioids, phenylephrine, pseudoephedrine, or their components; hyperthyroidism; narrow-angle glaucoma; prostatic hypertrophy; respiratory depression; severe asthma, coronary artery disease or hypertension; upper airway obstruction; urine retention; use of MAO inhibitors within 14 days

Mechanism of Action

Chlorpheniramine and pyrilamine competes with histamine for H_1 receptor sites, thereby antagonizing many histamine effects and reducing allergy signs and symptoms.

Hydrocodone suppresses cough by acting directly on opiate receptors in the medulla's cough center.

Phenylephrine stimulates alpha-adrenergic receptors and inhibits the intracellular enzyme adenyl cyclase, which then inhibits production of cAMP. Inhibition of cAMP causes arterial and venous constriction in nasal passages, which decreases blood flow and mucosal edema caused by allergic response.

Pseudoephedrine acts on $alpha_1$-adrenergic receptors in the mucosa of the respiratory tract to produce vasoconstriction. This process shrinks swollen nasal mucous membranes; reduces tissue hyperemia, edema, and nasal congestion; and increases nasal airway patency. It also may increase drainage of sinus secretions and open obstructed eustachian ostia.

Interactions

DRUGS

chlorpheniramine, pyrilamine, and hydrocodone
CNS depressants: Additive CNS effects
chlorpheniramine, hydrocodone, and pseudoephedrine
MAO inhibitors: Increased and prolonged cardiac stimulation, increased vasopressor effect, increased risk of severe cardiovascular and cerebrovascular effects, hyperpyrexia, and vomiting
chlorpheniramine and hydrocodone
anticholinergics, paregoric: Possibly intensified anticholinergic adverse effects
chlorpheniramine
phenytoin: Possibly increased serum phenytoin level and toxicity
hydrocodone
antihypertensives, diuretics: Potentiated hypotensive effects
buprenorphine: Decreased hydrocodone effectiveness
hydroxyzine: Increased hydrocodone analgesic effect; increased CNS depressant and hypotensive effects
metoclopramide: Antagonized metoclopramide effect on GI motility
naloxone: Anatagonized hydrocodone analgesic effect
naltrexone: Precipitated withdrawal symptoms in hydrocodone-dependent patients
neuromuscular blockers: Additive respiratory depressant effects
opioids: Additive CNS and respiratory depressants effects and hypotensive effects

phenylephrine

alpha blockers, haloperidol, loxapine, phenothiazines, thioxanthenes: Possibly decreased vasoconstrictor effect of phenylephrine

antihypertenisves, diuretics: Possibly decreased antihypertensive effects

atropine: Possibly enhanced vasopressor effect of phenylephrine

beta blockers: Decreased therapeutic effects of both drugs

bretylium: Possibly potentiated vaopressor effect and arrhythmias

doxapram: Increased vasopressor effect of both drugs

ergot alkaloids: Possibly cerebral blood vessel rupture, increased vasopressor effect, peripheral vascular ischemia, and gangrene (with ergotamine)

guanadrel, guanethidine: Increased vasopressor effect of phenylephrine; increased risk of severe hypertension and arrhythmias

hydrocarbon inhalation anesthetics: Increased risk of serious arrhythmias

maprotiline, tricyclic antidepressants: Increased risk of severe cardiovascular effects (including arrhythmias, hyperpyrexia, severe hypertension)

mecamylamine, methyldopa: Decreased hypotensive effects of these drugs, increased vasopressor effect of phenylephrine

nitrates: Possibly decreased vasopressor effect of phenylephrine and decreased antianginal effect of nitrates

oxytocin: Possibly severe, persistent hypertension

phenoxybenzamine: Decreased vasoconstrictor effect of phenylephrine, possibly hypotension and tachycardia

theophylline: Possibly enhanced toxicity (including cardiac toxicity)

thyroid hormones: Increased cardiovascular effects of each drug

pseudoephedrine

antacids: Increased pseudoephedrine absorption

antihypertensives, diuretics: Possibly decreased antihypertensive effects

beta blockers: Decreased therapeutic effects of both drugs

citrates: Possibly inhibited urinary excretion and prolonged duration of action of pseudoephedrine

CNS stimulant, other sympathomimetics: Possibly increased additive CNS stimulation to excessive levels

cocaine (mucosal-local): Possibly increased cardiovascular effects of either drug and CNS stimulation

digoxin, levodopa: Increased risk of cardiac arrhythmias

hydrocarbon inhalation anesthetics: Increased risk of serious arrhythmias

kaolin: Decreased pseudoephedrine absorption

nitrates: Reduced antianginal effects of nitrates
rauwolfia alkaloids: Possibly inhibited pseudoephedrine action
thyroid hormones: Increased cardiovascular effects of both drugs
ACTIVITIES
chlorpheniramine, pyrilamine, and hydrocodone
alcohol use: Additive CNS effects

Adverse Reactions

CNS: Anxiety, confusion, decreased mental and physical performance, depression, dizziness, drowsiness, euphoria, faintness, fear, headache, insomnia, light-headedness, mood changes, nervousness, paresthesia, restlessness, sedation, seizures, tiredness, trembling, weakness
CV: Angina, bradycardia, chest tightness, hypertension, hypotension, palpitations, tachycardia, ventricular arrhythmias
EENT: Blurred or double vision, dry mouth, laryngeal edema, laryngospasm, photophobia
GI: Anorexia, constipation, nausea, paralytic ileus, toxic megacolon, vomiting
GU: Dysuria, frequent urination, urinary hesitancy or retention
RESP: Dyspnea, shortness of breath, slow or irregular breathing, wheezing
Skin: Diaphoresis, facial flushing, pallor, pruritus, rash, uriticaria
Other: Angioedema, atelectasis, mental or physical dependence

Nursing Considerations

- Use cautiously in patients with a recent head injury and those with Addison's disease, asthma or other chronic respiratory disease, increased intraocular pressure, or liver or renal impairment.
- Monitor patients who may be more susceptible to dizziness, sedation, and hypotension, such as the elderly.
- Monitor renal function, as ordered, because pseudoephedrine is substantially excreted by the kidneys.
- Regularly evaluate effectiveness of chlorpheniramine, pyrilamine, hydrocodone, phenylephrine, and pseudoephedrine in reducing symptoms.
- Be aware that patient shouldn't have intradermal allergen tests within 72 hours of receiving drug because results may be altered.
PATIENT TEACHING
- Instruct patient to use a calibrated measuring device to ensure accurate dose.
- Urge patient to avoid alcohol and other antidepressants while taking drug.

- Instruct patient to avoid hazardous activities until drug's CNS effects are known.
- Suggest that patient relieve dry mouth with frequent rinsing and use of sugarless gum or hard candy.
- Tell patient to take last dose of the day a few hours before bedtime if drug makes her nervous or restless.

codeine polistirex and chlorpheniramine polistirex

Codeprex Pennkinetic

Class, Category, and Schedule

Chemical: Opioid and phenanthrene derivative (codeine), alkylamine (chlorpheniramine)
Therapeutic: Antitussive (codeine), antihistamine (chlorpheniramine),
Pregnancy category: C
Controlled substance schedule: III

Indications and Dosages

▶ *To relieve cough and upper respiratory symptoms due to hay fever, other upper respiratory allergies, or allergic rhinitis*
E.R. SUSPENSION
Adults and children age 12 and over. 40 mg codeine and 8 mg chlorpheniramine (10 ml) every 12 hr.
Children ages 6 to 12. 20 mg codeine and 4 mg chlorpheniramine (5 ml) every 12 hr.

Mechanism of Action

Codeine suppresses cough by directly acting on opiate receptors in the medulla's cough center.

Chlorpheniramine competes with histamine for H_1 receptor sites, thereby antagonizing many histamine effects and reducing allergy signs and symptoms.

Contraindications

Breast-feeding; constipation; hypersensitivity to codeine, chlorpheniramine, other opioids or their components; inflammatory bowel disease; prostatic hypertrophy; respiratory depression; severe asthma; upper airway obstruction, use of MAO inhibitors within 14 days

Interactions

DRUGS

codeine and chlorpheniramine

anticholinergics, paregoric: Possibly intensified adverse anticholinergic effects

CNS depressants: Additive CNS effects

MAO inhibitors: Increased and prolonged cardiac stimulation, increased vasopressor effect, increased risk of severe cardiovascular and cerebrovascular effects, hyperpyrexia, and vomiting

codeine

antihypertensives, diuretics: Potentiated hypotensive effects

buprenorphine: Decreased codeine effectiveness

hydroxyzine: Increased codeine analgesic effect; increased CNS depressant and hypotensive effects

metoclopramide: Antagonized effect of metoclopramide on GI motility

naloxone: Antagonized codeine analgesic effect

naltrexone: Precipitated withdrawal symptoms in codeine-dependent patients

neuromuscular blockers: Additive respiratory depressant effects

opioids: Additive CNS and respiratory depressants effects and hypotensive effects

tricyclic antidepressants: Possibly increased effect of either the antidepressant or codeine

chlorpheniramine

phenytoin: Possibly increased serum phenytoin level and toxicity

ACTIVITIES

codeine and chlorpheniramine

alcohol use: Additive CNS effects

Adverse Reactions

CNS: Asthenia, anxiety, confusion, dizziness, depression, drowsiness, dyskinesia, euphoria, excitability (especially in children) faintness, hallucinations, headache, impaired cognition, insomnia, irritability, light-headedness, nervousness, restlessness, sedation, syncope, tiredness, tremor, vertigo, weakness

CV: Bradycardia, hypertension, hypotension, orthostatic hypotension, palpitation, tachycardia

ENDO: Decreased lactation, early menses, gynecomastia, hyperglycemia, hypoglycemia

EENT: Blurred vision; diplopia; dry mouth, pharynx, and respiratory passages; hypermetropia; increased lacrimation; labyrinthitis; laryngismus; mydriasis; nasal stuffiness; photophobia; tinnitus

GI: Abdominal distention or pain, acute pancreatitis, anorexia, constipation, diarrhea, dyspepsia, epigastric distress, esophageal reflux, increased appetite, nausea, vomiting
GU: Decreased or increased libido, dysuria, urinary frequency or hesitancy, urine retention, ureteral spasm
RESP: Dyspnea, respiratory depression, wheezing
SKIN: Dermatitis, diaphoresis, erythema, flushing, pruritus, rash, urticaria
Other: Drug fever, emotional or physical dependence

Nursing Considerations

- Use cautiously in patients with a recent head injury and in those with Addison's disease, asthma or other chronic respiratory disease, increased intraocular pressure, hypothyroidism, or liver or renal impairment.
- **WARNING** Monitor respiratory function because codeine and chlorpheniramine may suppress the cough reflex and cause thickening of bronchial secretions, aggravating such conditions as asthma and COPD and, in rare cases, may depress respirations and induce apnea. Notify prescriber immediately if respiratory rate drops below 10 breaths/minute.
- Monitor children for excitation and elderly patients for dizziness, sedation, and hypotension; such patients may have an increased risk for these effects.
- Regularly evaluate effectiveness of codeine and chlorpheniramine in reducing symptoms.
- Patient shouldn't have intradermal allergen tests within 72 hours of receiving drug because results may be altered.
- **WARNING** Monitor patient closely for evidence of overdose, even at normal dosage, because some patients metabolize codeine quickly, causing a sudden rise in blood codeine level. This metabolic defect occurs in about 0.5 to 1% of Chinese, Japanese, and Hispanic people; 1 to 10% of Caucasians; 3% of African Americans; and 16 to 28% of North Africans, Ethiopians, and Arabs. Watch for extreme sleepiness, confusion, and shallow breathing after giving drug. If present, notify prescriber and be prepared to provide supportive care and discontinue drug, as ordered.

PATIENT TEACHING
- Instruct patient to shake suspension well before measuring dose and to use a calibrated device to ensure accurate dose.
- Tell patient that codeine and chlorpheniramine must not be diluted with fluids or mixed with other drugs.

- Urge patient to avoid alcohol and other antidepressants while taking codeine and chlorpheniramine.
- Instruct patient to avoid hazardous activities until drug's CNS effects are known.
- Suggest that patient relieve dry mouth with frequent rinsing and use of sugarless gum or hard candy.
- Tell patient to take last dose of the day a few hours before bedtime if drug makes him nervous or restless.
- Urge patient to notify prescriber if he develops trouble breathing or extreme sleepiness or confusion.

codeine phosphate, chlorpheniramine maleate, and pseudoephedrine sulfate

Decohistine DH, Dihistine DH, Novahistine DH, Ryna-C

Class, Category, and Schedule

Chemical: Opioid and phenanthrene derivative (codeine), alkylamine (chlorpheniramine), sympathomimetic amine (pseudoephedrine)

Therapeutic: Antitussive (codeine), antihistamine (chlorpheniramine), decongestant (pseudoephedrine)

Pregnancy category: C

Controlled substance schedule: V

Indications and Dosages

▶ *To relieve cough and upper respiratory symptoms of hay fever, other upper respiratory allergies, and allergic rhinitis*

ELIXIR, ORAL SOLUTION

Adults and children age 12 and over. 10 to 20 mg codeine, 2 to 4 mg chlorpheniramine, and 30 to 60 mg pseudoephedrine (5 to 10 ml depending on product) every 4 to 6 hr. *Maximum:* 40 ml daily.

Children ages 6 to 12. 10 mg codeine, 2 mg chlorpheniramine, and 30 mg peudoephedrine (5 ml) every 6 hr.

Contraindications

Constipation; hypersensitivity or idiosyncractic reactions to codeine, chlorpheniramine, other opioids, pseudoephedrine, or their components; hyperthyroidism; inflammatory bowel disease; narrow-angle glaucoma; prostatic hypertrophy; respiratory depression; severe asthma, corornary artery disease or hypertension; upper airway obstruction, urine retention; use of MAO inhibitors within 14 days

> ## Mechanism of Action
>
> Codeine suppresses cough by directly acting on opiate receptors in the medulla's cough center.
>
> Chlorpheniramine competes with histamine for H_1 receptor sites, thereby antagonizing many histamine effects and reducing allergy signs and symptoms.
>
> Pseudoephedrine acts on $alpha_1$-adrenergic receptors in the mucosa of the respiratory tract to produce vasoconstriction. This process shrinks swollen nasal mucous membranes; reduces tissue hyperemia, edema, and nasal congestion; and increases nasal airway patency. It also may increase drainage of sinus secretions and open obstructed eustachian ostia.

Interactions

DRUGS

codeine, chlorpheniramine, and pseudoephedrine

MAO inhibitors: Increased and prolonged cardiac stimulation, increased vasopressor effect, increased risk of severe cardiovascular and cerebrovascular effects, hyperpyrexia, vomiting

codeine and chlorpheniramine

anticholinergics, paregoric: Possibly intensified anticholinergic adverse effects

CNS depressants: Additive CNS effects

ACTIVITIES

alcohol use: Additive CNS effects

codeine

antihypertensives, diuretics: Potentiated hypotensive effects

buprenorphine: Decreased codeine effectiveness

hydroxyzine: Increased codeine analgesic effect; increased CNS depressant and hypotensive effects

metoclopramide: Antagonized effect of metoclopramide on GI motility

naloxone: Antagonized codeine analgesic effect

naltrexone: Precipitated withdrawal symptoms in codeine-dependent patients

neuromuscular blockers: Additive respiratory depressant effects

opioids: Additive CNS and respiratory depressants effects and hypotensive effects

tricyclic antidepressants: Possibly increased effect of either the antidepressant or codeine

chlorpheniramine

phenytoin: Possibly increased serum phenytoin levels and toxicity

pseudoephedrine

antacids: Increased absorption of pseudoephedrine
antihypertensives, diuretics: Possibly decreased antihypertensive effects
beta blockers: Decreased therapeutic effects of both drugs
citrates: Possibly inhibited urinary excretion and prolonged duration of pseudoephedrine action
CNS stimulant, other sympathomimetics: Possibly increased additive CNS stimulation to excessive levels
cocaine (mucosal-local): Possibly increased cardiovascular effects of either drug and CNS stimulation
digoxin, levodopa: Increased risk of cardiac arrhythmias
hydrocarbon inhalation anesthetics: Possibly serious arrhythmias
kaolin: Decreased pseudoephedrine absorption
nitrates: Reduced antianginal effects of nitrates
rauwolfia alkaloids: Possibly inhibited action of pseudoephedrine
thyroid hormones: Increased cardiovascular effects of both drugs

Adverse Reactions

CNS: Asthenia, anxiety, confusion, dizziness, depression, drowsiness, dyskinesia, euphoria, excitability, faintness, hallucinations, headache, impaired cognition, insomnia, irritability, light-headedness, nervousness, restlessness, sedation, syncope, tiredness, tremor, vertigo, weakness
CV: Bradycardia, hypertension, hypotension, orthostatic hypotension, palpitation, tachycardia
ENDO: Decreased lactation, early menses, gynecomastia, hyperglycemia, hypoglycemia
EENT: Blurred vision; diplopia; dry mouth, pharynx, and respiratory passages; hypermetropia; increased lacrimation; labyrinthitis; laryngismus; mydriasis; nasal stuffiness; photophobia; tinnitus
GI: Abdominal distention or pain, acute pancreatitis, anorexia, constipation, diarrhea, dyspepsia, epigastric distress, esophageal reflux, increased appetite, nausea, vomiting
GU: Decreased or increased libido, dysuria, urinary frequency or hesitancy, urine retention, ureteral spasm
RESP: Dyspnea, respiratory depression, wheezing
SKIN: Dermatitis, diaphoresis, erythema, flushing, pallor, pruritus, rash, urticaria
Other: Drug fever, emotional or physical dependence

Nursing Considerations

• Use cautiously in patients with a recent head injury and those with Addison's disease, asthma or other chronic respiratory disease, increased intraocular pressure, or liver or renal impairment.

- **WARNING** Monitor respiratory function because codeine, chlorpheniramine, and pseudoephedrine may suppress the cough reflex and cause thickening of bronchial secretions, aggravating such conditions as asthma and COPD. In rare cases, it may depress respirations and induce apnea. Notify prescriber immediately if respiratory rate drops below 10 breaths/ minute.
- Monitor patients who may be more susceptible to dizziness, sedation, and hypotension, such as the elderly.
- Monitor renal function, as ordered, because pseudoephedrine is substantially excreted by the kidneys.
- Regularly evaluate effectiveness of codeine, chlorpheniramine, and pseudoephedrine in reducing symptoms.
- Be aware that patient shouldn't have intradermal allergen tests within 72 hours of receiving drug because results may be altered.
- **WARNING** Monitor patient closely for evidence of overdose, even at normal dosage, because some patients metabolize codeine quickly, causing a sudden rise in blood codeine level. This metabolic defect occurs in about 0.5 to 1% of Chinese, Japanese, and Hispanic people; 1 to 10% of Caucasians; 3% of African Americans; and 16 to 28% of North Africans, Ethiopians, and Arabs. Watch for extreme sleepiness, confusion, and shallow breathing after giving drug. If present, notify prescriber and be prepared to provide supportive care and discontinue drug, as ordered.

PATIENT TEACHING
- Caution patient that codeine, chlorpheniramine, and pseudoephedrine must not be diluted with fluids or mixed with other drugs.
- Urge patient to avoid alcohol and other antidepressants while taking codeine, chlorpheniramine, and pseudoephedrine.
- Instruct patient to avoid hazardous activities until drug's CNS effects are known.
- Suggest that patient relieve dry mouth with frequent rinsing and use of sugarless gum or hard candy.
- Tell patient to take last dose of the day a few hours before bedtime if codeine, chlorpheniramine, and pseudoephedrine makes her nervous or restless.
- Urge patient to notify prescriber if she develops trouble breathing or extreme sleepiness or confusion.

codeine phosphate, phenylephrine hydrochloride, and pyrilamine maleate
Codimal PH

Class, Category, and Schedule
Chemical: Opioid and phenanthrene derivative (codeine), sympathomimetic amine (phenylephrine), ethylenediamine antihistamine (pyrilamine)
Therapeutic: Antitussive (codeine), decongestant (phenylephrine), antihistaminic (pyrilamine)
Pregnancy category: C
Schedule Category: V

Indications and Dosages
▶ *To relieve cough and upper respiratory symptoms of hay fever, other upper respiratory allergies, allergic rhinitis, and the common cold*
SYRUP
Adults. 10 to 20 mg codeine, 5 to 10 mg phenylephrine and 8.33 to 16.66 mg pyrilamine (5 to 10 ml) every 4 to 6 hr.
Children ages 6 to 12. 10 mg codeine, 5 mg phenylephrine, and 8.33 mg pyrilamine (5 ml) every 4 to 6 hr.

Mechanism of Action
Codeine suppresses cough by directly acting on opiate receptors in the medulla's cough center.

Phenylephrine stimulates alpha-adrenergic receptors and inhibits the intracellular enzyme adenyl cyclase, which then inhibits production of cAMP. Inhibition of cAMP causes arterial and venous constriction in nasal passages, which decreases blood flow and mucosal edema caused by allergic response.

Pyrilamine competes with histamine for H_1 receptor sites, thereby antagonizing many histamine effects to reduce allergy signs and symptoms.

Contraindications
Acute MI; angina; arrhythmias; breast-feeding, coronary artery disease; hypersensitivity to codeine, other opioids, phenylephrine, pyrilamine, or their components; irritable bowel syndrome; paralytic ileus; prostatic hypertrophy; respiratory depression; severe asthma; upper airway obstruction; use of MAO inhibitors within 14 days

Interactions
DRUGS
codeine and phenylephrine

MAO inhibitors: Increased and prolonged cardiac stimulation, increased vasopressor effect, increased risk of severe cardiovascular and cerebrovascular effects, hyperpyrexia, and vomiting

codeine and pyrilamine

anticholinergics, paregoric: Possibly intensified anticholinergic adverse effects

CNS depressants: Additive CNS effects

codeine

antihypertensives, diuretics: Potentiated hypotensive effects

antidiarrheals: Increased risk of severe constipation

buprenorphine: Decreased codeine effectiveness

hydroxyzine: Increased codeine analgesic effect; increased CNS depressant and hypotensive effects

metoclopramide: Antagonized effect of metoclopramide on GI motility

naloxone: Antagonized codeine analgesic effect

naltrexone: Precipitated withdrawal symptoms in codeine-dependent patients

neuromuscular blockers: Additive respiratory depressant effects

opioids: Additive CNS and respiratory depressants effects and hypotensive effects

tricyclic antidepressants: Possibly increased effect of either the antidepressant or codeine

phenylephrine

alpha blockers, haloperidol, loxapine, phenothiazines, thioxanthenes: Possibly decreased vasoconstrictor effect of phenylephrine

antihypertenisves, diuretics: Possibly decreased antihypertensive effects

atropine: Possibly enhanced vasopressor effect of phenylephrine

beta blockers: Decreased therapeutic effects of both drugs

bretylium: Possibly potentiated vaopressor effect and arrhythmias

doxapram: Increased vasopressor effect of both drugs

ergot alkaloids: Possibly cerebral blood vessel rupture, increased vasopressor effect, peripheral vascular ischemia, and gangrene (with ergotamine)

guanadrel, guanethidine: Increased vasopressor effect of phenylephrine; increased risk of severe hypertension and arrhythmias

hydrocarbon inhalation anesthetics: Increased risk of serious arrhythmias

maprotiline, tricyclic antidepressants: Increased risk of severe cardiovascular effects (including arrhythmias, hyperpyrexia, severe hypertension)

mecamylamine, methyldopa: Decreased hypotensive effects of these

drugs; increased vasopressor effect of phenylephrine
nitrates: Possibly decreased vasopressor effect of phenylephrine
and decreased antianginal effect of nitrates
oxytocin: Possibly severe, persistent hypertension
phenoxybenzamine: Decreased vasoconstrictor effect of phenylephrine; possibly hypotension and tachycardia
theophylline: Possibly enhanced toxicity (including cardiac toxicity)
thyroid hormones: Increased cardiovascular effects of each drug
ACTIVITIES
codeine and pyrilamine
alcohol use: Additive CNS effects

Adverse Reactions

CNS: Asthenia, anxiety, confusion, dizziness, depression, drowsiness, dyskinesia, euphoria, faintness, headache, insomnia, irritability, light-headedness, nervousness, paresthesia, restlessness,
sedation, syncope, tiredness, tremor, vertigo, weakness
CV: Angina, bradycardia, hypertension, hypotension, orthostatic
hypotension, palpitations, peripheral vasoconstriction that may
lead to necrosis or gangrene, tachycardia, ventricular arrhythmias
ENDO: Decreased lactation, early menses, gynecomastia, hyperglycemia, hypoglycemia
EENT: Blurred vision; diplopia; dry mouth, pharynx, and respiratory passages; hypermetropia; increased lacrimation; labyrinthitis;
laryngismus; mydriasis; nasal stuffiness; photophobia; tinnitus
GI: Abdominal distention or pain, acute pancreatitis, anorexia,
constipation, diarrhea, dyspepsia, epigastric distress, esophageal
reflux, increased appetite, nausea, vomiting
GU: Dysuria, increased libido, urinary frequency or hesitancy,
urine retention, ureteral spasm
RESP: Dyspnea, respiratory depression, wheezing
SKIN: Dermatitis, diaphoresis, erythema, flushing, pruritus, rash,
urticaria
Other: Drug fever, emotional or physical dependence

Nursing Considerations

- Use codeine, phenylephrine, and pyrilamine cautiously in patients with recent head injury and in those with Addison's disease, asthma or other chronic respiratory disease, cardiovascular
disease, diabetes, hypertension, liver or renal impairment, narrow-angle glaucoma, or thyroid imbalance.
- **WARNING** Monitor respiratory function because codeine,
phenylephrine, and pyrilamine may suppress the cough reflex
and cause thickening of bronchial secretions, aggravating

such conditions as asthma and COPD. In rare cases, it may depress respirations and induce apnea. Notify prescriber immediately if respiratory rate drops below 10 breaths/minute.

- Monitor patients who may be more susceptible to dizziness, sedation, and hypotension, such as the elderly.
- Regularly evaluate effectiveness of codeine, phenylephrine, and pyrilamine in reducing cough and upper respiratory symptoms.
- Patient shouldn't have allergen tests within 72 hours of receiving drug because results may be altered.
- **WARNING** Monitor patient closely for evidence of overdose, even at normal dosage, because some patients metabolize codeine quickly, causing a sudden rise in blood codeine level. This metabolic defect occurs in about 0.5 to 1% of Chinese, Japanese, and Hispanic people; 1 to 10% of Caucasians; 3% of African Americans; and 16 to 28% of North Africans, Ethiopians, and Arabs. Watch for extreme sleepiness, confusion, and shallow breathing after giving drug. If present, notify prescriber and be prepared to provide supportive care and discontinue drug, as ordered.

PATIENT TEACHING
- Instruct patient to use a calibrated measuring device to ensure accurate dose.
- Urge patient to avoid alcohol and other antidepressants while taking codeine, phenylephrine, and pyrilamine.
- Instruct patient to avoid hazardous activities until drug's CNS effects are known.
- Suggest that patient relieve dry mouth with frequent rinsing and use of sugarless gum or hard candy.
- Tell patient to take last dose of the day a few hours before bedtime if codeine, phenylephrine, and pyrilamine makes him nervous or restless.
- Urge patient to notify prescriber if he develops trouble breathing or extreme sleepiness or confusion.

codeine phosphate and pseudoephedrine hydrochloride
Cycofed, Nucofed

Class, Category, and Schedule
Chemical: Opioid and phenanthrene derivative (codeine), sympathomimetic amine (pseudoephedrine)

Therapeutic: Antitussive (codeine), decongestant (pseudo-ephedrine)
Pregnancy category: C
Controlled substance schedule: III

Indications and Dosages

▶ *To relieve cough and other symptoms of allergies and the common cold*

CAPSULES

Adults. 20 mg codeine and 60 mg pseudoephedrine (1 capsule) every 6 hr.

SYRUP

Adults and children age 12 and over. 20 mg codeine and 60 mg pseudoephedrine (5 ml) every 6 hr.

Children ages 6 to 12. 10 mg codeine and 30 mg pseudo-ephedrine (2.5 ml) every 6 hr.

Children ages 2 to 6. 5 mg codeine and 15 mg pseudoephedrine (1.25 ml) every 6 hr.

Mechanism of Action

Codeine suppresses cough by directly acting on opiate receptors in the medulla's cough center.

Pseudoephedrine acts on alpha$_1$-adrenergic receptors in the mucosa of the respiratory tract to produce vasoconstriction. This process shrinks swollen nasal mucous membranes; reduces tissue hyperemia, edema, and nasal congestion; and increases nasal airway patency. It also may increase drainage of sinus secretions and open obstructed eustachian ostia.

Contraindications

Hypersensitivity or idiosyncractic reactions to codeine, other opioids, pseudoephedrine, or their components; hyperthyroidism; irritable bowel syndrome; narrow-angle glaucoma; paralytic ileus; prostatic hypertrophy; respiratory depression; severe asthma, coronary artery disease, or hypertension; upper airway obstruction; urine retention; use of MAO inhibitors within 14 days

Interactions

DRUGS

codeine and pseudoephedrine

MAO inhibitors: Increased and prolonged cardiac stimulation, increased vasopressor effect, increased risk of severe cardiovascular and cerebrovascular effects, hyperpyrexia, and vomiting

codeine
anticholinergics, paregoric: Possibly intensified anticholinergic adverse effects
antidiarrheals: Increased risk for severe constipation
antihypertensives, diuretics: Potentiated hypotensive effects
buprenorphine: Decreased codeine effectiveness
CNS depressants: Additive CNS effects
hydroxyzine: Increased codeine analgesic effect; increased CNS depressant and hypotensive effects
metoclopramide: Antagonized effect of metoclopramide on GI motility
naloxone: Antagonized codeine analgesic effect
naltrexone: Precipitated withdrawal symptoms in codeine-dependent patients
neuromuscular blockers: Additive respiratory depressant effects
opioids: Additive CNS and respiratory depressants effects and hypotensive effects
tricyclic antidepressants: Possibly increased effect of either the antidepressant or codeine

pseudoephedrine
antacids: Increased pseudoephedrine absorption
antihypertensives, diuretics: Possibly decreased antihypertensive effects
beta blockers: Decreased therapeutic effects of both drugs
citrates: Possibly inhibited urinary pseudoephedrine excretion and prolonged duration of action
CNS stimulant, other sympathomimetics: Possibly increased additive CNS stimulation to excessive levels
cocaine (mucosal-local): Possibly increased cardiovascular effects of either drug and CNS stimulation
digoxin, levodopa: Increased risk of cardiac arrhythmias
hydrocarbon inhalation anesthetics: Increased risk of serious arrhythmias
kaolin: Decreased pseudoephedrine absorption
nitrates: Reduced antianginal effects of nitrates
rauwolfia alkaloids: Possibly inhibited action of pseudoephedrine
thyroid hormones: Increased cardiovascular effects of both drugs
ACTIVITIES
codeine
alcohol use: Additive CNS effects

Adverse Reactions
CNS: Confusion, dizziness, drowsiness, euphoria, faintness, hallu-

cinations, headache, insomnia, lack of coordination, lethargy, light-headedness, nervousness, restlessness, seizures, tiredness, trembling, weakness

CV: Angina, bradycardia, hypertension, hypotension, palpitations, tachycardia

EENT: Blurred or double vision, dry mouth, laryngeal edema, laryngospasm

GI: Abdominal cramps or pain, anorexia, constipation, nausea, paralytic ileus, toxic megacolon, vomiting

GU: Decreased libido, dysuria, frequent urination, impotence

RESP: Dyspnea, respiratory depression, shortness of breath, slow or irregular breathing, wheezing

Skin: Diaphoresis, facial flushing, pallor, pruritus, rash, uriticaria

Other: Angioedema, atelectasis

Nursing Considerations

- Use cautiously in patients with hypertension, diabetes mellitus, ischemic heart disease, increased intraocular pressure, or renal impairment because of pseudoephedrine.
- **WARNING** Monitor respiratory function because codeine may suppress the cough reflex and cause thickening of bronchial secretions, aggravating such conditions as asthma and COPD. In rare cases, it may depress respirations and induce apnea. Notify prescriber immediately if respiratory rate drops below 10 breaths/minute.
- Monitor renal function, as ordered, because pseudoephedrine is substantially excreted by the kidneys.
- Regularly evaluate effectiveness of codeine and pseudoephedrine in reducing cough and allergy symptoms.
- **WARNING** Monitor patient closely for evidence of overdose, even at normal dosage, because some patients metabolize codeine quickly, causing a sudden rise in blood codeine level. This metabolic defect occurs in about 0.5 to 1% of Chinese, Japanese, and Hispanic people; 1 to 10% of Caucasians; 3% of African Americans; and 16 to 28% of North Africans, Ethiopians, and Arabs. Watch for extreme sleepiness, confusion, and shallow breathing after giving drug. If present, notify prescriber and be prepared to provide supportive care and discontinue drug, as ordered.

PATIENT TEACHING

- Instruct patient to use a calibrated measuring device to ensure accurate dose of codeine and pseudoephedrine.
- Urge patient to avoid alcohol and other antidepressants while

taking codeine and pseudoephedrine.
- Instruct patient to avoid hazardous activities until drug's CNS effects are known.
- Suggest that patient relieve dry mouth with frequent rinsing and use of sugarless gum or hard candy.
- Tell patient to take last dose of the day a few hours before bedtime if drug makes her nervous or restless.
- Urge patient to notify prescriber if she develops trouble breathing or extreme sleepiness or confusion.

codeine phosphate, triprolidine hydrochloride, and pseudoephedrine hydrochloride

Triacin-C, Triafed w/Codeine

Class, Category, and Schedule

Chemical: Opioid and phenanthrene derivative (codeine), alkylamine antihistamine (triprolidine), sympathomimetic amine (pseudoephedrine)
Therapeutic: Antitussive (codeine), antihistamine (triprolidine), decongestant (pseudoephedrine)
Pregnancy category: C
Controlled substance schedule: V

Indications and Dosages

▶ *To relieve cough and upper respiratory symptoms of hay fever, other upper respiratory allergies, and allergic rhinitis*
SYRUP
Adults and children age 12 and over. 20 mg codeine, 2.5 mg triprolidine, and 60 mg pseudoephedrine (10 ml) every 4 to 6 hr.
Children ages 6 to 12. 10 mg codeine, 1.25 mg triprolidine, and 30 mg pseudoephedrine (5 ml) every 4 to 6 hr.
Children age 2 to 6. 5 mg codeine, 0.625 mg triprolidine, and 15 mg pseudoephedrine (2.5 ml) every 4 to 6 hr.

Contraindications

Acute MI; angina; hypersensitivity or idiosyncractic reactions to codeine, other opioids, triprolidine, pseudoephedrine, or their components; hyperthyroidism; narrow-angle glaucoma; paralytic ileus; prostatic hypertrophy; respiratory depression; severe asthma, corornary artery disease or hypertension; upper airway obstruction, urine retention; use of MAO inhibitors within 14 days

Mechanism of Action

Codeine suppresses cough by directly acting on opiate receptors in the medulla's cough center.

Triprolidine competes with histamine for H_1 receptor sites, thereby antagonizing many histamine effects and reducing allergy signs and symptoms.

Pseudoephedrine acts on alpha$_1$-adrenergic receptors in the mucosa of the respiratory tract to produce vasoconstriction. This process shrinks swollen nasal mucous membranes; reduces tissue hyperemia, edema, and nasal congestion; and increases nasal airway patency. It also may increase drainage of sinus secretions and open obstructed eustachian ostia.

Interactions

DRUGS

codeine and pseudoephedrine
MAO inhibitors: Increased and prolonged cardiac stimulation, increased vasopressor effect, increased risk of severe cardiovascular and cerebrovascular effects, hyperpyrexia, and vomiting

codeine and triprolidine
anticholinergics, paregoric: Possibly intensified anticholinergic adverse effects
CNS depressants: Additive CNS effects

codeine
antihypertensives, diuretics: Potentiated hypotensive effects
antidiarrheals: Increased risk of severe constipation
buprenorphine: Decreased codeine effectiveness
hydroxyzine: Increased codeine analgesic effect; increased CNS depressant and hypotensive effects
metoclopramide: Antagonized effect of metoclopramide on GI motility
naloxone: Anatagonized codeine analgesic effect
naltrexone: Precipitated withdrawal symptoms in codeine-dependent patients
neuromuscular blockers: Additive respiratory depressant effects
opioids: Additive CNS and respiratory depressants effects and hypotensive effects
tricyclic antidepressants: Possibly increased effect of either the antidepressant or codeine

triprolidine
MAO inhibitors: Prolonged and intensified anticholinergic (drying) effects of triprolidine

pseudoephedrine

antacids: Increased pseudoephedrine absorption

antihypertensives, diuretics: Possibly decreased antihypertensive effects

beta blockers: Decreased therapeutic effects of both drugs

citrates: Possibly inhibited urinary pseudoephedrine excretion and prolonged duration of action

CNS stimulant, other sympathomimetics: Possibly increased additive CNS stimulation to excessive levels

cocaine (mucosal-local): Possibly increased cardiovascular effects of either drug and CNS stimulation

digoxin, levodopa: Increased risk of cardiac arrhythmias

hydrocarbon inhalation anesthetics: Increased risk of serious arrhythmias

kaolin: Decreased pseudoephedrine absorption

nitrates: Reduced antianginal effects of nitrates

rauwolfia alkaloids: Possibly inhibited pseudoephedrine action

thyroid hormones: Increased cardiovascular effects of both drugs

ACTIVITIES

codeine and triprolidine

alcohol use: Additive CNS effects

Adverse Reactions

CNS: Asthenia, anxiety, confusion, dizziness, depression, drowsiness, dyskinesia, euphoria, excitability, faintness, headache, insomnia, irritability, light-headedness, nervousness, restlessness, sedation, syncope, tiredness, tremor, vertigo, weakness

CV: Bradycardia, hypertension, hypotension, orthostatic hypotension, palpitation, tachycardia

ENDO: Decreased lactation, early menses, gynecomastia, hyperglycemia, hypoglycemia

EENT: Blurred vision; diplopia; dry mouth, pharynx, and respiratory passages; hypermetropia; increased lacrimation; labyrinthitis; laryngismus; mydriasis; nasal stuffiness; photophobia; tinnitus

GI: Abdominal distention or pain, acute pancreatitis, anorexia, constipation, diarrhea, dyspepsia, epigastric distress, esophageal reflux, increased appetite, nausea, vomiting

GU: Decreased libido, dysuria, urinary frequency or hesitancy, urine retention, ureteral spasm

RESP: Dyspnea, respiratory depression, wheezing

SKIN: Dermatitis, diaphoresis, erythema, flushing, pallor, pruritus, rash, urticaria

Other: Drug fever, emotional or physical dependence

Nursing Considerations

- Use cautiously in patients with recent head injury and those with Addison's disease, asthma or other chronic respiratory disease, increased intraocular pressure, or liver or renal impairment.
- **WARNING** Monitor respiratory function because codeine, triprolidine, and pseudoephedrine may suppress cough reflex and cause thickening of bronchial secretions, aggravating such conditions as asthma and COPD. In rare cases, it may depress respirations and induce apnea. Notify prescriber immediately if respiratory rate drops below 10 breaths/minute.
- Monitor patients who may be more susceptible to dizziness, sedation, and hypotension, such as the elderly.
- Monitor renal function, as ordered, because pseudoephedrine is substantially excreted by the kidneys.
- Regularly evaluate effectiveness of codeine, triprolidine, and pseudoephedrine in reducing symptoms.
- Be aware that patient shouldn't have intradermal allergen tests within 72 hours of receiving drug because results may be altered.
- **WARNING** Monitor patient closely for evidence of overdose, even at normal dosage, because some patients metabolize codeine quickly, causing a sudden rise in blood codeine level. This metabolic defect occurs in about 0.5 to 1% of Chinese, Japanese, and Hispanic people; 1 to 10% of Caucasians; 3% of African Americans; and 16 to 28% of North Africans, Ethiopians, and Arabs. Watch for extreme sleepiness, confusion, and shallow breathing after giving drug. If present, notify prescriber and be prepared to provide supportive care and discontinue drug, as ordered.

PATIENT TEACHING

- Instruct patient to use a calibrated measuring device.
- Tell patient that codeine, triprolidine, and pseudoephedrine must not be diluted with fluids or mixed with other drugs.
- Urge patient to avoid alcohol and other antidepressants while taking codeine, triprolidine, and pseudoephedrine.
- Instruct patient to avoid hazardous activities until drug's CNS effects are known.
- Suggest that patient relieve dry mouth with frequent rinsing and use of sugarless gum or hard candy.
- Tell patient to take last dose of the day a few hours before bedtime if codeine, triprolidine, and pseudoephedrine makes him nervous or restless.
- Urge patient to notify prescriber if he develops trouble breathing or extreme sleepiness or confusion.

desloratadine and pseudoephedrine sulfate

Clarinex-D 12 Hour, Clarinex-D 24 Hour

Class and Category

Chemical: Active metabolite of loratadine a long-acting tricyclic histamine antagonist (desloratadine), sympathomimetic amine (pseudoephedrine)

Therapeutic: Antihistamine (desloratadine), decongestant (pseudo-ephedrine)

Pregnancy category: C

Indications and Dosages

▶ *To relieve nasal and non-nasal symptoms of seasonal allergic rhinitis, including nasal congestion*

E.R. TABLETS (CLARINEX-D 24 HOUR)

Adults and children age 12 and over. 5 mg desloratadine and 240 mg pseudoephedrine (1 tablet) daily.

DOSAGE ADJUSTMENT For patients with renal impairment, 5 mg desloratadine and 240 mg pseudoephedrine (1 tablet) every 48 hr.

E.R. TABLETS (CLARINEX-D 12 HOUR)

Adults and children age 12 and over. 2.5 mg desloratadine and 120 mg pseudoephedrine (1 tablet) b.i.d.

Mechanism of Action

Desloratadine is an active metabolite of loratadine that competes with free histamine for histamine H_1 receptor sites. Without histamine, vascular engorgement, mucosal edema, profuse watery secretion, local irritation, and sneezing that normally result from histamine action on afferent nerve terminals in nasal passages cannot occur.

Pseudoephedrine acts on alpha$_1$-adrenergic receptors in the mucosa of the respiratory tract to produce vasoconstriction. This process shrinks swollen nasal mucous membranes; reduces tissue hyperemia, edema, and nasal congestion; and increases nasal airway patency. It also may increase drainage of sinus secretions and open obstructed eustachian ostia.

Contraindications

Angina; hepatic insufficiency; hypersensitivity or idiosyncratic reactions to desloratadine, loratadine, pseudoephedrine, or their components; hyperthyroidism; narrow-angle glaucoma; prostatic hypertrophy; severe coronary artery disease or hypertension;

urine retention; use within 14 days of MAO inhibitor therapy

Interactions

DRUGS

desloratadine

barbiturates, CNS depressants, tricyclic antidepressants: Additive effects

pseudoephedrine

antacids: Increased pseudoephedrine absorption

beta blockers, diuretics, methyldopa, mecamylamine, reserpine, veratum alkaloids: Decreased antihypertensive effects of these drugs

citrates: Possibly inhibited urinary pseudoephedrine excretion and prolonged duration of action

CNS stimulant, other sympathomimetics: Possibly increased additive CNS stimulation to excessive levels

cocaine (mucosal-local): Possibly increased cardiovascular effects of either drug and CNS stimulation

digoxin, levodopa: Increased risk of cardiac arrhythmias

hydrocarbon inhalation anesthetics: Possibly serious arrhythmias

kaolin: Decreased pseudoephedrine absorption

MAO inhibitors: Increased and prolonged cardiac stimulation, increased vasopressor effect, increased risk of severe cardiovascular and cerebrovascular effects, hyperpyrexia, and vomiting

nitrates: Reduced antianginal effects of nitrates

rauwolfia alkaloids: Possibly inhibited pseudoephedrine action

ACTIVITIES

desloratadine

alcohol use: Additive effects

Adverse Reactions

CNS: Agitation, anxiety, dizziness, fatigue, headache, hyperactivity, insomnia, light-headedness, nervousness, restlessness, seizures, somnolence, trembling, weakness

CV: Angina, arrhythmia exacerbation, hypertension, palpitations, tachycardia

EENT: Dry mouth, pharyngitis, photophobia, ocular hypertension

ENDO: Dysmenorrhea

GI: Anorexia, nausea, vomiting

GU: Dysuria, urine retention

RESP: Bronchospasm, coughing, dyspnea

SKIN: Diaphoresis, pallor, pruritus, rash

Nursing Considerations

• Be aware that desloratadine and pseudodoephedrine therapy isn't recommended for patients with renal impairment.

- Use cautiously in patients with diabetes, hypertension, increased intraocular pressure, ischemic heart disease, or renal disease because of pseudoephedrine.
- Monitor elderly patients closely because they're more prone to developing adverse effects.
- Monitor renal function, as ordered, because pseudoephedrine is substantially excreted by the kidneys.
- Regularly evaluate effectiveness of desloratadine and pseudoephedrine in relieving seasonal and nonseasonal allergic rhinitis.
- Be aware that patient shouldn't have intradermal allergen tests within 4 days of receiving drug because results may be altered.

PATIENT TEACHING
- Instruct patients to take desloratadine and pseudoephedrine with a full glass of water and not to break or chew the tablet but to swallow it whole.
- Urge patient to avoid alcohol, other antidepressants, and OTC medication containing other antihistamines or sympathomimetics while taking desloratadine and pseudoephedrine.
- Instruct patient to avoid hazardous activities until drug's CNS effects are known.
- Suggest that patient relieve dry mouth with frequent rinsing and use of sugarless gum or hard candy.

dexchlorpheniramine tannate and pseudoephedrine tannate

Tanafed DP

Class and Category

Chemical: Alkylamine (dexchlorpheniramine), sympathomimetic amine (pseudoephedrine)
Therapeutic: Antihistamine (dexchlorpheniramine), decongestant (pseudoephedrine)
Pregnancy category: C

Indications and Dosages

▶ *To relieve persistent runny nose, sneezing and nasal congestion caused by upper respiratory infection, sinus inflammation, or hay fever; to relieve sinus pressure and drain sinuses*

SUSPENSION

Adults. 5 to 10 mg dexchlorpheniramine and 150 to 300 mg pseudoephedrine (10 to 20 ml) every 12 hr.

Mechanism of Action

Dexchlorpheniramine competes with histamine for H_1 receptor sites, antagonizing many histamine effects and reducing allergy signs and symptoms.

   Pseudoephedrine acts on $alpha_1$-adrenergic receptors in the mucosa of the respiratory tract to produce vasoconstriction. This process shrinks swollen nasal mucous membranes; reduces tissue hyperemia, edema, and nasal congestion; and increases nasal airway patency. It also may increase drainage of sinus secretions and open obstructed eustachian ostia.

Contraindications

Angina; breast-feeding; hypersensitivity or idiosyncractic reactions to dexchlorpheniramine, pseudoephedrine, or their components; hyperthyroidism; narrow-angle glaucoma; prostatic hypertrophy; severe coronary artery disease or hypertension; urine retention; use within 14 days of MAO inhibitor therapy

Interactions

DRUGS

dexchlorpheniramine

anticholinergics: Additive anticholinergic effects

CNS depressants: Additive CNS effects

MAO inhibitors: Prolonged and intensified anticholinergic (drying) effect of dexchlorpheniramine

phenytoin: Possibly increased serum phenytoin levels and toxicity

pseudoephedrine

antacids: Increased pseudoephedrine absorption

antihypertensives, diuretics: Possibly decreased antihypertensive effects

beta blockers: Decreased therapeutic effects of both drugs

citrates: Possibly inhibited urinary pseudoephedrine excretion and prolonged duration of action

CNS stimulant, other sympathomimetics: Possibly increased additive CNS stimulation to excessive levels

cocaine (mucosal-local): Possibly increased cardiovascular effects of either drug and CNS stimulation

digoxin, levodopa: Increased risk of cardiac arrhythmias

hydrocarbon inhalation anesthetics: Increased risk of serious arrhythmias

kaolin: Decreased pseudoephedrine absorption

MAO inhibitors: Increased and prolonged cardiac stimulation, increased vasopressor effect, increased risk of severe cardiovascular and cerebrovascular effects, hyperpyrexia, vomiting

nitrates: Reduced antianginal effects of nitrates
rauwolfia alkaloids: Possibly inhibited pseudoephedrine action
thyroid hormones: Increased cardiovascular effects of both drugs
ACTIVITIES
dexchlorpheniramine
alcohol use: Additive CNS effects

Adverse Reactions

CNS: Anxiety, chills, confusion, coordination disturbance, dizziness, drowsiness, excitation (children), fatigue, fear, hallucinations, headache, hysteria, insomnia, irritability, light-headedness, nervousness, numbness, restlessness, sedation, seizures, tenseness, trembling, vertigo, weakness
CV: Arrhythmias, chest tightness, hypertension, palpitations, tachycardia
EENT: Blurred or double vision; dry mouth, nose, and throat; nasal congestion, tinnitus
ENDO: Early menstruation
GI: Anorexia, constipation, diarrhea, nausea, stomach upset or pain, vomiting
GU: Dysuria, frequent urination, urinary hesitancy, urine retention
HEME: Anemia, unusual bleeding or bruising
RESP: Dyspnea, increased chest congestion, wheezing
SKIN: Diaphoresis, pallor, photosensitivity, rash, urticaria
Other: Anaphylaxis

Nursing Considerations

- Use cautiously in patients with asthma, cardiovascular disease, diabetes, emphysema or other chronic lung disease, hypertension, peptic ulcer, or narrow-angle glaucoma.
- Monitor patients who may be more susceptible to dizziness, sedation and hypotension, such as the elderly.
- Monitor renal function, as ordered, because pseudoephedrine is substantially excreted by the kidneys.
- Regularly evaluate effectiveness of dexchlorpheniramine and pseudoephedrine in reducing upper respiratory symptoms.
- Be aware that patient shouldn't undergo allergen tests within 72 hours of receiving drug because results may be altered.
PATIENT TEACHING
- Instruct patient to use a calibrated measuring device to ensure accurate dose.
- Urge patient to avoid alcohol and other antidepressants while taking dexchlorpheniramine and pseudoephedrine.

- Instruct patient to avoid hazardous activities until drug's CNS effects are known.
- Suggest that patient relieve dry mouth with frequent rinsing and use of sugarless gum or hard candy.
- Tell patient to take last dose of the day a few hours before bedtime if dexchlorpheniramine and pseudoephedrine makes him nervous or restless.

dextromethorphan hydrobromide, brompheniramine maleate, and phenylephrine hydrochloride
Alacol DM

Class and Category
Chemical: D-isomer codeine analog of levorphanol (dextromethorphan), alkylamine derivative (brompheniramine), sympathomimetic amine (phenylephrine)
Therapeutic: Antitussive (dextromethorphan), antihistaminic (brompheniramine), decongestant (phenylephrine)
Pregnancy category: C

Indications and Dosages
▶ *To relieve cough and nasal congestion in upper respiratory tract conditions*
SYRUP
Adults. 20 mg dextromethorphan, 4 mg brompheniramine, and 10 mg phenylephrine (10 ml) every 4 hr.

Mechanism of Action
Dextromethorphan suppresses cough by acting directly on the cough center in the medulla of the brain.

Brompheniramine competes with histamine for H_1 receptor sites, antagonizing many histamine effects and reducing allergy signs and symptoms.

Phenylephrine stimulates alpha-adrenergic receptors and inhibits the intracellular enzyme adenyl cyclase, which then inhibits production of cAMP. Inhibition of cAMP causes arterial and venous constriction in nasal passages, which decreases blood flow and mucosal edema caused by allergic response.

Contraindications
Asthma; breast-feeding; chronic bronchitis; emphysema; hypersensitivity to dextromethorphan, brompheniramine or phenyle-

phrine or their components; hyperthyroidism; narrow-angle glaucoma; productive cough; prostatic hypertrophy; severe hypertension; use of MAO inhibitors within 14 days

Interactions
DRUGS
dextromethorphan, brompheniramine and phenylephrine
MAO inhibitors: Possibly prolonged and intensified anticholinergic effects of brompheniramine and overall effects of dextromethorphan and phenylephrine
dextromethorphan and brompheniramine
CNS depressants: Additive CNS effects
dextromethorphan
amiodarone, fluoxetine, paroxetine, quinidine: Decreased dextromethorphan metabolism, which may result in increased plasma dextromethorphan level and adverse reactions
brompheniramine
anticholinergics: Potentiated anticholinergic effects
phenylephrine
alpha blockers, haloperidol, loxapine, phenothiazines, thioxanthenes: Possibly decreased vasoconstrictor effect of phenylephrine
antihypertenisves, diuretics: Possibly decreased antihypertensive effects
atropine: Possibly enhanced vasopressor effect of phenylephrine
beta blockers: Decreased therapeutic effects of both drugs
bretylium: Possibly potentiated vaopressor effect and arrhythmias
doxapram: Increased vasopressor effect of both drugs
ergot alkaloids: Possibly cerebral blood vessel rupture, increased vasopressor effect, peripheral vascular ischemia, and gangrene (with ergotamine)
guanadrel, guanethidine: Increased vasopressor effect of phenylephrine; increased risk of severe hypertension and arrhythmias
hydrocarbon inhalation anesthetics: Possibly serious arrhythmias
maprotiline, tricyclic antidepressants: Increased risk of severe cardiovascular effects (including arrhythmias, hyperpyrexia, severe hypertension)
mecamylamine, methyldopa: Decreased hypotensive effects of these drugs; increased vasopressor effect of phenylephrine
nitrates: Possibly decreased vasopressor effect of phenylephrine and decreased antianginal effect of nitrates
oxytocin: Possibly severe, persistent hypertension
phenoxybenzamine: Decreased vasoconstrictor effect of phenylephrine, possibly hypotension and tachycardia

theophylline: Possibly enhanced toxicity (including cardiac toxicity)
thyroid hormones: Increased cardiovascular effects of each drug
ACTIVITIES
dextromethorphan and brompheniramine
alcohol use: Additive CNS effects
dextromethorphan
smoking: Possibly increased respiratory secretion retention

Adverse Reactions

CNS: Confusion, dizziness, drowsiness, fever, hallucinations, headache, hyperactivity, insomnia, nervousness, paresthesia, restlessness, sedation, seizures, tiredness, tremor, weakness
CV: Angina, arrhythmias, bradycardia, edema, hypertension, hypotension, palpitations, peripheral vasoconstriction that may lead to necrosis or gangrene, tachycardia, ventricular arrhythmias
EENT: Dry mouth, sore throat
GI: Abdominal pain, constipation, nausea, vomiting
GU: Urinary hesitancy, urine retention
HEME: Unusual bleeding or bruising
RESP: Dyspnea, respiratory depression
Other: Anaphylaxis, emotional and physical dependence (prolonged use with high doses)

Nursing Considerations

- Use cautiously in patients with bladder neck obstruction, cardiovascular disease, hypertension, glaucoma, or urine retention.
- Also use cautiously in patient with diabetes because some products contain sugar, which may disrupt blood glucose control; in patients with impaired hepatic function because dextromethorphan is metabolized by the liver; and in patients with respiratory depression because dextromethorphan adversely affects respirations.
- Monitor patients who may be more susceptible to dizziness, sedation, and hypotension, such as the elderly.
- Assess patient regularly for bleeding or bruising abnormalities because of brompheniramine.
- Regularly evaluate effectiveness of dextromethorphan, brompheniramine, and phenylephrine in relieving cough and reducing nasal congestion.
- Be aware that patient shouldn't have intradermal allergen tests within 72 hours of receiving drug because results may be altered.
- **WARNING** Dextromethorphan has the potential for abuse because of its euphoric, hallucinogenic, and dissociative effects

when taken in doses higher than prescribed. Monitor patient closely.

PATIENT TEACHING
- Urge patient not to exceed prescribed dosage.
- Instruct patient to use a calibrated measuring device when measuring dextromethorphan, brompheniramine, and phenylephrine to ensure an accurate dose.
- Stress importance of taking drug exactly as prescribed and not increasing dose or frequency without consulting prescriber.
- Urge patient to avoid alcohol and other antidepressants while taking drug.
- Instruct patient to avoid hazardous activities until drug's CNS effects are known.
- Suggest that patient relieve dry mouth with frequent rinsing and use of sugarless gum or hard candy.

dextromethorphan hydrobromide, brompheniramine maleate, and pseudoephedrine hydrochloride

AccuHist DM, Anaplex-DM, Andehist-DM, Bromatane DX, Bromfed DM, Carbodex DM, Carbofed DM, Coldec DM, Dimetapp-DM, Robitussin Allergy & Cough, Rondamine DM, Rondec-DM, Sildec-DM

Class and Category

Chemical: D-isomer codeine analogue of levorphanol (dextromethorphan), propylamine derivative (brompheniramine), sympatho-mimetic amine (pseudoephedrine)
Therapeutic: Antitussive (dextromethorphan), antihistamine (brompheniramine), decongestant (pseudoephedrine)
Pregnancy category: C

Indications and Dosages

▶ *To relieve cough and persistent runny nose, sneezing, and nasal congestion caused by upper respiratory infections, sinus inflammation, or hay fever*

ORAL SOLUTION

Adults. 20 to 30 mg dextromethorphan, 4 mg brompheniramine, and 60 mg pseudoephedrine (5 or 10 ml depending on product) every 4 to 6 hr. Or, 15 mg dextromethorphan, 4 mg brompheniramine and 45 to 60 mg pseudoephedrine (5 ml) q.i.d. *Maximum:* 4 doses daily.

SYRUP

Adults and children age 12 and over. 20 to 30 mg dextromethorphan, 4 mg brompheniramine, and 60 mg pseudoephedrine (5 or 10 ml depending on product) every 4 to 6 hr. Or, 15 mg dextromethorphan, 4 mg brompheniramine, and 45 to 60 mg pseudoephedrine (5 ml) q.i.d. *Maximum:* 4 doses daily.

Children ages 6 to 12. 10 mg dextromethorphan, 2 mg brompheniramine, and 30 mg pseudoephedrine (5 ml) every 4 hr. *Maximum:* 4 doses daily.

Children ages 2 to 6. 5 mg dextromethorphan, 1 mg brompheniramine, and 15 mg pseudoephedrine (2.5 ml) every 4 hr. *Maximum:* 4 doses daily.

DROPS

Children ages 12 months to 24 months. 4 mg dextromethorphan, 1 mg brompheniramine, and 15 mg pseudoephedrine (1 ml) q.i.d.

Children ages 6 months to 12 months. 3 mg dextromethorphan, 0.75 mg brompheniramine, and 11.25 mg pseudoephedrine (0.75 ml) q.i.d.

Infants ages 3 months to 6 months. 2 mg dextromethorphan, 0.5 mg brompheniramine, and 7.5 mg pseudoephedrine (0.5 ml) q.i.d.

Infants ages 1 month to 3 months. 1 mg dextromethorphan, 0.25 mg brompheniramine, and 3.75 mg pseudoephedrine (0.25 ml) q.i.d.

Mechanism of Action

Dextromethorphan suppresses cough by acting directly on the cough center in the medulla of the brain.

Brompheniramine competes with histamine for H_1 receptor sites, antagonizing many histamine effects and reducing allergy signs and symptoms.

Pseudoephedrine acts on alpha$_1$-adrenergic receptors in the mucosa of the respiratory tract to produce vasoconstriction. This process shrinks swollen nasal mucous membranes; reduces tissue hyperemia, edema, and nasal congestion; and increases nasal airway patency. It also may increase drainage of sinus secretions and open obstructed eustachian ostia.

Contraindications

Asthma; breast-feeding; chronic bronchitis; emphysema; hypersensitivity or idiosyncractic reactions to dextromethorphan, brompheniramine, pseudoephedrine, or their components; hyperthyroidism; narrow-angle glaucoma; productive cough; prostatic hypertrophy; severe coronary artery disease or hypertension; urine retention; use within 14 days of MAO inhibitor therapy

Interactions
DRUGS
dextromethorphan and pseudoephedrine
MAO inhibitors: Increased and prolonged cardiac stimulation, increased vasopressor effect, increased risk of severe cardiovascular and cerebrovascular effects, hyperpyrexia, and vomiting
dextromethorphan and brompheniramine
CNS depressants: Additive CNS effects
dextromethorphan
amiodarone, fluoxetine, paroxetine, quinidine: Decreased metabolism of dextromethorphan, which may result in increased plasma dextromethorphan levels and adverse reactions
brompheniramine
anticholinergics: Additive anticholinergic effects
MAO inhibitors: Prolonged and intensified anticholinergic (drying) effects of brompheniramine
pseudoephedrine
antacids: Increased pseudoephedrine absorption
antihypertensives, diuretics: Possibly decreased antihypertensive effects
beta blockers: Decreased therapeutic effects of both drugs
citrates: Possibly inhibited urinary pseudoephedrine excretion and prolonged duration of action
CNS stimulant, other sympathomimetics: Possibly increased additive CNS stimulation to excessive levels
cocaine (mucosal-local): Possibly increased cardiovascular effects of either drug and CNS stimulation
digoxin, levodopa: Increased risk of cardiac arrhythmias
hydrocarbon inhalation anesthetics: Increased risk of serious arrhythmias
kaolin: Decreased pseudoephedrine absorption
nitrates: Reduced antianginal effects of nitrates
rauwolfia alkaloids: Possibly inhibited pseudoephedrine action
thyroid hormones: Increased cardiovascular effects of both drugs
ACTIVITIES
dextromethorphan and brompheniramine
alcohol use: Additive CNS effects
dextromethorphan
smoking: Possibly increased respiratory secretion retention

Adverse Reactions

CNS: Anxiety, chills, confusion, coordination disturbance, dizziness, drowsiness, fatigue, fear, hallucinations, headache, hyperactivity, hysteria, insomnia, irritability, light-headedness, nervousness, numbness, restlessness, sedation, seizures, tenseness, trembling, vertigo, weakness

CV: Arrhythmias, chest tightness, hypertension, palpitations, tachycardia

EENT: Blurred or double vision; dry mouth, nose, and throat; nasal congestion, tinnitus

ENDO: Early menstruation

GI: Abdominal pain, anorexia, constipation, diarrhea, nausea, stomach upset or pain, vomiting

GU: Dysuria, frequent urination, urinary hesitancy, urine retention

HEME: Anemia, unusual bleeding or bruising

RESP: Dyspnea, increased chest congestion, respiratory depression, wheezing

SKIN: Diaphoresis, pallor, photosensitivity, rash, urticaria

Other: Anaphylaxis, emotional and physical dependence (prolonged use with high doses)

Nursing Considerations

- Use cautiously in patients with asthma, cardiovascular disease, emphysema or other chronic lung disease, hypertension, or peptic ulcer.
- Also use cautiously in patients with diabetes because some products contain sugar, which may interfere with blood glucose control; in those with impaired hepatic function because dextromethorphan is metabolized by the liver; and in those with respiratory depression because dextromethorphan adversely affect respirations.
- Monitor patients who may be more susceptible to dizziness, sedation, and hypotension, such as the elderly.
- Monitor renal function, as ordered, because pseudoephedrine is substantially excreted by the kidneys.
- Regularly evaluate effectiveness of dextromethorphan, brompheniramine, and pseudoephedrine in relieving cough and reducing upper respiratory symptoms.
- Be aware that patient shouldn't have intradermal allergen tests within 72 hours of receiving drug because results may be altered.
- **WARNING** Dextromethorphan has the potential for abuse because of its euphoric, hallucinogenic, and dissociative effects

when taken in doses higher than prescribed. Monitor patient closely.

PATIENT TEACHING
• Urge patient not to exeed presribed dosage.
• Instruct patient to use a calibrated measuring device when using syrup or oral solution form to ensure accurate dose.
• Caution patient not to exceed prescribed dose or frequency without consulting prescriber.
• Urge patient to avoid alcohol and other antidepressants while taking drug.
• Instruct patient to avoid hazardous activities until drug's CNS effects are known.
• Suggest that patient relieve dry mouth with frequent rinsing and use of sugarless gum or hard candy.
• Tell patient to take last dose of the day a few hours before bedtime if dextromethorphan, brompheniramine and pseudoephedrine makes him nervous or restless.

dextromethorphan hydrobromide, carbinoxamine maleate, and pseudoephedrine hydrochloride

Andehist DM NR, Balamine DM, Carbinoxamine Compound, Carbodex DM, Carbofed DM, Cardec DM, C.P.-DM, Cydec-DM, Pediatex-DM, Pseudo-Car DM, Rondec-DM, Sildec-DM, Tussafed

Class and Category

Chemical: D-isomer codeine analogue of levorphanol (dextromethorphan), ethanolamine derivative (carbinoxamine), sympathomimetic amine (pseudoephedrine)
Therapeutic: Antitussive (dextromethorphan), antihistamine (carbinoxamine), decongestant (pseudoephedrine)
Pregnancy category: C

Indications and Dosages

▶ *To relieve cough, persistent runny nose, sneezing, and nasal congestion caused by upper respiratory tract infections, sinus inflammation, or hay fever*
ORAL SOLUTION
Adults and children age 6 and over. 15 mg dextromethorphan, 2 mg carbinoxamine, and 15 mg pseudoephedrine (5 ml) q.i.d.

Children ages 18 months to 6 years. 7.5 mg dextromethorphan, 1 mg carbinoxamine, and 7.5 mg psuedoephedrine (0.25 ml) q.i.d.

SYRUP

Adults and children age 6 and over. 12.5 or 15 mg dextromethorphan, 4 mg carbinoxamine, and 60 mg pseudoephedrine (5 ml) every 4 to 6 hr *Maximum:* 4 doses daily.

Children ages 18 months to 6 years. 6.25 to 7.5 mg dextromethorphan, 2 mg carbinoxamine, and 30 mg pseudoephedrine (2.5 ml) every 4 to 6 hr. *Maximum:* 4 doses daily.

DROPS (ANDEHIST DM NR, C.P.-DM, CARBOFED DM, RONDEC-DM)

Children ages 12 months to 24 months. 4 mg dextromethorphan, 1 mg carbinoxamine, and 15 mg pseudoephedrine (1 ml) q.i.d.

Children ages 6 months to 12 months. 3 mg dextromethorphan, 0.75 mg carbinoxamine, and 11.25 mg pseudoephedrine (0.75 ml) q.i.d.

Infants ages 3 months to 6 months. 2 mg dextromethorphan, 0.5 mg carbinoxamine, and 7.5 mg pseudoephedrine (0.5 ml) q.i.d.

Infants ages 1 month to 3 months. 1 mg dextromethorphan, 0.25 mg carbinoxamine, and 3.75 mg pseudoephedrine (0.25 ml) q.i.d.

DROPS (BALAMINE DM, CARBINOXAMINE COMPOUND, CARBODEX DM, CYDEC-DM, SILDEC-DM, TUSSAFED)

Children ages 9 months to 18 months. 3.5 or 4 mg dextromethorphan, 2 mg carbinoxamine, and 15 or 25 mg pseudoephedrine (1 ml) q.i.d.

Children ages 6 months to 9 months. 2.6 or 3 mg dextromethorphan, 1.5 mg carbinoxamine, and 18.75 or 11.25 mg pseudoephedrine (0.75 ml) q.i.d.

Infants ages 3 months to 6 months. 1.75 or 2 mg dextromethorphan, 1 mg carbinoxamine, and 12.5 or 7.5 mg pseudoephedrine (0.5 ml) q.i.d.

Infants ages 1 month to 3 months. 0.875 or 1 mg dextromethorphan, 0.5 mg carbinoxamine and 6.25 or 3.75 mg pseudoephedrine (0.25 ml) q.i.d.

Contraindications

Acute MI; angina; asthma; breast-feeding; chronic bronchitis; emphysema; hypersensitivity or idiosyncractic reactions to dextromethorphan, carbinoxamine, pseudoephedrine, or their components; hyperthyroidism; narrow-angle glaucoma; productive cough; severe coronary artery disease or hypertension; tachycardia; urine retention; use within 14 days of MAO inhibitor therapy

---

Mechanism of Action

Dextromethorphan suppresses cough by directly acting on the cough center in the medulla of the brain.

Carbinoxamine competes with histamine for H_1 receptor sites, thereby antagonizing many histamine effects and reducing allergy signs and symptoms.

Pseudoephedrine acts on $alpha_1$-adrenergic receptors in the mucosa of the respiratory tract to produce vasoconstriction. This process shrinks swollen nasal mucous membranes; reduces tissue hyperemia, edema, and nasal congestion; and increases nasal airway patency.

Interactions

DRUGS

dextromethorphan, carbinoxamine and pseudoephedrine

MAO inhibitors: Increased and prolonged cardiac stimulation, increased vasopressor effect, increased risk of severe cardiovascular and cerebrovascular effects, hyperpyrexia, and vomiting

dextromethorphan and carbinoxamine

CNS depressants: Additive CNS effects

dextromethorphan

amiodarone, fluoxetine, paroxetine, quinidine: Decreased metabolism of dextromethorphan which may result in increased plasma dextromethorphan levels and incidence of adverse reactions

carbinoxamine

anticholinergics: Additive anticholinergic effects

pseudoephedrine

antacids: Increased pseudoephedrine absorption

antihypertensives, diuretics: Possibly decreased antihypertensive effects

beta blockers: Decreased therapeutic effects of both drugs

citrates: Possibly inhibited urinary pseudoephedrine excretion and prolonged duration of action

CNS stimulant, other sympathomimetics: Possibly increased additive CNS stimulation to excessive levels

cocaine (mucosal-local): Possibly increased cardiovascular effects of either drug and CNS stimulation

digoxin, levodopa: Increased risk of cardiac arrhythmias

hydrocarbon inhalation anesthetics: Increased risk of serious arrhythmias

kaolin: Decreased pseudoephedrine absorption
nitrates: Reduced antianginal effects of nitrates
rauwolfia alkaloids: Possibly inhibited pseudoephedrine action
thyroid hormones: Increased cardiovascular effects of both drugs
ACTIVITIES
dextromethorphan and carbinoxamine
alcohol use: Additive CNS effects
dextromethorphan
smoking: Possibly increased respiratory secretion retention

Adverse Reactions

CNS: Anxiety, chills, confusion, coordination disturbance, dizziness, drowsiness, excitation (children), fatigue, fear, hallucinations, headache, hyperactivity, hysteria, insomnia, irritability, light-headedness, nervousness, numbness, restlessness, sedation, seizures, tenseness, trembling, vertigo, weakness
CV: Arrhythmias, chest tightness, hypertension, palpitations, tachycardia
EENT: Blurred or double vision; dry mouth, nose, and throat; nasal congestion, tinnitus
ENDO: Early menstruation
GI: Abdominal pain, anorexia, constipation, diarrhea, nausea, stomach upset or pain, vomiting
GU: Dysuria, frequent urination, urinary hesitancy, urine retention
HEME: Anemia, unusual bleeding or bruising
RESP: Dyspnea, increased chest congestion, respiratory depression, wheezing
SKIN: Diaphoresis, pallor, photosensitivity, rash, urticaria
Other: Anaphylaxis, emotional and physical dependence (prolonged use with high doses)

Nursing Considerations

- Use dextromethorphan, carbinoxamine, and pseudoephedrine cautiously in patients who have diabetes because some products contain sugar, which may disrupt blood glucose control; in those with impaired hepatic function because dextromethorphan is metabolized by the liver; and in those with respiratory depression because dextromethorphan adversely affects respirations.
- Monitor patients who may be more susceptible to dizziness, sedation, and hypotension, such as the elderly.
- Monitor renal function, as ordered, because pseudoephedrine is substantially excreted by the kidneys.

- Regularly evaluate effectiveness of dextromethorphan, carbinoxamine, and pseudoephedrine in reducing upper respiratory symptoms.
- Be aware that patient shouldn't have intradermal allergen tests within 72 hours of receiving drug because results may be altered.
- **WARNING** Dextromethorphan has the potential for abuse because of its euphoric, hallucinogenic, and dissociative effects when taken in doses higher than prescribed. Monitor patient closely.

PATIENT TEACHING
- Urge patient not to exceed prescribed dosage.
- Instruct patient to use a calibrated measuring device when measuring syrup to ensure accurate dose.
- Stress importance of taking drug exactly as prescribed and not increasing dose or frequency without consulting prescriber.
- Urge patient to avoid alcohol and other antidepressants while taking dextromethorphan, carbinoxamine, and pseudoephedrine.
- Instruct patient to avoid hazardous activities until drug's CNS effects are known.
- Suggest that patient relieve dry mouth with frequent rinsing and use of sugarless gum or hard candy.
- Tell patient to take last dose of the day a few hours before bedtime if dextromethorphan, carbinoxamine and pseudoephedrine makes her nervous or restless.

dextromethorphan hydrobromide, chlorpheniramine maleate, phenylephrine hydrochloride, and guaifenesin
Donatussin

Class and Category

Chemical: D-isomer codeine analog of levorphanol (dextromethorphan), propylamine derivative (chlorpheniramine), sympathomimetic amine (phenylephrine), glyceryl guaiacolate (guaifenesin)
Therapeutic: Antitussive (dextromethorphan), antihistaminic (chlorpheniramine), decongestant (phenylephrine), and expectorant (guaifenesin)
Pregnancy category: C

Indications and Dosages

▶ *To provide symptomatic relief of cough and nasal congestion associated with upper respiratory tract conditions*

SYRUP

Adults and children age 12 and over. 7.5 mg dextromethorphan, 2 mg chlorpheniramine, 10 mg phenylephrine, and 100 mg guaifenesin (5 ml) every 4 to 6 hr.

Children ages 6 to 12. 3.75 mg dextromethorphan, 1 mg chlorpheniramine, 5 mg phenylephrine, and 50 mg guaifenesin (2.5 ml) every 4 to 6 hr.

Children ages 2 to 6. 1.82 mg dextromethorphan, 0.5 mg chlorpheniramine, 2.5 mg phenylephrine, and 25 mg guaifenesin (1.25 ml) every 4 to 6 hr.

Mechanism of Action

Dextromethorphan suppresses cough by acting directly on the cough center in the medulla of the brain.

Chlorpheniramine competes with histamine for H_1 receptor sites, thereby antagonizing many histamine effects to reduce allergy signs and symptoms.

Phenylephrine stimulates alpha-adrenergic receptors and inhibits the intracellular enzyme adenyl cyclase, which then inhibits production of cAMP. Inhibition of cAMP causes arterial and venous constriction in nasal passages, which decreases blood flow and mucosal edema caused by allergic response.

Guaifenesin increases fluid and mucus removal from the upper respiratory tract by increasing the volume of secretions and reducing their adhesiveness and surface tension.

Contraindications

Asthma; breast-feeding; chronic bronchitis; emphysema; hypersensitivity to dextromethorphan, chlorpheniramine, phenylephrine, guaifenesin, or their components; productive cough; use of MAO inhibitors within 14 days

Interactions

DRUGS

dextromethorphan, chlorpheniramine and phenylephrine

MAO inhibitors: Increased and prolonged cardiac stimulation, increased vasopressor effect, increased risk of severe cardiovascular and cerebrovascular effects, hyperpyrexia, and vomiting

dextromethorphan and chlorpheniramine

CNS depressants: Additive CNS effects

dextromethorphan

amiodarone, fluoxetine, quinidine: Decreased metabolism of dextromethorphan, which may result in increased plasma dextromethorphan level and adverse reactions

chlorpheniramine

anticholinergics: Potentiated anticholinergic effects

phenytoin: Possibly increased serum phenytoin levels and toxicity

phenylephrine

alpha blockers, haloperidol, loxapine, phenothiazines, thioxanthenes: Possibly decreased vasoconstrictor effect of phenylephrine

antihypertenisves, diuretics: Possibly decreased antihypertensive effects

atropine: Possibly enhanced vasopressor effect of phenylephrine

beta blockers: Decreased therapeutic effects of both drugs

bretylium: Possibly potentiated vaopressor effect and arrhythmias

doxapram: Increased vasopressor effect of both drugs

ergot alkaloids: Possibly cerebral blood vessel rupture, increased vasopressor effect, peripheral vascular ischemia, and gangrene (with ergotamine)

guanadrel, guanethidine: Increased vasopressor effect of phenylephrine; increased risk of severe hypertension and arrhythmias

hydrocarbon inhalation anesthetics: Increased risk of serious arrhythmias

maprotiline, tricyclic antidepressants: Increased risk of severe cardiovascular effects (including arrhythmias, hyperpyrexia, severe hypertension)

mecamylamine, methyldopa: Decreased hypotensive effects of these drugs; increased vasopressor effect of phenylephrine

nitrates: Possibly decreased vasopressor effect of phenylephrine and decreased antianginal effect of nitrates

oxytocin: Possibly severe, persistent hypertension

phenoxybenzamine: Decreased vasoconstrictor effect of phenylephrine and possibly hypotension and tachycardia

theophylline: Possibly enhanced toxicity (including cardiac toxicity)

thyroid hormones: Increased cardiovascular effects of each drug

ACTIVITIES

dextromethorphan and chlorpheniramine

alcohol use: Additive CNS effects

dextromethorphan

smoking: Possibly increased respiratory secretion retention

Adverse Reactions

CNS: Confusion, dizziness, drowsiness, fever, hallucinations,

headache, hyperactivity, insomnia, nervousness, paresthesia, restlessness, sedation, seizures, tiredness, tremor, weakness
CV: Angina, arrhythmias, bradycardia, edema, hypertension, hypotension, palpitations, peripheral vasoconstriction that may lead to necrosis or gangrene, tachycardia, ventricular arrhythmias
EENT: Dry mouth, sore throat
GI: Abdominal pain, constipation, nausea, vomiting
GU: Urinary hesitancy, urine retention
RESP: Dyspnea, respiratory depression
SKIN: Rash, urticaria
Other: Anaphylaxis, emotional and physical dependence (prolonged use with high doses)

Nursing Considerations
- Use dextromethorphan, chlorpheniramine, phenylephrine, and guaifenesin cautiously in patients with bladder neck obstruction, cardiovascular disease, hypertension, hyperthyroidism, glaucoma, prostatic hypertrophy, or urine retention.
- Also use cautiously in patients with diabetes because products containing sugar may disrupt blood glucose control, in those with hepatic impairment because dextromethorphan is metabolized by the liver, and in those with respiratory depression because dextromethorphan adversely affect respirations.
- Monitor patients who may be more susceptible to experiencing dizziness, sedation, and hypotension, such as the elderly.
- Regularly evaluate effectiveness of dextromethorphan, chlorpheniramine, phenylephrine, and guaifenesin in relieving cough and reducing nasal congestion.
- Patient shouldn't have intradermal allergen tests within 72 hours of receiving drug because results may be altered.
- **WARNING** Dextromethorphan has the potential for abuse because of its euphoric, hallucinogenic, and dissociative effects when taken in doses higher than prescribed. Monitor patient closely.

PATIENT TEACHING
- Urge patient not to exceed prescribed dosage.
- Instruct patient to use a calibrated measuring device when measuring dextromethorphan, brompheniramine, phenylephrine, and guaifenesin to ensure accurate dose.
- Stress importance of taking drug exactly as prescribed and not increasing dose or frequency without consulting prescriber.
- Urge patient to avoid alcohol and other antidepressants while taking drug.

- Instruct patient to avoid hazardous activities until drug's CNS effects are known.
- Suggest that patient relieve dry mouth with frequent rinsing and use of sugarless gum or hard candy.

dextromethorphan tannate, chlorpheniramine tannate, and pseudoephedrine tannate
Tanafed DM

dextromethorphan tannate, dexchlorpheniramine tannate, and pseudoephedrine tannate
Tanafed DMX

Class and Category
Chemical: D-isomer codeine analogue of levorphanol (dextromethorphan), alkylamine (chlorpheniramine, dexchlorpheniramine), sympathomimetic amine (pseudoephedrine)
Therapeutic: Antitussive (dextromethorphan), antihistamine (chlorpheniramine, dexchlorpheniramine), decongestant (pseudoephedrine)
Pregnancy category: C

Indications and Dosages
▶ *To relieve cough, persistent runny nose, sneezing, and nasal congestion caused by upper respiratory infection, sinus inflammation or hay fever*
SUSPENSION (TANAFED DM)
Adults. 50 to 100 mg dextromethorphan, 9 to 18 mg chlorpheniramine, and 150 to 300 mg pseudoephedrine (10 to 20 ml) every 12 hr. *Maximum:* 40 ml daily.
SUSPENSION (TANAFED DMX)
Adults. 50 to 100 mg dextromethorphan, 5 to 10 mg chlorpheniramine, and 150 to 300 mg pseudoephedrine (10 to 20 ml) every 12 hr. *Maximum:* 40 ml daily.

Contraindications
Asthma; breast-feeding; chronic bronchitis; emphysema; hypersensitivity or idiosyncratic reactions to dextromethorphan, chlorpheniramine, dexchlorpheniramine, pseudoephedrine, or their components; hyperthyroidism; narrow-angle glaucoma; productive cough; severe coronary artery disease or hypertension; urine retention; use within 14 days of MAO inhibitor therapy

---

Mechanism of Action

Dextromethorphan suppresses cough by directly acting on the cough center in the medulla of the brain.

Chlorpheniramine and dexchlorpheniramine compete with histamine for H_1 receptor sites, thereby antagonizing many histamine effects and reducing allergy signs and symptoms.

Pseudoephedrine acts on $alpha_1$-adrenergic receptors in the mucosa of the respiratory tract to produce vasoconstriction. This process shrinks swollen nasal mucous membranes; reduces tissue hyperemia, edema, and nasal congestion; and increases nasal airway patency. It also may increase drainage of sinus secretions and open obstructed eustachian ostia.

Interactions

DRUGS

dextromethorphan, chlorpheniramine, dexchlorpheniramine, and pseudoephedrine

MAO inhibitors: Increased and prolonged cardiac stimulation, increased vasopressor effect, increased risk of severe cardiovascular and cerebrovascular effects, hyperpyrexia, and vomiting

dextromethorphan, chlorpheniramine, and dexchlorpheniramine

CNS depressants: Additive CNS effects

dextromethorphan

amiodarone, fluoxetine, quinidine: Decreased metabolism of dextromethorphan, which may result in increased plasma dextromethorphan level and adverse effects

chlorpheniramine and dexchlorpheniramine

anticholinergics: Additive anticholinergic effects

phenytoin: Possibly increased serum phenytoin level and toxicity

pseudoephedrine

antacids: Increased pseudoephedrine absorption

antihypertensives, diuretics: Possibly decreased antihypertensive effects

beta blockers: Decreased therapeutic effects of both drugs

citrates: Possibly inhibited urinary pseudoephedrine excretion and prolonged duration of action

CNS stimulant, other sympathomimetics: Possibly increased additive CNS stimulation to excessive levels

cocaine (mucosal-local): Possibly increased cardiovascular effects of either drug and CNS stimulation

digoxin, levodopa: Increased risk of cardiac arrhythmias

hydrocarbon inhalation anesthetics: Possibly serious arrhythmias
kaolin: Decreased pseudoephedrine absorption
nitrates: Reduced antianginal effects of nitrates
rauwolfia alkaloids: Possibly inhibited pseudoephedrine action
thyroid hormones: Increased cardiovascular effects of both drugs
ACTIVITIES

dextromethorphan, chlorpheniramine, and dexchlorpheniramine

alcohol use: Additive CNS effects

dextromethorphan

smoking: Possibly increased respiratory secretion retention

Adverse Reactions

CNS: Anxiety, chills, confusion, coordination disturbance, dizziness, drowsiness, fatigue, fear, hallucinations, headache, hyperactivity, hysteria, insomnia, irritability, light-headedness, nervousness, numbness, restlessness, sedation, seizures, tenseness, trembling, vertigo, weakness

CV: Arrhythmias, chest tightness, hypotension, palpitations, tachycardia

EENT: Blurred or double vision; dry mouth, nose, and throat; nasal congestion; tinnitus

ENDO: Early menstruation

GI: Abdominal pain, anorexia, constipation, diarrhea, nausea, stomach upset or pain, vomiting

GU: Dysuria, frequent urination, urinary hesitancy, urine retention

HEME: Anemia, unusual bleeding or bruising

RESP: Dyspnea, increased chest congestion, respiratory depression, wheezing

SKIN: Diaphoresis, pallor, photosensitivity, rash, urticaria

Other: Anaphylaxis, emotional and physical dependence (prolonged use with high doses)

Nursing Considerations

- Use cautiously in patients with cardiovascular disease or peptic ulcer.
- Also use cautiously in patient with diabetes because some products contain sugar, which may disrupt blood glucose control; in those with impaired hepatic function because dextromethorphan is metabolized by the liver; and in those with respiratory depression because dextromethorphan affects respiration.
- Monitor patients who may be more susceptible to dizziness, sedation, and hypotension, such as the elderly.

- Monitor renal function, as ordered, because pseudoephedrine is substantially excreted by the kidneys.
- Regularly evaluate effectiveness of drug in relieving cough and reducing upper respiratory symptoms.
- Be aware that patient shouldn't have intradermal allergen tests within 72 hours of receiving drug because results may be altered.
- **WARNING** Dextromethorphan has the potential for abuse because of its euphoric, hallucinogenic, and dissociative effects when taken in doses higher than prescribed. Monitor patient closely.

PATIENT TEACHING
- Urge patient not to exceed prescribed dosage.
- Instruct patient to use a calibrated measuring device to ensure accurate dose.
- Caution patient not to exceed dose or frequency without consulting prescriber.
- Urge patient to avoid alcohol and other antidepressants while taking drug.
- Instruct patient to avoid hazardous activities until drug's CNS effects are known.
- Suggest that patient relieve dry mouth with frequent rinsing and use of sugarless gum or hard candy.
- Tell patient to take last dose of the day a few hours before bedtime if drug makes her nervous or restless.

dextromethorphan hydrobromide, chlorpheniramine tannate, pseudoephedrine hydrochloride, guaifenesin, and potassium guaiacolsulfonate
Lemotussin-DM

Class and Category
Chemical: D-isomer codeine analog of levorphanol (dextromethorphan),
alkylamine (chlorpheniramine), sympathomimetic amine (pseudoephedrine), glyceryl guaiacolate (guaifenesin), unclassified (potassium guaiacolsulfonate)
Therapeutic: Antitussive (dextromethorphan), antihistamine

(chlorpheniramine), decongestant (pseudoephedrine), expectorants (guaifenesin, potassium guaiacolsulfonate)
Pregnancy category: C

Indications and Dosages

▶ *To relieve cough, persistent runny nose, sneezing, and nasal congestion caused by upper respiratory infection, sinus inflammation, or hay fever*

ORAL SOLUTION

Adults. 7.5 to 15 mg dextromethorphan, 2 to 4 mg chlorpheniramine, 10 to 20 mg pseudoephedrine, 50 to 100 mg guaifenesin and 50 to 100 mg potassium guaiacolsulfonate (5 to 10 ml) every 6 to 8 hr.

Mechanism of Action

Dextromethorphan suppresses cough by directly acting on the cough center in the medulla of the brain.

Chlorpheniramine competes with histamine for H_1 receptor sites, thereby antagonizing many histamine effects and reducing allergy effects.

Pseudoephedrine acts on $alpha_1$-adrenergic receptors in the mucosa of the respiratory tract to produce vasoconstriction. This process shrinks swollen nasal mucous membranes; reduces tissue hyperemia, edema, and nasal congestion; and increases nasal airway patency. It also may increase drainage of sinus secretions and open obstructed eustachian ostia.

Guaifenesin increases fluid and mucus removal from the upper respiratory tract by increasing the volume of secretions and reducing their adhesiveness and surface tension.

Contraindications

Acute MI; angina; asthma; breast-feeding; chronic bronchitis; emphysema; hyperkalemia, hypersensitivity or idiosyncratic reactions to dextromethorphan, chlorpheniramine, pseudoephedrine, guafenesin, potassium guaiacolsulfonate, or their components; hyperthyroidism; narrow-angle glaucoma; productive cough; severe coronary artery disease or hypertension; urine retention; use within 14 days of MAO inhibitor therapy

Interactions

DRUGS

dextromethorphan and pseudoephedrine

MAO inhibitors: Increased and prolonged cardiac stimulation, increased vasopressor effect, increased risk of severe cardiovascular

and cerebrovascular effects, hyperpyrexia, and vomiting
dextromethorphan and chlorpheniramine
CNS depressants: Additive CNS effects
dextromethorphan
amiodarone, fluoxetine, paroxetine, quinidine: Decreased metabolism of dextromethorphan, which may result in increased plasma dextromethorphan levels and adverse reactions
chlorpheniramine
anticholinergics: Additive anticholinergic effects
MAO inhibitors: Prolonged and intensified anticholinergic (drying) effects of chlorpheniramine
phenytoin: Possibly increased serum phenytoin level and toxicity
pseudoephedrine
antacids: Increased pseudoephedrine absorption
antihypertensives, diuretics: Possibly decreased antihypertensive effects
beta blockers: Decreased therapeutic effects of both drugs
citrates: Possibly inhibited urinary pseudoephedrine excretion and prolonged duration of action
CNS stimulant, other sympathomimetics: Possibly increased additive CNS stimulation to excessive levels
cocaine (mucosal-local): Possibly increased cardiovascular effects of either drug and CNS stimulation
digoxin, levodopa: Increased risk of cardiac arrhythmias
hydrocarbon inhalation anesthetics: Increased risk of serious arrhythmias
kaolin: Decreased pseudoephedrine absorption
nitrates: Reduced antianginal effects of nitrates
rauwolfia alkaloids: Possibly inhibited pseudoephedrine action
thyroid hormones: Increased cardiovascular effects of both drugs
potassium guaiacolsulfonate
potassium-sparing diuretics, potassium-containing drugs, potassium supplements: Increased risk of hyperkalemia
ACTIVITIES
dextromethorphan and chlorpheniramine
alcohol use: Additive CNS effects
dextromethorphan
smoking: Possibly increased respiratory secretion retention

Adverse Reactions

CNS: Anxiety, chills, confusion, coordination disturbance, dizziness, drowsiness, fatigue, fear, hallucinations, headache, hyperactivity, hysteria, insomnia, irritability, light-headedness, nervousness, numbness, restlessness, sedation, seizures, tenseness, trembling, vertigo, weakness

CV: Arrhythmias, chest tightness, hypertension, palpitations, tachycardia

EENT: Blurred or double vision; dry mouth, nose, and throat; nasal congestion; tinnitus

ENDO: Early menstruation

GI: Abdominal pain, anorexia, constipation, diarrhea, nausea, stomach upset or pain, vomiting

GU: Dysuria, frequent urination, urinary hesitancy, urine retention

HEME: Anemia, unusual bleeding or bruising

RESP: Dyspnea, increased chest congestion, respiratory depression, wheezing

SKIN: Diaphoresis, pallor, photosensitivity, rash, urticaria

Other: Anaphylaxis, emotional and physical dependence (prolonged use with high doses), hyperkalemia

Nursing Considerations

- Use cautiously in patients with cardiovascular disease, hypertension, or peptic ulcer.
- Also use cautiously in patients with diabetes because some products contain sugar, which may disrupt blood glucose control; in those with impaired hepatic function because dextromethorphan is metabolized by the liver; and in those with respiratory depression because dextromethorphan adversely affect respirations.
- Monitor patients who may be more susceptible to dizziness, sedation, and hypotension, such as the elderly.
- Monitor renal function, as ordered, because pseudoephedrine is substantially excreted by the kidneys.
- Regularly evaluate effectiveness of drug in relieving cough and reducing upper respiratory symptoms.
- Be aware that patient shouldn't have intradermal allergen tests within 72 hours of receiving drug because results may be altered.
- **WARNING** Dextromethorphan has the potential for abuse because of its euphoric, hallucinogenic, and dissociative effects when taken in doses higher than prescribed. Monitor patient closely.

PATIENT TEACHING

- Urge patient not to exceed prescribed dosage.
- Instruct patient to use a calibrated measuring device to ensure accurate dose.

- Caution patient not to exceed dose or frequency without consulting prescriber.
- Urge patient to avoid alcohol, CNS depressants, and potassium supplements while taking drug.
- Instruct patient to avoid hazardous activities until drug's CNS effects are known.
- Suggest that patient relieve dry mouth with frequent rinsing and use of sugarless gum or hard candy.
- Tell patient to take last dose of the day a few hours before bedtime if drug makes him nervous or restless.
- Advise patient to increase his fluid intake to help loosen mucus and thin secretions if not contraindicated by a fluid-restrictive condition such as heart failure or liver or renal disease.

dextromethorphan hydrobromide and guaifenesin

Allfen-DM, Aquatab DM, Dex GG TR, Duratuss DM,
Gani-Tuss-DM NR, GFN 1000/DM 60, GFN 1200/DM 60,
Guaifenesin DM, Guaifenesin-DM NR, Guaifenex DM,
Guiadrine DM, Humibid DM, Hydro-Tussin DM, Iobid DM,
Maxi-tuss DM, Muco-Fen DM, Respa-DM, Robitussin-DM,
Sudal-DM, SU-TUSS DM, Touro DM, TUSS-bid,
Tussi-Organidin-DM NR, Z-Cof LA

Class and Category

Chemical: D-isomer codeine analog of levorphanol (dextromethorphan), glyceryl guaiacolate (guaifenesin)
Therapeutic: Antitussive (dextromethorphan), expectorant (guaifenesin)
Pregnancy category: C

Indications and Dosages

▶ *To relieve cough caused by minor throat and bronchial irritation, especially when secretions are thick*
ELIXIR, ORAL LIQUID
Adults and children age 12 and over. 20 mg dextromethorphan and 200 mg guaifenesin (5 or 10 ml depending on product) every 4 hr.
Children ages 6 to 12. 10 mg dextromethorphan and 100 mg guaifenesin (5 ml) every 4 hr.
Children ages 2 to 6. 5 mg dextromethorphan and 50 mg guaifenesin (2.5 ml) every 4 hr.

Children ages 6 months to 2 years. 1.25 to 2.5 mg dextromethorphan and 12.5 to 25 mg guaifenesin (0.6 to 1.25 ml) every 4 hr.
E.R. TABLETS
Adults and children age 12 and over. 28 to 60 mg dextromethorphan and 600 to 1,300 mg guaifenesin (1 or 2 tablets depending on product) every 12 hr.
Children ages 6 to 12. 30 mg dextromethorphan and 575 or 600 mg guaifenesin (1 tablet) every 12 hr.
Children ages 2 to 6. 15 mg dextromethorphan and 287.5 or 300 mg guaifenesin (½ tablet) every 12 hr.

Mechanism of Action
Dextromethorphan suppresses cough by acting directly on the cough center in the medulla of the brain.
   Guaifenesin increases fluid and mucus removal from the upper respiratory tract by increasing the volume of secretions and reducing their adhesiveness and surface tension.

Contraindications
Asthma; chronic bronchitis; emphysema; hypersensitivity to dextromethorphan, guaifenesin, or their components; productive cough

Interactions
DRUGS
dextromethorphan
amiodarone, fluoxetine, paroxetine, quinidine: Decreased metabolism of dextromethorphan, which may result in increased plasma dextromethorphan level and adverse effects
CNS depressants: Additive CNS effects
MAO inhibitors: Increased and prolonged cardiac stimulation, increased vasopressor effect, increased risk of severe cardiovascular and cerebrovascular effects, hyperpyrexia, and vomiting
ACTIVITIES
dextromethorphan
smoking: Possibly increased respiratory secretion retention

Adverse Reactions
CNS: Confusion, dizziness, drowsiness, hallucinations, headache, hyperactivity
GI: Abdominal pain, constipation, nausea, vomiting
RESP: Respiratory depression

SKIN: Rash, urticaria

Other: Emotional and physical dependence (prolonged use with high doses), serotonin syndrome

Nursing Considerations

- Use cautiously in patients with diabetes because some products contain sugar, which may disrupt blood glucose control.
- Also use cautiously in patients with impaired hepatic function because dextromethorphan is metabolized by the liver and in those with respiratory depression because dextromethorphan adversely affect respirations.
- **WARNING** Dextromethorphan has the potential for abuse because of its euphoric, hallucinogenic, and dissociative effects when taken in doses higher than prescribed. Monitor patient closely.

PATIENT TEACHING

- Urge patient not to exceed prescribed dosage.
- Stress importance of taking dextromethorphan and guaifenesin exactly as prescribed and not increasing dose or frequency without consulting prescriber.
- Instruct patient to use a calibrated measuring device to ensure accurate dose when using liquid or elixir form of drug.
- Caution patient not to use other CNS depressants while taking dextromethorphan and guaifenesin.
- Caution patient to avoid hazardous activities until drug's CNS effects are known.
- To prevent constipation, encourage patient to consume plenty of fluids and high-fiber foods, if not contraindicated by another condition.
- Advise patient to notify prescriber if she becomes short of breath or has difficulty breathing.
- Advise patient to increase her fluid intake to help loosen mucus and thin secretions if not contraindicated by a fluid-restrictive condition such as heart failure or liver or renal disease

dextromethorphan hydrobromide, phenylephrine hydrochloride, and guaifenesin

Tussafed Ex

Class and Category

Chemical: D-isomer codeine analog of levorphanol (dextromethor-

phan), sympathomimetic amine (phenylephrine), glyceryl guaiacolate (guaifenesin)
Therapeutic: Antitussive (dextromethorphan), decongestant
(phenylephrine), expectorant (guaifenesin)
Pregnancy category: C

Indications and Dosages

▶ *To relieve cough and other upper respiratory symptoms of the
common cold and allergies*
SYRUP
Adults. 30 mg dextromethorphan, 10 mg phenylephrine, and
200 mg guaifenesin (5 ml) q.i.d.

Mechanism of Action

Dextromethorphan suppresses cough by acting directly on the cough center
in the medulla of the brain.

Phenylephrine stimulates alpha-adrenergic receptors and inhibits the intracellular enzyme adenyl cyclase, which then inhibits production of cAMP. Inhibition of cAMP causes arterial and venous constriction in nasal passages,
which decreases blood flow and mucosal edema caused by allergic response.

Guaifenesin increases fluid and mucus removal from the upper respiratory
tract by increasing the volume of secretions and reducing their adhesiveness
and surface tension.

Contraindications

Angina; asthma; chronic bronchitis; emphysema; hypersensitivity
to dextromethorphan, bisulfites, guaifenesin, phenylephrine, or
their components; severe coronary artery disease or hypertension;
use within 14 days of MAO inhibitor therapy; urine retention;
ventricular tachycardia

Interactions

DRUGS
dextromethorphan and phenylephrine
MAO inhibitors: Increased and prolonged cardiac stimulation, increased vasopressor effect, increased risk of severe cardiovascular
and cerebrovascular effects, hyperpyrexia, and vomiting
dextromethorphan
amiodarone, fluoxetine, paroxetine, quinidine: Decreased dextromethorphan metabolism, which may result in increased plasma
dextromethorphan level and adverse effects
CNS depressants: Additive CNS effects

phenylephrine

alpha blockers, haloperidol, loxapine, phenothiazines, thioxanthenes: Possibly decreased vasoconstrictor effect of phenylephrine

antihypertenisves, diuretics: Possibly decreased antihypertensive effects

atropine: Possibly enhanced vasopressor effect of phenylephrine

beta blockers: Decreased therapeutic effects of both drugs

bretylium: Possibly potentiated vaopressor effect and arrhythmias

doxapram: Increased vasopressor effect of both drugs

ergot alkaloids: Possibly cerebral blood vessel rupture, increased vasopressor effect, peripheral vascular ischemia, and gangrene (with ergotamine)

guanadrel, guanethidine: Increased vasopressor effect of phenylephrine; increased risk of severe hypertension and arrhythmias

hydrocarbon inhalation anesthetics: Possibly serious arrhythmias

maprotiline, tricyclic antidepressants: Increased risk of severe cardiovascular effects (including arrhythmias, hyperpyrexia, severe hypertension)

mecamylamine, methyldopa: Decreased hypotensive effects of these drugs; increased vasopressor effect of phenylephrine

nitrates: Possibly decreased vasopressor effect of phenylephrine and decreased antianginal effect of nitrates

oxytocin: Possibly severe, persistent hypertension

phenoxybenzamine: Decreased vasoconstrictor effect of phenylephrine, possibly hypotension and tachycardia

theophylline: Possibly enhanced toxicity (including cardiac toxicity)

thyroid hormones: Increased cardiovascular effects of each drug

ACTIVITIES

dextromethorphan

smoking: Possibly increased respiratory secretion retention

Adverse Reactions

CNS: Anxiety, confusion, dizziness, drowsiness, hallucinations, headache, hyperactivity, insomnia, nervousness, paresthesia, restlessness, tremor, weakness

CV: Angina, bradycardia, hypertension, palpitations, peripheral vasoconstriction that may lead to necrosis or gangrene, tachycardia, ventricular arrhythmia

GI: Abdominal pain, constipation, nausea, vomiting

RESP: Dyspnea, respiratory depression

SKIN: Pallor, rash, urticaria

Other: Allergic reaction, emotional and physical dependence (prolonged use with high doses), serotonin syndrome

Nursing Considerations

- Assess patient for signs and symptoms of angina, arrhythmias, and hypertension because phenylephrine may increase myocardial oxygen demand and the risk of proarrhythmias and blood pressure changes.
- Use cautiously in patients with diabetes because some products contain sugar, which may disrupt blood glucose control; in those with impaired hepatic function because dextromethorphan is metabolized by the liver; and in those with respiratory depression because dextromethorphan affects respirations.
- **WARNING** Monitor patient with thyroid disease for increased sensitivity to catecholamines and possibly thyrotoxicity or cardiotoxicity.
- Regularly evaluate effectiveness of dextromethorphan, phenylephrine, and guaifenesin in relieving upper respiratory symptoms. Notify prescriber if symptoms persist or worsen.
- **WARNING** Dextromethorphan has the potential for abuse because of its euphoric, hallucinogenic, and dissociative effects when taken in doses higher than prescribed. Monitor patient closely.

PATIENT TEACHING

- Urge patient not to exceed prescribed dosage.
- Stress importance of taking this drug exactly as prescribed and not increasing the dose or frequency without consulting prescriber.
- Caution patient not to use other CNS depressants while taking dextromethorphan, phenylephrine, and guaifenesin.
- Instruct patient to increase fluid intake (unless contraindicated) to help thin secretions.
- Caution patient to avoid hazardous activities until drug's CNS effects are known.

dextromethorphan, pseudoephedrine hydrochloride, and guaifenesin

Aquatab C, GFN 600/PSE 60/DM 30, GFN 1200/CM 60/PSE 120, Maxifed DM, Medent-DM, PanMist-DM, Profen Forte DM, Profen II DM, Protuss DM, Robitussin-CF, Robitussin Cough and Cold, Touro CC, Tussafed-LA, Z-Cof DM

Class and Category

Chemical: D-isomer codeine analog of levorphanol (dextromethor-

phan), sympathomimetic amine (pseudoephedrine), glyceryl guaiacolate (guaifenesin)
Therapeutic: Antitussive (dextromethomethorphan), decongestant (pseudoephedrine), expectorant (guaifenesin)
Pregnancy category: C

Indications and Dosages

▶ *To treat nasal congestion and cough, especially nonproductive cough caused by the common cold, acute respiratory infections, acute and chronic bronchitis, hay fever, and sinusitis*
SYRUP
Adults. 15 to 30 mg dextromethorphan, 40 to 80 mg pseudo-ephedrine, and 100 to 400 mg guaifenesin (5 to 10 ml depending on product) every 4 to 6 hr. *Maximum:* 4 doses daily.
E.R. TABLETS
Adults. 30 to 64 mg dextromethorphan, 45 to 120 mg pseudo-ephedrine, and 550 to 1,200 mg guaifenesin (1 or 2 tablets depending on product) every 12 hr.

Mechanism of Action

Dextromethorphan suppresses cough by acting directly on the cough center in the medulla of the brain.

Pseudoephedrine acts on alpha$_1$-adrenergic receptors in respiratory mucosa, producing vasoconstriction that shrinks swollen nasal mucous membranes; reduces tissue hyperemia, edema, and nasal congestion; and increases nasal airway patency. It also may increase sinus drainage and open obstructed eustachian ostia.

Guaifenesin increases fluid and mucus removal from the upper respiratory tract by increasing the volume of secretions and reducing their adhesiveness and surface tension.

Contraindications

Acute MI; angina; asthma; cardiac arrhythmias; chronic bronchitis; emphysema; hypersensitivity or idiosyncratic reactions to dextromethorphan, pseudoephedrine, guaifenesin, or their components; hyperthyroidism; narrow-angle glaucoma; prostatic hypertrophy; severe coronary artery disease or hypertension; urine retention; use within 14 days of MAO inhibitor therapy

Interactions
DRUGS
dextromethorphan and pseudoephedrine

MAO inhibitors: Increased and prolonged cardiac stimulation, increased vasopressor effect, increased risk of severe cardiovascular and cerebrovascular effects, hyperpyrexia, and vomiting

dextromethorphan

amiodarone, fluoxetine,paroxetine, quinidine: Decreased dextromethorphan metabolism, which may result in increased plasma dextromethorphan level and adverse effects

CNS depressants: Additive CNS effects

pseudoephedrine

antacids: Increased pseudoephedrine absorption

antihypertensives, diuretics: Possibly decreased antihypertensive effects

beta blockers: Decreased therapeutic effects of both drugs

citrates: Possibly inhibited urinary pseudoephedrine excretion and prolonged duration of action

CNS stimulant, other sympathomimetics: Possibly increased additive CNS stimulation to excessive levels

cocaine (mucosal-local): Possibly increased cardiovascular effects of either drug and CNS stimulation

digoxin, levodopa: Increased risk of cardiac arrhythmias

hydrocarbon inhalation anesthetics: Possibly serious arrhythmias

kaolin: Decreased pseudoephedrine absorption

nitrates: Reduced antianginal effects of nitrates

rauwolfia alkaloids: Possibly inhibited pseudoephedrine action

thyroid hormones: Increased cardiovascular effects of both drugs

ACTIVITIES

dextromethorphan

smoking: Possibly increased respiratory secretion retention

Adverse Reactions

CNS: Anxiety, confusion, dizziness, drowsiness, excitability, hallucinations, headache, hyperactivity, insomnia, irritability, lightheadedness, nervousness, restlessness, trembling, weakness

CV: Angina, hypertension, palpitations, tachycardia

GI: Abdominal pain, constipation, nausea, vomiting

GU: Dysuria

RESP: Respiratory depression

SKIN: Diaphoresis, pallor, rash, urticaria

Other: Emotional and physical dependence (prolonged use with high doses), serotonin syndrome

Nursing Considerations

• Use cautiously in patients with diabetes, hypertension, increased intraocular pressure, ischemic heart disease, stenosing

peptic ulcer, or pyloroduodenal obstruction because of the vaso-constictive action of pseudoephedrine.
- Evaluate therapeutic response. Notify prescriber if cough and other symptoms persist or worsen despite use of dextromethorphan, pseudoephedrine, and guaifenesin.
- Monitor renal function, as ordered, because pseudoephedrine is substantially excreted by the kidneys.
- **WARNING** Dextromethorphan has the potential for abuse because of its euphoric, hallucinogenic, and dissociative effects when taken in doses higher than prescribed. Monitor patient closely.

PATIENT TEACHING
- Urge patient not to exceed prescribed dosage.
- Instruct patient to take dextromethorphan, pseudoephedrine, and guaifenesin exactly as prescribed and not to increase dose or frequency without consulting prescriber.
- Instruct patient to use a calibrated measuring device to ensure accurate dose of syrup.
- To minimize nausea, suggest that patient take drug with food and a full glass of water.
- Advise patient not to break, crush, or chew E.R. tablets but to swallow them whole.
- Advise patient to avoid alcohol or other CNS depressants while taking drug.
- Caution patient to avoid hazardous activities until drug's CNS effects are known.
- Instruct patient to increase fluid intake (unless contraindicated) to help thin secretions.

ephedrine hydrochloride and guaifenesin

Broncholate, Bronkaid, Primatene

Class and Category

Chemical: Sympathomimetic amine (ephedrine), glyceryl guaiacolate (guaifenesin)
Therapeutic: Bronchodilator (ephedrine), expectorant (guaifenesin)
Pregnancy category: C

Indications and Dosages

▶ *To relieve upper respiratory symptoms of the common cold and seasonal allergies*

SYRUP
Adults and children age 12 and over. 12.5 to 25 mg
ephedrine and 200 to 400 mg guaifenesin (10 to 20 ml) every
4 hr.
Children ages 6 to 12. 6.25 to 12.5 mg ephedrine and 100 to
200 mg guaifenesin (5 to 10 ml) every 4 hr.
Children ages 2 to 6. 3.125 to 6.25 mg ephedrine and 50 to
100 mg guaifenesin (2.5 to 5 ml) every 4 hr.

Mechanism of Action
Ephedrine stimulates beta-adrenergic receptors in the lungs to relax
bronchial smooth muscle, which relieves bronchospasm. It also stimulates
alpha-adrenergic receptors in nasal passages to produce vasoconstriction and
a drying effect on nasal mucous membranes.
   Guaifenesin increases fluid and mucus removal from the upper respiratory
tract by increasing the volume of secretions and reducing their adhesiveness
and surface tension.

Contraindications
Breast-feeding; cardiac disease, including arrhythmias; hypersensitivity to ephedrine, guaifenesin, or their components; hypertension; hyperthyroidism; pregnancy; prostatic hypertrophy; uncontrolled seizure disorder; use within 14 days of MAO inhibitor
therapy

Interactions
DRUGS
ephedrine
alpha blockers, haloperidol, loxapine, phenothiazines, thioxanthenes:
Possibly decreased vasoconstrictor effect of ephedrine
beta blockers: Decreased therapeutic effects of each drug
ergot alkaloids: Possibly cerebral blood vessel rupture, increased vasopressor effect, peripheral vascular ischemia, and gangrene (with
ergotamine)
guanadrel, guanethidine: Possibly decreased hypotensive effects of
these agents
guanethidine, methyldopa, reserpine: Reduced pressor response of
ephedrine
hydrocarbon inhalation anesthetics: Possibly serious arrhythmias
MAO inhibitors: Increased pressor effect of ephedrine; possibly increased risk of severe hypertensive crisis

theophylline: Possibly enhanced toxicity, especially increased nausea, nervousness and insomnia
thyroid hormones: Increased cardiovascular effects of each drug
tricyclic antidepressants: Possibly increased pressor response
urinary acidifers: May decrease half-life of ephedrine, which may lead to decreased effects
urinary alkalizers: May increase half-life of ephedrine, which may lead to increased effects

Adverse Reactions

CNS: Anxiety, confusion, dizziness, headache, insomnia, nervousness, seizures, tremor, vertigo
CV: Arrhythmias, hypertension, palpitations, tachycardia
ENDO: Hyperglycemia
GI: Abdominal pain, anorexia, diarrhea, nausea, vomiting
MS: Muscle cramps
SKIN: Diaphoresis, rash, urticaria

Nursing Considerations

• Evaluate effectiveness of ephedrine in relieving respiratory symptoms, and notify prescriber if symptoms worsen.
• Monitor patient's blood glucose level closely because ephedrine can cause hyperglycemia.

PATIENT TEACHING

• Caution patient to take drug exactly as prescribed and not to increase dose or frequency without consulting prescriber.
• Instruct patient to avoid hazardous activities until drug's CNS effects are known.
• Tell patient to take last dose of the day a few hours before bedtime if drug makes her nervous.
• Instruct patient with diabetes to monitor blood glucose level closely during drug therapy.
• Advise patient to increase fluid intake (if not contraindicated) to help loosen mucus and thin secretions.

fexofenadine hydrochloride and pseudoephedrine hydrochloride

Allegra-D 12 Hour, Allegra-D 24 Hour

Class and Category

Chemical: Terfenadine metabolite (fexofenadine), (sympatho-mimetic amine (pseudoephedrine)

Therapeutic: Antihistaminic (fexofenadine), decongestant (pseudo-ephedrine)
Pregnancy category: C

Indications and Dosages

▶ *To relieve symptoms of seasonal allergic rhinitis*
TABLETS (ALLEGRA-D 12 HOUR)
Adults and children age 12 and over. 60 mg fexofenadine and 120 mg pseudoephedrine (1 tablet) b.i.d.
DOSAGE ADJUSTMENT For patients with renal impairment, dosage frequency decreased to once daily.
TABLETS (ALLEGRA-D 24 HOUR)
Adults and children age 12 and over. 180 mg fexofenadine and 240 mg pseudoephedrine (1 tablet) daily.

Mechanism of Action

Fexofenadine competes with histamine for histamine H_1 receptor sites on effector cells and antagonizes the vasodilator effect of endogenously released histamine. This prevents vascular engorgement, mucosal edema, sneezing, and profuse watery secretion and irritation that normally result from histamine action on peripheral afferent nerve terminals.

Pseudoephedrine acts on $alpha_1$-adrenergic receptors in the mucosa of the respiratory tract to produce vasoconstriction. This process shrinks swollen nasal mucous membranes; reduces tissue hyperemia, edema, and nasal congestion; and increases nasal airway patency. It also may increase drainage of sinus secretions and open obstructed eustachian ostia.

Contraindications

Hypersensitivity or idiosyncratic reactions to fexofenadine, pseudoephedrine, or their components; hyperthyroidism; narrow-angle glaucoma; severe coronary artery disease or hypertension; urine retention; use within 14 days of MAO inhibitor therapy

Interactions

DRUGS
fexofenadine
aluminum and magnesium containing antacids: Decreased fexofenadine absorption
erythromycin, ketoconazole: Enchanced fexofenadine absorption which increased plasma fexofenadine levels
psuedoephedrine
antacids: Increased pseudoephedrine absorption

antihypertensives, diuretics: Possibly decreased antihypertensive effects

beta blockers: Decreased therapeutic effects of both drugs

citrates: Possibly inhibited urinary pseudoephedrine excretion and prolonged duration of action

CNS stimulant, other sympathomimetics: Possibly increased additive CNS stimulation to excessive levels

cocaine (mucosal-local): Possibly increased cardiovascular effects of either drug and CNS stimulation

digoxin, levodopa: Increased risk of cardiac arrhythmias

hydrocarbon inhalation anesthetics: Increased risk of serious arrhythmias

kaolin: Decreased pseudoephedrine absorption

MAO inhibitors: Increased and prolonged cardiac stimulation, increased vasopressor effect, increased risk of severe cardiovascular and cerebrovascular effects, hyperpyrexia, vomiting

nitrates: Reduced antianginal effects of nitrates

rauwolfia alkaloids: Possibly inhibited pseudoephedrine action

thyroid hormones: Increased cardiovascular effects of both drugs

FOODS

fexofenadine

all foods: Decreased fexofenadine absorption

fruit juices: Possibly decreased fexofenadine absorption

Adverse Reactions

CNS: Anxiety, excitability, dizziness, drowsiness, fear, hallucinations, headache, insomnia, light-headedness, nervousness, paranoia, restlessness, seizures, sleep disturbances, trembling, weakness

CV: Arrhythmias, hypertension, palpitations, tachycardia

EENT: Dry mouth, throat irritation

GI: Abdominal pain, nausea, vomiting

GU: Dysuria

MS: Back pain

RESP: Dyspnea, upper respiratory tract infection

SKIN: Pallor, pruritus, rash, urticaria

Other: Anaphylaxis, angioedema

Nursing Considerations

- Be aware that Allegra-D 24 Hour isn't recommended for patients with renal insufficiency.
- Use cautiously in patients with diabetes, hypertension, increased intraocular pressure, ischemic heart disease, prostatic

hypertrophy, stenosing peptic ulcer, or pyloroduodenal obstruction because of the vasoconstrictive action of pseudoephedrine.

• Monitor elderly patients closely for CNS effects because they're more likely to develop these adverse effects.

• Monitor renal function, as ordered, because pseudoephedrine is substantially excreted by the kidneys.

• Evaluate effectiveness of fexofenadine and pseudoephedrine in relieving symptoms of seasonal allergic rhinitis, such as sneezing, rhinorrhea, pruritus, lacrimation, and nasal congestion.

• Be aware that patient shouldn't have intradermal allergen tests within 4 days of receiving drug because results may be altered.

PATIENT TEACHING

• Instruct patient to take fexofenadine and pseudoephedrine only with water on an empty stomach and to swallow the tablet whole without crushing or chewing it.

• Caution patient not to exceed dosage prescribed.

• Advise patient that if she experiences nervousness, dizziness, or sleeplessness, she should stop taking fexofenadine and pseudoephedrine and consult the prescriber.

• Urge patient to avoid alcohol, other antidepressants, and OTC drugs containing other antihistamines or sympathomimetics while taking fexofenadine and pseudoephedrine.

• Instruct patient to avoid hazardous activities until drug's CNS effects are known.

fluticasone propionate and salmeterol

Advair Diskus 100/50, Advair Diskus 250/50,
Advair Diskus 500/50, Advair HFA 45/21, Advair HFA 115/21,
Advair HFA 230/21

Class and Category

Chemical: Corticorsteroid (fluticasone), beta$_2$-adrengeric receptor agonist (salmeterol)

Therapeutic: Anti-inflammatory agent (fluticasone), bronchodilator (salmeterol)

Pregnancy category: C

Indications and Dosages

▶ *To provide long-term maintenance treatment of asthma*
INHALATION (DISKUS)

Adults and children age 12 and over not using an inhaled corticosteroid. One inhalation of 100 mcg fluticasone and 50 mcg salmeterol b.i.d.

Adults and children age 12 and over taking beclometha-sone dipropionate or triamcinolone acetonide by inhalation. One inhalation of 100 or 250 mcg fluticasone and 50 mcg salmeterol b.i.d.

Adults and children age 12 and over taking budesonide or fluticasone propionate by inhalation. One inhalation of 100, 250, or 500 mcg fluticasone and 50 mcg salmeterol b.i.d.

Adults and children age 12 and over taking flunisolide. One inhalation of 100 or 250 mcg fluticasone and 50 mcg salmeterol b.i.d.

Children ages 4 to 12 who are symptomatic despite using an inhaled corticosteroid. One inhalation of 100 mcg fluticasone and 50 mcg salmeterol b.i.d.

INHALATION (HFA)

Adults and children age 12 and over not using an inhaled corticosteroid. *Initial:* Two inhalations of 45 or 115 mcg fluticasone and 21 mcg salmeterol b.i.d. *Maximum:* Two inhalations of 230 mcg fluticasone and 21 mcg salmeterol b.i.d.

Adults and children age 12 and over using an inhaled corticosteroid. *Initial:* Two inhalations of 45 to 230 mcg fluticasone and 21 mcg salmeterol b.i.d. *Maximum:* Two inhalations of 230 mcg fluticasone and 21 mcg salmeterol b.i.d.

▶ *To provide maintenance treatment of COPD with chronic bronchitis, emphysema, or both*

INHALATION (DISKUS)

Adults. One inhalation of 250 mcg fluticasone and 50 mcg salmeterol b.i.d.

Mechanism of Action

Fluticasone inhibits cells involved in the inflammatory response of asthma, such as mast cells, eosinophils, basophils, lymphocytes, macrophages, and neutrophils. It also inhibits production or secretion of chemical mediators, such as histamine, eicosanoids, leukotrienes, and cytokines.

Salmeterol attaches to beta$_2$ receptors on bronchial cell membranes, stimulating the intracellular enzyme adenylate cyclase to convert adenosine triphosphate to cAMP. The resulting increase in intracellular cAMP level relaxes bronchial smooth-muscle cells, stabilizes mast cells, and inhibits histamine release.

Contraindications

Hypersensitivity to fluticasone, salmeterol, or their components;

primary treatment of status asthmaticus or other acute asthma or COPD episodes that require intensive measures; severe hypersensitivity to milk proteins; untreated nasal mucosal infection (nasal suspension)

Interactions

DRUGS

fluticasone

ketoconazole, ritonavir, and other strong CYP 3A4 inhibitors (long-term use): Possibly increased blood fluticasone level and decreased serum cortisol level

salmeterol

atazanavir, clarithromycin, indinavir, itraconazole, ketoconazole, nefazodone, nelfinavir, ritonavir, saquinavir, telithromycin, other strong CYP 3A4 inhibitors: Increased risk of serious cardiovascular adverse effects

beta blockers: Mutual inhibition of therapeutic effects

loop or thiazide diuretics: Increased risk of hypokalemia and potentially life-threatening arrhythmias

MAO inhibitors, tricyclic antidepressants: Potentiated adverse vascular effects, such as hypertensive crisis

Adverse Reactions

CNS: Aggressiveness, agitation, depression, difficulty speaking, dizziness, fatigue, fever, headache, hyperactivity, insomnia, irritability, malaise, nervousness, paresthesia, restlessness, tremor

CV: Arrhythmias, chest pain, palpitations, tachycardia, ventricular tachycardia

EENT: Allergic rhinitis; cataracts; conjunctivitis; dry mouth, nose, and throat; eye irritation; glaucoma; laryngitis; laryngeal spasm, irritation, or swelling; loss of voice; nasal congestion or discharge; oropharyngeal candidiasis; otitis media; pharyngitis; sinus problems; tonsillitis

ENDO: Adrenal insufficiency, cushingoid symptoms, hypercorticism, hyperglycemia, reduced growth velocity in children and adolescents

GI: Abdominal pain, diarrhea, indigestion, nausea, vomiting

GU: Dysmenorrhea

HEME: Easy bruising

MS: Arthralgia, muscle cramps and spasms, myalgia, myositis, osteoporosis

RESP: Asthma exacerbation, bronchitis, chest congestion and tightness, cough, dyspnea, paradoxical bronchospasm, respiratory tract infection, wheezing

SKIN: Dermatitis, ecchymosis, eczema, pallor, photodermatitis, rash, urticaria

Other: Anaphylaxis, angioedema, flulike symptoms, generalized aches and pains, weight gain

Nursing Considerations

- **WARNING** Be aware that fluticasone and salmeterol should not be started in a patient with rapidly deteriorating asthma control, as evidenced by decreased responsiveness to the usual drugs; increased need for inhaled, short-acting beta$_2$-agonists or systemic corticosteroids; significant increase in symptoms with recent emergency room visits; or sudden or progressive deterioration in pulmonary function. These patients are at risk for serious or life-threatening reactions to salmeterol, including death.

- Use fluticasone and salmeterol cautiously in patients with ocular herpes simplex, pulmonary tuberculosis, or untreated systemic bacterial, fungal, parasitic, or viral infection because fluticasone can mask signs and symptoms and severity of condition.

- Use drug cautiously in patients with hepatic impairment because fluticasone and salmeterol are both metabolized in the liver.

- Be aware that fluticasone and salmeterol shouldn't be used to relieve bronchospasm quickly because of its prolonged onset of action. As prescribed, give a fast-acting inhaled bronchodilator if bronchospsm occurs.

- Monitor effectiveness of fluticasone and salmeterol. Notify prescriber if patient needs more short-acting inhalations than usual or the patient develops a significant decrease in lung function. Have patient reassessed, and expect his medication regimen to change, which may include increasing the strength of fluticasone and salmeterol combination (never the number of inhalations) or adding an inhaled or systemic corticosteroid.

- **WARNING** Be aware that a recent study suggests asthma-related deaths may be increased in African-American patients taking salmeterol. Monitor this patient population closely throughout therapy, and notify prescriber immediately of any changes in patient's respiratory status.

- Watch for arrhythmias and changes in blood pressure after use in patients with cardiovascular disorders, including ischemic cardiac disease, hypertension, and arrhythmias, because of drug's beta-adrengeric effects.

- Monitor patient for immediate hypersensitivity reaction after giving fluticasone and salmeterol. Reaction may include urticaria, rash, angioedema, bronchospasm, or laryngeal spasm, irritation, or swelling. Notify prescriber immediately, and expect to provide supportive care and to discontinue drug.

• Assess patient for risk factors for decreased bone mineral content, such as smoking, advanced age, sedentary lifestyle, poor nutrition, family history of osteoporosis, or chronic use of drugs that can reduce bone mass, such as anticonvulsants and corticosteroids. If present, have the patient undergo a bone mineral density study, as prescribed, because chronic use of any drug containing fluticasone may adversely affect bone density.

• Be aware that systemic absorption may occur with inhalation of fluticasone and salmeterol with the potential to suppress the hypothalamic-pituitary-adrenal axis with long-term use. Don't stop drug abruptly but withdraw gradually, as prescribed, to prevent acute adrenal insufficiency.

PATIENT TEACHING

• Before fluticasone and salmeterol therapy starts, explain the risk of potentially life-threatening adverse effects.

• Advise patient to take doses 12 hours apart for optimum effect. Caution against using fluticasone and salmeterol more than every 12 hours or stopping it abruptly.

• Teach patient how to use the diskus by instructing him to slide the lever only once when preparing dose to avoid wasting doses. Advise him to exhale immediately before using the diskus and then to place the mouthpiece to his lips, holding it in a level, horizontal position, and inhale through his mouth, not his nose. Then he should remove the mouthpiece from his mouth, hold his breath for at least 10 seconds, and exhale slowly. Then tell patient to close the diskus, which will also reset the dose lever for the next scheduled dose.

• Advise patient to discard diskus 1 month after removing it from the foil overwrap or when dose indicator reads zero, whichever comes first.

• Teach patient how to use the HFA aerosol form, if prescribed, by instructing him to prime the canister before the first use by releasing four test sprays into the air away from his face, shaking the canister well for 5 seconds before each spray. If the canister has not been used for more than 4 weeks or it has been dropped, instruct patient to reprime the canister by shaking well before each spray and releasing two test sprays into the air away from his face.

- Remind patient using HFA aerosol form to shake the canister well for 5 seconds before each inhalation and to clean the inhaler at least once weekly after the evening dose, according to manufacturer instructions, to prevent drug buildup.
- To minimize dry mouth, advise patient to rinse his mouth with water after each dose and to spit the water without swallowing.
- Warn patient not to use fluticasone and salmeterol to treat acute bronchospasm but instead to use a short-acting bronchodilator as prescribed.
- Urge patient to carry medical identification indicating the need for supplemental systemic corticosteroids during stress or severe asthma attack.
- Caution patient to report exposure to chickenpox, measles, or other infectious diseases because prophylactic treatment may be required.
- Explain that drug commonly causes palpitations, rapid heart rate, tremor, or nervousness and that these effects should be reported if severe or they persist. Also, tell patient that although chest pain may occur with fluticasone and salmeterol use, he should always seek prompt medical care if chest pain occurs.
- Stress the importance of routine eye examinations because cataracts or glaucoma may occur with fluticasone and salmeterol.
- Instruct woman of childbearing age to notify prescriber ifshe is or could be pregnant.

guaifenesin and codeine phosphate

Brontex, Cheracol, Endal, Gani-Tuss NR, Guiatuss AC Syrup, Halotussin AC Liquid, Mytussin AC Cough Syrup, Robafen AC, Robitussin A-C Syrup, Romilar AC Liquid, Tussi-Organidin NR Liquid, Tussi-Organidin-S NR Liquid

Class, Category, and Schedule

Chemical: Glyceryl guaiacolate (guaifenesin), phenanthrene derivative (codeine)
Therapeutic: Expectorant (guaifenesin), antitussive (codeine)
Pregnancy category: C
Controlled substance schedule: V (oral solution), III (tablets)

Indications and Dosages

▶ *To relieve cough and chest congestion*
ORAL SOLUTION, SYRUP (ALL BRANDS EXCEPT BRONTEX)
Adults and children age 12 and over. 100 to 200 mg guaifen-

esin and 10 to 20 mg codeine (5 or 10 ml depending on product) every 4 to 6 hr. *Maximum:* 6 doses daily.

Children ages 6 to 12. 50 to 100 mg guaifenesin and 5 to 10 mg codeine (5 ml) every 6 to 8 hr. *Maximum:* 6 doses daily.

Children ages 2 to 6. 50 mg guaifenesin and 5 mg codeine (2.5 ml) every 6 to 8 hr.

ORAL SOLUTION (BRONTEX)

Adults and children age 12 and over. 300 mg guaifenesin and 10 mg codeine (20 ml) every 4 hr. *Maximum:* 6 doses daily.

Children ages 6 to 12. 150 mg guaifenesin and 5 mg codeine (10 ml) every 4 hr.

TABLETS (BRONTEX)

Adults and children age 12 and over. 300 mg guaifenesin and 10 mg codeine (1 tablet) every 4 hr.

Mechanism of Action

Guaifenesin increases fluid and mucus removal from the upper respiratory tract by increasing the volume of secretions and reducing their adhesiveness and surface tension.

Codeine suppresses cough by directly acting on opiate receptors in the medulla's cough center.

Contraindications

Hypersensitivity to guaifenesin, codeine, other opioids, or their components; irritable bowel syndrome; paralytic ileus; significant respiratory depression

Interactions

DRUGS

codeine

anticholinergics, paregoric: Possibly intensified anticholinergic adverse effects

antidiarrheals: Increased risk of severe constipation

antihypertensives, diuretics: Potentiated hypotensive effects

buprenorphine: Decreased codeine effectiveness

CNS depressants: Additive CNS depression

hydroxyzine: Increased codeine analgesic effect; increased CNS depressant and hypotensive effects

MAO inhibitors: Increased risk of unpredictable, severe, and sometimes fatal reactions with codeine

metoclopramide: Antagonized effect of metoclopramide on GI motility

naloxone: Anatagonized codeine analgesic effect
naltrexone: Precipitated withdrawal symptoms in codeine-dependent patients
neuromuscular blockers: Additive respiratory depressant effects
opioids: Additive CNS and respiratory depressants effects and hypotensive effects
ACTIVITIES
codeine
alcohol use: Additive CNS depression

Adverse Reactions

CNS: Coma, delirium, depression, disorientation, dizziness, drowsiness, euphoria, hallucinations, headache, lack of coordination, lethargy, light-headedness, mental and physical impairment, mood changes, restlessness, sedation, seizures, tremor
CV: Bradycardia, heart block, hypertension, orthostatic hypotension, palpitations, tachycardia
EENT: Altered taste, blurred vision, diplopia, dry mouth, laryngeal edema, laryngospasm, miosis
GI: Abdominal cramps and pain, anorexia, constipation, flatulence, gastroesophageal reflux, ileus, indigestion, nausea, vomiting
GU: Decreased libido, difficult ejaculation, dysuria, impotence, oliguria, ureteral spasm, urinary incontinence, urine retention
MS: Muscle rigidity
RESP: Apnea, bronchoconstriction, bronchospasm, depressed cough reflex, respiratory depression
SKIN: Diaphoresis, flushing, pallor, pruritus, rash, urticaria
Other: Anaphylaxis, facial edema, physical and psychological dependence

Nursing Considerations

- Evaluate patient for therapeutic response, including decreased cough. Notify prescriber if symptoms persist or worsen despite use of guaifenesin and codeine.
- Take safety precautions, if needed, because codeine can cause excessive drowsiness.
- Monitor respiratory depth, effort, and rate. Notify prescriber immediately if respiratory rate drops below 10 breaths/minute.
- Assess urine output; decreasing output may signal urine retention.
- **WARNING** Assess patient for evidence of physical and psychological dependence.
- **WARNING** Monitor patient closely for evidence of overdose,

even at normal dosage, because some patients metabolize codeine quickly, causing a sudden rise in blood codeine level. This metabolic defect occurs in about 0.5 to 1% of Chinese, Japanese, and Hispanic people; 1 to 10% of Caucasians; 3% of African Americans; and 16 to 28% of North Africans, Ethiopians, and Arabs. Watch for extreme sleepiness, confusion, and shallow breathing after giving drug. If present, notify prescriber and be prepared to provide supportive care and discontinue drug, as ordered.

PATIENT TEACHING
- Instruct patient to take guaifenesin and codeine exactly as prescribed and not to increase dose or frequency without consulting prescriber.
- Tell patient to take drug with a full glass of water.
- Advise patient to avoid alcohol or other CNS depressants while taking drug.
- To minimize nausea, suggest that patient take drug with food.
- Caution patient to avoid hazardous activities until drug's CNS effects are known.
- Caution patient to get up slowly from a sitting or lying position.
- To prevent constipation, encourage patient to consume plenty of fluids and high-fiber foods, if not contraindicated.
- Advise patient to notify prescriber if she becomes short of breath or has difficulty breathing.
- Urge patient to notify prescriber if she has trouble breathing or develops extreme sleepiness or confusion.

guaifenesin, codeine phosphate, and pseudoephedrine hydrochloride

Cycofed, Dihistine Expectorant, Guiatuss DAC, Halotussin DAC, KG-Fed Expectorant, Mytussin DAC, Novagest Expectorant with Codeine, Nucofed Expectorant, Nucofed Pediatric Expectorant, Nucotuss Expectorant, Nucotuss Pediatric Expectorant, Robitussin DAC, Ryna-CX

Class, Category, and Schedule

Chemical: Glyceryl guaiacolate (guaifenesin), phenanthrene derivative (codeine), sympathomimetic amine (pseudoephedrine)
Therapeutic: Expectorant (guaifenesin), antitussive (codeine), decongestant (pseudoephedrine)
Pregnancy category: C

Controlled substance schedule: V (all except Nucofed and Nucotuss Expectorant Syrup), III (Nucofed and Nucotuss Expectorant Syrup)

Indications and Dosages

▶ *To relieve cough and chest congestion*

ORAL SOLUTION, SYRUP

Adults and children age 12 and over. 200 mg guaifenesin, 20 mg codeine, and 60 mg pseudoephedrine (available as either 5 ml or 10 ml depending on brand) every 4 to 6 hr. *Maximum:* 4 doses daily

Children ages 6 to 12. 100 mg guaifenesin, 10 mg codeine, and 30 mg pseudoephedrine (5 ml) every 6 hr. *Maximum:* 4 doses daily.

Children ages 2 to 6. 50 mg guaifenesin, 5 mg codeine, and 15 mg pseudoephedrine (2.5 ml) every 6 hr. *Maximum:* 4 doses daily.

Mechanism of Action

Guaifenesin increases fluid and mucus removal from the upper respiratory tract by increasing the volume of secretions and reducing their adhesiveness and surface tension.

Codeine suppresses cough by directly acting on opiate receptors in the medulla's cough center.

Pseudoephedrine acts on alpha$_1$-adrenergic receptors in the mucosa of the respiratory tract to produce vasoconstriction. This process shrinks swollen nasal mucous membranes; reduces tissue hyperemia, edema, and nasal congestion; and increases nasal airway patency. It also may increase drainage of sinus secretions and open obstructed eustachian ostia.

Contraindications

Hypersensitivity or idiosyncratic reactions to guaifenesin, codeine, pseudoephedrine, other opioids, or their components; hyperthyroidism; narrow-angle glaucoma; prostatic hypertrophy; severe coronary artery disease or hypertension; significant respiratory depression; urine retention; use within 14 days of MAO inhibitor therapy

Interactions

DRUGS

codeine and pseudoephedrine

MAO inhibitors: Increased and prolonged cardiac stimulation, in-

creased vasopressor effect, increased risk of severe cardiovascular and cerebrovascular effects, hyperpyrexia, vomiting

codeine

anticholinergics, paregoric: Possibly intensified anticholinergic adverse effects

antidiarrheals: Increased risk of severe constipation

antihypertensives, diuretics: Potentiated hypotensive effects

buprenorphine: Decreased codeine effectiveness

CNS depressants: Additive CNS depression

hydroxyzine: Increased codeine analgesic effect; increased CNS depressant and hypotensive effects

metoclopramide: Antagonized effect of metoclopramide on GI motility

naloxone: Anatagonized codeine analgesic effect

naltrexone: Precipitated withdrawal symptoms in codeine-dependent patients

neuromuscular blockers: Additive respiratory depressant effects

opioids: Additive CNS and respiratory depressants effects and hypotensive effects

pseudoephedrine

antacids: Increased pseudoephedrine absorption

antihypertensives, diuretics: Possibly decreased antihypertensive effects

beta blockers: Decreased therapeutic effects of both drugs

citrates: Possibly inhibited urinary pseudoephedrine excretion and prolonged duration of action

CNS stimulant, other sympathomimetics: Possibly increased additive CNS stimulation to excessive levels

cocaine (mucosal-local): Possibly increased cardiovascular effects of either drug and CNS stimulation

digoxin, levodopa: Increased risk of cardiac arrhythmias

hydrocarbon inhalation anesthetics: Increased risk of serious arrhythmias

kaolin: Decreased pseudoephedrine absorption

nitrates: Reduced antianginal effects of nitrates

rauwolfia alkaloids: Possibly inhibited pseudoephedrine action

thyroid hormones: Increased cardiovascular effects of both drugs

ACTIVITIES

codeine

alcohol use: Additive CNS depression

Adverse Reactions

CNS: Coma, delirium, depression, disorientation, dizziness, drowsiness, euphoria, hallucinations, headache, insomnia, lack of coordination, lethargy, light-headedness, mental and physical impairment, mood changes, nervousness, restlessness, sedation, seizures, tremor, weakness

CV: Bradycardia, heart block, hypertension, orthostatic hypotension, palpitations, tachycardia

EENT: Altered taste, blurred vision, diplopia, dry mouth, laryngeal edema, laryngospasm, miosis

GI: Abdominal cramps and pain, anorexia, constipation, flatulence, gastroesophageal reflux, ileus, indigestion, nausea, vomiting

GU: Decreased libido, difficult ejaculation, dysuria, impotence, oliguria, ureteral spasm, urinary incontinence, urine retention

MS: Muscle rigidity

RESP: Apnea, bronchoconstriction, bronchospasm, depressed cough reflex, respiratory depression

SKIN: Diaphoresis, flushing, pallor, pruritus, rash, urticaria

Other: Anaphylaxis, facial edema, physical and psychological dependence

Nursing Considerations

- Use cautiously in patients with diabetes, hypertension, hyperthyroidism, increased intraocular pressure, ischemic heart disease, prostatic hypertrophy, stenosing peptic ulcer or pyloroduodenal obstruction because of the vasoconstictive action of pseudoephedrine.
- Watch for therapeutic response, including decreased cough. Notify prescriber if symptoms persist or worsen despite use of guaifenesin, codeine, and pseudoephedrine.
- Monitor renal function, as ordered, because pseudoephedrine is substantially excreted by the kidneys.
- Take safety precautions, if needed, because codeine can cause excessive drowsiness.
- Monitor respiratory depth, effort, and rate. Notify prescriber immediately if respiratory rate drops below 10 breaths/minute.
- Assess urine output; decreasing output may signal urine retention.
- **WARNING** Assess patient for evidence of physical and psychological dependence.
- **WARNING** Monitor patient closely for evidence of overdose, even at normal dosage, because some patients metabolize codeine quickly, causing a sudden rise in blood codeine level. This metabolic defect occurs in about 0.5 to 1% of Chinese,

Japanese, and Hispanic people; 1 to 10% of Caucasians; 3% of African Americans; and 16 to 28% of North Africans, Ethiopians, and Arabs. Watch for extreme sleepiness, confusion, and shallow breathing after giving drug. If present, notify prescriber and be prepared to provide supportive care and discontinue drug, as ordered.

PATIENT TEACHING
• Instruct patient to take guaifenesin, codeine, and pseudo-ephedrine exactly as prescribed and not to increase dosage or frequency without consulting prescriber.
• Tell patient to take each dose with a full glass of water.
• Advise patient to avoid alcohol or other CNS depressants while taking drug.
• To minimize nausea, suggest that patient take drug with food.
• Caution patient to avoid hazardous activities until drug's CNS effects are known.
• Caution patient to get up slowly from a sitting or lying position.
• To prevent constipation, encourage patient to consume plenty of fluids and high-fiber foods, if not contraindicated.
• Advise patient to notify prescriber if he becomes short of breath or has difficulty breathing.
• Urge patient to notify prescriber if he has trouble breathing or develops extreme sleepiness or confusion.

guaifenesin and hydrocodone bitartrate

Codiclear DH, Co-Tuss V, Hycosin Expectorant,
Hycotuss Expectorant, Hydrocodone GF, Kwelcof, Pneumotussin,
Vicodin Tuss, Vitussin

Class, Category, and Schedule

Chemical: Glyceryl guaiacolate (guaifenesin), opioid and phenan-threne derivative (hydrocodone)
Therapeutic: Expectorant (guaifenesin), antitussive (hydrocodone)
Pregnancy category: C
Controlled substance schedule: III

Indications and Dosages

▶ *To relieve cough and other symptoms of allergies and the common cold*

ORAL SOLUTION, SYRUP
Adults and children age 12 and over. 100 to 400 mg guaifen-esin and 5 mg hydrocodone (5 or 10 ml) every 4 to 6 hr.

Children ages 2 to 12. 50 to 100 mg guaifenesin and 2.5 to 5 mg hydrocodone (2.5 or 5 ml) every 4 to 6 hr.
TABLETS
Adults. 300 to 600 mg guaifenesin and 2.5 to 5 mg hydrocodone (1 or 2 tablets) every 4 to 6 hr. *Maximum:* 4 doses daily.

Mechanism of Action
Guaifenesin increases fluid and mucus removal from the upper respiratory tract by increasing the volume of secretions and reducing their adhesiveness and surface tension.

Hydrocodone suppresses cough by directly acting on opiate receptors in the medulla's cough center.

Contraindications
Hypersensitivity or idiosyncractic reactions to guaifenesin, hydrocodone, other opioids, or their components; respiratory depression

Interactions
DRUGS
hydrocodone
anticholinergics, paregoric: Possibly intensified anticholinergic adverse effects
antidiarrheals: Increased risk of severe constipation or paralytic ileus
antihypertensives, diuretics: Potentiated hypotensive effects
buprenorphine: Decreased hydrocodone effectiveness
CNS depressants: Additive CNS depression
hydroxyzine: Increased hydrocodone analgesic effect; increased CNS depressant and hypotensive effects
MAO inhibitors: Increased and prolonged cardiac stimulation, increased vasopressor effect, increased risk of severe cardiovascular and cerebrovascular effects, hyperpyrexia, vomiting
metoclopramide: Antagonized effect of metoclopramide on GI motility
naloxone: Antagonized hydrocodone analgesic effect
naltrexone: Precipitated withdrawal symptoms in hydrocodone-dependent patients
neuromuscular blockers: Additive respiratory depressant effects
opioids: Additive CNS and respiratory depressants effects and hypotensive effects

ACTIVITIES
hydrocodone
alcohol use: Additive CNS effects

Adverse Reactions

CNS: Coma, delirium, depression, disorientation, dizziness, drowsiness, euphoria, hallucinations, headache, lack of coordination, lethargy, light-headedness, mental and physical impairment, mood changes, restlessness, sedation, seizures, tremor

CV: Bradycardia, heart block, hypertension, orthostatic hypotension, palpitations, tachycardia

EENT: Altered taste, blurred vision, diplopia, dry mouth, laryngeal edema, laryngospasm, miosis

GI: Abdominal cramps and pain, anorexia, constipation, flatulence, gastroesophageal reflux, ileus, indigestion, nausea, vomiting

GU: Decreased libido, difficult ejaculation, dysuria, impotence, oliguria, ureteral spasm, urinary incontinence, urine retention

MS: Muscle rigidity

RESP: Apnea, bronchoconstriction, bronchospasm, depressed cough reflex, respiratory depression

SKIN: Diaphoresis, flushing, pallor, pruritus, rash, urticaria

Other: Anaphylaxis, facial edema, physical and psychological dependence

Nursing Considerations

- Watch for therapeutic response, including decreased cough. Notify prescriber if symptoms persist or worsen despite use of guaifenesin and hydrocodone.
- Monitor respiratory depth, effort, and rate. Notify prescriber immediately if respiratory rate drops below 10 breaths/minute.
- Assess urine output; decreasing output may signal retention.
- **WARNING** Assess patient for evidence of physical and psychological dependence.

PATIENT TEACHING

- Instruct patient to take guaifenesin and hydrocodone exactly as prescribed and not to increase dose or frequency without consulting prescriber.
- Instruct patient to use a calibrated measuring device to ensure accurate dose when using liquid form of drug.
- Tell patient to take each dose with a full glass of water.
- Advise patient to avoid alcohol or other CNS depressants while taking drug.
- To minimize nausea, suggest that patient take drug with food.

- Caution patient to avoid hazardous activities until drug's CNS effects are known.
- Caution patient to get up slowly from a sitting or lying position.
- Advise patient to notify prescriber if she becomes short of breath or has difficulty breathing.

guaifenesin and hydromorphone hydrochloride

Dilaudid Cough Syrup

Class, Category, and Schedule

Chemical: Glyceryl guaiacolate (guaifenesin), opioid and phenan-threne derivative (hydromorphone)
Therapeutic: Expectorant (guaifenesin), antitussive (hydromorphone)
Pregnancy category: C
Controlled substance schedule: II

Indications and Dosages

▶ *To relieve cough and other symptoms of allergies and the common cold*

SYRUP

Adults. 1 mg hydromorphone and 100 guaifenesin (5 ml) every 3 to 4 hr.

Mechanism of Action

Guaifenesin increases fluid and mucus removal from the upper respiratory tract by increasing the volume of secretions and reducing their adhesiveness and surface tension.

Hydromorphone suppresses cough by acting directly on opiate receptors in the medulla's cough center.

Contraindications

Hypersensitivity or idiosyncractic reactions to guaifenesin, hydro-morphone, other opioids, or their components; respiratory depression

Interactions

DRUGS

hydromorphone

anticholinergics, paregoric: Possibly intensified anticholinergic adverse effects

antihypertensives, diuretics: Potentiated hypotensive effects
buprenorphine: Decreased hydromorphone effectiveness
CNS depressants: Additive CNS depression
hydroxyzine: Increased hydromorphone analgesic effect; increased CNS depressant and hypotensive effects
MAO inhibitors: Increased and prolonged cardiac stimulation, increased vasopressor effect, increased risk of severe cardiovascular and cerebrovascular effects, hyperpyrexia, vomiting
metoclopramide: Antagonized effect of metoclopramide on GI motility
naloxone: Antagonized hydromorphone analgesic effect
naltrexone: Precipitated withdrawal symptoms in hydromorphone-dependent patients
neuromuscular blockers: Additive respiratory depressant effects
opioids: Additive CNS and respiratory depressants effects and hypotensive effects
ACTIVITIES
hydromorphone
alcohol use: Additive CNS effects

Adverse Reactions

CNS: Coma, delirium, depression, disorientation, dizziness, drowsiness, euphoria, hallucinations, headache, lack of coordination, lethargy, light-headedness, mental and physical impairment, mood changes, restlessness, sedation, seizures, tremor
CV: Bradycardia, heart block, hypertension, orthostatic hypotension, palpitations, tachycardia
EENT: Altered taste, blurred vision, diplopia, dry mouth, laryngeal edema, laryngospasm, miosis
GI: Abdominal cramps and pain, anorexia, constipation, flatulence, gastroesophageal reflux, ileus, indigestion, nausea, vomiting
GU: Decreased libido, difficult ejaculation, dysuria, impotence, oliguria, ureteral spasm, urinary incontinence, urine retention
MS: Muscle rigidity
RESP: Apnea, bronchoconstriction, bronchospasm, depressed cough reflex, respiratory depression
SKIN: Diaphoresis, flushing, pallor, pruritus, rash, urticaria
Other: Anaphylaxis, facial edema, physical and psychological dependence

Nursing Considerations

• Evaluate therapeutic response, including decreased cough. If symptoms persist or worsen despite use of guaifenesin and hydromorphone, notify prescriber.

- Monitor respiratory depth, effort, and rate. If respiratory rate drops below 10 breaths/minute, notify prescriber immediately.
- Assess urine output; decreasing output may signal retention.
- **WARNING** Assess patient for evidence of physical and psychological dependence.

PATIENT TEACHING
- Instruct patient to take guaifenesin and hydromorphone exactly as prescribed and not to increase dose or frequency without consulting prescriber.
- Instruct patient to use a calibrated measuring device to ensure accurate dose.
- Advise patient to avoid alcohol or other CNS depressants while taking drug.
- To minimize nausea, suggest that patient take drug with food.
- Caution patient to avoid hazardous activities until drug's CNS effects are known.
- Caution patient to get up slowly from a sitting or lying position.
- Advise patient to notify prescriber if he becomes short of breath or has difficulty breathing.

guaifenesin and pseudoephedrine hydrochloride

Anatussin LA, AquatabD, Coldmist JR, Coldmist LA, Congess SR, Deconsal II, Defen-LA, Durasal II, Duratuss, Duratuss GP, Dynex, Entex PSE, GP-500, GFN/PSE, GP-500, GP 1200/60, Guaifed, Guaifenex GP, Guaifenex PSE, Guaifenex PSE 60, Guaifenex PSE 120, Guaifenex-Rx, GuaiMAX-D, Guaipax PSE, Guai-Vent/PSE, Guiatuss PE, H 9600 SR, Iosal II, Maxifed, Maxifed-G, Miraphen PSE, Nasatab LA, PanMist JR, PanMist LA, PanMist-S, Profen II, Profen Forte, Pseudovent, Pseudovent-PED, Respa-1st, Respaire-60 SR, Respaire-120 SR, Robafen PE, Robitussin PE, Robitussin Severe Congestion, Ru-Tuss, Ru-Tuss DE, Severe Congestion Tussin, Sinufed Timecelles, Sinutab Non-Drying, Stamoist E, Sudafed Non-Drowsy Non-Drying Sinus, Sudal 60/500, Sudal 120/600, Thera-Hist Expectorant Chest Congestion, Touro LA, Triacting, Triaminic Chest Congestion, Tuss-LA, V-Dec M, Versacaps, Zephrex, Zephrex-LA

Class and Category

Chemical: Sympathomimetic amine (pseudoephedrine), glyceryl guaiacolate (guaifenesin)

Therapeutic: Decongestant (pseudoephedrine), expectorant (guaifenesin)
Pregnancy category: C

Indications and Dosages

▶ *To relieve symptoms of seasonal allergic rhinitis*
SYRUP
Adults and children age 12 and over. 100 to 400 mg guaifenesin and 30 to 80 mg pseudoephrine (5 to 10 ml depending on product) q.i.d.
Children ages 6 to 12. 100 to 200 mg guaifenesin and 30 mg pseudoephedrine (2.5 to 5 ml depending on product) every 4 to 6 hr. *Maximum:* 4 doses daily.
Children ages 2 to 6. 50 to 100 mg and 15 mg pseudoephedrine (1.25 to 2.5 ml depending on product) every 4 to 6 hr. *Maximum:* 4 doses daily.
ORAL SOLUTION
Adults and children age 12 and over. 200 mg guaifenesin and 60 mg pseudoephedrine (10 ml) every 4 hr. *Maximum:* 4 doses daily.
Children ages 6 to 12. 30 mg pseudoephedrine and 100 mg guaifenesin (10 ml) every 4 to 6 hr. *Maximum:* 4 doses daily.
Children ages 2 to 6. 50 mg guaifenesin and 15 mg pseudoephedrine (5 ml) every 4 to 6 hr. *Maximum:* 4 doses daily.
E.R. CAPSULES
Adults and children age 12 and over. 200 to 600 mg guaifenesin and 60 to 120 mg pseudoephrine (1 or 2 capsules depending on product) every 12 hr.
Children ages 6 to 12. 300 mg quaifenesin and 60 mg pseudoephedrine (1 capsule) every 12 hr.
LIQUID CAPSULES
Adults. 240 to 400 mg guaifenesin and 60 mg pseudoephedrine (2 capsules) every 4 hr. *Maximum:* 8 capsules daily.
E.R. TABLETS
Adults and children age 12 and over. 400 to 1,200 mg guaifenesin and 45 to 120 mg pseudoephedrine (1 or 2 tablets depending on product) every 12 hr.
Children ages 6 to 12. 200 to 600 mg guaifenesin and 30 to 60 mg pseudoephedrine (½ to 2 tablets depending on product) every 12 hr.
Children ages 2 to 6. 150 to 300 mg guaifenesin and 15 to 30 mg pseudoephedrine (½ to 1 tablet depending on product) every 12 hr.

TABLETS
Adults. 400 mg guaifenesin and 60 mg pseudoephedrine
(1 tablet) every 6 hr.

Mechanism of Action

Guaifenesin increases fluid and mucus removal from the upper respiratory tract by increasing the volume of secretions and reducing their adhesiveness and surface tension.

Pseudoephedrine acts on alpha$_1$-adrenergic receptors in the mucosa of the respiratory tract to produce vasoconstriction. This process shrinks swollen nasal mucous membranes; reduces tissue hyperemia, edema, and nasal congestion; and increases nasal airway patency. It also may increase drainage of sinus secretions and open obstructed eustachian ostia.

Contraindications

Hypersensitivity or idiosyncractic reactions to pseudoephedrine, guaifenesin, or their components; hyperthyroidism; narrow-angle glaucoma; prostatic hypertrophy; severe coronary artery disease or hypertension; urine retention; use within 14 days of MAO inhibitor therapy

Interactions

DRUGS

pseudoephedrine
antacids: Increased pseudoephedrine absorption
antihypertensives, diuretics: Possibly decreased antihypertensive effects
beta blockers: Decreased therapeutic effects of both drugs
citrates: Possibly inhibited urinary pseudoephedrine excretion and prolonged duration of action
CNS stimulant, other sympathomimetics: Possibly increased additive CNS stimulation to excessive levels
cocaine (mucosal-local): Possibly increased cardiovascular effects of either drug and CNS stimulation
digoxin, levodopa: Increased risk of cardiac arrhythmias
hydrocarbon inhalation anesthetics: Possibly serious arrhythmias
kaolin: Decreased pseudoephedrine absorption
MAO inhibitors: Increased and prolonged cardiac stimulation, increased vasopressor effect, increased risk of severe cardiovascular and cerebrovascular effects, hyperpyrexia, vomiting
nitrates: Reduced antianginal effects of nitrates
rauwolfia alkaloids: Possibly inhibited pseudoephedrine action

thyroid hormones: Increased cardiovascular effects of both drugs

Adverse Reactions

CNS: Dizziness, headache, insomnia, light-headedness, nervousness, restlessness, trembling, weakness

CV: Angina, hypertension, palpitations, tachycardia

GI: Nausea, vomiting

GU: Dysuria

SKIN: Diaphoresis, pallor, rash, urticaria

Nursing Considerations

- Use drug cautiously in patients with diabetes, hypertension, increased intraocular pressure, ischemic heart disease, stenosing peptic ulcer, or pyloroduodenal obstruction because of vasoconstrictive action of pseudoephedrine.
- Evaluate therapeutic response. Notify prescriber if symptoms persist or worsen despite drug therapy.
- Monitor renal function, as ordered, because pseudoephedrine is substantially excreted by the kidneys.

PATIENT TEACHING

- Instruct patient to take drug exactly as prescribed and not to increase dose or frequency without consulting prescriber.
- To minimize nausea, suggest that patient take drug with food and to take each dose with a full glass of water.
- Advise patient not to break, crush, or chew E.R. tablets or capsules but to swallow them whole.
- Advise patient to avoid alcohol or other CNS depressants while taking drug.
- Caution patient to avoid hazardous activities until drug's CNS effects are known.
- Instruct patient to increase fluid intake (unless contraindicated) to help thin secretions.

hydrocodone bitartrate, brompheniramine maleate, and pseudoephedrine hydrochloride

Anaplex HD

Class, Category, and Schedule

Chemical: Opioid and phenanthrene derivative (hydrocodone), alkylamine (brompheniramine), sympathomimetic amine (pseudoephedrine)

Therapeutic: Antitussive (hydrocodone), antihistamine
(brompheniramine), decongestant (pseudoephedrine)
Pregnancy category: C
Controlled substance schedule: III

Indications and Dosages

▶ *To relieve cough and upper respiratory symptoms caused by hay*
fever, other upper respiratory allergies, or allergic rhinitis
ORAL SOLUTION
Adults. 3.4 mg hydrocodone, 4 mg brompheniramine, and 60 mg
pseudoephedrine (10 ml) t.i.d. or q.i.d. *Maximum:* 40 ml daily.

Mechanism of Action

Hydrocodone suppresses cough by directly acting on opiate receptors in the
medulla's cough center.

Brompheniramine competes with histamine for H_1 receptor sites, thereby
antagonizing many histamine effects and reducing allergy effects.

Pseudoephedrine acts on alpha$_1$-adrenergic receptors in mucosa of the respiratory tract to produce vasoconstriction. This process shrinks swollen nasal
mucous membranes; reduces tissue hyperemia, edema, and nasal congestion;
and increases nasal airway patency. It also may increase drainage of sinus
secretions and open obstructed eustachian ostia.

Contraindications

Hypersensitivity or idiosyncractic reactions to hydrocodone, other
opioids, brompheniramine, pseudoephedrine, or their components; hyperthyroidism; narrow-angle glaucoma; prostatic hypertrophy; respiratory depression; severe asthma or coronary artery
disease; severe or uncontrolled hypertension; upper airway obstruction, urine retention; use of MAO inhibitors within 14 days

Interactions

DRUGS

hydrocodone, bromheniramine, and pseudoephedrine

MAO inhibitors: Increased and prolonged cardiac stimulation, increased vasopressor effect, increased risk of severe cardiovascular
and cerebrovascular effects, hyperpyrexia, and vomiting

hydrocodone and brompheniramine

anticholinergics, paregoric: Possibly intensified anticholinergic adverse effects

CNS depressants: Additive CNS effects

hydrocodone

antihypertensives, diuretics: Potentiated hypotensive effects
buprenorphine: Decreased hydrocodone effectiveness
hydroxyzine: Increased hydrocodone analgesic effect; increased CNS depressant and hypotensive effects
metoclopramide: Antagonized effect of metoclopramide on GI motility
naloxone: Anatagonized hydrocodone analgesic effect
naltrexone: Precipitated withdrawal symptoms in hydrocodone-dependent patients
neuromuscular blockers: Additive respiratory depressant effects
opioids: Additive CNS and respiratory depressants effects and hypotensive effects
tricyclic antidepressants: Possibly increased effect of either the antidepressant or hydrocodone

pseudoephedrine

antacids: Increased pseudoephedrine absorption
antihypertensives, diuretics: Possibly decreased antihypertensive effects
beta blockers: Decreased therapeutic effects of both drugs
citrates: Possibly inhibited urinary pseudoephedrine excretion and prolonged duration of action
CNS stimulant, other sympathomimetics: Possibly increased additive CNS stimulation to excessive levels
cocaine (mucosal-local): Possibly increased cardiovascular effects of either drug and CNS stimulation
digoxin, levodopa: Increased risk of cardiac arrhythmias
hydrocarbon inhalation anesthetics: Possibly serious arrhythmias
kaolin: Decreased pseudoephedrine absorption
nitrates: Reduced antianginal effects of nitrates
rauwolfia alkaloids: Possibly inhibited pseudoephedrine action
thyroid hormones: Increased cardiovascular effects of both drugs
ACTIVITIES

hydrocodone and brompheniramine

alcohol use: Additive CNS effects

Adverse Reactions

CNS: Asthenia, anxiety, confusion, dizziness, depression, drowsiness, dyskinesia, euphoria, excitability, faintness, headache, insomnia, irritability, light-headedness, nervousness, restlessness, sedation, syncope, tiredness, tremor, vertigo, weakness
CV: Bradycardia, hypertension, hypotension, orthostatic hypotension, palpitation, tachycardia

ENDO: Decreased lactation, early menses, gynecomastia, hyperglycemia, hypoglycemia
EENT: Blurred vision; diplopia; dry mouth, pharynx, and respiratory passages; hypermetropia; increased lacrimation; labyrinthitis; laryngismus; mydriasis; nasal stuffiness; photophobia; tinnitus
GI: Abdominal distention or pain, acute pancreatitis, anorexia, constipation, diarrhea, dyspepsia, epigastric distress, esophageal reflux, increased appetite, nausea, vomiting
GU: Dysuria, increased libido, urinary frequency or hesitancy, urine retention, ureteral spasm
RESP: Dyspnea, respiratory depression, wheezing
SKIN: Dermatitis, diaphoresis, erythema, flushing, pallor, pruritus, rash, urticaria
Other: Drug fever, emotional or physical dependence

Nursing Considerations

- Use cautiously in patients with recent head injury and those with Addison's disease, mildly to moderately severe asthma or other chronic respiratory disease, increased intraocular pressure, or liver or renal impairment.
- **WARNING** Monitor patient's respiratory function because hydrocodone, brompheniramine, and pseudoephedrine may suppress cough reflex and cause thickening of bronchial secretions, aggravating such conditions as asthma and COPD. Rarely, it may depress respirations and induce apnea. Notify prescriber immediately if respiratory rate drops below 10 breaths/minute.
- Monitor patients who may be more susceptible to dizziness, sedation, and hypotension, such as the elderly.
- Monitor renal function, as ordered, because pseudoephedrine is substantially excreted by the kidneys.
- Regularly evaluate effectiveness of hydrocodone, brompheniramine, and pseudoephedrine in reducing symptoms.
- Be aware that patient shouldn't have intradermal allergen tests within 72 hours of receiving drug because results may be altered.

PATIENT TEACHING
- Tell patient that hydrocodone, brompheniramine, and pseudoephedrine must not be diluted with fluids or mixed with other drugs.
- Urge patient to avoid alcohol and other antidepressants while taking hydrocodone, brompheniramine, and pseudoephedrine.
- Instruct patient to avoid hazardous activities until drug's CNS effects are known.

- Suggest that patient relieve dry mouth with frequent rinsing and use of sugarless gum or hard candy.
- Tell patient to take last dose of the day a few hours before bedtime if hydrocodone, brompheniramine, and pseudoephedrine makes him nervous or restless.

hydrocodone bitartrate, carbinoxamine maleate, and pseudoephedrine hydrochloride

Histex HC

Class, Category, and Schedule

Chemical: Opioid and phenanthrene derivative (hydrocodone), ethanolamine derivative (carbinoxamine), sympathomimetic amine (pseudoephedrine)

Therapeutic: Antitussive (hydrocodone), antihistamine (carbinoxamine), decongestant (pseudoephedrine)

Pregnancy category: C

Controlled substance schedule: III

Indications and Dosages

▶ *To relieve cough and upper respiratory symptoms caused by hay fever, other upper respiratory allergies, or allergic rhinitis*

ORAL SOLUTION

Adults. 5 to 10 mg hydrocodone, 2 to 4 mg carbinoxamine, and 30 to 60 mg pseudoephedrine (5 to 10 ml) every 4 to 6 hr.

Mechanism of Action

Hydrocodone suppresses cough by acting directly on opiate receptors in the medulla's cough center.

Carbinoxaminecompetes with histamine for H_1 receptor sites, thereby antagonizing many histamine effects and reducing allergy signs and symptoms.

Pseudoephedrine acts on alpha$_1$-adrenergic receptors in the mucosa of the respiratory tract to produce vasoconstriction. This process shrinks swollen nasal mucous membranes; reduces tissue hyperemia, edema, and nasal congestion; and increases nasal airway patency. It also may increase drainage of sinus secretions and open obstructed eustachian ostia.

Contraindications

Hypersensitivity or idiosyncractic reactions to hydrocodone, other opioids, carbinoxamine, pseudoephedrine, or their components; hyperthyroidism; narrow-angle glaucoma; prostatic hypertrophy; respiratory depression; severe asthma or coronary artery disease; severe or uncontrolled hypertension; upper airway obstruction, urine retention; use of MAO inhibitors within 14 days

Interactions
DRUGS
hydrocodone, carbinoxamine and pseudoephedrine
MAO inhibitors: Increased and prolonged cardiac stimulation, increased vasopressor effect, increased risk of severe cardiovascular and cerebrovascular effects, hyperpyrexia, and vomiting
hydrocodone and carbinoxamine
anticholinergics, paregoric: Possibly intensified anticholinergic adverse effects
CNS depressants: Additive CNS effects
hydrocodone
antihypertensives, diuretics: Potentiated hypotensive effects
buprenorphine: Decreased hydrocodone effectiveness
hydroxyzine: Increased hydrocodone analgesic effect; increased CNS depressant and hypotensive effects
metoclopramide: Antagonized effect of metoclopramide on GI motility
naloxone: Antagonized hydrocodone analgesic effect
naltrexone: Precipitated withdrawal symptoms in hydrocodone-dependent patients
neuromuscular blockers: Additive respiratory depressant effects
opioids: Additive CNS and respiratory depressants effects and hypotensive effects
tricyclic antidepressants: Possibly increased effect of either the antidepressant or hydrocodone
pseudoephedrine
antacids: Increased pseudoephedrine absorption
antihypertensives, diuretics: Possibly decreased antihypertensive effects
beta blockers: Decreased therapeutic effects of both drugs
citrates: Possibly inhibited urinary pseudoephedrine excretion and prolonged duration of action
CNS stimulant, other sympathomimetics: Possibly increased additive CNS stimulation to excessive levels
cocaine (mucosal-local): Possibly increased cardiovascular effects of either drug and CNS stimulation
digoxin, levodopa: Increased risk of cardiac arrhythmias

hydrocarbon inhalation anesthetics: Possibly serious arrhythmias
kaolin: Decreased pseudoephedrine absorption
nitrates: Reduced antianginal effects of nitrates
rauwolfia alkaloids: Possibly inhibited pseudoephedrine action
thyroid hormones: Increased cardiovascular effects of both drugs
ACTIVITIES
hydrocodone and carbinoxamine
alcohol use: Additive CNS effects

Adverse Reactions

CNS: Asthenia, anxiety, confusion, dizziness, depression, drowsiness, dyskinesia, euphoria, excitability, faintness, headache, insomnia, irritability, light-headedness, nervousness, restlessness, sedation, syncope, tiredness, tremor, vertigo, weakness
CV: Bradycardia, hypertension, hypotension, orthostatic hypotension, palpitation, tachycardia
ENDO: Decreased lactation, early menses, gynecomastia, hyperglycemia, hypoglycemia
EENT: Blurred vision; diplopia; dry mouth, pharynx, and respiratory passages; hypermetropia; increased lacrimation; labyrinthitis; laryngismus; mydriasis; nasal stuffiness; photophobia; tinnitus
GI: Abdominal distention or pain, acute pancreatitis, anorexia, constipation, diarrhea, dyspepsia, epigastric distress, esophageal reflux, increased appetite, nausea, vomiting
GU: Dysuria, increased libido, urinary frequency or hesitancy, urine retention, ureteral spasm
RESP: Dyspnea, respiratory depression, wheezing
SKIN: Dermatitis, diaphoresis, erythema, flushing, pallor, pruritus, rash, urticaria
Other: Drug fever, emotional or physical dependence

Nursing Considerations

- Use cautiously in patients with recent head injury and those with Addison's disease, mildly to moderately severe asthma or other chronic respiratory disease, increased intraocular pressure, or liver or renal impairment.
- **WARNING** Monitor respiratory function because hydrocodone, carbinoxamine, and pseudoephedrine may suppress cough reflex and cause thickening of bronchial secretions, aggravating such conditions as asthma and COPD. Rarely, it may depress respirations and induce apnea. Notify prescriber immediately if respiratory rate drops below 10 breaths/minute.
- Monitor patients who may be more susceptible to dizziness, sedation, and hypotension, such as the elderly.

- Monitor renal function, as ordered, because pseudoephedrine is substantially excreted by the kidneys.
- Regularly evaluate effectiveness of hydrocodone, carbinoxamine, and pseudoephedrine in reducing symptoms.
- Be aware that patient shouldn't have intradermal allergen tests within 72 hours of receiving drug because results may be altered.

PATIENT TEACHING
- Instruct patient to use calibrated measuring spoon to ensure accurate dosage.
- Tell patient that hydrocodone, carbinoxamine, and pseudoephedrine must not be diluted with fluids or mixed with other drugs.
- Urge patient to avoid alcohol and other antidepressants while taking hydrocodone, carbinoxamine, and pseudoephedrine.
- Instruct patient to avoid hazardous activities until drug's CNS effects are known.
- Suggest that patient relieve dry mouth with frequent rinsing and use of sugarless gum or hard candy.
- Tell patient to take last dose of the day a few hours before bedtime if hydrocodone, carbinoxamine, and pseudoephedrine makes her nervous or restless.

hydrocodone bitartrate, chlorpheniramine maleate, phenylephrine hydrochloride, acetaminophen, and caffeine

Hycomine Compound

Class, Category, and Schedule

Chemical: Opioid and phenanthrene derivative (hydrocodone), alkylamine (chlorpheniramine), sympathomimetic amine (phenylephrine), acetamide (acetaminophen), and methylxantine derivative (caffeine)

Therapeutic: Antitussive (hydrocodone), antihistamine (chlorpheniramine), decongestant (phenylephrine), analgesic and antipyretic (acetaminophen), and centrally acting stimulant (caffeine)

Pregnancy category: C

Controlled substance schedule: III

Indications and Dosages

▶ *To relieve cough, nasal congestion, and discomfort from upper respiratory tract infections*

TABLETS
Adults and children age 12 and over. 5 mg hydrocodone, 2 mg chlorpheniramine, 10 mg phenylephrine, 250 mg acetaminophen, and 30 mg caffeine (1 tablet) q.i.d.
Children ages 6 to 12. 2.5 mg hydrocodone, 1 mg chlorpheniramine, 5 mg phenylephrine, 125 mg acetaminophen, and 15 mg caffeine (½ tablet) q.i.d.

Mechanism of Action

Hydrocodone suppresses cough by acting directly on opiate receptors in the medulla's cough center.

Chlorpheniramine competes with histamine for H_1 receptor sites, thereby antagonizing many histamine effects and reducing allergy signs and symptoms.

Phenylephrine stimulates alpha-adrenergic receptors and inhibits the intracellular enzyme adenyl cyclase, which then inhibits production of cAMP. Inhibition of cAMP causes arterial and venous constriction in nasal passages, which decreases blood flow and mucosal edema caused by allergic response.

Acetaminophen inhibits the enzyme cyclooxygenase, thereby blocking prostaglandin production and interfering with pain impulse generation in the peripheral nervous system.

Caffeine is a competitive, nonselective antagonist of adenosine receptor sites that stimulates the CNS and counteracts the sedative properties of hydrocodone and chlorpheniramine.

Contraindications

Breast-feeding; diabetes mellitus; heart disease; hypersensitivity to hydrocodone, other opioids, chlorpheniramine, other antihistamines, phenylephrine, other sympathomimetic amines, acetaminophen, caffeine, or their components; hypertension; hyperthyroidism; presence of intracranial lesion and increased intracranial pressure; respiratory depression; severe asthma or hepatic impairment; upper airway obstruction, use of MAO inhibitor within 14 days

Interactions

DRUGS

hydrocodone, chlorpheniramine, and acetaminophen
anticholinergics: Possibly intensified anticholinergic adverse effects (hydrocondone, chlorpheniramine, phenylephrine); decreased onset of acetaminophen action

CNS depressants: Additive CNS effects

hydrocodone, chlorpheniramine, and phenylephrine

MAO inhibitors: Increased and prolonged cardiac stimulation, increased vasopressor effect, increased risk of severe cardiovascular and cerebrovascular effects, hyperpyrexia, and vomiting

hydrocodone

antihypertensives, diuretics: Potentiated hypotensive effects

buprenorphine: Decreased hydrocodone effectiveness

hydroxyzine: Increased hydrocodone analgesic effect; increased CNS depressant and hypotensive effects

metoclopramide: Antagonized metoclopramide effects on GI motility

naloxone: Antagonized hydrocodone analgesic effect

naltrexone: Precipitated withdrawal symptoms in hydrocodone-dependent patients

neuromuscular blockers: Additive respiratory depressant effects

opioids: Additive CNS and respiratory depressants effects and hypotensive effects

chlorpheniramine

phenytoin: Possibly increased serum phenytoin levels and toxicity

phenylephrine

alpha blockers, haloperidol, loxapine, phenothiazines, thioxanthenes: Possibly decreased vasoconstrictor effect of phenylephrine

antihypertenisves, diuretics: Possibly decreased antihypertensive effects

atropine: Possibly enhanced vasopressor effect of phenylephrine

beta blockers: Decreased therapeutic effects of both drugs

bretylium: Possibly potentiated vaopressor effect and arrhythmias

doxapram: Increased vasopressor effect of both drugs

ergot alkaloids: Possibly cerebral blood vessel rupture, increased vasopressor effect, peripheral vascular ischemia, and gangrene (with ergotamine)

guanadrel, guanethidine: Increased vasopressor effect of phenylephrine, increased risk of severe hypertension and arrhythmias

hydrocarbon inhalation anesthetics: Increased risk of serious arrhythmias

maprotiline, tricyclic antidepressants: Increased risk of severe cardiovascular effects (including arrhythmias, hyperpyrexia, severe hypertension)

mecamylamine, methyldopa: Decreased hypotensive effects of these drugs, increased vasopressor effect of phenylephrine

nitrates: Possibly decreased vasopressor effect of phenylephrine and decreased antianginal effect of nitrates

oxytocin: Possibly severe, persistent hypertension
phenoxybenzamine: Decreased vasoconstrictor effect of phenylephrine, possibly hypotension and tachycardia
theophylline: Possibly enhanced toxicity (including cardiac toxicity)
thyroid hormones: Increased cardiovascular effects of each drug
acetaminophen
*barbiturates, carbamazepine, hydantoins, isoniazid, rifampin, sulfinpyra-
zone:* Decreased therapeutic effects and increased hepatotoxic effects of acetaminophen
lamotrigine, loop diuretics: Possibly decreased therapeutic effects of
these drugs
oral contraceptives: Decreased effectiveness of acetaminophen
probenecid: Possibly increased therapeutic effects of acetaminophen
propranolol: Possibly increased action of acetaminophen
zidovudine: Possibly decreased effects of zidovudine
caffeine
beta-adrenergic agonists: Possibly enhanced cardiac inotropic effects
of beta-adrenergic agonists
disulfiram: Decreased blood clearance of caffeine
ACTIVITIES
hydrocodone, chlorpheniramine, and acetaminophen
alcohol use: Additive CNS effects; increased risk of hepatotoxicity
(acetaminophen)

Adverse Reactions

CNS: Anxiety, coma, confusion, decreased mental and physical
performance, delirium, depression, disorientation, dizziness,
drowsiness, excitation (children), euphoria, faintness, fear, hallucinations, headache, insomnia, lack of coordination, lethargy,
light-headedness, mental and physical impairment, mood
changes, nervousness, paresthesia, restlessness, sedation, seizures,
tiredness, tremor, weakness
CV: Angina, bradycardia, chest tightness, heart block, hypertension, hypotension, palpitations, peripheral vasoconstriction, tachycardia, ventricular arrhythmias
EENT: Altered taste, blurred vision, diplopia, dry mouth, laryngeal edema, laryngospasm, miosis
ENDO: Hypoglycemic coma
GI: Abdominal cramps and pain, anorexia, constipation, flatulence, gastroesophageal reflux, jaundice, hepatotoxicity, indigestion, nausea, paralytic ileus, toxic megacolon, vomiting
GU: Decreased libido, difficult ejaculation, dysuria, frequent urination, impotence, oliguria, ureteral spasm, urinary hesitancy,

urinary incontinence, urine retention
HEME: Hemolytic anemia (with long-term use), leukopenia, neutropenia, pancytopenia, thrombocytopenia
MS: Muscle rigidity
RESP: Apnea, bronchoconstriction, bronchospasm, depressed cough reflex, dyspnea, respiratory depression, shortness of breath, slow or irregular breathing, wheezing
Skin: Diaphoresis, facial flushing, pallor, pruritus, rash, uriticaria
Other: Angioedema, anaphylaxis, physical or psychological dependence

Nursing Considerations

- Use cautiously in patients with recent head injury and in those with Addison's disease, mildly to moderately severe asthma or other chronic respiratory disease, increased intraocular pressure, or liver or renal impairment.
- Monitor children for excitation and elderly patients for dizziness, sedation, and hypotension; such patients may have an increased risk for these effects.
- Regularly evaluate effectiveness of hydrocodone, chlorpheniramine, phenylephrine, acetaminophen, and caffeine in reducing cough and upper respiratory symptoms.
- Know that the daily dose of acetaminophen shouldn't exceed 4 grams.
- **WARNING** Assess patient for evidence of physical and psychological dependence.
- Monitor urine output; decreasing output may signal retention.
- Be aware that patient shouldn't have intradermal allergen tests within 72 hours of receiving drug because results may be altered.

PATIENT TEACHING

- Instruct patient to take drug with food or after meals to minimize stomach upset.
- Instruct patient to take drug exactly as prescribed and not to adjust dose or frequency without consulting prescriber because drug can become habit-forming.
- Urge patient to avoid alcohol and other antidepressants while taking drug and also to contact prescriber before taking other prescription or OTC drugs that may contain similar ingredients, possibly causing toxicity.
- Advise patient to notify prescriber if he becomes short of breath or has difficulty breathing.
- Instruct patient to avoid hazardous activities until drug's CNS effects are known.

- Suggest that patient relieve dry mouth with frequent rinsing and use of sugarless gum or hard candy.
- Tell patient to take last dose of the day a few hours before bedtime if drug makes him nervous or restless.

hydrocodone bitartrate, guaifenesin, and pseudoephedrine hydrochloride

Duratuss HD, Hydro-Tussin HD, Nalex Expectorant, Pancof-XP, Su-Tuss HD

Class, Category, and Schedule

Chemical: Opioid and phenanthrene derivative (hydrocodone), glyceryl guaiacolate (guaifenesin), sympathomimetic amine (pseudoephedrine)

Therapeutic: Antitussive (hydrocodone), expectorant (guaifenesin), decongestant (pseudoephedrine)

Pregnancy category: C

Controlled substance schedule: III

Indications and Dosages

▶ *To relieve cough and other symptoms caused by allergies and the common cold*

ORAL SOLUTION

Adults. 3 to 5 mg hydrocodone, 100 to 200 mg guaifenesin, and 15 to 60 mg pseudoephedrine (5 to 10 ml depending on product) every 4 to 6 hr. Or, doses may be given q.i.d.

ELIXIR

Adults. 5 mg hydrocodone, 200 mg guaifenesin, and 60 mg pseudoephedrine (10 ml) every 4 to 6 hr. *Maximum:* 4 doses daily.

Mechanism of Action

Hydrocodone suppresses cough by acting directly on opiate receptors in the medulla's cough center.

Guaifenesin increases fluid and mucus removal from the upper respiratory tract by increasing the volume of secretions and reducing their adhesiveness and surface tension.

Pseudoephedrine acts on alpha$_1$-adrenergic receptors in the mucosa of the respiratory tract to produce vasoconstriction. This process shrinks swollen nasal mucous membranes; reduces tissue hyperemia, edema, and nasal congestion; and increases nasal airway patency. It also may increase drainage of sinus secretions and open obstructed eustachian ostia.

Contraindications

Hypersensitivity or idiosyncractic reactions to hydrocodone, other opioids, guaifenesin, pseudoephedrine, or their components; hyperthyroidism; narrow-angle glaucoma; respiratory depression; severe asthma, coronary artery disease or hypertension; upper airway obstruction; urine retention; use of MAO inhibitors within 14 days

Interactions

DRUGS

hydrocodone and pseudoephedrine

MAO inhibitors: Increased and prolonged cardiac stimulation, increased vasopressor effect, increased risk of severe cardiovascular and cerebrovascular effects, hyperpyrexia, vomiting

hydrocodone

anticholinergics, paregoric: Possibly intensified anticholinergic adverse effects

antihypertensives, diuretics: Potentiated hypotensive effects

buprenorphine: Decreased hydrocodone effectiveness

CNS depressants: Additive CNS depression

hydroxyzine: Increased hydrocodone analgesic effect; increased CNS depressant and hypotensive effects

metoclopramide: Antagonized effect of metoclopramide on GI motility

naloxone: Antagonized hydrocodone analgesic effect

naltrexone: Precipitated withdrawal symptoms in hydrocodone-dependent patients

neuromuscular blockers: Additive respiratory depressant effects

opioids: Additive CNS and respiratory depressants effects and hypotensive effects

pseudoephedrine

antacids: Increased pseudoephedrine absorption

antihypertensives, diuretics: Possibly decreased antihypertensive effects

beta blockers: Decreased therapeutic effects of both drugs

citrates: Possibly inhibited urinary pseudoephedrine excretion and prolonged duration of action

CNS stimulant, other sympathomimetics: Possibly increased additive CNS stimulation to excessive levels

cocaine (mucosal-local): Possibly increased cardiovascular effects of either drug and CNS stimulation

digoxin, levodopa: Increased risk of cardiac arrhythmias

hydrocarbon inhalation anesthetics: Possibly serious arrhythmias

kaolin: Decreased pseudoephedrine absorption
nitrates: Reduced antianaginal effects of nitrates
rauwolfia alkaloids: Possibly inhibited pseudoephedrine action
thyroid hormones: Increased cardiovascular effects of both drugs
ACTIVITIES
hydrocodone
alcohol use: Additive CNS effects

Adverse Reactions

CNS: Confusion, dizziness, drowsiness, euphoria, faintness, head-ache, insomnia, light-headedness, nervousness, restlessness, seizures, tiredness, trembling, weakness
CV: Bradycardia, hypotension, palpitations, tachycardia
EENT: Blurred or double vision, dry mouth, laryngeal edema, laryngospasm
GI: Anorexia, constipation, nausea, paralytic ileus, toxic mega-colon, vomiting
GU: Dysuria, frequent urination
RESP: Dyspnea, shortness of breath, slow or irregular breathing, wheezing
Skin: Diaphoresis, facial flushing, pallor, pruritus, rash, uriticaria
Other: Angioedema, atelectasis

Nursing Considerations

- Use cautiously in patients with hypertension, diabetes mellitus, ischemic heart disease, increased intraocular pressure, or renal impairment because of pseudoephedrine.
- Monitor renal function, as ordered, because pseudoephedrine is substantially excreted by the kidneys.
- Regularly evaluate effectiveness of hyrdocodone, guaifenesin, and pseudoephedrine in reducing patient's cough and allergy symptoms.
- Be aware that patient shouldn't have intradermal allergen tests within 72 hours of receiving drug because results may be al-tered.

PATIENT TEACHING
- Instruct patient to use a calibrated measuring device to ensure an accurate dose.
- Urge patient to avoid alcohol and other antidepressants while taking hydrocodone, guaifenesin, and pseudoephedrine.
- Instruct patient to avoid hazardous activities until drug's CNS effects are known.
- Suggest that patient relieve dry mouth with frequent rinsing and use of sugarless gum or hard candy.

• Tell patient to take last dose of the day a few hours before bedtime if hydrocodone, guaifenesin, and pseudoephedrine makes her nervous or restless.

hydrocodone bitartrate and homatropine methylbromide
Hycodan, Hydromet, Hydromide, Hydropane, Tussigon

Class, Category, and Schedule
Chemical: Opioid and phenanthrene derivative (hydrocodone), quaternary ammonium compound (homatropine)
Therapeutic: Antitussive (hydrocodone), anticholinergic (homatropine)
Pregnancy category: C
Controlled substance schedule: III

Indications and Dosages
▶ *To relieve cough, persistent runny nose, and nasal congestion caused by upper respiratory infections, sinus inflammation, or hay fever*
SYRUP, TABLETS
Adults and children age 12 and over. 5 mg hydrocodone and 1.5 mg homatropine (5 ml or 1 tablet) every 4 to 6 hr.
Children age 6 to 12. 2.5 mg hydrocodone and 0.75 mg homatropine (2.5 ml or ½ tablet) every 4 to 6 hr.

Mechanism of Action
Hydrocodone suppresses cough by acting directly on opiate receptors in the medulla's cough center.

Homatropine competitively inhibits acetylcholine at autonomic postganglionic cholinergic receptors. Because the most sensitive receptors are in the salivary, bronchial, and sweat glands, this action reduces secretions from these glands. It also reduces nasal, oropharyngeal, and bronchial secretions and decreases airway resistance by relaxing smooth muscles in the bronchi and bronchioles.

Contraindications
Cardiac disease, such as arrhythmias, severe hypertension, and mitral stenosis; esophageal reflux; hemorrhage with hemodynamic instability; hypersensitivity to hydrocodone, other opioids, homatropine, or their components; ileus; intestinal atony; myasthenia gravis; narrow-angle glaucoma; obstructive GI or uropathic

disease; significant respiratory depression; ulcerative colitis; urine retention

Interactions
DRUGS

hydrocodone and homatropine

anticholinergics, paregoric: Possibly intensified anticholinergic adverse effects

metoclopramide: Possibly antagonized metoclopramide effects on GI motility

hydrocodone

antihypertensives, diuretics: Potentiated hypotensive effects

buprenorphine: Decreased hydrocodone effectiveness

CNS depressants: Additive CNS effects

hydroxyzine: Increased hydrocodone analgesic effect; increased CNS depressant and hypotensive effects

MAO inhibitors: Increased and prolonged cardiac stimulation, increased vasopressor effect, increased risk of severe cardiovascular and cerebrovascular effects, hyperpyrexia, and vomiting

naloxone: Antagonized hydrocodone analgesic effect

naltrexone: Precipitated withdrawal symptoms in hydrocodone-dependent patients

neuromuscular blockers: Additive respiratory depressant effects

opioids: Additive CNS and respiratory depressants effects and hypotensive effects

homatropine

antacids, adsorbent antidiarrheals: Possibly reduced absorption of anticholinergics

antimyasthenics: Possibly reduced intestinal motility

haloperidol: Possibly decreased antipsychotic effectiveness of haloperidol

ketoconazole: Possibly significant decreased ketoconazole absorption

opioid analgesics: Increased risk of severe constipation, paralytic ileus, and urine retention

potassium chloride: Possibly increased severity of potassium chloride induced GI lesions

urinary alkalizers such as calcium and or magnesium-containing antacids, carbonic anhydrase inhibitors, citrates, and sodium bicarbonate: Delayed urinary excretion of homatropine with increased therapeutic effects and incidence of adverse reactions

ACTIVITIES

hydrocodone

alcohol use: Additive CNS effects

Adverse Reactions

CNS: Confusion, dizziness, drowsiness, euphoria, faintness, hallucinations, headache, insomnia, light-headedness, mania, mood changes, nervousness, restlessness, seizures, tiredness, weakness
CV: Bradycardia, hypotension, palpitations, tachycardia
EENT: Blurred or double vision; dry eyes, mouth, nose, and throat; laryngeal edema; laryngospasm
GI: Anorexia, constipation, nausea, paralytic ileus, toxic megacolon, vomiting
GU: Dysuria, frequent urination, urinary hesitancy, urine retention
RESP: Dyspnea, shortness of breath, slow or irregular breathing, wheezing
Skin: Decreased sweating, diaphoresis, dry skin, facial flushing, pruritus, rash, uriticaria
Other: Angioedema, anaphylaxis

Nursing Considerations

• Regularly evaluate effectiveness of hydrocodone and homatropine in relieving cough and upper respiratory symptoms.
• Take safety precautions as needed.
• Monitor respiratory depth, effort, and rate. Notify prescriber immediately if respiratory rate drops below 10 breaths/minute.
• Assess urine output; decreasing output may signal retention.
• **WARNING** Assess patient for evidence of physical and psychological dependence.

PATIENT TEACHING

• Instruct patient to use a calibrated measuring device to ensure accurate dose of syrup form.
• Caution patient to take drug exactly as prescribed and not to adjust dose or frequency without consulting prescriber.
• Urge patient to avoid alcohol and other antidepressants while taking hydrocodone and homatropine.
• Instruct patient to avoid hazardous activities until drug's CNS effects are known.
• Suggest that patient relieve dry mouth with frequent rinsing and use of sugarless gum or hard candy and to use lubricating eye drops for dry eyes.
• To prevent constipation, urge patient to consume plenty of fluids and high-fiber foods, if not contraindicated.
• Advise patient to notify prescriber if he becomes short of breath or has difficulty breathing or if he develops persistent or severe diarrhea, constipation, or has difficulty urinating.

hydrocodone bitartrate and phenylephrine hydrochloride

Lortus-HD, Nalex DH, Tusdec HC

Class, Category, and Schedule

Chemical: Opioid and phenanthrene derivative (hydrocodone), sympathomimetic amine (phenylephrine)
Therapeutic: Antitussive (hydrocodone), decongestant (phenylephrine)
Pregnancy category: C
Controlled substance schedule: III

Indications and Dosages

▶ *To relieve cough and other upper respiratory symptoms caused by the common cold and allergies*

ELIXIR

Adults and children age 12 and over. 3.75 to 5 mg hydrocodone and 7.5 to 10 mg phenylephrine (10 ml) every 4 to 6 hr. *Maximum:* 4 doses daily.

Children ages 6 to 12. 1.67 mg hydrocodone and 5 mg phenylephrine (5 ml) every 4 to 6 hr. *Maximum:* 4 doses daily.

Children ages 2 to 6. 0.84 to 1.67 mg hydrocodone and 2.5 to 5 mg phenylephrine (2.5 to 5 ml) every 4 to 6 hr. *Maximum:* 4 doses daily.

Mechanism of Action

Hydrocodone suppresses cough by acting directly on opiate receptors in the medulla's cough center.

Phenylephrine stimulates alpha-adrenergic receptors and inhibits the intracellular enzyme adenyl cyclase, which then inhibits production of cAMP. Inhibition of cAMP causes arterial and venous constriction in nasal passages, which decreases blood flow and mucosal edema caused by allergic response.

Contraindications

Hypersensitivity to hydrocodone, other opioids, bisulfites, phenylephrine, or their components; severe coronary artery disease or hypertension; significant respiratory depression; use of an MAO inhibitor within 14 days; ventricular tachycardia

Interactions

DRUGS

hydrocodone and phenylephrine

MAO inhibitors: Increased and prolonged cardiac stimulation, in-

creased vasopressor effect, increased risk of severe cardiovascular and cerebrovascular effects, hyperpyrexia, and vomiting

hydrocodone

anticholinergics, paregoric: Possibly intensified anticholinergic adverse effects

antihypertensives, diuretics: Potentiated hypotensive effects

buprenorphine: Decreased hydrocodone effectivess

CNS depressants: Additive CNS effects

hydroxyzine: Increased hydrocodone analgesic effect; increased CNS depressant and hypotensive effects

metoclopramide: Possibly antagonized metoclopramide effects on GI motility

naloxone: Antagonized hydrocodone analgesic effect

naltrexone: Precipitated withdrawal symptoms in hydrocodone-dependent patients

neuromuscular blockers: Additive respiratory depressant effects

opioids: Additive CNS and respiratory depressants effects and hypotensive effects

phenylephrine

alpha blockers, haloperidol, loxapine, phenothiazines, thioxanthenes: Possibly decreased vasoconstrictor effect of phenylephrine

antihypertenisves, diuretics: Possibly decreased antihypertensive effects

atropine: Possibly enhanced vasopressor effect of phenylephrine

beta blockers: Decreased therapeutic effects of both drugs

bretylium: Possibly potentiated vaopressor effect and arrhythmias

doxapram: Increased vasopressor effect of both drugs

ergot alkaloids: Possibly cerebral blood vessel rupture, increased vasopressor effect, peripheral vascular ischemia, and gangrene (with ergotamine)

guanadrel, guanethidine: Increased vasopressor effect of phenylephrine; increased risk of severe hypertension and arrhythmias

hydrocarbon inhalation anesthetics: Possibly serious arrhythmias

maprotiline, tricyclic antidepressants: Increased risk of severe cardiovascular effects (including arrhythmias, hyperpyrexia, severe hypertension)

mecamylamine, methyldopa: Decreased hypotensive effects of these drugs; increased vasopressor effect of phenylephrine

nitrates: Possibly decreased vasopressor effect of phenylephrine and decreased antianginal effect of nitrates

oxytocin: Possibly severe, persistent hypertension

phenoxybenzamine: Decreased vasoconstrictor effect of phenylephrine, possibly hypotension and tachycardia

theophylline: Possibly enhanced toxicity (including cardiac toxicity)
thyroid hormones: Increased cardiovascular effects of each drug
ACTIVITIES
hydrocodone
alcohol use: Additive CNS effects

Adverse Reactions

CNS: Confusion, dizziness, drowsiness, euphoria, faintness, headache, insomnia, light-headedness, nervousness, paresthesia, restlessness, seizures, tiredness, tremor, weakness
CV: Angina, bradycardia, hypertension, hypotension, palpitations, peripheral vasoconstriction that may lead to necrosis or gangrene, tachycardia, ventricular arrhythmia
EENT: Blurred or double vision, dry mouth, laryngeal edema, laryngospasm
GI: Anorexia, constipation, nausea, paralytic ileus, toxic megacolon, vomiting
GU: Dysuria, frequent urination
RESP: Dyspnea, shortness of breath, slow or irregular breathing, wheezing
SKIN: Diaphoresis, facial flushing, pallor, pruritus
Other: Angioedema, anaphylaxis

Nursing Considerations

- Assess patient for signs and symptoms of angina, arrhythmias, and hypertension because phenylephrine may increase myocardial oxygen demand and the risk of proarrhythmias and blood pressure changes.
- **WARNING** Monitor patient with thyroid disease for increased sensitivity to catecholamines and possible thyrotoxicity or cardiotoxicity.
- Regularly evaluate effectiveness of hydrocodone and phenylephrine in relieving upper respiratory symptoms. Notify prescriber if symptoms persist or worsen.
- Take safety precautions as needed.
- Monitor patient's respiratory depth, effort, and rate. Notify prescriber immediately if respiratory rate drops below 10 breaths/ minute.
- **WARNING** Assess patient for evidence of physical and psychological dependence.

PATIENT TEACHING
- Instruct patient to use a calibrated measuring device to ensure accurate dose.
- Caution patient to take drug exactly as prescribed and not to

adjust dose or frequency without consulting prescriber.
- Urge patient to avoid alcohol and other antidepressants while taking hydrocodone and phenylephrine.
- Instruct patient to avoid hazardous activities until drug's CNS effects are known.
- Suggest that patient relieve dry mouth with frequent rinsing and use of sugarless gum or hard candy.
- To prevent constipation, encourage patient to consume plenty of fluids and high-fiber foods, if not contraindicated.
- Advise patient to notify prescriber if she becomes short of breath or has difficulty breathing or if she develops persistent or severe diarrhea, constipation or has difficulty urinating.
- Instruct patient to increase fluid intake (unless contraindicated) to help thin secretions.

hydrocodone bitartrate, phenylephrine hydrochloride, and guaifenesin

Atuss-G, Donatussin DC, Entex HC, Levall 5.0, Tussafed HC, Tussafed HCG

Class, Category, and Schedule

Chemical: Opioid and phenanthrene derivative (hydrocodone), sympathomimetic amine (phenylephrine), glyceryl guaiacolate (guaifenesin)
Therapeutic: Antitussive (hydrocodone), decongestant (phenyl-ephrine), expectorant (guaifenesin)
Pregnancy category: C
Controlled substance schedule: III

Indications and Dosages

▶ *To relieve cough and other upper respiratory symptoms related to the common cold and allergies*
SYRUP
Adults. 4 to 5 mg hydrocodone, 12 to 20 mg phenylephrine, and 100 to 200 mg guaifenesin (10 ml) every 4 to 6 hr.
ORAL SOLUTION
Adults. 5 to 10 mg hydrocodone, 7.5 to 20 mg phenylephrine, and 100 to 450 mg guaifenesin (5 or 10 ml depending on product) every 4 to 6 hr.

Contraindications

Hypersensitivity to hydrocodone, other opioids, bisulfites, phenyl-ephrine, guaifenesin, or their components; severe coronary artery disease or hypertension; significant respiratory depression; use within 14 days of MAO inhibitor therapy; ventricular tachycardia

---

Mechanism of Action

Hydrocodone suppresses cough by acting directly on opiate receptors in the medulla's cough center.

Phenylephrine stimulates alpha-adrenergic receptors and inhibits the intracellular enzyme adenyl cyclase, which in turn inhibits production of cAMP. Inhibition of cAMP causes arterial and venous constriction in the nasal passages, which decreases blood flow and mucosal edema caused by allergic response.

Guaifenesin increases fluid and mucus removal from the upper respiratory tract by increasing the volume of secretions and reducing their adhesiveness and surface tension.

Interactions

DRUGS

hydrocodone and phenylephrine

MAO inhibitors: Increased and prolonged cardiac stimulation, increased vasopressor effect, increased risk of severe cardiovascular and cerebrovascular effects, hyperpyrexia, and vomiting

hydrocodone

anticholinergics, paregoric: Possibly intensified anticholinergic adverse effects

antihypertensives, diuretics: Potentiated hypotensive effects

buprenorphine: Decreased effectiveness of hydrocodone

CNS depressants: Additive CNS effects

hydroxyzine: Increased hydrocodone analgesic effect; increased CNS depressant and hypotensive effects

metoclopramide: Possibly antagonized metoclopramide effects on GI *motility naloxone:* Anatagonized hydrocodone analgesic effect

naltrexone: Precipitated withdrawal symptoms in hydrocodone-dependent patients

neuromuscular blockers: Additive respiratory depressant effects

opioids: Additive CNS and respiratory depressants effects and hypotensive effects

phenylephrine

alpha blockers, haloperidol, loxapine, phenothiazines, thioxanthenes: Possibly decreased vasoconstrictor effect of phenylephrine

antihypertenisves, diuretics: Possibly decreased antihypertensive effects

atropine: Possibly enhanced vasopressor effect of phenylephrine
beta blockers: Decreased therapeutic effects of both drugs
bretylium: Possibly potentiated vaopressor effect and arrhythmias
doxapram: Increased vasopressor effect of both drugs
ergot alkaloids: Possibly cerebral blood vessel rupture, increased vasopressor effect, peripheral vascular ischemia, and gangrene (with ergotamine)
guanadrel, guanethidine: Increased vasopressor effect of phenylephrine, increased risk of severe hypertension and arrhythmias
hydrocarbon inhalation anesthetics: Increased risk of serious arrhythmias
maprotiline, tricyclic antidepressants: Increased risk of severe cardiovascular effects (including arrhythmias, hyperpyrexia, severe hypertension)
mecamylamine, methyldopa: Decreased hypotensive effects of these drugs, increased vasopressor effect of phenylephrine
nitrates: Possibly decreased vasopressor effect of phenylephrine and decreased antianginal effect of nitrates
oxytocin: Possibly severe, persistent hypertension
phenoxybenzamine: Decreased vasoconstrictor effect of phenylephrine, possibly hypotension and tachycardia
theophylline: Possibly enhanced toxicity (including cardiac toxicity)
thyroid hormones: Increased cardiovascular effects of each drug
ACTIVITIES
hydrocodone
alcohol use: Additive CNS effects

Adverse Reactions

CNS: Confusion, dizziness, drowsiness, euphoria, faintness, headache, insomnia, light-headedness, nervousness, paresthesia, restlessness, seizures, tiredness, tremor, weakness
CV: Angina, bradycardia, hypertension, hypotension, palpitations, peripheral vasoconstriction that may lead to necrosis or gangrene, tachycardia, ventricular arrhythmia
EENT: Blurred or double vision, dry mouth, laryngeal edema, laryngospasm
GI: Anorexia, constipation, nausea, paralytic ileus, toxic megacolon, vomiting
GU: Dysuria, frequent urination
RESP: Dyspnea, shortness of breath, slow or irregular breathing, wheezing
SKIN: Diaphoresis, facial flushing, pallor, pruritus, rash, urticaria
Other: Angioedema, anaphylaxis

Nursing Considerations

- Assess patient for signs and symptoms of angina, arrhythmias, and hypertension because phenylephrine may increase myocardial oxygen demand and the risk of proarrhythmias and blood pressure changes.
- **WARNING** Monitor patient with thyroid disease for increased sensitivity to catecholamines and possible thyrotoxicity or cardiotoxicity.
- Regularly evaluate effectiveness of hydrocodone, phenylephrine, and guaifenesin in relieving upper respiratory symptoms. Notify prescriber if symptoms persist or worsen.
- Take safety precautions as needed.
- Monitor respiratory depth, effort, and rate. Notify prescriber immediately if respiratory rate drops below 10 breaths/minute.
- Assess urine output; decreasing output may signal retention.
- **WARNING** Assess patient for evidence of physical and psychological dependence.

PATIENT TEACHING

- Instruct patient to use a calibrated measuring device to ensure accurate dose.
- Caution patient to take drug exactly as prescribed and not to adjust dose or frequency without consulting prescriber.
- Urge patient to avoid alcohol and other antidepressants while taking hydrocodone, phenylephrine, and guaifenesin.
- Instruct patient to avoid hazardous activities until drug's CNS effects are known.
- Suggest that patient relieve dry mouth with frequent rinsing and use of sugarless gum or hard candy.
- To help thin secretions and prevent constipation, urge patient to consume plenty of fluids and high-fiber foods, if not contraindicated.
- Advise patient to notify prescriber if he becomes short of breath or has difficulty breathing or if he develops persistent or severe diarrhea, constipation, or trouble urinating.

hydrocodone bitartrate, phenylephrine hydrochloride, and pyrilamine maleate
Codal-DH, Codimal DH, Dicomal-DH, Mintuss MR

Class, Category, and Schedule
Chemical: Opioid and phenanthrene derivative (hydrocodone),

sympathomimetic amine (phenylephrine), ethylenediamine derivative (pyrilamine)
Therapeutic: Antitussive (hydrocodone), decongestant (phenylephrine), antihistaminic (pyrilamine)
Pregnancy category: C
Schedule Category: III

Indications and Dosages
▶ *To relieve cough and upper respiratory symptoms caused by hay fever, other upper respiratory allergies, or allergic rhinitis*
SYRUP
Adults. 1.66 to 10 mg hydrocodone, 5 to 10 mg phenylephrine and 5 to 16.66 mg pyrilamine (5 to 10 ml depending on product) every 4 hr.

Mechanism of Action
Hydrocodone suppresses cough by acting directly on opiate receptors in the medulla's cough center.

Phenylephrine stimulates alpha-adrenergic receptors and inhibits the intracellular enzyme adenyl cyclase, which then inhibits production of cAMP. Inhibition of cAMP causes arterial and venous constriction in nasal passages, which decreases blood flow and mucosal edema caused by allergic response.

Pyrilamine competes with histamine for H_1 receptor sites, thereby antagonizing many histamine effects to reduce allergy signs and symptoms.

Contraindications
Breast-feeding; hypersensitivity to hydrocodone, other opioids, phenylephrine, pyrilamine, or their components; respiratory depression; severe asthma; upper airway obstruction; use of an MAO inhibitor within 14 days

Interactions
DRUGS
hydrocodone, phenylephrine, and pyrilamine
MAO inhibitors: Increased and prolonged cardiac stimulation, increased vasopressor effect, increased risk of severe cardiovascular and cerebrovascular effects, hyperpyrexia, and vomiting
hydrocodone and pyrilamine
anticholinergics, paregoric: Possibly intensified anticholinergic adverse effects
CNS depressants: Additive CNS effects
hydrocodone
antihypertensives, diuretics: Potentiated hypotensive effects

buprenorphine: Decreased hydrocodone effectiveness
hydroxyzine: Increased hydrocodone analgesic effect; increased CNS depressant and hypotensive effects
metoclopramide: Antagonized metoclopramide effect on GI motility
naloxone: Antagonized hydrocodone analgesic effect
naltrexone: Precipitated withdrawal symptoms in hydrocodone-dependent patients
neuromuscular blockers: Additive respiratory depressant effects
opioids: Additive CNS and respiratory depressants effects and hypotensive effects
tricyclic antidepressants: Possibly increased effect of either the antidepressant or hydrocodone

phenylephrine
alpha blockers, haloperidol, loxapine, phenothiazines, thioxanthenes: Possibly decreased vasoconstrictor effect of phenylephrine
antihypertenisves, diuretics: Possibly decreased antihypertensive effects
atropine: Possibly enhanced vasopressor effect of phenylephrine
beta blockers: Decreased therapeutic effects of both drugs
bretylium: Possibly potentiated vaopressor effect and arrhythmias
doxapram: Increased vasopressor effect of both drugs
ergot alkaloids: Possibly cerebral blood vessel rupture, increased vasopressor effect, peripheral vascular ischemia, and gangrene (with ergotamine)
guanadrel, guanethidine: Increased vasopressor effect of phenylephrine; increased risk of severe hypertension and arrhythmias
hydrocarbon inhalation anesthetics: Possibly serious arrhythmias
maprotiline, tricyclic antidepressants: Increased risk of severe cardiovascular effects (including arrhythmias, hyperpyrexia, severe hypertension)
mecamylamine, methyldopa: Decreased hypotensive effects of these drugs; increased vasopressor effect of phenylephrine
nitrates: Possibly decreased vasopressor effect of phenylephrine and decreased antianginal effect of nitrates
oxytocin: Possibly severe, persistent hypertension
phenoxybenzamine: Decreased vasoconstrictor effect of phenylephrine, possibly hypotension and tachycardia
theophylline: Possibly enhanced toxicity (including cardiac toxicity)
thyroid hormones: Increased cardiovascular effects of each drug

ACTIVITIES
hydrocodone and pyrilamine
alcohol use: Additive CNS effects

Adverse Reactions

CNS: Asthenia, anxiety, confusion, dizziness, depression, drowsiness, dyskinesia, euphoria, faintness, headache, insomnia, irritability, light-headedness, nervousness, paresthesia, restlessness, sedation, syncope, tiredness, tremor, vertigo, weakness

CV: Angina, bradycardia, hypertension, hypotension, orthostatic hypotension, palpitations, peripheral vasoconstriction that may lead to necrosis or gangrene, tachycardia, ventricular arrhythmias

ENDO: Decreased lactation, early menses, gynecomastia, hyperglycemia, hypoglycemia

EENT: Blurred vision; diplopia; dry mouth, pharynx, and respiratory passages; hypermetropia; increased lacrimation; labyrinthitis; laryngismus; mydriasis; nasal stuffiness; photophobia; tinnitus

GI: Abdominal distention or pain, acute pancreatitis, anorexia, constipation, diarrhea, dyspepsia, epigastric distress, esophageal reflux, increased appetite, nausea, vomiting

GU: Dysuria, increased libido, urinary frequency or hesitancy, urine retention, ureteral spasm

RESP: Dyspnea, respiratory depression, wheezing

SKIN: Dermatitis, diaphoresis, erythema, flushing, pruritus, rash, urticaria

Other: Drug fever, emotional or physical dependence

Nursing Considerations

- Use cautiously in patients with recent head injury and those with Addison's disease, mildly to moderately severe asthma or other chronic respiratory disease, cardiovascular disease, diabetes, hypertension, liver or renal impairment, narrow-angle glaucoma, prostatic hypertrophy, or thyroid imbalance.
- **WARNING** Monitor respiratory function because hydrocodone, phenylephrine, and pyrilamine may suppress cough reflex and cause thickening of bronchial secretions, aggravating such conditions as asthma and COPD. Rarely, it may depress respirations and induce apnea. Notify prescriber immediately if respiratory rate drops below 10 breaths/minute.
- Monitor patients who may be more susceptible to dizziness, sedation, and hypotension, such as the elderly.
- Regularly evaluate effectiveness of hydrocodone, phenylephrine, and pyrilamine in reducing cough and upper respiratory symptoms.
- Be aware that patient shouldn't have intradermal allergen tests within 72 hours of receiving drug because results may be altered.

PATIENT TEACHING
- Instruct patient to use a calibrated measuring device to ensure accurate dose.
- Urge patient to avoid alcohol and other antidepressants while taking hydrocodone, phenylephrine, and pyrilamine.
- Instruct patient to avoid hazardous activities until drug's CNS effects are known.
- Suggest that patient relieve dry mouth with frequent rinsing and use of sugarless gum or hard candy.
- Tell patient to take last dose of the day a few hours before bedtime if drug makes her nervous or restless.

hydrocodone bitartrate and potassium guaiacolsulfonate

Cotuss EX, Entuss, Hydron EX, Hydron KGS, Marcof Expectorant, Prolex DH

Class, Category, and Schedule

Chemical: Opioid and phenanthrene derivative (hydrocodone), unclassified (potassium guaiacolsulfonate)
Therapeutic: Antitussive (hydrocodone), expectorant (potassium guaiacolsulfonate
Pregnancy category: C
Controlled substance schedule: III

Indications and Dosages

▶ *To relieve cough caused by minor throat and bronchial irritation, especially when secretions are thick*
ORAL SOLUTION, SYRUP
Adults. 4.5 mg hydrocodone and 120 to 450 mg potassium guaiacolsulfonate (5 to 15 ml depending on product) every 4 to 6 hr or q.i.d. (depending on product).

Contraindications

Hyperkalemia; hypersensitivity or idiosyncractic reactions to hydrocodone, potassium guaiacolsulfonate, other opioids, or their components; respiratory depression

Interactions

DRUGS
hydrocodone
anticholinergics, paregoric: Possibly intensified anticholinergic adverse effects

antihypertensives, diuretics: Potentiated hypotensive effects
buprenorphine: Decreased hydrocodone effectiveness
CNS depressants: Additive CNS depression
hydroxyzine: Increased hydrocodone analgesic effect; increased
CNS depressant and hypotensive effects
MAO inhibitors: Increased and prolonged cardiac stimulation, increased vasopressor effect, increased risk of severe cardiovascular
and cerebrovascular effects, hyperpyrexia, vomiting
metoclopramide: Antagonized effect of metoclopramide on GI
motility
naloxone: Antagonized hydrocodone analgesic effect
naltrexone: Precipitated withdrawal symptoms in hydrocodone-
dependent patients
neuromuscular blockers: Additive respiratory depressant effects
opioids: Additive CNS and respiratory depressants effects and hypotensive effects
potassium guaiacolsulfonate
*drugs that increase potassium levels such as ACE inhibitors, potassium-
sparing diuretics, potassium-containing drugs, potassium supplements:* Increased risk of hyperkalemia
ACTIVITIES
hydrocodone
alcohol use: Additive CNS effects

Mechanism of Action
Hydrocodone suppresses cough by acting directly on opiate receptors in the
medulla's cough center.

  Potassium guaiacolsulfonate is thought to act by increasing the fluid volume in respiratory tract secretions. This decreases the viscosity of bronchial
secretions, making it easier to remove them from the respiratory tract.

Adverse Reactions
CNS: Coma, delirium, depression, disorientation, dizziness,
drowsiness, euphoria, hallucinations, headache, lack of coordination, lethargy, light-headedness, mental and physical impairment,
mood changes, restlessness, sedation, seizures, tremor
CV: Bradycardia, heart block, hypertension, orthostatic hypotension, palpitations, tachycardia
EENT: Altered taste, blurred vision, diplopia, dry mouth, laryngeal edema, laryngospasm, miosis
GI: Abdominal cramps and pain, anorexia, constipation, flatu-

lence, gastroesophageal reflux, ileus, indigestion, nausea, vomiting

GU: Decreased libido, difficult ejaculation, dysuria, impotence, oliguria, ureteral spasm, urinary incontinence, urine retention

MS: Muscle rigidity

RESP: Apnea, bronchoconstriction, bronchospasm, depressed cough reflex, respiratory depression

SKIN: Diaphoresis, flushing, pallor, pruritus, rash, urticaria

Other: Anaphylaxis, facial edema, hyperkalemia, physical and psychological dependence

Nursing Considerations

- Evaluate for therapeutic response, such as decreased cough. Notify prescriber if symptoms persist or worsen despite use of hydrocodone and potassium guaiacolsulfonate.
- Monitor respiratory depth, effort, and rate. Notify prescriber immediately if respiratory rate drops below 10 breaths/minute.
- Assess urine output; decreasing output may signal retention.
- **WARNING** Assess patient for evidence of physical and psychological dependence.

PATIENT TEACHING

- Instruct patient to take hydrocodone and potassium guaiacolsulfonate exactly as prescribed and not to increase dose or frequency without consulting prescriber.
- Advise patient to avoid alcohol or other CNS depressants while taking drug.
- To minimize nausea, suggest that patient take drug with food.
- Instruct patient to avoid hazardous activities until drug's CNS effects are known.
- Caution patient to get up slowly from a sitting or lying position.
- Advise patient to notify prescriber if she becomes short of breath or has difficulty breathing.

hydrocodone bitartrate and pseudoephedrine hydrochloride

Detussin, Histussin D, Pancof HC, P-V Tussin Tablets, Tyrodone

Class, Category, and Schedule

Chemical: Opioid and phenanthrene derivative (hydrocodone), sympathomimetic amine (pseudoephedrine)

Therapeutic: Antitussive (hydrocodone), decongestant (pseudoephedrine)

Pregnancy category: C
Controlled substance schedule: III

Indications and Dosages

▶ *To relieve cough and other symptoms caused by allergies and the common cold*

SYRUP

Adults. 3 to 6 mg hydrocodone and 15 to 60 mg pseudo-ephedrine (5 to 10 ml depending on product) q.i.d.

TABLETS

Adults. 5 mg hydrocodone and 60 mg pseudoephedrine (1 tablet) every 4 to 6 hr. *Maximum:* 4 doses daily.

Mechanism of Action

Hydrocodone suppresses cough by acting directly on opiate receptors in the medulla's cough center.

Pseudoephedrine acts on alpha$_1$-adrenergic receptors in the mucosa of the respiratory tract to produce vasoconstriction. This process shrinks swollen nasal mucous membranes; reduces tissue hyperemia, edema, and nasal congestion; and increases nasal airway patency. It also may increase drainage of sinus secretions and open obstructed eustachian ostia.

Contraindications

Hypersensitivity or idiosyncractic reactions to hydrocodone, other opioids, pseudoephedrine, or their components; hyperthyroidism; narrow-angle glaucoma; prostatic hypertrophy; respiratory depression; severe asthma, coronary artery disease or hypertension; upper airway obstruction; urine retention; use of an MAO inhibitor within 14 days

Interactions

DRUGS

hydrocodone and pseudoephedrine

MAO inhibitors: Increased and prolonged cardiac stimulation, increased vasopressor effect, increased risk of severe cardiovascular and cerebrovascular effects, hyperpyrexia, and vomiting

hydrocodone

anticholinergics, paregoric: Possibly intensified anticholinergic adverse effects

antidiarrheals: Increased risk of severe constipation

antihypertensives, diuretics: Potentiated hypotensive effects

buprenorphine: Decreased hydrocodone effectiveness

CNS depressants: Additive CNS depression

hydroxyzine: Increased hydrocodone analgesic effect; increased CNS depressant and hypotensive effects

metoclopramide: Antagonized effect of metoclopramide on GI motility

naloxone: Antagonized hydrocodone analgesic effect

naltrexone: Precipitated withdrawal symptoms in hydrocodone-dependent patients

neuromuscular blockers: Additive respiratory depressant effects

opioids: Additive CNS and respiratory depressants effects and hypotensive effects

pseudoephedrine

antacids: Increased pseudoephedrine absorption

antihypertensives, diuretics: Possibly decreased antihypertensive effects

beta blockers: Decreased therapeutic effects of both drugs

citrates: Possibly inhibited urinary pseudoephedrine excretion and prolonged duration of action

CNS stimulant, other sympathomimetics: Possibly increased additive CNS stimulation to excessive levels

cocaine (mucosal-local): Possibly increased cardiovascular effects of either drug and CNS stimulation

digoxin, levodopa: Increased risk of cardiac arrhythmias

hydrocarbon inhalation anesthetics: Increased risk of serious arrhythmias

kaolin: Decreased absorption of pseudoephedrine

nitrates: Reduced antianginal effects of nitrates

rauwolfia alkaloids: Possibly inhibited action of pseudoephedrine

thyroid hormones: Increased cardiovascular effects of both drugs

ACTIVITIES

hydrocodone

alcohol use: Additive CNS effects

Adverse Reactions

CNS: Confusion, dizziness, drowsiness, euphoria, faintness, headache, insomnia, light-headedness, nervousness, restlessness, seizures, tiredness, trembling, weakness

CV: Bradycardia, hypotension, palpitations, tachycardia

EENT: Blurred or double vision, dry mouth, laryngeal edema, laryngospasm

GI: Anorexia, constipation, nausea, paralytic ileus, toxic megacolon, vomiting

GU: Dysuria, frequent urination

RESP: Dyspnea, shortness of breath, slow or irregular breathing, wheezing
Skin: Diaphoresis, facial flushing, pallor, pruritus, rash, uriticaria
Other: Angioedema, atelectasis

Nursing Considerations

- Use cautiously in patients with hypertension, diabetes mellitus, ischemic heart disease, increased intraocular pressure, or renal impairment because of pseudoephedrine.
- Monitor renal function, as ordered, because pseudoephedrine is substantially excreted by the kidneys.
- Regularly evaluate effectiveness of hyrdocodone and pseudoephedrine in reducing cough and allergy symptoms.

PATIENT TEACHING

- Instruct patient to use a calibrated measuring device to ensure accurate dose of hydrocodone and pseudoephedrine.
- Urge patient to avoid alcohol and other antidepressants while taking hydrocodone and pseudoephedrine.
- Instruct patient to avoid hazardous activities until drug's CNS effects are known.
- Suggest that patient relieve dry mouth with frequent rinsing and use of sugarless gum or hard candy.
- Tell patient to take last dose of the day a few hours before bedtime if drug makes him nervous or restless.

hydrocodone bitartrate, pseudoephedrine hydrochloride, and potassium guaiacolsulfonate
Protuss-D

Class, Category, and Schedule
Chemical: Opioid and phenanthrene derivative (hydrocodone), sympathomimetic amine (pseudoephedrine), unclassified (potassium guaiacolsulfonate)
Therapeutic: Antitussive (hydrocodone), decongestant (pseudoephedrine), expectorant (potassium guaiacolsulfonate)
Pregnancy category: C
Controlled substance schedule: III

Indications and Dosages
▶ *To relieve cough and other symptoms caused by allergies and the common cold*

ORAL SOLUTION
Adults and children age 12 and over. 5 to 7.5 mg hydrocodone, 30 to 45 mg pseudoephedrine, and 300 to 450 mg potassium guaiacolsulfonate (5 to 7.5 ml) every 6 hr.
Children ages 6 to 12. 2.5 to 5 mg hydrocodone, 15 to 30 mg pseudoephedrine, and 150 to 300 mg potassium guaiacolsulfonate (2.5 to 5 ml) every 6 hr.
Children ages 2 to 6. 1.25 to 2.5 mg hydrocodone, 7.5 to 15 mg pseudoephedrine, and 75 to 150 mg potassium guaiacolsulfonate (1.25 to 2.5 ml) every 6 hr.

Mechanism of Action
Hydrocodone suppresses cough by directly acting on opiate receptors in the medulla's cough center.

Pseudoephedrine acts on alpha$_1$-adrenergic receptors in the mucosa of the respiratory tract to produce vasoconstriction. This process shrinks swollen nasal mucous membranes; reduces tissue hyperemia, edema, and nasal congestion; and increases nasal airway patency. It also may increase drainage of sinus secretions and open obstructed eustachian ostia.

Potassium guaiacolsulfonate is thought to act by increasing the fluid volume contained in respiratory tract secretions. This decreases the viscosity of bronchial secretions making it easier to remove them from the respiratory tract.

Contraindications
Hypersensitivity or idiosyncractic reactions to hydrocodone, other opioids, pseudoephedrine, potassium guaiacolsulfonate, or their components; hyperkalemia; hyperthyroidism; narrow-angle glaucoma; prostatic hypertrophy; respiratory depression; severe asthma, coronary artery disease or hypertension; upper airway obstruction, urine retention; use of an MAO inhibitor within 14 days

Interactions
DRUGS
hydrocodone and pseudoephedrine
MAO inhibitors: Increased and prolonged cardiac stimulation, increased vasopressor effect, increased risk of severe cardiovascular and cerebrovascular effects, hyperpyrexia, vomiting
hydrocodone
anticholinergics, paregoric: Possibly intensified anticholinergic adverse effects

antihypertensives, diuretics: Potentiated hypotensive effects

buprenorphine: Decreased hydrocodone effectiveness

CNS depressants: Additive CNS depression

hydroxyzine: Increased hydrocodone analgesic effect; increased CNS depressant and hypotensive effects

metoclopramide: Antagonized effect of metoclopramide on GI motility

naloxone: Antagonized hydrocodone analgesic effect

naltrexone: Precipitated withdrawal symptoms in hydrocodone-dependent patients

neuromuscular blockers: Additive respiratory depressant effects

opioids: Additive CNS and respiratory depressants effects and hypotensive effects

pseudoephedrine

antacids: Increased pseudoephedrine absorption

antihypertensives, diuretics: Possibly decreased antihypertensive effects

beta blockers: Decreased therapeutic effects of both drugs

citrates: Possibly inhibited urinary pseudoephedrine excretion and prolonged duration of action

CNS stimulant, other sympathomimetics: Possibly increased additive CNS stimulation to excessive levels

cocaine (mucosal-local): Possibly increased cardiovascular effects of either drug and CNS stimulation

digoxin, levodopa: Increased risk of cardiac arrhythmias

hydrocarbon inhalation anesthetics: Increased risk of serious arrhythmias

kaolin: Decreased absorption of pseudoephedrine

nitrates: Reduced antianginal effects of nitrates

rauwolfia alkaloids: Possibly inhibited action of pseudoephedrine

thyroid hormones: Increased cardiovascular effects of both drugs

potassium guaiacolsulfonate

drugs that increase potassium levels, such as ACE inhibitors, potassium-sparing diuretics, potassium-containing drugs, potassium supplements: Increased risk of hyperkalemia

ACTIVITIES

hydrocodone

alcohol use: Additive CNS effects

Adverse Reactions

CNS: Confusion, dizziness, drowsiness, euphoria, faintness, headache, insomnia, light-headedness, nervousness, restlessness, seizures, tiredness, trembling, weakness

CV: Bradycardia, hypotension, palpitations, tachycardia
EENT: Blurred or double vision, dry mouth, laryngeal edema, laryngospasm
GI: Anorexia, constipation, nausea, paralytic ileus, toxic megacolon, vomiting
GU: Dysuria, frequent urination
RESP: Dyspnea, shortness of breath, slow or irregular breathing, wheezing
Skin: Diaphoresis, facial flushing, pallor, pruritus, rash, uriticaria
Other: Angioedema, atelectasis, hyperkalemia

Nursing Considerations

- Use cautiously in patients with hypertension, diabetes mellitus, ischemic heart disease, increased intraocular pressure, or renal impairment because of pseudoephedrine.
- Monitor renal function, as ordered, because pseudoephedrine is substantially excreted by the kidneys.
- Regularly evaluate effectiveness of hyrdocodone, pseudoephedrine, and potassium guaiacolsulfonate in reducing cough and allergy symptoms.

PATIENT TEACHING

- Instruct patient to use a calibrated measuring device to ensure accurate dose of hydrocodone, pseudoephedrine, and potassium guaiacolsulfonate.
- Urge patient to avoid alcohol and other antidepressants while taking drug.
- Instruct patient to avoid hazardous activities until drug's CNS effects are known.
- Suggest that patient relieve dry mouth with frequent rinsing and use of sugarless gum or hard candy.
- Tell patient to take last dose of the day a few hours before bedtime if hydrocodone, pseudoephedrine, and potassium guaiacolsulfonate makes her nervous or restless.

ipratropium bromide and albuterol sulfate

Combivent, DuoNeb

Class and Category

Chemical: Quarternary N-methyl isopropyl derivative of noratropine (ipratropium); selective beta$_2$-adrenergic agonist, sympathomimetic (albuterol)

Therapeutic: Bronchodilator
Pregnancy category: C

Indications and Dosages

▶ *To treat bronchospasm in patients with COPD who need more than one bronchodilator*

INHALATION AEROSOL (COMBIVENT)

Adults. 2 inhalations (36 mcg ipratropium, 180 mcg albuterol base) q.i.d. and as needed. *Maximum:* 12 inhalations (216 mcg ipratropium, 1.08 grams albuterol base) in 24 hr.

INHALATION SOLUTION FOR NEBULIZER (DUONEB)

Adults. 3 ml (0.5 mg ipratropium, 2.5 mg albuterol base) q.i.d. *Maximum:* 2 additional 3-ml doses in 24 hr, p.r.n.

Mechanism of Action

Ipratropium prevents acetylcholine (after its release from cholinergic fibers) from attaching to muscarinic receptors on membranes of smooth-muscle cells. By blocking acetylcholine's effects in the bronchi and bronchioles, ipratropium relaxes smooth muscles and causes bronchodilation.

Albuterol attaches to beta$_2$ receptors on bronchial cell membranes, which stimulates the intracellular enzyme adenylate cyclase to convert adenosine triphosphate to cyclic adenosine monophosphate (cAMP). This reaction decreases intracellular calcium and increases intracellular cAMP. Together, these effects relax bronchial smooth-muscle cells and inhibit histamine release.

Contraindications

Hypersensitivity to albuterol, ipratropium, or their components; hypersensitivity to atropine or its derivatives; hypersensitivity to peanuts, soya lecithin, soybeans, or related products (with aerosol inhaler)

Interactions

DRUGS

anticholinergics, such as atropine: Possibly additive effects of ipratropium

beta blockers: Possibly mutual inhibition of therapeutic effects

MAO inhibitors, tricyclic antidepressants: Possibly potentiation of albuterol's adverse cardiovascular effects

non–potassium-sparing diuretics, such as loop and thiazide diuretics: Increased risk of hypokalemia

sympathomimetic bronchodilators, such as theophylline: Increased risk of adverse cardiovascular effects

Adverse Reactions

CNS: Drowsiness, headache, nervousness, tremor
CV: Chest pain, increased heart rate, palpitations
EENT: Acute eye pain, altered taste, blurred vision, dry mouth, pharyngitis, sinusitis, sore throat, voice alterations, worsened angle-closure glaucoma
GI: Constipation, diarrhea, indigestion, nausea
GU: UTI
MS: Back pain, leg cramps, muscle aches
RESP: Bronchitis, cough, exacerbation of COPD, paradoxical bronchospasm, pneumonia, upper respiratory tract infection, wheezing
SKIN: Flushing
Other: Hypokalemia

Nursing Considerations

- Prime the aerosol inhaler with three priming sprays if using it for the first time or if it hasn't been used for more than 24 hours.
- As prescribed, administer nebulized dose using a mouthpiece or properly fitted face mask attached to a jet nebulizer connected to an air compressor with adequate airflow.
- **WARNING** Avoid spraying drug directly into patient's eyes because it may cause vision disturbances. In a patient with angle-closure glaucoma, spraying drug directly into his eyes may precipitate an acute attack or worsen the condition.
- Monitor urine output if patient has a history of prostatic hyperplasia or bladder-neck obstruction because drug may aggravate these conditions and cause urine retention.
- Monitor heart rate and rhythm and blood pressure often in patients with a history of arrhythmias, coronary artery insufficiency, or hypertension because the drug may cause adverse cardiovascular effects in these patients. If adverse cardiovascular effects occur, expect to discontinue drug.
- Monitor serum potassium level because drug may cause transient hypokalemia.
- Although immediate hypersensitivity reactions are rare, monitor patient for angioedema, bronchospasm, oropharyngeal edema, pruritus, rash, urticaria, and anaphylaxis.

PATIENT TEACHING

- Teach patient how to use inhaler or nebulizer properly. Instruct him to shake aerosol inhaler vigorously for 10 seconds before each inhalation and to wait 1 minute between inhalations.

- Instruct patient to rinse mouth after each nebulizer or inhaler treatment to help minimize throat dryness and irritation.
- Advise patient to keep drug out of his eyes because it may cause irritation or blurred vision. If drug contacts his eyes, instruct patient to flush them with cool tap water and to contact prescriber immediately.
- Caution patient not to exceed prescribed dose because of possible serious adverse reactions or death. Advise patient to contact prescriber immediately if doses become less effective.
- Advise patient to contact prescriber before using other inhaled drugs.

loratadine and pseudoephedrine sulfate

Claritin-D 12 Hour, Claritin-D 24 Hour

Class and Category

Chemical: Azatadine devirative (loratadine), sympathomimetic amine (pseudoephedrine)
Therapeutic: Antihistamine (loratadine), decongestant (pseudoephedrine)
Pregnancy category: B

Indications and Dosages

▶ *To relieve symptoms of seasonal allergic rhinitis*
E.R. TABLETS (CLARITIN-D 12)
Adults and children age 12 and over. 5 mg loratadine and 120 mg pseudoephedrine (1 tablet) every 12 hr.
DOSAGE ADJUSTMENT For patients with renal impairment (creatinine clearance less than 30 ml/min/1.73 m^2) dosage reduced to 5 mg loratadine and 120 mg psuedoephedrine (1 tablet) every 24 hr.
E.R. TABLETS (CLARITIN-D 24)
Adults and children age 12 and over. 10 mg loratadine and 240 mg pseudoephedrine (1 tablet) every 24 hr.
DOSAGE ADJUSTMENT For patients with renal impairment (creatinine clearance less than 30 ml/min/1.73 m^2) dosage reduced to 10 mg loratadine and 240 mg psuedoephedrine (1 tablet) every 48 hr.

Contraindications

Hepatic insufficiency; history of dysphagia or abnormal esophageal peristalsis; hypersensitivity or idiosyncractic reactions to loratadine, pseudoephedrine, or their components; narrow-angle glaucoma; severe coronary artery disease or hypertension; urine retention; use of an MAO inhibitor within 14 days

---

Mechanism of Action

Loratadine competes with histamine for histamine H_1 receptor sites on effector cells and antagonizes the vasodilator effect of endogenously released histamine. This prevents vascular engorgement, mucosal edema, profuse watery secretion, local irritation, and sneezing that normally result from histamine action on afferent nerve terminals in nasal passages.

Pseudoephedrine acts on alpha$_1$-adrenergic receptors in the mucosa of the respiratory tract to produce vasoconstriction. This process shrinks swollen nasal mucous membranes; reduces tissue hyperemia, edema, and nasal congestion; and increases nasal airway patency. It also may increase drainage of sinus secretions and open obstructed eustachian ostia.

Interactions
DRUGS
loratadine
barbiturates, CNS depressants, tricyclic antidepressants: Additive effects
pseudoephedrine
antacids: Increased pseudoephedrine absorption
beta blockers, diuretics, methyldopa, mecamylamine, reserpine, veratum alkaloids: Decreased antihypertensive effects of these agents
citrates: Possibly inhibited urinary excretion and prolonged duration of action of pseudoephedrine
CNS stimulant, other sympathomimetics: Possibly increased additive CNS stimulation to excessive levels
cocaine (mucosal-local): Possibly increased cardiovascular effects of either drug and CNS stimulation
digoxin, levodopa: Increased risk of cardiac arrhythmias
hydrocarbon inhalation anesthetics: POssibly serious arrhythmias
kaolin: Decreased pseudoephedrine absorptino
MAO inhibitors: Increased and prolonged cardiac stimulation, increased vasopressor effect, increased risk of severe cardiovascular and cerebrovascular effects, hyperpyrexia, vomiting
nitrates: Reduced antianginal effects of nitrates
rauwolfia alkaloids: Possibly inhibited pseudoephedrine action
thyroid hormones: Increased cardiovascular effects of both drugs
ACTIVITIES
loratadine
alcohol use: Additive effects

Adverse Reactions

CNS: Dizziness, fatigue, headache, insomnia, light-headedness, nervousness, restlessness, seizures, somnolence, trembling, weakness

CV: Palpitations, tachycardia

EENT: Dry mouth, pharyngitis

ENDO: Dysmenorrhea

GI: Anorexia, nausea, vomiting

GU: Dysuria, urine retention

RESP: Bronchospasm, coughing, dyspnea

SKIN: Diaphoresis, pallor

Nursing Considerations

- Be aware that because a previously marketed formulation of loratadine and pseudoephedrine caused esophageal obstruction and perforation, the current formulation of the drug isn't recommended for patients who have a history of trouble swallowing tablets or who have been diagnosed with upper-GI narrowing or abnormal esophageal peristalsis.
- Use fexofenadine and pseudoephedrine cautiously in patients who have diabetes, hypertension, hyperthyroidism, increased intraocular pressure, ischemic heart disease, prostatic hypertrophy, or renal disease because of the effects of pseudoephedrine.
- Monitor elderly patients closely because they are more prone to developing adverse effects.
- Monitor renal function, as ordered, because pseudoephedrine is substantially excreted by the kidneys.
- Regularly evaluate effectiveness of loratadine and pseudoephedrine in relieving seasonal allergic rhinitis.
- Be aware that patient shouldn't have intradermal allergen tests within 4 days of receiving drug because test results may be altered.

PATIENT TEACHING

- Instruct patients to take loratadine and pseudoephedrine with a full glass of water.
- Urge patient to avoid alcohol, other antidepressants, and OTC drugs containing other antihistamines or sympathomimetics while taking loratadine and pseudoephedrine.
- Instruct patient to avoid hazardous activities until drug's CNS effects are known.
- Suggest that patient relieve dry mouth with frequent rinsing and use of sugarless gum or hard candy.

phenylephrine hydrochloride and chlorpheniramine maleate
Dallergy-JR, Ed A-Hist

phenylephrine tannate and chlorpheniramine tannate
Ed A-Hist, Rescon JR, Rynatan, Rynatan Pediatric

Class and Category
Chemical: Sympathomimetic amine (phenylephrine), propylamine derivative (chlorpheniramine)
Therapeutic: Decongestant (phenylephrine), antihistaminic (chlorpheniramine)
Pregnancy category: C

Indications and Dosages
▶ *To provide symptomatic relief of nasal congestion caused by the common cold, sinusitis, allergic rhinitis, and other upper respiratory tract conditions*

ER CAPSULES (DALLERGY-JR)
Adults and children age 12 and over. 40 mg phenylephrine and 8 mg chlorpheniramine (1 capsule) every 12 hr.
Children ages 6 to 12. 20 mg phenylephrine and 4 mg chlorpheniramine (1 capsule) every 12 hr.

E.R. TABLETS (ED A-HIST, RESCON JR)
Adults and children age 12 and over. 20 to 40 mg phenylephrine and 4 to 8 mg chlorpheniramine (1 to 2 tablets) every 12 hr.
Children ages 6 to 12. 20 mg phenylephrine and 4 mg chlorpheniramine (1 tablet) every 12 hr.

SUSPENSION (RYNATAN, RYNATAN PEDIATRIC)
Adults and children age 6 and over. 5 to 10 mg phenylephrine and 4.5 to 9 mg chlorpheniramine (5 to 10 ml) every 12 hr.
Children ages 2 to 6. 2.5 to 5 mg phenylephrine and 2.25 to 4.5 mg chlorpheniramine (2.5 to 5 ml) every 12 hr.

Contraindications
Breast-feeding, hypersensitivity to phenylephrine, chlorpheniramine or their components; use of an MAO inhibitor within 14 days

Mechanism of Action

Phenylephrine stimulates alpha-adrenergic receptors and inhibits activity of the intracellular enzyme adenyl cyclase, which then inhibits production of cAMP. The inhibition of cAMP causes arterial and venous constriction in nasal passages, which decreases blood flow and mucosal edema caused by an allergic response.

Chlorpheniramine competes with histamine for H_1 receptor sites, thereby antagonizing many histamine effects to reduce allergy signs and symptoms.

Interactions
DRUGS
phenylephrine and chlorpheniramine
MAO inhibitors: Possibly prolonged and intensified anticholinergic effects of chlorpheniramine and overall effects of phenylephrine
phenylephrine
alpha blockers, haloperidol, loxapine, phenothiazines, thioxanthenes: Possibly decreased vasoconstrictor effect of phenylephrine
antihypertenisves, diuretics: Possibly decreased antihypertensive effects
atropine: Possibly enhanced vasopressor effect of phenylephrine
beta blockers: Decreased therapeutic effects of both drugs
bretylium: Possibly potentiated vaopressor effect and arrhythmias
doxapram: Increased vasopressor effect of both drugs
ergot alkaloids: Possibly cerebral blood vessel rupture, increased vasopressor effect, peripheral vascular ischemia, and gangrene (with ergotamine)
guanadrel, guanethidine: Increased vasopressor effect of phenylephrine, increased risk of severe hypertension and arrhythmias
hydrocarbon inhalation anesthetics: Increased risk of serious arrhythmias
maprotiline, tricyclic antidepressants: Increased risk of severe cardiovascular effects (including arrhythmias, hyperpyrexia, severe hypertension)
mecamylamine, methyldopa: Decreased hypotensive effects of these drugs; increased vasopressor effect of phenylephrine
nitrates: Possibly decreased vasopressor effect of phenylephrine and decreased antianginal effect of nitrates
oxytocin: Possibly severe, persistent hypertension
phenoxybenzamine: Decreased vasoconstrictor effect of phenylephrine, possibly hypotension, and tachycardia

theophylline: Possibly enhanced toxicity (including cardiac toxicity)

thyroid hormones: Increased cardiovascular effects of each drug

chlorpheniramine

CNS depressants: Additive CNS effects

phenytoin: Possibly increased serum phenytoin levels and toxicity

ACTIVITIES

chlorpheniramine

alcohol use: Additive CNS effects

Adverse Reactions

CNS: Dizziness, drowsiness, excitation (children), headache, insomnia, nervousness, paresthesia, restlessness, sedation, somnolence, tremor, weakness

CV: Angina, bradycardia, hypertension, hypotension, palpitations, peripheral vasoconstriction that may lead to necrosis or gangrene, tachycardia, ventricular arrhythmias

EENT: Dry mouth

GI: Anorexia, constipation, nausea, vomiting

GU: Urinary hesitancy, urine retention

RESP: Asthma exacerbation, dyspnea

Nursing Considerations

- Use cautiously in patients with cardiovascular disease, diabetes, hypertension, hyperthyroidism, narrow-angle glaucoma, and prostatic hypertrophy.
- Monitor children for excitation and elderly patients for dizziness, sedation, and hypotension; such patients may have an increased risk for these effects.
- Regularly evaluate effectiveness of phenylephrine and chlorpheniramine in reducing nasal congestion.
- Be aware that patient shouldn't have intradermal allergen tests within 72 hours of receiving drug because results may be altered.

PATIENT TEACHING

- Instruct patient to use a calibrated measuring device when using suspension form of phenylephrine and chlorpheniramine to ensure accurate dose.
- Urge patient to avoid alcohol and other antidepressants while taking phenylephrine and chlorpheniramine.
- Instruct patient to avoid hazardous activities until drug's CNS effects are known.
- Suggest that patient relieve dry mouth with frequent rinsing and use of sugarless gum or hard candy.

phenylephrine hydrochloride, chlorpheniramine tannate, and guaifenesin
Decolate, Donatussin

Class and Category
Chemical: Sympathomimetic amine (phenylephrine), propylamine derivative (chlorpheniramine), glyceryl guaiacolate (guaifenesin)
Therapeutic: Decongestant (phenylephrine), antihistaminic (chlorpheniramine), expectorant (guaifenesin)
Pregnancy category: C

Indications and Dosages
▶ *To provide symptomatic relief of upper respiratory symptoms caused by the common cold, sinusitis, allergic rhinitis, and other upper respiratory tract conditions*
TABLETS
Adults. 5 mg phenylephrine, 4 mg chlorpheniramine, and 100 mg guaifenesin (1 tablet) t.i.d. or q.i.d.
ORAL SOLUTION (DROPS)
Children ages 1 to 2. 2 to 4 mg phenylephrine, 1 to 2 mg chlorpheniramine, and 20 to 40 mg guaifenesin (1 to 2 ml) every 4 to 6 hr.
Children ages 6 months to 1 year. 1 to 2 mg phenylephrine, 0.6 to 1 mg chlorpheniramine, and 10 to 20 mg guaifenesin (0.6 to 1 ml) every 4 to 6 hr.
Infants ages 3 to 6 months. 0.3 to 0.6 ml (1 ml, containing 2 mg phenylephrine, 1 mg chlorpheniramine, and 20 mg guaifenesin) every 4 to 6 hr.
Infants under age 3 months. 2 to 3 drops/month of age (1 ml containing 2 mg phenylephrine, 1 mg chlorpheniramine, and 20 mg guaifenesin) every 4 to 6 hr.

Mechanism of Action
Phenylephrine stimulates alpha-adrenergic receptors and inhibits the intracellular enzyme adenyl cyclase, which then inhibits production of cAMP. Inhibition of cAMP causes arterial and venous constriction in nasal passages, which decreases blood flow and mucosal edema caused by allergic response.

Chlorpheniramine competes with histamine for H_1 receptor sites, thereby antagonizing many histamine effects to reduce allergy signs and symptoms.

Guaifenesin increases fluid and mucus removal from upper respiratory tract by increasing secretions and reducing their adhesiveness and surface tension.

Contraindications

Breast-feeding, hypersensitivity to phenylephrine, chlorpheniramine, guaifenesin, or their components; use of MAO inhibitors
within 14 days

Interactions

DRUGS

phenylephrine and chlorpheniramine

MAO inhibitors: Possibly prolonged and intensified anticholinergic
effects of chlorpheniramine and overall effects of phenylephrine

phenylephrine

alpha blockers, haloperidol, loxapine, phenothiazines, thioxanthenes:
Possibly decreased vasoconstrictor effect of phenylephrine

antihypertenisves, diuretics: Possibly decreased antihypertensive effects

atropine: Possibly enhanced vasopressor effect of phenylephrine

beta blockers: Decreased therapeutic effects of both drugs

bretylium: Possibly potentiated vaopressor effect and arrhythmias

doxapram: Increased vasopressor effect of both drugs

ergot alkaloids: Possibly cerebral blood vessel rupture, increased vasopressor effect, peripheral vascular ischemia, and gangrene (with
ergotamine)

guanadrel, guanethidine: Increased vasopressor effect of phenylephrine, increased risk of severe hypertension and arrhythmias

hydrocarbon inhalation anesthetics: Possibly serious arrhythmias

maprotiline, tricyclic antidepressants: Increased risk of severe cardiovascular effects (including arrhythmias, hyperpyrexia, severe hypertension)

mecamylamine, methyldopa: Decreased hypotensive effects of these
drugs, increased vasopressor effect of phenylephrine

nitrates: Possibly decreased vasopressor effect of phenylephrine
and decreased antianginal effect of nitrates

oxytocin: Possibly severe, persistent hypertension

phenoxybenzamine: Decreased vasoconstrictor effect of phenylephrine, possibly hypotension and tachycardia

theophylline: Possibly enhanced toxicity (including cardiac toxicity)

thyroid hormones: Increased cardiovascular effects of each drug

chlorpheniramine

CNS depressants: Additive CNS effects

phenytoin: Possibly increased serum phenytoin levels and toxicity

ACTIVITIES

chlorpheniramine

alcohol use: Additive CNS effects

Adverse Reactions

CNS: Dizziness, drowsiness, excitation (children), headache, insomnia, nervousness, paresthesia, restlessness, sedation, tremor, weakness

CV: Angina, bradycardia, hypertension, hypotension, palpitations, peripheral vasoconstriction that may lead to necrosis or gangrene, tachycardia, ventricular arrhythmias

EENT: Dry mouth

GI: Constipation, nausea, vomiting

GU: Urinary hesitancy, urine retention

RESP: Dyspnea

SKIN: Rash, urticaria

Nursing Considerations

- Use cautiously in patients with cardiovascular disease, diabetes, hypertension, hyperthyroidism, narrow-angle glaucoma, or prostatic hypertrophy.
- Monitor patients who may be more susceptible to dizziness, sedation, and hypotension, such as the elderly.
- Regularly evaluate effectiveness of phenylephrine, chlorpheniramine, and guaifenesin in reducing upper respiratory symptoms.
- Be aware that patient shouldn't have intradermal allergen tests within 72 hours of receiving drug because results may be altered.

PATIENT TEACHING

- Instruct patient to take each dose with a full glass of water.
- Urge patient to avoid alcohol and other antidepressants while taking phenylephrine, chlorpheniramine, and guaifenesin.
- Instruct patient to avoid hazardous activities until drug's CNS effects are known.
- Suggest that patient relieve dry mouth with frequent rinsing and use of sugarless gum or hard candy.
- Instruct patient to increase fluid intake (unless contraindicated) to help thin secretions.

phenylephrine hydrochloride, chlorpheniramine maleate, and methscopolamine nitrate

AH-Chew, D.A. Chewable, Dallergy, Dehistine Syrup, DriHist SR, Duradryl, Duradryl JR, Dura-Vent/DA, Ex-Histine, Extendryl, Extendryl JR, Extendryl SR, Hista-Vent DA, OMNhist L.A., Pre-Hist-D

Class and Category

Chemical: Sympathomimetic amine (phenylephrine), alkylamine derivative (chlorpheniramine), hyoscine methobromide (methscopolamine)

Therapeutic: Decongestant (phenylephrine), antihistaminic (chlorpheniramine), anticholinergic (methscopolamine)

Pregnancy category: C

Indications and Dosages

▶ *To relieve nasal congestion caused by the common cold, sinusitis, allergic rhinitis, and other upper respiratory tract conditions*

SYRUP

Adults and children age 12 and over. 10 to 20 mg phenylephrine, 2 to 4 mg chlorpheniramine, and 1.25 or 2.5 mg methscopolamine (5 or 10 ml depending on product) every 4 to 6 hr. *Maximum:* 4 doses daily.

Children ages 6 to 12. 10 mg phenylephrine, 2 mg chlorpheniramine, and 0.625 mg methscopolamine (5 ml) every 4 to 6 hr.

CHEWABLE TABLETS

Adults and children age 12 and over. 10 to 20 mg phenylephrine, 4 to 8 mg chlorpheniramine and 1.25 to 2.5 mg methscopolamine (1 or 2 tablets depending on product) every 4 hr.

Children age 6 to 12. 10 mg phenylephrine, 4 mg chlorpheniramine, and 1.25 mg methscopolamine (1 tablet) every 4 hr.

TABLETS

Adults and children age 12 and over. 10 mg phenylephrine, 4 mg chlorpheniramine, and 1.25 mg methscopolamine (1 tablet) every 4 to 6 hr. *Maximum:* 4 tablets daily.

Children ages 6 to 12. 5 mg phenylephrine, 2 mg chlorpheniramine, and 0.625 mg methscopolamine (½ tablet) every 4 to 6 hr.

E.R. TABLETS

Adults. 20 mg phenylephrine, 8 to 12 mg chlorpheniramine, and 2.5 mg methscopolamine (1 tablet) every 12 hr.

Children ages 6 to 12. 10 mg phenylephrine, 4 to 6 mg chlorpheniramine, and 1.25 mg methscopolamine (½ tablet) every 12 hr.

E.R. CAPSULES

Adults and children age 12 and over. 20 mg phenylephrine, 8 to 12 mg chlorpheniramine, and 2.5 mg methscopolamine (1 capsule) every 12 hr.

Contraindications

Angle-closure glaucoma; breast-feeding; cardiac disease, such as arrhythmias, congestive heart failure, coronary artery disease, and mitral stenosis; hemorrhage with hemodynamic instability; hepatic dysfunction; hypersensitivity to phenylephrine, chlorpheniramine, methscopolamine, or their components; ileus; intestinal atony; myasthenia gravis; myocardial ishcemia; obstructive GI or uropathic disease; prostatic hypertrophy; reflux esophagitis; renal impairment; tachycardia; toxic megacolon; ulcerative colitis; use of an MAO inhibitor within 14 days

---

Mechanism of Action

Phenylephrine stimulates alpha-adrenergic receptors and inhibits the intracellular enzyme adenyl cyclase, which then inhibits production of cAMP. Inhibition of cAMP causes arterial and venous constriction in nasal passages, which decreases blood flow and mucosal edema caused by allergic response.

Chlorpheniramine competes with histamine for H_1 receptor sites, thereby antagonizing many histamine effects to reduce allergy signs and symptoms.

Methscopolamine competitively inhibits acetylcholine at autonomic postganglionic cholinergic receptors. Because the most sensitive receptors are in the salivary, bronchial, and sweat glands, this action reduces secretions from these glands. It also reduces nasal, oropharyngeal, and bronchial secretions and decreases airway resistance by relaxing smooth muscles in the bronchi and bronchioles.

Interactions

DRUGS

phenylephrine and chlorpheniramine

MAO inhibitors: Possibly prolonged and intensified anticholinergic effects of chlorpheniramine and overall effects of phenylephrine

chlorpheniramine and methscopolamine

anticholinergics (other): Possibly intensified anticholinergic effects
CNS depressants: Additive CNS effects

phenylephrine

alpha blockers, haloperidol, loxapine, phenothiazines, thioxanthenes: Possibly decreased vasoconstrictor effect of phenylephrine
antihypertenisves, diuretics: Possibly decreased antihypertensive effects
atropine: Possibly enhanced vasopressor effect of phenylephrine
beta blockers: Decreased therapeutic effects of both drugs
bretylium: Possibly potentiated vaopressor effect and arrhythmias
doxapram: Increased vasopressor effect of both drugs
ergot alkaloids: Possibly cerebral blood vessel rupture, increased va-

sopressor effect, peripheral vascular ischemia, and gangrene (with ergotamine)

guanadrel, guanethidine: Increased vasopressor effect of phenylephrine; increased risk of severe hypertension and arrhythmias

hydrocarbon inhalation anesthetics: Increased risk of serious arrhythmias

maprotiline, tricyclic antidepressants: Increased risk of severe cardiovascular effects (including arrhythmias, hyperpyrexia, severe hypertension)

mecamylamine, methyldopa: Decreased hypotensive effects of these drugs, increased vasopressor effect of phenylephrine

nitrates: Possibly decreased vasopressor effect of phenylephrine and decreased antianginal effect of nitrates

oxytocin: Possibly severe, persistent hypertension

phenoxybenzamine: Decreased vasoconstrictor effect of phenylephrine; possibly hypotension and tachycardia

theophylline: Possibly enhanced toxicity (including cardiac toxicity)

thyroid hormones: Increased cardiovascular effects of each drug

chlorpheniramine

phenytoin: Possibly increased serum phenytoin level and toxicity

methscopolamine

adsorbent antidiarrheals, antacids: Decreased absorption and therapeutic effects of methscopolamine

antimyasthenics: Possibly reduced intestinal motility

haloperidol: Decreased antipsychotic effect of haloperidol

ketoconazole: Decreased ketoconazole absorption

lorazepam (parenteral): Possibly hallucinations, irrational behavior, and sedation

metoclopramide: Possibly antagonized effect of metoclopramide on GI motility

opioid analgesics: Increased risk of severe constipation and ileus

potassium chloride: Possibly increased severity of potassium chloride–induced GI lesions

sildenafil, tadalafil, vardenafil: Possibly increased risk of hypotension

urinary alkalizers (antacids, carbonic anhydrase inhibitors, citrates, sodium bicarbonate): Delayed excretion of methscopolamine, possibly leading to increased therapeutic and adverse effects

ACTIVITIES

chlorpheniramine and methscopolamine

alcohol use: Additive CNS effects

Adverse Reactions

CNS: Anxiety, dizziness, drowsiness, euphoria, fear, headache, in-

somnia, irritability, memory loss, nervousness, paradoxical stimu-
lation, paresthesia, restlessness, sedation, tremor, weakness
CV: Angina, bradycardia, hypertension, hypotension, palpitations,
peripheral vasoconstriction that may lead to necrosis or gangrene,
tachycardia, ventricular arrhythmias
EENT: Blurred vision; dry eyes, mouth, nose, and throat; mydria-
sis
GI: Constipation, dysphagia, nausea, vomiting
GU: Urinary hesitancy, urine retention
RESP: Dyspnea
SKIN: Decreased sweating, dry skin, flushing

Nursing Considerations

• Use phenylephrine, chlorpheniramine, and methoscopolamine
  cautiously in patients with diabetes, hypertension, and hyperthyroidism.
• Monitor patients who may be more susceptible to dizziness, sedation, and hypotension, such as the elderly.
• Assess patient for bladder distention and monitor urine output
  because methscopolamine's antimuscarinic effects can cause
  urine retention.
• Regularly evaluate drug effects on upper respiratory symptoms.
• Be aware that patient shouldn't have intradermal allergen tests
  within 72 hours of receiving drug because results may be altered.

PATIENT TEACHING
• Instruct patient to use a calibrated measuring device when using liquid form of phenylephrine, chlorpheniramine, and methscopolamine to ensure accurate dose.
• Urge patient to avoid alcohol, other antidepressants, and OTC
  cough and cold preparations without consulting prescriber first
  while taking drug.
• Instruct patient to avoid hazardous activities until drug's CNS
  effects are known.
• Suggest that patient relieve dry mouth with frequent rinsing
  and use of sugarless gum or hard candy and to use lubricating
  eye drops for dry eyes.

phenylephrine hydrochloride, chlorpheniramine maleate, and phenyltoloxamine citrate

Comhist, Nalex-A

Class and Category

Chemical: Sympathomimetic amine (phenylephrine), propylamine derivative (chlorpheniramine), ethanolamine derivative (phenyltoloxamine)

Therapeutic: Decongestant (phenylephrine), antihistamines (chlorpheniramine, phenyltoloxamine)

Pregnancy category: C

Indications and Dosages

▶ *To relieve nasal congestion caused by the common cold, sinusitis, allergic rhinitis, and other upper respiratory tract conditions*

TABLETS

Adults. 10 to 20 mg phenylephrine, 2 to 4 mg chlorpheniramine, and 25 to 50 mg phenyltoloxamine (1 to 2 tablets) every 8 hr.

E.R. TABLETS

Adults and children age 12 and over. 10 to 20 mg phenylephrine, 2 to 4 mg chlorpheniramine, and 20 to 40 mg phenyltoloxamine (½ to 1 tablet) every 8 to 12 hr.

Children ages 6 to 12. 10 mg phenylephrine, 2 mg chlorpheniramine, and 20 mg phenyltoloxamine (½ tablet) every 8 to 12 hr.

SOLUTION (NALEX A)

Adults and children age 12 and over. 10 mg phenylephrine, 5 mg chlorpheniramine, and 15 mg phenyltoloxamine (10 ml) every 4 hr.

Children ages 6 to 12. 5 mg phenylephrine, 2.5 mg chlorpheniramine, and 7.5 mg phenyltoloxamine (5 ml) every 4 hr.

Children up to age 6. 1.25 to 2.5 mg phenylephrine, 0.625 to 1.25 mg chlorpheniramine, and 1.87 to 3.75 mg phenyltoloxamine (1.25 to 2.5 ml) every 4 hr.

Mechanism of Action

Phenylephrine stimulates alpha-adrenergic receptors and inhibits the intracellular enzyme adenyl cyclase, which then inhibits production of cAMP. Inhibition of cAMP causes arterial and venous constriction in nasal passages, which decreases blood flow and mucosal edema caused by allergic response.

Chlorpheniramine and phenyltoloxamine compete with histamine for H_1 receptor sites, thereby antagonizing many histamine effects to reduce allergy signs and symptoms.

Contraindications

Breast-feeding, hypersensitivity to phenylephrine, chlorpheniramine, phenyltoloxamine, or their components; use of an MAO inhibitor within 14 days

Interactions

phenylephrine, chlorpheniramine, and phenyltoloxamine

MAO inhibitors: Increased and prolonged cardiac stimulation, increased vasopressor effect, increased risk of severe cardiovascular and cerebrovascular effects, hyperpyrexia, and vomiting

chlorpheniramine and phenyltoloxamine

CNS depressants: Additive CNS effects

phenytoin: Possibly increased serum phenytoin levels and toxicity

phenylephrine

alpha blockers, haloperidol, loxapine, phenothiazines, thioxanthenes: Possibly decreased vasoconstrictor effect of phenylephrine

antihypertenisves, diuretics: Possibly decreased antihypertensive effects

atropine: Possibly enhanced vasopressor effect of phenylephrine

beta blockers: Decreased therapeutic effects of both drugs

bretylium: Possibly potentiated vaopressor effect and arrhythmias

doxapram: Increased vasopressor effect of both drugs

ergot alkaloids: Possibly cerebral blood vessel rupture, increased vasopressor effect, peripheral vascular ischemia, and gangrene (with ergotamine)

guanadrel, guanethidine: Increased vasopressor effect of phenylephrine, increased risk of severe hypertension and arrhythmias

hydrocarbon inhalation anesthetics: Increased risk of serious arrhythmias

maprotiline, tricyclic antidepressants: Increased risk of severe cardiovascular effects (including arrhythmias, hyperpyrexia, severe hypertension)

mecamylamine, methyldopa: Decreased hypotensive effects of these drugs, increased vasopressor effect of phenylephrine

nitrates: Possibly decreased vasopressor effect of phenylephrine and decreased antianginal effect of nitrates

oxytocin: Possibly severe, persistent hypertension

phenoxybenzamine: Decreased vasoconstrictor effect of phenylephrine, possibly hypotension and tachycardia

theophylline: Possibly enhanced toxicity (including cardiac toxicity)

thyroid hormones: Increased cardiovascular effects of each drug

chlorpheniramine and phenyltoloxamine

alcohol use: Additive CNS effects

Adverse Reactions

CNS: Dizziness, drowsiness, excitation (children), headache, insomnia, nervousness, paresthesia, restlessness, sedation, tremor, weakness

CV: Angina, bradycardia, hypertension, hypotension, palpitations, peripheral vasoconstriction that may lead to necrosis or gangrene, tachycardia, ventricular arrhythmias

EENT: Dry mouth

GI: Constipation, nausea, vomiting

GU: Urinary hesitancy, urine retention

RESP: Dyspnea

Nursing Considerations

- Use cautiously in patients with cardiovascular disease, diabetes, hypertension, hyperthyroidism, narrow-angle glaucoma, or prostatic hypertrophy.
- Monitor patients who may be more susceptible to dizziness, sedation, and hypotension, such as the elderly.
- Regularly evaluate effectiveness of phenylephrine, chlorpheniramine, and phenyltoloxamine in reducing nasal congestion.
- Be aware that patient shouldn't have intradermal allergen tests within 72 hours of receiving drug because results may be altered.

PATIENT TEACHING

- Instruct patient to take drug exactly as prescribed and not to increase dosage or frequency without consulting prescriber.
- Urge patient to avoid alcohol and other antidepressants while taking phenylephrine, chlorpheniramine, and phenyltoloxamine.
- Instruct patient to avoid hazardous activities until drug's CNS effects are known.
- Suggest that patient relieve dry mouth with frequent rinsing and use of sugarless gum or hard candy.

phenylephrine tannate, chlorpheniramine tannate, and pyrilamine tannate

AlleRx, Atrohist Pediatric, Rhinatate Pediatric, R-Tannamine, R-Tannamine Pediatric, R-Tannate, Triotann, Triotann Pediatric, Triotann-S Pediatric, Tri-Tannate

Class and Category

Chemical: Sympathomimetic amine (phenylephrine), propylamine derivative (chlorpheniramine), ethylenediamine derivative (pyrilamine)

Therapeutic: Decongestant (phenylephrine), antihistaminic (chlorpheniramine, pyrilamine)

Pregnancy category: C

Indications and Dosages

▶ *To relieve nasal congestion caused by the common cold, sinusitis, allergic rhinitis, and other upper respiratory tract conditions*

SUSPENSION

Adults. 30 mg phenylephrine, 10 to 12 mg chlorpheniramine, and 62.5 to 75 mg pyrilamine (30 ml) every 12 hr.

Children age 6 and over. 5 to 10 mg phenylephrine, 2 to 4 mg chlorpheniramine, and 12.5 to 25 mg pyrilamine (5 to 10 ml) every 12 hr.

Children ages 2 to 6. 2.5 to 5 mg phenylephrine, 1 to 2 mg chlorpheniramine, and 6.25 to 12.5 mg pyrilamine (2.5 to 5 ml) every 12 hr.

TABLETS

Adults. 25 to 50 mg phenylephrine, 8 to 16 mg chlorpheniramine, and 25 to 50 mg pyrilamine (1 to 2 tablets) every 12 hr.

Mechanism of Action

Phenylephrine stimulates alpha-adrenergic receptors and inhibits the intracellular enzyme adenyl cyclase, which then inhibits production of cAMP. Inhibition of cAMP causes arterial and venous constriction in nasal passages, which decreases blood flow and mucosal edema caused by allergic response.

Chlorpheniramine and pyrilamine compete with histamine for H_1 receptor sites, antagonizing many histamine effects and reducing allergy effects.

Contraindications

Breast-feeding, hypersensitivity to phenylephrine, chlorpheniramine, pyrilamine or their components; use of MAO inhibitors within 14 days

Interactions

DRUGS

phenylephrine, chlorpheniramine and pyrilamine

MAO inhibitors: Possibly prolonged and intensified anticholinergic effects of chlorpheniramine and overall effects of phenylephrine

phenylephrine

alpha blockers, haloperidol, loxapine, phenothiazines, thioxanthenes:

Possibly decreased vasoconstrictor effect of phenylephrine

antihypertenisves, diuretics: Possibly decreased antihypertensive effects

atropine: Possibly enhanced vasopressor effect of phenylephrine

beta blockers: Decreased therapeutic effects of both drugs

bretylium: Possibly potentiated vaopressor effect and arrhythmias

doxapram: Increased vasopressor effect of both drugs

ergot alkaloids: Possibly cerebral blood vessel rupture, increased vasopressor effect, peripheral vascular ischemia, and gangrene (with ergotamine)

guanadrel, guanethidine: Increased vasopressor effect of phenylephrine, increased risk of severe hypertension and arrhythmias

hydrocarbon inhalation anesthetics: Increased risk of serious arrhythmias

maprotiline, tricyclic antidepressants: Increased risk of severe cardiovascular effects (including arrhythmias, hyperpyrexia, severe hypertension)

mecamylamine, methyldopa: Decreased hypotensive effects of these drugs; increased vasopressor effect of phenylephrine

nitrates: Possibly decreased vasopressor effect of phenylephrine and decreased antianginal effect of nitrates

oxytocin: Possibly severe, persistent hypertension

phenoxybenzamine: Decreased vasoconstrictor effect of phenylephrine; possibly hypotension and tachycardia

theophylline: Possibly enhanced toxicity (including cardiac toxicity)

thyroid hormones: Increased cardiovascular effects of each drug

chlorpheniramine

CNS depressants: Additive CNS effects

phenytoin: Possibly increased serum phenytoin levels and toxicity

ACTIVITIES

chlorpheniramine

alcohol use: Additive CNS effects

Adverse Reactions

CNS: Dizziness, drowsiness, headache, insomnia, nervousness, paresthesia, restlessness, sedation, tremor, weakness

CV: Angina, bradycardia, hypertension, hypotension, palpitations, peripheral vasoconstriction that may lead to necrosis or gangrene, tachycardia, ventricular arrhythmias

EENT: Dry mouth

GI: Constipation, nausea, vomiting

GU: Urinary hesitancy, urine retention

RESP: Dyspnea

Nursing Considerations

- Use cautiously in patients with cardiovascular disease, diabetes, hypertension, hyperthyroidism, narrow-angle glaucoma, or prostatic hypertrophy.
- Monitor patients who may be more susceptible to dizziness, sedation, and hypotension, such as the elderly.
- Regularly evaluate effectiveness of phenylephrine, chlorpheniramine, and pyrilamine in reducing nasal congestion.
- Be aware that patient shouldn't have intradermal allergen tests within 72 hours of receiving drug because results may be altered.

PATIENT TEACHING

- Instruct patient to use a calibrated device when measuring dose of phenylephrine, chlorpheniramine, and pyrilamine to ensure accurate dose.
- Urge patient to avoid alcohol and other antidepressants while taking phenylephrine, chlorpheniramine, and pyrilamine.
- Instruct patient to avoid hazardous activities until drug's CNS effects are known.
- Suggest that patient relieve dry mouth with frequent rinsing and use of sugarless gum or hard candy.

phenylephrine hydrochloride and guaifenesin

Crantex ER, Deconsall II, Endal, Entex, Entex ER, Entex LA, GFN 600/Phenylephrine 20, Guaifed, Guaifed-PD, Liquibid-D, Liquibid PD, PhenaVent LA, SINUvent PE

Class and Category

Chemical: Sympathomimetic amine (phenylephrine), glyceryl guaiacolate (guaifenesin)
Therapeutic: Decongestant (phenylephrine), expectorant (guaifenesin)
Pregnancy category: C

Indications and Dosages

▶ *To relieve upper respiratory symptoms caused by the common cold or allergies*

ORAL SOLUTION

Adults. 7.5 to 15 mg phenylephrine and 100 to 200 mg guaifenesin (5 to 10 ml) every 4 to 6 hr. *Maximum:* 40 ml daily.

E.R. CAPSULES

Adults. 7.5 to 20 mg phenylephrine and 200 to 800 mg guaifen-

esin (1 or 2 capsules depending on product) every 12 hr.
Children age 12 and over. 10 mg phenylephrine and 300 mg guaifenesin (1 capsule) every 12 hr.
Children ages 6 to 12. 7.5 mg phenylephrine and 200 mg guaifenesin (1 capsule) every 12 hr.
E.R. TABLETS
Adults and children age 12 and over. 20 to 50 mg phenylephrine and 275 to 1200 mg guaifenesin (1 or 2 tablets depending on product) every 12 hr.
Children ages 6 to 12. 12.5 to 25 mg phenylephrine and 275 to 600 mg guaifenesin (½ tablet) every 12 hr.

Mechanism of Action

Phenylephrine stimulates alpha-adrenergic receptors and inhibits the intracellular enzyme adenyl cyclase, which then inhibits production of cAMP. Inhibition of cAMP causes arterial and venous constriction in nasal passages, which decreases blood flow and mucosal edema caused by allergic response.

Guaifenesin increases fluid and mucus removal from the upper respiratory tract by increasing the volume of secretions and reducing their adhesiveness and surface tension.

Contraindications

Hypersensitivity to bisulfites, guaifenesin, phenylephrine, or their components; severe coronary artery disease or hypertension; use within 14 days of MAO inhibitor therapy; ventricular tachycardia

Interactions

DRUGS

phenylephrine

alpha blockers, haloperidol, loxapine, phenothiazines, thioxanthenes: Possibly decreased vasoconstrictor effect of phenylephrine
antihypertenisves, diuretics: Possibly decreased antihypertensive effects
atropine: Possibly enhanced vasopressor effect of phenylephrine
beta blockers: Decreased therapeutic effects of both drugs
bretylium: Possibly potentiated vaopressor effect and arrhythmias
doxapram: Increased vasopressor effect of both drugs
ergot alkaloids: Possibly cerebral blood vessel rupture, increased vasopressor effect, peripheral vascular ischemia, and gangrene (with ergotamine)
guanadrel, guanethidine: Increased vasopressor effect of phenylephrine; increased risk of severe hypertension and arrhythmias

hydrocarbon inhalation anesthetics: Increased risk of serious arrhythmias

MAO inhibitors: Increased and prolonged cardiac stimulation, increased vasopressor effect, increased risk of severe cardiovascular and cerebrovascular effects, hyperpyrexia, vomiting

maprotiline, tricyclic antidepressants: Increased risk of severe cardiovascular effects (including arrhythmias, hyperpyrexia, severe hypertension)

mecamylamine, methyldopa: Decreased hypotensive effects of these drugs; increased vasopressor effect of phenylephrine

nitrates: Possibly decreased vasopressor effect of phenylephrine and decreased antianginal effect of nitrates

oxytocin: Possibly severe, persistent hypertension

phenoxybenzamine: Decreased vasoconstrictor effect of phenylephrine; possibly hypotension and tachycardia

theophylline: Possibly enhanced toxicity (including cardiac toxicity)

thyroid hormones: Increased cardiovascular effects of each drug

Adverse Reactions

CNS: Dizziness, hallucinations, headache, insomnia, nervousness, paresthesia, restlessness, seizures, tremor, weakness

CV: Angina, bradycardia, hypertension, hypotension, palpitations, peripheral vasoconstriction that may lead to necrosis or gangrene, tachycardia, ventricular arrhythmia

GI: Nausea, vomiting

RESP: Dyspnea

SKIN: Pallor, rash, urticaria

Other: Allergic reaction

Nursing Considerations

- Assess patient for signs and symptoms of angina, arrhythmias, and hypertension because phenylephrine may increase myocardial oxygen demand and the risk of proarrhythmias and blood pressure changes.
- **WARNING** Monitor patient with thyroid disease for increased sensitivity to catecholamines and possible thyrotoxicity or cardiotoxicity.
- Regularly evaluate effectiveness of phenylephrine and guaifenesin in relieving upper respiratory symptoms. Notify prescriber if symptoms persist or worsen.
- Watch for signs of more serious condition, such as cough that lasts longer than 1 week, fever, persistent headache, and rash.

PATIENT TEACHING

- Instruct patient to take each dose with a full glass of water.

- Advise patient not to break, crush, or chew E.R. tablets or capsules but to swallow them whole.
- Instruct patient to increase fluid intake (unless contraindicated) to help thin secretions.
- Caution patient to avoid hazardous activities until drug's CNS effects are known.

phenylephrine tannate and pyrilamine tannate

Duonate-12, P-Tanna 12, R-Tannic-S A/D, Ryna-12, Viravan-S

Class and Category

Chemical: Sympathomimetic amine (phenylephrine), ethylene-diamine derivative (pyrilamine)

Therapeutic: Decongestant (phenylephrine), antihistaminic (pyrilamine)

Pregnancy category: C

Indications and Dosages

▶ *To relieve nasal congestion caused by the common cold, sinusitis, allergic rhinitis, and other upper respiratory tract conditions*

SUSPENSION

Adults. 12.5 mg phenylephrine and 30 mg pyrilamine or 25 mg phenylephrine and 60 mg pyrilamine (5 or 10 ml) every 12 hr.

Children age 6 and over. 5 to 10 mg phenylephrine and 30 to 60 mg pyrilamine (5 or 10 ml) every 12 hr.

Children ages 2 to 6. 2.5 to 5 mg phenylephrine and 15 to 30 mg pyrilamine (2.5 ml or 5 ml) every 12 hr.

CHEWABLE TABLETS

Adults. 25 mg phenylephrine and 30 mg pyrilamine (1 tablet) every 12 hr.

Children ages 6 to 12. 12.5 mg phenylephrine and 15 mg pyrilamine (½ tablet) every 12 hr.

TABLETS

Adults. 25 to 50 mg phenylephrine and 60 to 120 mg pyrilamine (1 or 2 tablets) every 12 hr.

Children ages 6 to 12. 12.5 to 25 mg phenylephrine and 30 to 60 mg pyrilamine (½ to 1 tablet) every 12 hr.

Contraindications

Breast-feeding; hypersensitivity to phenylephrine, pyrilamine, or their components; use of an MAO inhibitor within 14 days

Mechanism of Action

Phenylephrine stimulates alpha-adrenergic receptors and inhibits the intracellular enzyme adenyl cyclase, which then inhibits production of cAMP. Inhibition of cAMP causes arterial and venous constriction in nasal passages, which decreases blood flow and mucosal edema caused by allergic response.

Pyrilamine competes with histamine for H_1 receptor sites, thereby antagonizing many histamine effects to reduce allergy signs and symptoms.

Interactions

DRUGS

phenylephrine and pyrilamine

MAO inhibitors: Possibly prolonged and intensified anticholinergic effects of pyrilamine and overall effects of phenylephrine

phenylephrine

alpha blockers, haloperidol, loxapine, phenothiazines, thioxanthenes: Possibly decreased vasoconstrictor effect of phenylephrine

antihypertenisves, diuretics: Possibly decreased antihypertensive effects

atropine: Possibly enhanced vasopressor effect of phenylephrine

beta blockers: Decreased therapeutic effects of both drugs

bretylium: Possibly potentiated vaopressor effect and arrhythmias

doxapram: Increased vasopressor effect of both drugs

ergot alkaloids: Possibly cerebral blood vessel rupture, increased vasopressor effect, peripheral vascular ischemia, and gangrene (with ergotamine)

guanadrel, guanethidine: Increased vasopressor effect of phenylephrine; increased risk of severe hypertension and arrhythmias

hydrocarbon inhalation anesthetics: Increased risk of serious arrhythmias

maprotiline, tricyclic antidepressants: Increased risk of severe cardiovascular effects (including arrhythmias, hyperpyrexia, severe hypertension)

mecamylamine, methyldopa: Decreased hypotensive effects of these drugs; increased vasopressor effect of phenylephrine

nitrates: Possibly decreased vasopressor effect of phenylephrine and decreased antianginal effect of nitrates

oxytocin: Possibly severe, persistent hypertension

phenoxybenzamine: Decreased vasoconstrictor effect of phenylephrine; possibly hypotension and tachycardia

theophylline: Possibly enhanced toxicity (including cardiac toxicity)

thyroid hormones: Increased cardiovascular effects of each drug
pyrilamine
CNS depressants: Additive CNS effects
ACTIVITIES
pyrilamine
alcohol use: Additive CNS effects

Adverse Reactions

CNS: Dizziness, drowsiness, excitation (children), headache, insomnia, nervousness, paresthesia, restlessness, sedation, tremor, weakness
CV: Angina, bradycardia, hypertension, hypotension, palpitations, peripheral vasoconstriction that may lead to necrosis or gangrene, tachycardia, ventricular arrhythmias
EENT: Dry mouth
GI: Constipation, nausea, vomiting
GU: Urinary hesitancy, urine retention
RESP: Dyspnea

Nursing Considerations

- Use cautiously in patients with cardiovascular disease, diabetes, hypertension, hyperthyroidism, narrow-angle glaucoma, or prostatic hypertrophy.
- Monitor children for excitation and elderly patients for dizziness, sedation, and hypotension; such patients may have an increased risk for these effects.
- Regularly evaluate effectiveness of phenylephrine and pyrilamine in reducing nasal congestion.
- Be aware that patient shouldn't have intradermal allergen tests within 72 hours of receiving drug because results may be altered.

PATIENT TEACHING
- Instruct patient to use a calibrated measuring device to ensure an accurate dose of phenylephrine and pyrilamine drug suspension.
- Tell patient to swallow nonchewable tablets whole.
- Urge patient to avoid alcohol and other antidepressants while taking phenylephrine and pyrilamine.
- Instruct patient to avoid hazardous activities until drug's CNS effects are known.
- Suggest that patient relieve dry mouth with frequent rinsing and use of sugarless gum or hard candy.

promethazine hydrochloride and codeine phosphate

Phenergan with Codeine, Prometh with Codeine

Class, Category, and Schedule

Chemical: Phenothiazine derivative (promethazine), phenanthrene derivative (codeine)
Therapeutic: Antihistamine (promethazine), analgesic and antitussive (codeine)
Pregnancy category: C
Controlled substance schedule: V

Indications and Dosages

▶ *To relieve cough and other symptoms caused by allergies and the common cold*

SYRUP

Adults and children age 12 and over. 6.25 mg promethazine and 10 mg codeine (5 ml) every 4 to 6 hr. *Maximum:* 30 ml daily.
Children ages 6 to 12. 3.125 to 6.25 mg promethazine and 5 to 10 mg codeine (2.5 to 5 ml) every 4 to 6 hr. *Maximum:* 30 ml daily.
Children ages 2 to 6. 1.56 to 3.125 promethazine and 2.5 to 5 mg codeine (1.25 to 2.5 ml) every 4 to 6 hr. *Maximum:* 0.5 ml/kg/day for children weighing 12 to 18 kg (26 to 40 lb); 6 ml/day for children weighing less than 12 kg.
DOSAGE ADJUSTMENT For patient with renal insufficiency (creatinine clearance of 10 to 50 ml/min/1.73 m^2), dosage reduced by 75%.

Mechanism of Action

Promethazine competes with histamine for H_1 receptor sites, thereby antagonizing many histamine effects and reducing allergy signs and symptoms.

Codeine suppresses cough by directly acting on opiate receptors in the medulla's cough center.

Contraindications

Angle-closure glaucoma; benign prostatic hyperplasia; bladder neck obstruction; bone marrow depression; breast-feeding; children under age 2; coma; hypersensitivity to promethazine, codeine, other opioids, or their components; hypertensive crisis; pyloroduodenal obstruction; stenosing peptic ulcer; significant respiratory depression; use of CNS depressants in large quantities

Interactions

DRUGS

promethazine and codeine

anticholinergics: Possibly intensified anticholinergic adverse effects

CNS depressants: Additive CNS depression

MAO inhibitors: Possibly prolonged and intensified anticholinergic and CNS depressant effects of promethazine; increased risk of unpredictable, severe, and sometimes fatal reactions with codeine

promethazine

amphetamines: Decreased stimulant effect of amphetamines

anticonvulsants: Lowered seizure threshold

appetite suppressants: Possibly antagonized anorectic effect of appetite suppressants

beta blockers: Increased risk of additive hypotensive effects, irreversible retinopathy, arrhythmias, and tardive dyskinesia

bromocriptine: Decreased bromocriptine effectiveness

dopamine: Possibly antagonized peripheral vasoconstriction with high doses of dopamine

ephedrine, metaraminol, methoxamine: Decreased vasopressor response to these drugs

epinephrine: Blocked alpha-adrenergic effects of epinephrine; increased risk of hypotension

guanadrel, guanethidine: Decreased antihypertensive effects

hepatotoxic drugs: Increased risk of hepatotoxicity

hypotension-producing drugs: Possibly severe hypotension with syncope

levodopa: Inhibited antidyskinetic effects of levodopa

metrizamide: Increased risk of seizures

ototoxic drugs: Possibly masking of some symptoms of ototoxicity, such as dizziness, tinnitus, and vertigo

quinidine: Additive cardiac effects

riboflavin: Increased riboflavin requirements

codeine

antihypertensives, diuretics: Potentiated hypotensive effects

buprenorphine: Decreased codeine effectiveness

hydroxyzine: Increased codeine analgesic effect; increased CNS depressant and hypotensive effects

metoclopramide: Antagonized effect of metoclopramide on GI motility

naloxone: Antagonized codeine analgesic effect

naltrexone: Precipitated withdrawal symptoms in codeine-dependent patients

neuromuscular blockers: Additive respiratory depressant effects
opioids: Additive CNS and respiratory depressant effects and hypotensive effects
paregoric: Increased risk of severe constipation
ACTIVITIES
promethazine and codeine
alcohol use: Additive CNS depression

Adverse Reactions

CNS: Akathisia, CNS stimulation, coma, confusion, delirium, depression, disorientation, dizziness, drowsiness, dystonia, euphoria, excitation, fatigue, hallucinations, headache, hysteria, insomnia, irritability, lack of coordination, lethargy, light-headedness, mental and physical impairment, mood changes, nervousness, neuroleptic malignant syndrome, paradoxical stimulation, pseudoparkinsonism, restlessness, sedation, seizures, syncope, tardive dyskinesia, tremor
CV: Bradycardia, heart block, hypertension, orthostatic hypotension, palpitations, tachycardia
EENT: Altered taste; blurred vision; diplopia; dry mouth, nose, and throat; laryngeal edema; laryngospasm; miosis; nasal congestion; tinnitus; vision changes
ENDO: Hyperglycemia
GI: Abdominal cramps and pain, anorexia, constipation, flatulence, gastroesophageal reflux, ileus, indigestion, nausea, vomiting
GU: Decreased libido, difficult ejaculation, dysuria, impotence, oliguria, ureteral spasm, urinary incontinence, urine retention
HEME: Agranulocytosis, leukopenia, thrombocytopenia, thrombocytopenic purpura
MS: Muscle rigidity
RESP: Apnea, bronchoconstriction, bronchospasm, depressed cough reflex, respiratory depression, tenacious bronchial secretions
SKIN: Dermatitis, diaphoresis, flushing, jaundice, pallor, photosensitivity, pruritus, rash, urticaria
Other: Anaphylaxis, angioedema, paradoxical reactions, physical and psychological dependence

Nursing Considerations

- Use cautiously in patients with head injury, peptic ulcer, abdominal obstruction (except pyloroduodenal obstruction, which is a contraindication), cardiovascular disease, liver or kidney impairment, fever, seizures, hypothyroidism, intestinal inflammation, or Addison's disease.

- Use cautiously in children age 2 and over because of risk for respiratory depression.
- Also use cautiously in patients who have recently had stomach, intestinal, or urinary tract surgery.
- Monitor effectiveness of promethazine and codeine in relieving allergy symptoms and cough. Notify prescriber if symptoms persist or worsen.
- **WARNING** Monitor respiratory function because promethazine and codeine may suppress the cough reflex and cause thickening of bronchial secretions, aggravating such conditions as asthma and COPD. Rarely, it may depress respirations and induce apnea. Notify prescriber immediately if respiratory rate drops below 10 breaths/minute.
- Monitor patient's hematologic status, as ordered, because promethazine may cause bone marrow depression. Assess patient for signs and symptoms of infection or bleeding.
- **WARNING** Monitor patient for evidence of neuroleptic malignant syndrome, such as fever, hypertension or hypotension, involuntary motor activity, mental changes, muscle rigidity, tachycardia, and tachypenia. Be prepared to provide supportive treatment and additional drug therapy, as needed and prescribed.
- Take safety precautions, if needed, because promethazine and codeine can cause considerable drowsiness and many other adverse CNS effects.
- Be aware that patient shouldn't have intradermal allergen tests within 72 hours of receiving promethazine and codeine because drug may significantly alter flare response.
- **WARNING** Monitor patient closely for evidence of overdose, even at normal dosage, because some patients metabolize codeine quickly, causing a sudden rise in blood codeine level. This metabolic defect occurs in about 0.5 to 1% of Chinese, Japanese, or Hispanic people; 1 to 10% of Caucasians; 3% of African Americans; and 16 to 28% of North Africans, Ethiopians, and Arabs. Watch for extreme sleepiness, confusion, and shallow breathing after giving drug. If present, notify prescriber and be prepared to provide supportive care and discontinue the drug, as ordered.

PATIENT TEACHING

- Tell patient to take only the dosage prescribed and not to increase dose or frequency without consulting prescriber.

- Instruct patient to use a calibrated measuring device to ensure accurate dose of liquid form.
- Advise patient to contact prescriber if symptoms, including cough, aren't better after 5 days of therapy.
- Instruct patient to avoid hazardous activities until drug's CNS effects are known.
- Warn patient to avoid alcoholic beverages, OTC antihistamine, and CNS depressants while taking promethazine and codeine.
- Caution patient to drink plenty of fluids and increase dietary fiber because codeine can cause or worsen constipation.
- Tell patient to rise slowly from a lying or sitting position to minimize dizziness or light-headedness.
- Alert female patients that promethazine and codeine may affect pregnancy test results.
- Instruct diabetic patient to monitor her blood glucose level closely while taking promethazine and codeine.
- Tell patient to report any involuntary muscle movements or unusual sensitivity to sunlight to the prescriber because drug may need to be discontinued.
- Advise patient to avoid excessive sun exposure and to use sunscreen when outdoors.
- Urge patient to notify prescriber if she has trouble breathing or develops extreme sleepiness or confusion.

promethazine hydrochloride and dextromethorphan hydrobromide

Phenergan with Dextromethorphan, Promethazine DM

Class and Category

Chemical: Phenothiazine derivative (promethazine), D-isomer codeine analogue of levorphanol (dextromethorphan)
Therapeutic: Antihistamine (promethazine), antitussive (dextromethorphan)
Pregnancy category: C

Indications and Dosages

▶ *To relieve cough and allergic signs and symptoms caused by upper respiratory conditions such as the common cold and seasonal allergies*
SYRUP

Adults and children age 12 and over. 6.25 mg promethazine and 15 mg dextromethorphan (5 ml) every 4 to 6 hr. *Maximum:* 30 ml every 24 hr.

Children ages 6 to 12. 3.125 to 6.25 mg promethazine and
7.5 to 15 mg dextromethorphan (2.5 to 5 ml) every 4 to 6 hr.
Maximum: 20 ml every 24 hr.
Children ages 2 to 6. 1.5 to 3.125 mg promethazine and 3.75 to
7.5 mg dextromethorphan (1.25 to 2.5 ml) every 4 to 6 hr. *Maximum:* 10 ml every 24 hr.
ORAL SOLUTION
Adults. 6.25 mg promethazine and 15 mg dextromethorphan
(5 ml) every 4 to 6 hr. *Maximum:* 30 ml every 24 hr.

Mechanism of Action
Promethazine competes with histamine for H$_1$ receptor sites, thereby antagonizing many histamine effects and reducing allergy signs and symptoms.
 Dextromethorphan suppresses cough by directly acting on the cough center in the medulla of the brain.

Contraindications
Angle-closure glaucoma; asthma; benign prostatic hyperplasia;
bladder neck obstruction; bone marrow depression; breast-
feeding; chronic bronchitis; coma; emphysema; hypersensitivity to
promethazine, dextromethorphan, or their components; hypertensive crisis; productive cough; pyloroduodenal obstruction;
stenosing peptic ulcer; use of large quantities of CNS depressants;
use of an MAO inhibitor within 14 days

Interactions
DRUGS
promethazine and dextromethorphan
CNS depressants: Additive CNS depression
MAO inhibitors: Possibly prolonged and intensified anticholinergic
and CNS depressant effects of promethazine; increased risk of unpredictable, severe, and sometimes fatal reactions with dextromethorphan
promethazine
amphetamines: Decreased stimulant effect of amphetamines
anticonvulsants: Lowered seizure threshold
anticholinergics: Possibly intensified anticholinergic adverse effects
appetite suppressants: Possibly antagonized anorectic effect of appetite suppressants
beta blockers: Increased risk of additive hypotensive effects, irreversible retinopathy, arrhythmias, and tardive dyskinesia
bromocriptine: Decreased effectiveness of bromocriptine

dopamine: Possibly antagonized peripheral vasoconstriction (with high doses of dopamine

ephedrine, metaraminol, methoxamine: Decreased vasopressor response to these drugs

epinephrine: Blocked alpha-adrenergic effects of epinephrine; increased risk of hypotension

guanadrel, guanethidine: Decreased antihypertensive effects of these drugs

hepatotoxic drugs: Increased risk of hepatotoxicity

hypotension-producing drugs: Possibly severe hypotension with syncope

levodopa: Inhibited antidyskinetic effects of levodopa

metrizamide: Increased risk of seizures

ototoxic drugs: Possibly masking of some symptoms of ototoxicity, such as dizziness, tinnitus, and vertigo

quinidine: Additive cardiac effects

riboflavin: Increased riboflavin requirements

dextromethorphan

amiodarone, fluoxetine, quinidine: Decreased metabolism of dextromethorphan, which may increase plasma dextromethorphan levels and adverse reactions

CNS depressants: Additive CNS effects

ACTIVITIES

promethazine and dextromethorphan

alcohol use: Additive CNS depression

dextromethorphan

smoking: Possibly increased respiratory secretion retention

Adverse Reactions

CNS: Akathisia, CNS stimulation, confusion, dizziness, drowsiness, dystonia, euphoria, excitation, fatigue, hallucinations, hyperactivity, hysteria, insomnia, irritability, nervousness, neuroleptic malignant syndrome, paradoxical stimulation, pseudoparkinsonism, restlessness, sedation, seizures, syncope, tardive dyskinesia, tremor

CV: Bradycardia, hypertension, hypotension, tachycardia

EENT: Blurred vision; diplopia; dry mouth, nose, and throat; nasal congestion; tinnitus; vision changes

GI: Abdominal pain, anorexia, constipation, ileus, nausea, vomiting

GU: Dysuria

HEME: Agranulocytosis, leukopenia, thrombocytopenia, thrombocytopenic purpura

RESP: Apnea, respiratory depression, tenacious bronchial secretions

SKIN: Dermatitis, diaphoresis, jaundice, photosensitivity, rash, urticaria

Other: Angioedema, emotional and physical dependence (prolonged use with high doses), paradoxical reactions

Nursing Considerations

- Use promethazine and dextromethorphan cautiously in patients with cardiovascular disease or hepatic dysfunction because of potential adverse effects.
- Use cautiously in children age 2 and over because of risk of respiratory depression.
- Also use cautiously in patients with diabetes because some products contain sugar, which may disrupt blood glucose control; in those with impaired hepatic function because dextromethorphan is metabolized by the liver; in those with respiratory depression because dextromethorphan adversely affects respirations; and in those with seizure disorders or those who take medication that affects seizure threshold because promethazine may lower the seizure threshold.
- **WARNING** Dextromethorphan has the potential for abuse because of its euphoric, hallucinogenic, and dissociative effects when taken in doses higher than prescribed. Monitor patient closely.
- **WARNING** Monitor respiratory function because drug may suppress cough reflex and cause thickening of bronchial secretions. It also may depress respirations and induce apnea.
- Monitor patient's hematologic status, as ordered, because promethazine may cause bone marrow depression, especially when used with other marrow-toxic agents. Assess patient for signs and symptoms of infection or bleeding.
- **WARNING** Monitor patient for evidence of neuroleptic malignant syndrome, such as fever, hypertension or hypotension, involuntary motor activity, mental changes, muscle rigidity, tachycardia, and tachypenia. Be prepared to provide supportive treatment and additional drug therapy, as prescribed.
- Take safety precautions, if needed, because promethazine and dextromethorphan can cause drowsiness and many other adverse CNS effects.
- Patient shouldn't have intradermal allergen tests within 72 hours of receiving promethazine and dextromethorphan because drug may significantly alter flare response.

PATIENT TEACHING
- Advise patient not to exceed prescribed dosage.
- Instruct patient to use a calibrated measuring device to ensure an accurate dose.
- Stress importance of taking promethazine and dextromethorphan exactly as prescribed and not increasing dose or frequency without consulting prescriber.
- Warn patient to avoid alcoholic beverages and OTC antihistamines and CNS depressants while taking promethazine and dextromethorphan.
- Tell patient to rise slowly from a lying or sitting position to minimize dizziness or light-headedness.
- Instruct diabetic patient to monitor his blood glucose level closely while taking promethazine and dextromethorphan.
- Tell patient to report involuntary muscle movements or unusual sensitivity to sunlight because drug may need to be stopped.
- Advise patient to avoid excessive sun exposure and to use sunscreen when outdoors.

promethazine hydrochloride and phenylephrine hydrochloride

Phenameth VC, Phenergan VC, Prometh VC Plain, Promethazine VC

Class and Category

Chemical: Phenothiazine derivative (promethazine), sympathomimetic amine (phenylephrine)
Therapeutic: Antihistamine (promethazine), decongestant (phenylephrine)
Pregnancy category: C

Indications and Dosages

▶ *To relieve cough and other symptoms caused by allergies and the common cold*
SYRUP
Adults and children age 12 and over. 6.25 mg promethazine and 5 mg phenylephrine (5 ml) every 4 to 6 hr. *Maximum:* 30 ml every 24 hr.
Children ages 6 to 12. 3.125 to 6.25 mg promethazine and 2.5 to 5 mg phenylephrine (2.5 to 5 ml) every 4 to 6 hr. *Maximum:* 15 ml every 24 hr
Children ages 2 to 6. 1.56 to 3.125 promethazine and 1.25 to

2.5 mg phenylephrine (1.25 to 2.5 ml) every 4 to 6 hr. *Maximum:* 7.5 ml every 24 hr.

Mechanism of Action

Promethazine competes with histamine for H_1 receptor sites, thereby antagonizing many histamine effects and reducing allergy signs and symptoms.

Phenylephrine stimulates alpha-adrenergic receptors, constricting local vessels and decreasing blood flow and mucosal edema to relieve nasal congestion.

Contraindications

Angle-closure glaucoma; benign prostatic hyperplasia; bladder neck obstruction; bone marrow depression; breast-feeding; children under age 2; coma; hypersensitivity to bisulfites, promethazine, phenylephrine, or their components; lower respiratory disorders (including asthma); pyloroduodenal obstruction; severe coronary artery disease or hypertension; stenosing peptic ulcer; use of large quantities of CNS depressants; use of MAO inhibitor within 14 days; ventricular tachycardia

Interactions

DRUGS

promethazine and phenylephrine

guanadrel, guanethidine: Decreased antihypertensive effects of these drugs; increased risk of severe hypertension and arrhythmias; increased vasopressor effect of phenylephrine

MAO inhibitors: Possibly prolonged and intensified anticholinergic and CNS depressant effects of promethazine; increased and prolonged cardiac stimulation, increased vasopressor effect, increased risk of severe cardiovascular and cerebrovascular effects, hyperpyrexia, and vomiting with phenylephrine

promethazine

amphetamines: Decreased stimulant effect of amphetamines

anticholinergics: Possibly intensified anticholinergic adverse effects

anticonvulsants: Lowered seizure threshold

appetite suppressants: Possibly antagonized anorectic effect of appetite suppressants

beta blockers: Increased risk of additive hypotensive effects, irreversible retinopathy, arrhythmias, and tardive dyskinesia

bromocriptine: Decreased effectiveness of bromocriptine

CNS depressants: Additive CNS depression

dopamine: Possibly antagonized peripheral vasoconstriction (with high doses of dopamine

ephedrine, metaraminol, methoxamine: Decreased vasopressor response to these drugs

epinephrine: Blocked alpha-adrenergic effects of epinephrine; increased risk of hypotension

hepatotoxic drugs: Increased risk of hepatotoxicity

hypotension-producing drugs: Possibly severe hypotension with syncope

levodopa: Inhibited antidyskinetic effects of levodopa

metrizamide: Increased risk of seizures

ototoxic drugs: Possibly masking of some symptoms of ototoxicity, such as dizziness, tinnitus, and vertigo

quinidine: Additive cardiac effects

riboflavin: Increased riboflavin requirements

phenylephrine

alpha blockers, haloperidol, loxapine, phenothiazines, thioxanthenes: Possibly decreased vasoconstrictor effect of phenylephrine

antihypertenisves, diuretics: Possibly decreased antihypertensive effects

atropine: Possibly enhanced vasopressor effect of phenylephrine

beta blockers: Decreased therapeutic effects of both drugs

bretylium: Possibly potentiated vaopressor effect and arrhythmias

doxapram: Increased vasopressor effect of both drugs

ergot alkaloids: Possibly cerebral blood vessel rupture, increased vasopressor effect, peripheral vascular ischemia, and gangrene (with ergotamine)

hydrocarbon inhalation anesthetics: Increased risk of serious arrhythmias

maprotiline, tricyclic antidepressants: Increased risk of severe cardiovascular effects (including arrhythmias, hyperpyrexia, severe hypertension)

mecamylamine, methyldopa: Decreased hypotensive effects of these drugs, increased vasopressor effect of phenylephrine

nitrates: Possibly decreased vasopressor effect of phenylephrine and decreased antianginal effect of nitrates

oxytocin: Possibly severe, persistent hypertension

phenoxybenzamine: Decreased vasoconstrictor effect of phenylephrine, possibly hypotension and tachycardia

theophylline: Possibly enhanced toxicity (including cardiac toxicity)

thyroid hormones: Increased cardiovascular effects of each drug

ACTIVITIES

promethazine

alcohol use: Additive CNS depression

Adverse Reactions

CNS: Akathisia, CNS stimulation, confusion, dizziness, drowsiness, dystonia, euphoria, excitation, fatigue, hallucinations, headache, hysteria, insomnia, irritability, lack of coordination, nervousness, neuroleptic malignant syndrome, paradoxical stimulation, pseudoparkinsonism, restlessness, sedation, seizures, syncope, tardive dyskinesia, tremor, weakness

CV: Angina, bradycardia, hypertension, orthostatic hypotension, palpitations, peripheral vasoconstriction, tachycardia, ventricular arrhythmias

EENT: Blurred vision; diplopia; dry mouth, nose, and throat; nasal congestion; tinnitus; vision changes

ENDO: Hyperglycemia

GI: Anorexia, ileus, nausea, vomiting

GU: Dysuria

HEME: Agranulocytosis, leukopenia, thrombocytopenia, thrombocytopenic purpura

RESP: Apnea, dyspnea, respiratory depression, tenacious bronchial secretions

SKIN: Dermatitis, diaphoresis, jaundice, pallor, photosensitivity, rash, urticaria

Other: Angioedema, paradoxical reactions

Nursing Considerations

- Use cautiously in patients with cardiovascular disease, hepatic dysfunction, or sleep apnea because of potential adverse effects.
- Use cautiously in children age 2 and over because of risk of respiratory depression.
- Use cautiously in patients who have seizure disorders or receive drugs that lower the seizure threshold, such as opioids and anesthetics.
- Monitor effectiveness of promethazine and phenylephrine in relieving allergy symptoms. Notify prescriber if symptoms persist or worsen.
- **WARNING** Monitor respiratory function because promethazine and phenylephrine may suppress cough reflex and cause thickening of bronchial secretions, aggravating such conditions as asthma and COPD. Rarely, it may depress respirations and induce apnea. Notify prescriber immediately if respiratory rate drops below 10 breaths/minute.
- Monitor patient's hematologic status as ordered because promethazine may cause bone marrow depression. Assess patient for signs and symptoms of infection or bleeding.

- **WARNING** Monitor patient for evidence of neuroleptic malignant syndrome, such as fever, hypertension or hypotension, involuntary motor activity, mental changes, muscle rigidity, tachycardia, and tachypenia. Be prepared to provide supportive treatment and additional drug therapy, as prescribed.
- Take safety precautions, if needed, because promethazine and phenylephrine can cause considerable drowsiness and multiple other adverse CNS effects.
- Be aware that patient shouldn't have intradermal allergen tests within 72 hours of receiving promethazine and phenylephrine because drug may significantly alter flare response.

PATIENT TEACHING
- Tell patient to take only the dosage prescribed and not to increase dose or frequency without consulting prescriber.
- Instruct patient to use a calibrated measuring device to ensure accurate dose.
- Advise patient to contact prescriber if signs and symptoms persist after 5 days of therapy.
- Instruct patient to avoid hazardous activities until drug's CNS effects are known.
- Warn patient to avoid alcoholic beverages, OTC decongestants, and CNS depressants while taking drug.
- Tell patient to rise slowly from a lying or sitting position to minimize dizziness or light-headness.
- Instruct diabetic patient to monitor her blood glucose level closely while taking promethazine and phenylephrine.
- Tell patient to report involuntary muscle movements or unusual sensitivity to sunlight because drug may need to be stopped.
- Advise patient to avoid excessive sun exposure and to use sunscreen when outdoors.

promethazine hydrochloride, phenylephrine hydrochloride, and codeine phosphate
Phenergan VC with Codeine, Prometh VC with Codeine, Promethazine VC with Codeine

Class, Category, and Schedule
Chemical: Phenothiazine derivative (promethazine), sympathomimetic amine (phenylephrine), and phenanthrene alkaloid of opium (codeine)

Therapeutic: Antihistamine (promethazine), decongestant (phenylephrine) and analgesic and antiussive (codeine)
Pregnancy category: C
Controlled substance schedule: V

Indications and Dosages

▶ *To relieve cough and other symptoms caused by allergies and the common cold*
SYRUP
Adults and children age 12 and over. 6.25 mg promethazine, 5 mg phenylephrine, and 10 mg codeine (5 ml) every 4 to 6 hr. *Maximum:* 30 ml every 24 hr.
Children ages 6 to 12. 3.125 to 6.25 mg promethazine, 2.5 to 5 mg phenylephrine, and 5 to 10 mg codeine (2.5 to 5 ml) every 4 to 6 hr. *Maximum:* 15 ml every 24 hr.
Children ages 2 to 6. 1.56 to 3.125 promethazine, 1.25 to 2.5 mg phenylephrine, and 2.5 to 5 mg codeine (1.25 to 2.5 ml) every 4 to 6 hr. *Maximum:* 9 ml every 24 hr for children weighing 18 kg (40 lb) or more, 8 ml every 24 hr for children weighing 16 to 18 kg (35 to 40 lb), 7 ml every 24 hr for children weighing 14 to 16 kg (30 to 35 lb), and 6 ml every 24 hr for children weighing 12 to 14 kg (25 to 30 lb).

Mechanism of Action

Promethazine competes with histamine for H_1 receptor sites, thereby antagonizing many histamine effects and reducing allergy signs and symptoms.

Phenylephrine stimulates alpha-adrenergic receptors, constricting local vessels and decreasing blood flow and mucosal edema to relieve nasal congestion.

Codeine suppresses cough by acting on opiate receptors in the medulla.

Contraindications

Angle-closure glaucoma; benign prostatic hyperplasia; bladder neck obstruction; bone marrow depression; breast-feeding; children under age 2; coma; hypersensitivity to bisulfites, promethazine, phenylephrine, codeine, other opioids, or their components; lower respiratory tract disorders (including asthma); pyloroduodenal obstruction; severe coronary artery disease or hypertension; stenosing peptic ulcer; significant respiratory depression; use of large quantities of CNS depressants; use of an MAO inhibitor within 14 days; ventricular tachycardia

Interactions
DRUGS
promethazine, phenylephrine, and codeine
MAO inhibitors: With promethazine, possibly prolonged and intensified anticholinergic and CNS depressant effects; with phenylephrine and codeine, increased and prolonged cardiac stimulation, increased vasopressor effect, increased risk of severe cardiovascular and cerebrovascular effects (including hypertensive crisis), hyperpyrexia, and vomiting
promethazine and phenylephrine
guanadrel, guanethidine: Decreased antihypertensive effects of these drugs; increased risk of severe hypertension and arrhythmias; increased vasopressor effect of phenylephrine
promethazine and codeine
anticholinergics: Possibly intensified anticholinergic adverse effects
CNS depressants: Additive CNS depression
promethazine
amphetamines: Decreased stimulant effect of amphetamines
anticonvulsants: Lowered seizure threshold
appetite suppressants: Possibly antagonized anorectic effect of appetite suppressants
beta blockers: Increased risk of additive hypotensive effects, irreversible retinopathy, arrhythmias, and tardive dyskinesia
bromocriptine: Decreased effectiveness of bromocriptine
dopamine: Possibly antagonized peripheral vasoconstriction with high doses of dopamine
ephedrine, metaraminol, methoxamine: Decreased vasopressor response to these drugs
epinephrine: Blocked alpha-adrenergic effects of epinephrine; increased risk of hypotension
hepatotoxic drugs: Increased risk of hepatotoxicity
hypotension-producing drugs: Possibly severe hypotension and syncope
levodopa: Inhibited antidyskinetic effects of levodopa
metrizamide: Increased risk of seizures
ototoxic drugs: Possibly masking of some symptoms of ototoxicity, such as dizziness, tinnitus, and vertigo
quinidine: Additive cardiac effects
riboflavin: Increased riboflavin requirements
phenylephrine
alpha blockers, haloperidol, loxapine, phenothiazines, thioxanthenes: Possibly decreased vasoconstrictor effect of phenylephrine

antihypertenisves, diuretics: Possibly decreased antihypertensive effect

atropine: Possibly enhanced vasopressor effect of phenylephrine

beta blockers: Decreased therapeutic effects of both drugs

bretylium: Possibly potentiated vaopressor effect and arrhythmias

doxapram: Increased vasopressor effect of both drugs

ergot alkaloids: Possibly cerebral blood vessel rupture, increased vasopressor effect, peripheral vascular ischemia, and gangrene (with ergotamine)

hydrocarbon inhalation anesthetics: Increased risk of serious arrhythmias

maprotiline, tricyclic antidepressants: Increased risk of severe cardiovascular effects (including arrhythmias, hyperpyrexia, severe hypertension)

mecamylamine, methyldopa: Decreased hypotensive effects of these drugs; increased vasopressor effect of phenylephrine

nitrates: Possibly decreased vasopressor effect of phenylephrine and decreased antianginal effect of nitrates

oxytocin: Possibly severe, persistent hypertension

phenoxybenzamine: Decreased vasoconstrictor effect of phenylephrine, possibly hypotension and tachycardia

theophylline: Possibly enhanced toxicity (including cardiac toxicity)

thyroid hormones: Increased cardiovascular effects of each drug

codeine

antihypertensives, diuretics: Potentiated hypotensive effects

buprenorphine: Decreased effectiveness of codeine

hydroxyzine: Increased codeine analgesic effect; increased CNS depressant and hypotensive effects

metoclopramide: Antagonized effect of metoclopramide on GI motility

naloxone: Antagonized codeine analgesic effect

naltrexone: Precipitated withdrawal symptoms in codeine-dependent patients

neuromuscular blockers: Additive respiratory depressant effects

opioids: Additive CNS and respiratory depressant and hypotensive effects

paregoric: Increased risk of severe constipation

ACTIVITIES

promethazine and codeine

alcohol use: Additive CNS depression

Adverse Reactions

CNS: Akathisia, CNS stimulation, coma, confusion, delirium, depression, disorientation, dizziness, drowsiness, dystonia, euphoria, excitation, fatigue, hallucinations, headache, hysteria, insomnia, irritability, lack of coordination, lethargy, light-headedness, mental and physical impairment, mood changes, nervousness, neuroleptic malignant syndrome, paradoxical stimulation, paresthesia, pseudoparkinsonism, restlessness, sedation, seizures, syncope, tardive dyskinesia, tremor, weakness

CV: Angina, bradycardia, heart block, hypertension, orthostatic hypotension, palpitations, peripheral vasoconstriction, tachycardia, ventricular arrhythmias

EENT: Altered taste; blurred vision; diplopia; dry mouth, nose, and throat; laryngeal edema; laryngospasm; miosis; nasal congestion; rhinitis; tinnitus; vision changes

ENDO: Hyperglycemia

GI: Abdominal cramps and pain, anorexia, constipation, flatulence, gastroesophageal reflux, ileus, indigestion, nausea, vomiting

GU: Decreased libido, difficult ejaculation, dysuria, impotence, oliguria, ureteral spasm, urinary incontinence, urine retention

HEME: Agranulocytosis, leukopenia, thrombocytopenia, thrombocytopenic purpura

MS: Muscle rigidity

RESP: Apnea, bronchoconstriction, bronchospasm, depressed cough reflex, dyspnea, respiratory depression, tenacious bronchial secretions

SKIN: Dermatitis, diaphoresis, flushing, jaundice, pallor, photosensitivity, pruritus, rash, urticaria

Other: Anaphylaxis, angioedema, paradoxical reactions, physical and psychological dependence

Nursing Considerations

- Use cautiously in children age 2 and over because of risk for respiratory depression.
- Use cautiously in patients with a head injury or who have cardiovascular disease, liver or kidney impairment, fever, seizures, hypothyroidism, intestinal inflammation, or Addison's disease.
- Also use cautiously in patients who have recently had stomach, intestinal, or urinary tract surgery.
- Monitor effectiveness of promethazine, phenylephrine, and codeine in relieving allergy symptoms and cough. Notify prescriber if symptoms persist or worsen.
- **WARNING** Monitor respiratory function because promethazine, phenylephrine, and codeine may suppress cough reflex

and cause thickening of bronchial secretions, aggravating such conditions as asthma and COPD. In rare cases, it may depress respirations and induce apnea. Notify prescriber immediately if respiratory rate drops below 10 breaths/minute.

• Monitor patient's hematologic status, as ordered, because promethazine may cause bone marrow depression. Assess patient for signs and symptoms of infection or bleeding.

• **WARNING** Monitor patient for evidence of neuroleptic malignant syndrome, such as fever, hypertension or hypotension, involuntary motor activity, mental changes, muscle rigidity, tachycardia, and tachypenia. Be prepared to provide supportive treatment and additional drug therapy, as prescribed.

• Take safety precautions, if needed, because promethazine, phenylephrine, and codeine can cause considerable drowsiness and many other adverse CNS effects.

• Patient shouldn't have intradermal allergen tests within 72 hours of receiving promethazine, phenylephrine, and codeine because drug may significantly alter flare response.

• **WARNING** Monitor patient closely for signs of overdose, even at normal dosage, because some patients metabolize codeine quickly, leading to a sudden rise in blood codeine level. This metabolic defect occurs in about 0.5 to 1% of Chinese, Japanese, and Hispanic people; 1 to 10% of Caucasians; 3% of African Americans; and 16 to 28% of North Africans, Ethiopians, and Arabs. Watch for extreme sleepiness, confusion, and shallow breathing after giving drug. If present, notify prescriber and be prepared to provide supportive care and discontinue drug, as ordered.

PATIENT TEACHING

• Tell patient to take only the dosage prescribed and not to increase dose or frequency without consulting prescriber.

• Instruct patient to use a calibrated measuring device to ensure accurate dose.

• Advise patient to contact prescriber if symptoms, including cough, are not better after 5 days of therapy.

• Instruct patient to avoid hazardous activities until drug's CNS effects are known.

• Warn patient to avoid alcoholic beverages and OTC antihistamine and CNS depressant drugs while taking promethazine, phenylephrine, and codeine.

• Caution patient to drink plenty of fluids and increase dietary fiber because codeine can cause or worsen constipation.

- Tell patient to rise slowly from a lying or sitting position to minimize dizziness or light-headedness.
- Alert female patients that promethazine, phenylephrine, and codeine may affect pregnancy test results.
- Instruct diabetic patient to monitor his blood glucose level closely while taking promethazine, phenylephrine, and codeine.
- Tell patient to report involuntary muscle movements or unusual sensitivity to sunlight because drug may need to be stopped.
- Advise patient to avoid excessive sun exposure and to use sunscreen when outdoors.
- Urge patient to notify prescriber if he has trouble breathing or develops extreme sleepiness or confusion.

pseudoephedrine hydrochloride and methscopolamine nitrate

AlleRx-D, PSE 120/MSC 2.5

Class and Category

Chemical: Sympathomimetic amine (pseudoephedrine), hyoscine methobromide (methscopolamine)
Therapeutic: Decongestant (pseudoephedrine), anticholinergic (methscopolamine)
Pregnancy category: C

Indications and Dosages

▶ *To relieve nasal congestion caused by the common cold, sinusitis, allergic rhinitis, and other upper respiratory tract conditions*
E. R. TABLETS
Adults. 120 mg pseudoephedrine and 2.5 mg methscopolamine (1 tablet) every 12 hr.

Contraindications

Breast-feeding; cardiac disease, such as arrhythmias, heart failure, coronary artery disease, and mitral stenosis; hemorrhage with hemodynamic instability; hepatic dysfunction; hypersensitivity or idiosyncractic reactions to pseudoephedrine, methscopolamine, or their components; hyperthyroidism; ileus; intestinal atony; myasthenia gravis; myocardial ischemia; narrow-angle glaucoma; obstructive GI or uropathic disease; renal impairment; tachycardia; toxic megacolon; ulcerative colitis; severe coronary artery disease or hypertension; urine retention; use of an MAO inhibitor within 14 days

---

Mechanism of Action

Pseudoephedrine acts on alpha$_1$-adrenergic receptors in the mucosa of the respiratory tract to produce vasoconstriction. This process shrinks swollen nasal mucous membranes; reduces tissue hyperemia, edema, and nasal congestion; and increases nasal airway patency. It also may increase drainage of sinus secretions and open obstructed eustachian ostia.

Methscopolamine competitively inhibits acetylcholine at autonomic postganglionic cholinergic receptors. Because the most sensitive receptors are in the salivary, bronchial, and sweat glands, this action reduces secretions from these glands. It also reduces nasal, oropharyngeal, and bronchial secretions and decreases airway resistance by relaxing smooth muscles in the bronchi and bronchioles.

Interactions

DRUGS

pseudoephedrine

antacids: Increased pseudoephedrine absorption

antihypertensives, diuretics: Possibly decreased antihypertensive effect

beta blockers: Decreased therapeutic effects of both drugs

citrates: Possibly inhibited urinary pseudoephedrine excretion and prolonged duration of action

CNS stimulant, other sympathomimetics: Possibly increased additive CNS stimulation to excessive levels

cocaine (mucosal-local): Possibly increased cardiovascular effects of either drug and CNS stimulation

digoxin, levodopa: Increased risk of cardiac arrhythmias

hydrocarbon inhalation anesthetics: Increased risk of serious arrhythmias

kaolin: Decreased pseudoephedrine absorption

MAO inhibitors: Increased and prolonged cardiac stimulation; increased vasopressor effect; increased risk of severe cardiovascular and cerebrovascular effects, such as hypertensive crisis, hyperpyrexia, and vomiting

nitrates: Reduced antianginal effects of nitrates

rauwolfia alkaloids: Possibly inhibited pseudoephedrine action

thyroid hormones: Increased cardiovascular effects of both drugs

methscopolamine

adsorbent antidiarrheals, antacids: Decreased absorption and therapeutic effects of methoscopolamine

anticholinergics (other): Possibly intensified anticholinergic effects

antimyasthenics: Possibly reduced intestinal motility
CNS depressants: Possibly potentiated effects of either drug, resulting in additive sedation
haloperidol: Decreased antipsychotic effect of haloperidol
ketoconazole: Decreased ketoconazole absorption
lorazepam (parenteral): Possibly hallucinations, irrational behavior, and sedation
metoclopramide: Possibly antagonized effect of metoclopramide on GI motility
opioid analgesics: Increased risk of severe constipation and ileus
potassium chloride: Possibly increased severity of potassium chloride-induced GI lesions,
urinary alkalizers (antacids, carbonic anhydrase inhibitors, citrates, sodium bicarbonate): Delayed excretion of methscopolamine, possibly leading to increased therapeutic and adverse effects
ACTIVITIES
methscopolamine
alcohol use: Additive CNS effects

Adverse Reactions

CNS: Dizziness, drowsiness, euphoria, headache, insomnia, lightheadedness, memory loss, nervousness, paradoxical stimulation, restlessness, trembling, weakness
CV: Palpitations, tachycardia
EENT: Blurred vision; dry eyes, mouth, nose, and throat; mydriasis
GI: Constipation, dysphagia, nausea, vomiting
GU: Dysuria, urinary hesitancy, urine retention
SKIN: Decreased sweating, diaphoresis, dry skin, flushing, pallor

Nursing Considerations

- Monitor renal function, as ordered, because pseudoephedrine is substantially excreted by the kidneys.
- Monitor patients who may be more susceptible to dizziness, drowsiness, and weakness, such as the elderly.
- Monitor renal function, as ordered, because pseudoephedrine is substantially excreted by the kidneys.
- Regularly evaluate effectiveness of pseudoephedrine and methscopolamine in reducing upper respiratory symptoms.

PATIENT TEACHING
- Tell patient to take last dose of the day a few hours before bedtime if drug makes her nervous or restless.
- Instruct patient to swallow tablets whole and not to break, crush, or chew them.

- Urge patient to avoid alcohol, other antidepressants, or OTC preparations without consulting prescriber while taking pseudoephedrine and methscopolamine.
- Instruct patient to avoid hazardous activities until drug's CNS effects are known.
- Suggest frequent rinsing and use of sugarless gum or hard candy for dry mouth; suggest lubricating drops for dry eyes.

theophylline and guaifenesin
Bronchial, Glyceryl-T, Mudrane GG-2, Quibron, Quibron-300, Slo-Phyllin GG
dyphylline and guaifenesin
Dilor-G, Dyflex-G, Dyline GG, Lyfyllin-GG, Panfil G

Class and Category
Chemical: Xanthine derivative (theophylline, dyphylline), glyceryl guaiacolate (guaifenesin)
Therapeutic: Bronchodilator (theophylline, dyphylline), expectorant (guaifenesin)
Pregnancy category: C

Indications and Dosages
▶ *To treat or prevent bronchial spasm; to treat chronic bronchitis and emphysema*
CAPSULES (BRONCHIAL, QUIBRON-300, QUIBRON)
Adults. Highly individualized based on theophylline need. 150 or 300 mg theophylline and 90 or 180 mg guaifenesin per capsule, depending on product used. Number of capsules based on individual dosage calculated to provide 16 mg/kg/day or 400 mg theophylline/day (whichever is less) in divided doses every 6 to 8 hr.
CAPSULES (GLYCERYL-T)
Adults. 150 to 300 mg theophylline and 90 to 180 mg guaifenesin (1 or 2 capsules) b.i.d. or t.i.d.
CAPSULES (SLO-PHYLLIN GG)
Adults. Highly individualized based on theophylline need. 150 mg theophylline and 90 mg guaifenesin per capsule. Number of capsules based on individual dosage calculated to provide 3 mg/kg of theophylline in divided doses every 6 to 8 hr.
TABLETS (MUDRANE GG-2)
Adults. 111 mg theophylline and 100 mg guaifenesin t.i.d. or q.i.d.
TABLETS (DYFLEX-G, DYLINE G.G., LUFYLLIN-GG, PANFIL G)
Adults. 200 to 400 mg dyphylline and 100 to 400 mg guaifen-

esin (1 to 2 tablets depending on product used) t.i.d. or q.i.d.
ORAL SOLUTION (THEOLATE, GLYCERYL-T)
Adults. 150 mg theophylline and 90 mg guaifenesin (15 ml)
every 6 to 8 hr.
ORAL SOLUTION (SLO-PHYLLIN, SYNOPHYLATE-GG)
Adults. Highly individualized based on theophylline need.
150 mg theophylline and 90 or 100 mg guaifenesin per 15 ml.
Number of ml based on individual dosage calculated to provide
3 mg/kg of theophylline in divided doses every 8 hr.
ORAL SOLUTION (ELIXOPHYLLIN GG)
Adults. Highly individualized based on theophylline need.
100 mg theophylline and 100 mg guaifenesin per 15 ml. Number
of ml prescribed based on individual dosage calculated to provide
3 mg/kg of theophylline in divided doses every 8 hr.
ORAL SOLUTION (DILOR-G, DYLINE-GG)
Adults. 100 mg dyphylline and 100 mg guaifenesin per 5 ml or
200 mg dyphylline and 200 mg guaifenesin per 10 ml t.i.d. or q.i.d.
ORAL SOLUTION (PANFIL G)
Adults. 200 mg dyphylline and 100 mg guaifenesin/10 ml t.i.d.
or q.i.d.
ORAL SOLUTION (DYPHYLLINE-GG)
Adults. 200 mg dyphylline and 200 mg guaifenesin (30 ml) q.i.d.

Mechanism of Action
Theophylline and dyphylline inhibit phosphodiesterase enzymes, causing
bronchodilation. Normally, these enzymes inactivate cAMP and cGMP, which
are responsible for bronchial smooth muscle relaxation. These agents also
may cause calcium translocation, antagonize prostaglandins and adenosine
receptors, stimulate catecholamines, and inhibit cGMP metabolism.

    Guaifenesin increases fluid and mucus removal from the upper respiratory
tract by increasing the volume of secretions and reducing their adhesiveness
and surface tension.

Contraindications
Hypersensitivity to theophylline, dyphylline, guaifenesin or their
components; peptic ulcer disease; uncontrolled seizure disorder

Interactions
DRUGS
theophylline and dyphylline
adenosine: Decreased adenosine effectiveness

allopurinol, cimetidine, ciprofloxacin, clarithromycin, disulfiram, enoxacin, erythromycin, fluvoxamine, interferon alpha (human recombinant), methotrexate, mexiletine, pentoxifylline, propafenone, propranolol, tacrine, thiabendazole, ticlopidine, troleandomycin, verapamil: Increased blood theophylline or dyphylline level and risk of toxicity
aminoglutethimide, carbamazepine, isoproterenol (I.V.), moricizine, oral contraceptives (containing estrogen), phenobarbital, phenytoin, rifampin: Decreased blood theophylline or dyphylline level and possibly drug effectiveness
benzodiazepines: Possibly reversal of benzodiazepine sedation
beta blockers: Possibly decreased bronchodilator effect of theophylline or dyphylline
ephedrine: Increased adverse effects, including insomnia, nausea, and nervousness
halothane anesthetics: Increased risk of ventricular arrhythmias
ketamine: Lowered seizure threshold
lithium: Decreased lithium effectiveness
neuromuscular blockers: Possibly antagonized neuromuscular blockage
sucralfate: Decreased absorption of theophylline or dyphylline
FOODS
theophylline and dyphylline
caffeine (large amounts): Possibly increased risk of adverse reactions
high-carbohydrate, low-protein diet: Possibly decreased theophylline or dyphylline elimination
low-carbohydrate, high-protein diet; daily intake of charbroiled beef: Possibly increased theophyllin or dyphylline elimination
ACTIVITIES
theophylline and dyphylline
alcohol use: Increased blood theophylline or dyphylline level and risk of toxicity
smoking: Increased drug clearance, decreased drug effectiveness

Adverse Reactions
CNS: Agitation, behavioral changes, confusion, disorientation, dizziness, headache, insomnia, nervousness, seizures, tremor
CV: Hypotension, tachycardia, ventricular arrhythmias
ENDO: Hyperglycemia
GI: Abdominal pain, diarrhea, heartburn, nausea, vomiting
GU: Increased urine output
SKIN: Rash, urticaria

Nursing Considerations
- Be aware that ideal body weight is used to calculate theophylline and dyphylline dosages; drug doesn't bind well in body fat.

- Be aware that E.R. capsules and tablets shouldn't be used for oral loading doses.
- Monitor blood theophylline (dyphylline) levels as ordered to gauge therapeutic level and detect toxicity.
- Suspect toxicity if patient develops nausea, vomiting, irritability, and restlessness, and be prepared to obtain blood theophylline (dyphylline) level.
- Assess heart rate and rhythm often because theophylline and dyphylline can worsen existing arrhythmias.
- Be especially alert for signs of toxicity in patient with acute pulmonary edema, hypothyroidism, influenza vaccination, prolonged fever, sepsis with multiple organ failure, shock, or viral pulmonary infection because of decreased drug clearance. Also monitor patients with uncorrected acidemia because they have an increased risk of toxicity.
- Evaluate drug's effectiveness in relieving respiratory symptoms, and notify prescriber if symptoms worsen.

PATIENT TEACHING

- Instruct patient prescribed oral solution or syrup to use a calibrated measuring device to ensure accurate dose.
- Teach patient to swallow theophylline or dyphylline and guaifenesin tablets whole and not to chew or crush them, unless scored for breaking.
- Explain that patient may open capsules and mix contents with soft food but that he shouldn't chew or crush granules.
- Instruct patient to take drug with a full glass of water on an empty stomach (30 to 60 minutes before meals or 2 hours after meals). If he develops GI distress, suggest taking drug with food or antacids.
- Encourage patient to take drug at the same times every day.
- Stress importance of not interchanging brands because concentration of drug varies among manufacturers.
- Urge patient to avoid alcohol while taking drug.
- Instruct patient to avoid hazardous activities until drug's CNS effects are known.
- Tell patient to take last dose of the day a few hours before bedtime if drug makes him nervous.
- Advise patient to notify prescriber if he develops a fever, makes a significant dietary change, or starts or stops smoking or taking other drugs because these factors may alter blood theophylline and dyphylline level.
- Instruct patient to notify prescriber if his underlying respiratory condition worsens.

theophylline and potassium iodide
Elixophyllin-KI, Theophylline KI

Class and Category
Chemical: Xanthine derivative (theophylline), iodine (potassium iodide)
Therapeutic: Bronchodilator (theophylline), expectorant (potassium iodide
Pregnancy category: D

Indications and Dosages
▶ *To relieve bronchospasm caused by asthma, bronchitis, or emphysema; to treat chronic bronchitis and emphysema*
ELIXIR
Adults. Highly individualized based on theophylline need. 80 mg theophylline and 130 mg potassium iodide per 15 ml. Number of ml prescribed based on individual dosage calculated to provide 3 mg/kg of theophylline in divided doses every 8 hr.

Mechanism of Action
Theophylline inhibits phosphodiesterase enzymes, causing bronchodilation. Normally, these enzymes inactivate cAMP and cGMP, which are responsible for bronchial smooth muscle relaxation. These agents also may cause calcium translocation, antagonize prostaglandins and adenosine receptors, stimulate catecholamines, and inhibit cGMP metabolism.

Potassium iodide increases fluid and mucus removal from the upper respiratory tract by increasing the volume of secretions and reducing their adhesiveness and surface tension.

Contraindications
Acute bronchitis; Addison's disease; dehydration; heat cramps; hyperkalemia; hyperthyroidism; hypersensitivity to theophylline, iodide, or their components; peptic ulcer disease; iodism; renal impairment; tuberculosis; uncontrolled seizure disorder

Interactions
DRUGS
theophylline
adenosine: Decreased adenosine effectiveness
allopurinol, cimetidine, ciprofloxacin, clarithromycin, disulfiram, enoxacin, erythromycin, fluvoxamine, interferon alfa (human recombinant), methotrexate, mexiletine, pentoxifylline, propafenone, propranolol,

tacrine, thiabendazole, ticlopidine, troleandomycin, verapamil: Increased blood theophylline level and risk of toxicity

aminoglutethimide, carbamazepine, hormonal contraceptives (containing estrogen), isoproterenol (I.V.), moricizine, phenobarbital, phenytoin, rifampin: Decreased blood theophylline level and possibly effects

benzodiazepines: Possibly reversal of benzodiazepine sedation

beta blockers: Possibly decreased bronchodilator effect

ephedrine: Increased adverse effects, including insomnia, nausea, and nervousness

halothane anesthetics: Increased risk of ventricular arrhythmias

ketamine: Lowered seizure threshold

lithium: Decreased lithium effectiveness

neuromuscular blockers: Possibly antagonized neuromuscular blockage

sucralfate: Decreased absorption of theophylline

potassium iodide

antithyroid drugs, lithium: Increased risk of hypothyroidism and goiter

captopril, enalapril, lisinopril, potassium-sparing diuretics: Increased risk of hyperkalemia

FOODS

theophylline

caffeine (high amounts): Increased risk of adverse reactions

high-carbohydrate, low-protein diet: Possibly decreased theophylline elimination

low-carbohydrate, high-protein diet; daily intake of charbroiled beef: Possibly increased theophyllin elimination

ACTIVITIES

theophylline

alcohol use: Increased blood theophylline level and risk of toxicity

smoking: Increased drug clearance, decreased drug effectiveness

Adverse Reactions

CNS: Agitation, behavioral changes, confusion, disorientation, dizziness, fatigue, headache, heaviness or weakness in legs, insomnia, nervousness, paresthesia, seizures, tremor

CV: Hypotension, irregular heartbeat, tachycardia, ventricular arrhythmias

ENDO: Hyperglycemia

EENT: Burning in mouth or throat, increased salivation, metallic taste, sore teeth or gums

GI: Abdominal pain, diarrhea, epigastric pain, heartburn, indigestion, nausea, vomiting

GU: Increased urine output

HEME: Eosinophilia

MS: Arthralgia
SKIN: Acneiform lesions, urticaria
Other: Angioedema, lymphadenopathy

Nursing Considerations

- Use with caution in pregnant or breast-feeding mothers because potassium iodide can cause hypothyroidism and goiter in the fetus and newborn or rash and thyroid suppression in the nursing infant because it is excreted in breast milk.
- Be aware that ideal body weight is used to calculate theophylline dosages because drug doesn't bind well in body fat.
- Monitor blood theophylline levels, as ordered, to gauge therapeutic level and detect toxicity.
- Suspect theophylline toxicity if patient has nausea, vomiting, irritability, or restlessness; expect to obtain blood drug level.
- Monitor serum potassium level regularly in patients with renal impairment because of the risk of hyperkalemia.
- Assess heart rate and rhythm often because theophylline and potassium iodide may worsen existing arrhythmias.
- Be especially alert for signs of toxicity in patient with acute pulmonary edema, hypothyroidism, influenza vaccination, prolonged fever, sepsis with multiple organ failure, shock, or viral pulmonary infection because of decreased drug clearance. Uncorrected acidemia increases the risk of toxicity.
- Evaluate effectiveness of drug in relieving respiratory symptoms; notify prescriber if symptoms worsen.

PATIENT TEACHING

- Instruct patient to use a calibrated measuring device to ensure accurate dose.
- Instruct patient to take drug with a full glass of water on an empty stomach (30 to 60 minutes before meals or 2 hours after meals). If she develops GI distress, suggest taking drug with food or antacids.
- Encourage patient to take drug at the same times every day.
- Urge patient to avoid alcohol while taking drug.
- Instruct patient to avoid hazardous activities until drug's CNS effects are known.
- Tell patient to take last dose of the day a few hours before bedtime if drug makes her nervous.
- Urge patient to notify prescriber if she develops a fever, makes a significant dietary change, or starts or stops smoking or taking other drugs; these factors may alter blood theophylline level.
- Instruct patient to report worsening respiratory condition.

APPENDICES

ANTINEOPLASTIC COMBINATION THERAPY FOR SELECTED COMMON CANCERS

This table lists common cancers for which combination chemotherapy is standard therapy. Specific regimens, dosages, and protocols depend on the stage of the cancer, presence of metastasis, and the patient's physical condition at the time of therapy.

Cancer Type	Combination Therapy Used
Breast (Female)	**Node-Negative Patients** • CMF: cyclophosphamide, methotrexate, and fluorouracil • FAC/CAF: fluorouracil, doxorubicin, and cyclophosphamide • AC: doxorubicin and cyclophosphamide **Node-Positive Patients** • FAC (CAF): fluorouracil, doxorubicin, and cyclophosphamide • CEF: cyclophosphamide, epirubicin, and fluorouracil • AC: doxorubicin and cyclophosphamide • EC: epirubicin and cyclophosphamide • TAC: docetaxel, doxorubicin, cyclophosphamide, with or without filgrastim support • CMF: cyclophosphamide, methotrexate, and fluorouracil • A-CMF: doxorubicin followed by cyclophosphamide, methotrexate, and fluorouracil • AC-T: doxorubicin and cyclophosphamide followed by paclitaxel or docetaxel • A-T-C: doxorubicin followed by paclitaxel followed by cyclophosphamide
Lung	**General Combinations** • paclitaxel and carboplatin • cisplatin and vinorelbine • cisplatin and etoposide • carboplatin and etoposide **Non–Small-Cell Lung Cancer** • gemcitabine, cisplatin, and vinorelbine • etoposide, cisplatin **Small-Cell Lung Cancer (limited stage)** • etoposide, cisplatin • etoposide, cisplatin, and vincristine

(continued)

ANTINEOPLASTIC COMBINATION THERAPY FOR SELECTED COMMON CANCERS *(continued)*

Cancer Type	Combination Therapy Used
Lung *(continued)*	**Small-Cell Lung Cancer (extensive stage)** • cyclophosphamide, doxorubicin, and vincristine • cyclophosphamide, doxorubicin, and etoposide • etoposide and cisplatin or carboplatin • ifosfamide, carboplatin, and etoposide • cyclophosphamide, methotrexate, and lomustine • cyclophosphamide, methotrexate, lomustine, and vincristine • cyclophosphamide, etoposide, and vincristine • cyclophosphamide, doxorubicn, etoposide, and vincristine • cyclophosphamide, doxorubicin, etoposide, and vincristine
Colon	• irinotecan, fluorouracil, leucovorin • folic acid, fluorouracil, irinotecan • oxaliplatin, leucovorin, fluorouracil • fluorouracil, levamisole • fluorouracil, leucovorin
Melanoma	• dacarbazine, carmustine, cisplatin, and tamoxifen • dacarbazine, carmustine and cisplatin • cisplatin, vinblastine, and dacarbazine
Bladder (invasive)	• MVAC: methotrexate, vinblastine, doxorubicin [adriamycin], and cisplatin • CMV: cisplatin, methotrexate, and vincristine • CISCA: cisplatin, cyclophosphamide, and doxorubicin • GC: gemcitabine and cisplatin

ANTINEOPLASTIC COMBINATION THERAPY FOR SELECTED COMMON CANCERS (continued)

Cancer Type	Combination Therapy Used
Non-Hodgkin's Lymphoma	• CHOP: cyclophosphamide, doxorubin or hydroxydoxorubicin, vincristine, and prednisone • CHOP-R: cyclophosphamide, doxorubin or hydroxydoxorubicin, vincristine, and prednisone plus rituxan • CVP: cyclophosphamide, vincristine, and prednisolone • BACOD: bleomycin, doxorubicin, cyclophosphamide, vincristine, and dexamethasone • MACOP-B: methotrexate, doxorubicin, cyclophosphamide, vincristine, prednisone, and bleomycin • Pro-MACE-CytaBOM: prednisone, methotrexate (with leucovorin rescuer), doxorubicin, cyclophosphamide, etoposide, cytarabine, bleomycin, vincristine • EPOCH: etoposide, prednisone, vincristine, cyclophosphamide, fluoxymesterone
Pancreatic	• gemcitabine and erlotinib

COMBINATION ORAL CONTRACEPTIVES

Combination oral contraceptives (COCs) prevent pregnancy mainly by preventing ovulation. They also thicken the cervical mucus, which helps prevent sperm from passing through the cervix. COCs contain estrogen and progesterone in varying amounts and delivery sequence, depending on the manufacturer.

Minor adverse reactions to COCs include spotting or bleeding between menstrual periods, headache, nausea, vomiting, breast tenderness, dizziness, weight or mood changes, and facial acne or melasma. Most of these reactions resolve after the first few months of use. Serious adverse reactions to estrogen-containing contraceptive pills include blood clots, MI, and stroke. Women who smoke have a higher risk of these complications. Therefore, women who smoke should not consider using COCs.

There are several contraindications to COCs, including being age 35 or over, a smoker, or pregnant; being diabetic for 20 years or more; having complications of diabetes; or having a history of active thromboembolic or CV disease, known or suspected breast cancer, active liver disease or tumors, or migraine headaches with visual abnormalities, such as blurring or loss of vision.

Familiarize yourself with the many COCs by reviewing the table that appears on the following pages. Also, give patients the following detailed instructions on how to take prescribed COCs correctly and safely.

GENERAL INSTRUCTIONS
• Take the first pill on any of the first 7 days of your menstrual period (day 1 is the first day of bleeding). Many women find it easiest to take the first pill on the first day of bleeding.
• During the first cycle of pills, use a backup contraceptive method, such as a condom, until you have taken the pills for 2 consecutive days.
• Swallow 1 pill each day at the same time of day, whether or not you have sexual intercourse.
• If you're using a 28-day or 84-day extended cycle packet, don't skip a single day between packets, even if you are still menstruating. Always start a new packet the day after finishing the last packet. If you're using a 21-day packet, wait 7 days after finishing a packet before starting a new packet of pills.
• If this is your first time taking COCs and you have no problems, return to your healthcare provider when you need a new supply of pills. Bring the empty pill packets with you when you return.
• If you've just delivered a baby and you aren't breastfeeding, you may start taking the pill after the third postpartum week, or

COMBINATION ORAL CONTRACEPTIVES *(continued)*

any time you and your healthcare provider confirm that you aren't pregnant.

• If you've just had an abortion, you may start taking the pill on the same day as the abortion or any time you and your healthcare provider confirm that you aren't pregnant.

• If you're ill and have severe vomiting or diarrhea, your pills may not work effectively. Use another contraceptive method or avoid sexual intercourse until you're better and have taken the pills for 7 consecutive days without severe vomiting or diarrhea.

• Some medications interfere with the pill's effectiveness. Check with your healthcare provider if you start taking medication for seizures or convulsions, or you begin taking rifampin (rifampicin)—a drug used to treat tuberculosis. Bring the pill packets with you when you visit your healthcare provider, and explain that you're taking a COC.

If you miss taking a pill

• If you miss day 1, take a pill as soon as you remember. Take the next pill at the regular time, even if this means taking 2 pills on the same day.

• If you miss taking a pill 2 or more days in a row, take a pill as soon as you remember, and continue taking a pill each day. Wait to have sexual intercourse, or use an additional contraceptive method (such as condoms), until you have taken 1 COC pill daily for 7 consecutive days. This will give the pills time to protect you fully against pregnancy.

• If you have trouble remembering to take a pill every day, talk with your healthcare provider about using another method of family planning.

OTHER INSTRUCTIONS

• Usually, your period will start while you're taking the fourth week of pills. If you don't have a period, keep taking the pills as prescribed.

• If you think you could be pregnant, contact your healthcare provider.

• Go to the hospital immediately if you have any of the following signs and symptoms: severe pain in your belly; severe pain in your chest; severe headache, dizziness, weakness, or numbness; blurred or reduced vision; speech problems; yellowing of the skin or eyes (jaundice); severe pain in your leg (calf or thigh).

(continued)

COMBINATION ORAL CONTRACEPTIVES *(continued)*

Trade Names	Estrogen Content*	Synthetic Progesterone Content
Monophasic Contraceptives		
LoSeasonique (extended cycle of 84 days)	*84 tablets:* 2 mcg ethinyl estradiol *7 tabets:* 1 mcg ethinyl estradiol	*84 tablets:* 100 mcg levonorgestrel *7 tablets:* no levonorgestrel
Alesse, Levline, Lutera	*21 tablets:* 20 mcg ethinyl estradiol *7 tablets:* placebo	*21 tablets:* 100 mcg levonoregestrel *7 tablets:* placebo
Loestrin 1/20 Fe, Loestrin 24 Fe, Microgestin 1/20	*21 tablets:* 20 mcg ethinyl estradiol *7 tablets:* placebo	*21 tablets:* 1,000 mcg norethindrone *7 tablets:* placebo
Levlen, Levora, Nordette	*21 tablets:* 30 mcg ethinyl estradiol *7 tablets:* placebo	*21 tablets:* 150 mcg levonoregestrel *7 tablets:* placebo
Seasonale, Quasense (extended cycle of 84 days)	*84 tablets:* 30 mcg ethinyl estradiol	*84 tablets:* 150 mcg levonorgestrel
Seasonique (extended cycle of 84 days)	*84 tablets:* 30 mcg ethinyl estradiol *7 tablets:* 10 mcg ethinyl estradiol	*84 tablets:* 150 mcg levonorgestrel *7 tablets:* no levonorgestrel
Lo-Ovral	*21 tablets:* 30 mcg ethinyl estradiol *7 tablets:* placebo	*21 tablets:* 300 mcg norgestrel *7 tablets:* placebo
Desogen, Ortho-Cept	*21 tablets:* 30 mcg ethinyl estradiol *7 tablets:* placebo	*21 tablets:* 150 mcg desogestrel *7 tablets:* placebo
Loestrin 1.5/30, Microgestin 1.5/30	*21 tablets:* 30 mcg ethinyl estradiol *7 tablets:* placebo	*21 tablets:* 1,500 mcg norethindrone *7 tablets:* placebo

* Products organized by amount of estrogen provided.

COMBINATION ORAL CONTRACEPTIVES *(continued)*

Trade Names	Estrogen Content	Synthetic Progesterone Content
Monophasic Contraceptives *(continued)*		
Yasmin	*21 tablets:* 30 mcg ethinyl estradiol *7 tablets:* placebo	*21 tablets:* 3,000 mcg drospirenone *7 tablets:* placebo
Ortho-Cyclen	*21 tablets:* 35 mcg ethinyl estradiol *7 tablets:* placebo	*21 tablets:* 250 mcg norgestimate *7 tablets:* placebo
Femcon Fe, Ovcon-35	*21 tablets:* 35 mcg ethinyl estradiol *7 tablets:* placebo (Ovcon-35), ferrous fumarate (Femcon Fe)	*21 tablets:* 400 mcg norethindrone *7 tablets:* placebo (Ovcon-35), ferrous fumarate (Femcon Fe)
Brevicon, Modicon	*21 tablets:* 35 mcg ethinyl estradiol *7 tablets:* placebo	*21 tablets:* 500 mcg norethindrone *7 tablets:* placebo
Ortho-Novum 1/35, Necon, Norethin, Norinyl 1/35	*21 tablets:* 35 mcg ethinyl estradiol *7 tablets:* placebo	*21 tablets:* 1,000 mcg norethindrone *7 tablets:* placebo
Demulen 1/35, Zovia 1/35	*21 tablets:* 35 mcg ethinyl estradiol *7 tablets:* placebo	*21 tablets:* 1,000 mcg ethynodiol diacetate *7 tablets:* placebo
Ovcon 50	*21 tablets:* 50 mcg ethinyl estradiol *7 tablets:* placebo	*21 tablets:* 1,000 mcg norethindrone *7 tablets:* placebo
Ogestrel, Ovral	*21 tablets:* 50 mcg ethinyl estradiol *7 tablets:* placebo	*21 tablets:* 500 mcg norgestrel *7 tablets:* placebo
Demulen 1/50, Zovia 1/50	*21 tablets:* 50 mcg ethinyl estradiol *7 tablets:* placebo	*21 tablets:* 1,000 mcg ethynodiol diacetate *7 tablets:* placebo

(continued)

COMBINATION ORAL CONTRACEPTIVES *(continued)*

Trade Names	Estrogen Content	Synthetic Progesterone Content
Monophasic Contraceptives *(continued)*		
Necon 1/50, Norinyl 1/50, Ortho-Novum 1/50	*21 tablets:* 50 mcg mestraol *7 tablets:* placebo	*21 tablets:* 1,000 mcg norethindrone *7 tablets:* placebo
Multiphasic Contraceptives		
Kariva, Mircette	*21 tablets:* 20 mcg ethinyl estradiol *5 tablets:* 10 mcg ethinyl estradiol *2 tablets:* placebo	*21 tablets:* 150 mcg desogestrel *5 tablets:* 0 mcg desogestrel *2 tablets:* placebo
Estrostep Fe	*5 tablets:* 20 mcg ethinyl estradiol *7 tablets:* 30 mcg ethinyl estradiol *9 tablets:* 35 mcg ethinyl estradiol *7 tablets:* ferrous fumarate	*21 tablets:* 1,000 mcg ethinyl estradiol *7 tablets:* ferrous fumarate
Cyclessa, Velivet	*7 tablets:* 25 mcg ethinyl estradiol *7 tablets:* 25 mcg ethinyl estradiol *7 tablets:* 25 mcg ethinyl estradiol *7 tablets:* ferric oxide	*7 tablets:* 100 mcg desogestrel *7 tablets:* 125 mcg desogestrel *7 tablets:* 150 mcg desogestrel *7 tablets:* ferric oxide
TriLevelen, Triphasil, Trivora	*6 tablets:* 30 mcg ethinyl estradiol *5 tablets:* 40 mcg ethinyl estradiol *10 tablets:* 30 mcg ethinyl estradiol *7 tablets:* placebo	*6 tablets:* 50 mcg levonorgestrel *5 tablets:* 75 mcg levonorgestrel *10 tablets:* 125 mcg levonorgestrel *7 tablets:* placebo

COMBINATION ORAL CONTRACEPTIVES *(continued)*

Trade Names	Estrogen Content	Synthetic Progesterone Content
Multiphasic Contraceptives *(continued)*		
Ortho-Novum 10/11	*10 tablets:* 35 mcg ethinyl estradiol *11 tablets:* 35 mcg ethinyl estradiol *7 tablets:* placebo	*10 tablets:* 500 mcg norethindrone *11 tablets:* 1,000 mcg norethindrone *7 tablets:* placebo
Ortho-Novum 7/7/7	*7 tablets:* 35 mcg ethinyl estradiol *7 tablets:* 35 mcg ethinyl estradiol *7 tablets:* 35 mcg ethinyl estradiol *7 tablets:* placebo	*7 tablets:* 500 mcg norethindrone *7 tablets:* 750 mcg norethindrone *7 tablets:* 1,000 mcg norethindrone *7 tablets:* placebo
Ortho Tri Cyclen	*7 tablets:* 35 mcg ethinyl estradiol *7 tablets:* 35 mcg ethinyl estradiol *7 tablets:* 35 mcg ethinyl estadiol *7 tablets:* placebo	*7 tablets:* 180 mcg norgestimate *7 tablets:* 215 mcg norgestimate *7 tablets:* 250 mcg norgestimate *7 tablets:* placebo
Ortho Tri Cyclen Lo	*7 tablets:* 25 mcg ethinyl estradiol *7 tablets:* 25 mcg ethinyl estradiol *7 tablets:* 25 mcg ethinyl estradiol *7 tablets:* placebo	*7 tablets:* 180 mcg norgestimate *7 tablets:* 215 mcg norgestimate *7 tablets:* 250 mcg norgestimate *7 tablets:* placebo
Continuous Contraceptives		
Lybrel	*28 tablets:* 20 mcg ethinyl estradiol	*28 tablets:* 90 mcg levonorgestrel

COMPATIBLE DRUGS IN A SYRINGE

The chart below lets you know at a glance whether listed drugs are compatible for at least 15 minutes when mixed together in a syringe for immediate administration. However, keep in mind that drugs listed as compatible when mixed in a syringe may not be compatible when prepared for other routes of administration. Drug combinations pre-

	atropine	chlorpromazine	dexamethasone	diazepam	diphenhydramine	droperidol	furosemide	glycopyrrolate	haloperidol	heparin	hydromorphone
atropine		C	n/a	n/a	C	C	n/a	C	I	n/a	C
chlorpromazine	C		n/a	n/a	C	C	n/a	C	n/a	I	C
dexamethasone	n/a	n/a		n/a	I	n/a	n/a	n/a	n/a	n/a	C
diazepam	n/a	n/a	n/a		n/a	n/a	n/a	I	n/a	I	n/a
diphenhydramine	C	C	I	n/a		C	n/a	C	I	n/a	C
droperidol	C	C	n/a	n/a	C		I	C	n/a	I	n/a
furosemide	n/a	n/a	n/a	n/a	n/a	I		n/a	n/a	C	n/a
glycopyrrolate	C	C	I	C	C	C	n/a		C	n/a	C
haloperidol	n/a	n/a	n/a	n/a	C	n/a	n/a	n/a		I	C
heparin	C	I	n/a	I	n/a	I	C	n/a	I		n/a
hydromorphone	C	C	n/a	n/a	C	n/a	n/a	C	C	n/a	
hydroxyzine	C	C	n/a	n/a	C	C	n/a	C	I	n/a	C
ketorolac	n/a	n/a	n/a	I	n/a	n/a	n/a	n/a	I	n/a	I
lidocaine	n/a	n/a	n/a	n/a	n/a	n/a	n/a	C	n/a	C	n/a
lorazepam	n/a	n/a	n/a	n/a	n/a	n/a	n/a	n/a	n/a	n/a	C
meperidine	C	C	n/a	C	C	C	n/a	C	n/a	I	n/a
metoclopramide	C	C	n/a	n/a	C	C	I	n/a	n/a	C	C
midazolam	C	C	n/a	n/a	C	n/a	n/a	C	C	n/a	C
morphine	C	C	n/a	n/a	C	C	n/a	C	I	C*	n/a
pentobarbital	C	I	n/a	n/a	I	I	n/a	I	n/a	n/a	C
prochlorperazine	C	n/a	n/a	n/a	C	C	n/a	C	n/a	n/a	I
ranitidine	C	I	C	n/a	C	n/a	n/a	C	n/a	n/a	C
scopolamine	C	C	n/a	n/a	C	C	n/a	C	n/a	n/a	C

* Compatible only with morphine doses of 1 mg, 2 mg, and 5 mg.

pared for immediate administration usually require a more concentrated solution than those prepared for infusion.

Key: C = compatible; I = Incompatible; n/a = Compatibility information not available; n = No recommendations can be given

	hydroxyzine	ketorolac	lidocaine	lorazepam	meperidine	metoclopramide	midazolam	morphine	pentobarbital	prochlorperazine	ranitidine	scopolamine
	C	n/a	n/a	n/a	C	C	C	C	C	C	C	C
	C	n/a	n/a	n/a	C	C	C	I	I	C	C	C
	n/a	n/a	n/a	n/a	n/a	C	n/a	n/a	n/a	n/a	C	n/a
	n/a	I	n/a	n/a	n/a	n/a	n/a	n/a	n/a	n/a	I	n/a
	C	n/a	n/a	n/a	C	C	C	C	I	C	C	C
	C	n/a	n/a	n/a	C	C	C	C	I	C	n/a	C
	n/a	n/a	n/a	n/a	n/a	I	n/a	n/a	n/a	n/a	n	n/a
	C	n/a	C	n/a	C	n/a	C	C	I	C	C	C
	I	I	n/a	n/a	n/a	n/a	n/a	I	n/a	n/a	n/a	n/a
	n/a	n/a	C	n/a	I	C	n/a	C	n/a	n/a	n	n/a
	C	I	n/a	C	n/a	n/a	C	n/a	C	I	C	C
		I	C	n/a	C	C	C	C	I	C	C	C
	I		n/a	n/a	n/a	n/a	n/a	n/a	n/a	I	n/a	n/a
	C	n/a		n/a	n/a	C	n/a	n/a	n/a	n/a	n/a	n/a
	n/a	n/a	n/a		n/a	n/a	n/a	n/a	n/a	n/a	I	n/a
	C	n/a	n/a	n/a		C	C	I	I	C	C	C
	n/a	n/a	C	n/a	C		C	C	n/a	C	C	C
	C	n/a	n/a	n/a	C	C		C	I	I	I	C
	C	n/a	n/a	n/a	n/a	C	C		I	C	C	C
	I	n/a	n/a	n/a	I	I	I	I		I	I	C
	C	I	n/a	n/a	C	C	I	C	I		C	C
	I	n/a	n/a	I	C	C	I	C	I	C		C
	C	n/a	n/a	n/a	C	C	C	C	C	C	C	

DRUG FORMULAS AND CALCULATIONS

When administering drugs, you must be familiar with drug formulas and calculation methods to ensure that your patient receives the prescribed drug in the correct dosage, strength, or flow rate. This appendix will provide you with a quick review of how to calculate solution strengths, drug dosages, and I.V. flow rates.

CALCULATING THE STRENGTH OF A SOLUTION

Most solutions come prepared in the required strength by the pharmacy or medical supply source. But sometimes only the concentrated form is available, and you'll need to dilute the solution or solid to administer the prescribed strength.

When a solid form of a drug is used to prepare a solution, the drug must be completely dissolved. Solid forms, such as tablets, crystals, and powders, are considered 100% strength. (An exception is boric acid, which is only 5% at full strength.) The final diluted solution is stated in terms of liquid measurement. To prepare a solution, you'll need to add the prescribed solid or liquid form of the drug (the solute) to the prescribed amount of diluent (the solvent). Two of the most common diluents used in the clinical setting are normal saline solution and sterile water.

You can use either of two formulas to calculate the strength of a solution, as shown in the examples below.

Method 1: Calculating percentage and volume

Use the following formula:

$$\frac{\text{Weaker solution}}{\text{Stronger solution}} = \frac{\text{Solute}}{\text{Solvent}}$$

Example: You need to dilute a stock solution of 100% strength to a 5% solution. How much solute will you need to add to obtain 500 ml of the 5% solution?

Calculate as follows:

$$\frac{5\ (\%)\ \text{(Weaker solution)}}{100\ (\%)\ \text{(Stronger solution)}} = \frac{\text{X (g) (Solute)}}{500\ \text{ml (Solvent)}}$$

$$100\ \text{X} = (500)(5)\ \text{or } 2{,}500$$

$$\text{X} = 25\ \text{g}$$

Answer: You'll need to add 25 g of solute to each 500 ml of solvent to prepare a 5% solution.

CALCULATING THE STRENGTH OF A SOLUTION *(continued)*

Method 2: Calculating percentage and volume

Use the following formula:

$$\frac{\text{(Desired strength)}}{\text{(Available strength)}} \times \begin{matrix}\text{Total amount}\\\text{of desired}\\\text{solution}\end{matrix} = X \begin{matrix}\text{(Amount of undiluted}\\\text{drug needed to}\\\text{make solution)}\end{matrix}$$

Example: You need to make 100 ml of a 20% solution, using an 80% solution. How much of the 80% solution must you add to the sterile water to yield a final volume of 100 ml of a 20% solution?

Calculate as follows:

$$\frac{20\ (\%)\ \text{(Desired strength)}}{80\ (\%)\ \text{(Available strength)}} \times 100\ \text{ml} \begin{matrix}\text{(Total amount of}\\\text{desired solution)}\end{matrix} = X$$

$$\frac{0.20}{0.80} = 0.25$$

$$0.25 \times 100\ \text{(ml)} = X$$

$$X = 25\ \text{ml of 80\% solution}$$

Answer: You'll need to add 25 ml of the 80% solution to the water to yield a final volume of 100 ml of a 20% solution.

CALCULATING DRUG DOSAGES

You may be required to calculate drug dosages when you need to administer a drug that's available only in one measure, but prescribed in another. You should also be prepared to convert various units of measure, such as milligrams (mg) to grains (gr), and dry measurements to liquid. You can use three common methods of ratio and proportion to calculate drug dosages, as shown in the examples on the next five pages.

(continued)

DRUG FORMULAS AND CALCULATIONS
(continued)

CALCULATING ORAL DRUG DOSAGES
Example: You need to give a patient 0.25 mg of digoxin, which comes only in 0.125-mg tablets. How many tablets will you need to give him to attain the proper dosage?

Method 1: Using labeled amount of drug
In this method, true proportions between the drug label and the prescribed dose are used to determine ratio and proportion. The drug label, which states the amount of drug in one unit of measurement—in this case, 0.125-mg in each tablet of digoxin—is the first ratio, expressed as follows:

milligrams : tablets = milligrams : tablets

0.125 mg (amount of drug) : 1 tablet (unit of measure)

The prescribed dose—in this case, 0.25-mg—is the second ratio; it must be stated in the same order and units of measure as the first, as follows:

0.125 mg : 1 tablet = 0.25 mg : X (tablets)

Calculate as follows:

$$0.125 X = 0.25$$

$$X = \frac{0.25}{0.125}$$

$$X = 2$$

Answer: You'll need to give the patient 2 tablets of digoxin 0.125 mg.

Be sure to use critical thinking to assess whether your answer is correct. Because the amount of drug prescribed is greater than the amount of drug in one tablet, it's reasonable to expect the required number of tablets to be greater than one.

CALCULATING ORAL DRUG DOSAGES *(continued)*

Method 2: Using an established formula
To determine the correct number of digoxin tablets to give using this method, use the following formula:

$$\frac{\text{Prescribed dose}}{\text{Dose available}} \times \text{Quantity (unit of measure)} = \text{X (unknown quantity to be given)}$$

Calculate as follows:

$$\frac{0.25 \text{ mg}}{0.125 \text{ mg}} \times 1 \text{ tablet} = \text{X (number of 0.125-mg tablets)}$$

$$\frac{0.25}{0.125} = 2\text{X}$$

$$2 = \text{X}$$

Answer: You'll need to give the patient 2 tablets of digoxin 0.125 mg.

Method 3: Calculating according to proportion size
This method uses the same components as method #1, but the ratio is based on proportions according to size. To determine the correct number of digoxin tablets to give using this method, use the following formula:

$$\frac{\text{smaller}}{\text{larger}} = \frac{\text{smaller}}{\text{larger}}$$

Substitute 0.125 into the smaller part and 0.25 into the greater part of the first ratio. Critical thinking leads us to believe that you'll need more than 1 tablet of the weaker 0.125-mg strength to equal the stronger 0.25 mg. Set up the proportion as follows:

$$\frac{0.125 \text{ mg}}{0.25 \text{ mg}} = \frac{1 \text{ (tablet)}}{\text{X (tablets)}}$$

Calculate as follows:

$$0.125 \text{ X} = 0.25$$

$$\text{X} = \frac{0.25}{0.125}$$

$$\text{X} = 2 \text{ tablets}$$

Answer: You'll need to give the patient 2 tablets of digoxin 0.125 mg.

(continued)

DRUG FORMULAS AND CALCULATIONS
(continued)

CALCULATING PARENTERAL DRUG DOSAGES
The same methods used for calculating oral drugs and solutions can be used for preparing parenteral injections.
Example: You need to administer a prescribed dose of 1 mg morphine sulfate from a unit-dose cartridge containing 4 mg per 2 ml. How many milliliters will you need to give to equal the prescribed dose of 1 mg?

Method 1: Using labeled amount of drug
Using the same ratio as for oral drugs, the drug label—in this case, 4 mg—is the first ratio, and the prescribed dose—in this case, 1 mg—is the second ratio, expressed as follows:

4 mg (the amount of drug) : 2 ml (the unit of measure)

Calculate as follows:

$$4 \text{ mg} : 2 \text{ ml} = 1 \text{ mg} : X \text{ ml}$$
$$4X = 2$$
$$X = \frac{2}{4}$$
$$X = 0.5 \text{ ml}$$

Answer: You'll need to give 0.5 ml of morphine sulfate to equal the prescribed dose of 1 mg.

Method 2: Using an established formula
Use this formula:

$$\frac{\text{Prescribed dose}}{\text{Dose available}} \times \text{Quantity (unit of measure)} = X \text{ (unknown quantity to be given)}$$

Calculate as follows:

$$\frac{1 \text{ mg}}{4 \text{ mg}} \times 2 \text{ ml} = X \text{ (number of ml)}$$

$$\frac{4}{2} = 0.5$$

Answer: You'll need to give 0.5 ml of morphine sulfate to equal the prescribed dose of 1 mg.

CALCULATING PARENTERAL DRUG DOSAGES *(continued)*

Method 3: Calculating according to proportion size
To determine the correct amount of morphine sulfate to give using this method, use the following formula:

smaller : greater = smaller : greater
milligrams : milligrams = milliliters : milliliters

Critical thinking leads us to believe that 1 mg is less than 4 mg and that you'll need less than 2 ml to give 1 mg of the drug; therefore, 1 mg goes into the smaller part of the first ratio, and X goes into the smaller part of the second ratio. Set up the proportion as follows:

$$1 \text{ mg} : 4 \text{ mg} = X \text{ (ml)} : 2 \text{ ml}$$
$$4X = 2$$
$$X = \frac{2}{4}$$
$$X = 0.5$$

Answer: You'll need to give 0.5 ml of morphine sulfate to equal the prescribed dose of 1 mg.

CALCULATING I.V. FLOW RATES
When an I.V. solution is delivered by gravity, you must calculate the number of drops needed per minute for proper infusion. To calculate I.V. flow rates, you need to know three things:
• the drip factor—or the number of drops contained in 1 ml for the type of I.V. set you'll be using. This information is provided on the individual package label.
• the amount and type of fluid that you'll infuse as prescribed on the physician's order sheet
• the infusion duration time in minutes.
    Once you've gathered this information, you can calculate the I.V. flow rate using the following equation:

$$\frac{\text{Total number of ml}}{\text{Total number of minutes}} \times \text{drip factor (gtt/ml)} = \text{flow rate (gtt/min)}$$

(continued)

DRUG FORMULAS AND CALCULATIONS
(continued)

CALCULATING I.V. FLOW RATES *(continued)*
Example 1: If the physician prescribes 1,000 ml of D_5W to infuse over 10 hours, and the drip rate for your administration set delivers 15 drops (gtt) per ml, calculate as follows:

$$\frac{1,000 \text{ ml}}{10 \text{ hours x 60 minutes}} \times 15 \text{ gtt/ml} = X \text{ gtt/minute}$$

$$\frac{1,000 \text{ ml}}{600 \text{ minutes}} \times 15 \text{ gtt/ml} = X \text{ gtt/minute}$$

$$1.67 \text{ ml/minute} \times 15 \text{ gtt/ml} = X \text{ gtt/minute}$$

$$25.05 \text{ gtt/minute} = X$$

Answer: To infuse, round off 25.05 to 25 gtt/minute or according to your institution's policy.

Example 2: If the physician prescribes 500 ml of 0.45% NS to infuse over 2 hours, and the drip rate for your administration set delivers 10 gtt/ml, calculate as follows:

$$\frac{500 \text{ ml}}{2 \text{ hours} \times 60 \text{ minutes}} \times 10 \text{ gtt/ml} = X \text{ gtt/minute}$$

$$\frac{500 \text{ ml}}{120 \text{ minutes}} \times 10 \text{ gtt/ml} = X \text{ gtt/minute}$$

$$4.17 \text{ ml/minute} \times 10 \text{ gtt/ml} = X \text{ gtt/minute}$$

$$41.7 \text{ gtt/minute} = X$$

Answer: To infuse, round off 41.7 to 42 gtt/minute or according to your institution's policy.

Note: When preparing for I.V. administration using a controlled infusion device, the electronic flow-regulator will either count drops using an electronic eye or use a controlled pumping action to deliver the fluid in milliliters. Your final calculation will be based on the unit of measure used by the device: drops per minute or ml per hour.

WEIGHTS AND EQUIVALENTS

Table 1: Liquid Equivalents Among Household Apothecaries', and Metric Systems

Household	Apothecaries'	Metric
1 teaspoon (tsp)	1 fluid dram	5 milliliters (ml)
1 tablespoon (tbs)	0.5 fluid ounce	15 ml
2 tbs (1 ounce [1 oz])	1 fluid ounce	30 ml
1 cupful	8 fluid ounces	240 ml
1 pint (pt)	16 fluid ounces	473 ml
1 quart (qt)	32 fluid ounces	946 ml (1 liter)

Table 2: Solid Equivalents Among Apothecaries' and Metric Systems

Apothecaries'	Metric
15 grains (gr)	1 gram (g) (1,000 milligrams [mg])
10 gr	0.5 g (500 mg)
7.5 gr	0.5 g (500 mg)
5 gr	0.3 g (300 mg)
3 gr	0.2 g (200 mg)
1.5 gr	0.1 g (100 mg)
1 gr	0.06 g (60 mg) or 0.065 g (65 mg)
0.75 gr	0.05 g (50 mg)
0.5 gr	0.03 g (30 mg)
0.25 gr	0.015 g (15 mg)
1/60 gr	0.001 g (1 mg)
1/100 gr	0.5 mg
1/120 gr	0.5 mg
1/150 gr	0.4 mg

(continued)

WEIGHTS AND EQUIVALENTS (continued)

Table 3: Solid Equivalents Among Avoirdupois Apothecaries', and Metric Systems

Avoirdupois	Apothecaries'	Metric
1 gr	1 gr	0.065 g
15.4 gr	15 gr	1 g
1 ounce (1 oz)	480 gr	28.35 g
437.5 gr	1 oz	31 g
1 pound (lb)	1.33 lb	454 g
0.75 lb	1 lb	373 g
2.2 lb	2.7 lb	1 kilogram (kg)

ABBREVIATIONS

The following abbreviations, which are common to nursing practice, are used throughout the book.

ABG	arterial blood gas
a.c.	before meals
ACE	angiotensin-converting enzyme
ADH	antidiuretic hormone
AIDS	acquired immunodeficiency syndrome
ALT	alanine aminotransferase
ANA	antinuclear antibodies
APTT	activated partial thromboplastin time
AST	aspartate aminotransferase
ATP	adenosine triphosphate
AV	atrioventricular
b.i.d.	twice a day
BUN	blood urea nitrogen
°C	degrees Celsius
cAMP	cyclic adenosine monophosphate
(CAN)	Canadian drug trade name
cap	capsule
CBC	complete blood count
cGMP	cyclic guanosine monophosphate
CK	creatine kinase
Cl	chloride
cm	centimeter
CMV	cytomegalovirus
CNS	central nervous system
COPD	chronic obstructive pulmonary disease
C.R.	controlled-release
CSF	cerebrospinal fluid
CV	cardiovascular
CVA	cerebrovascular accident
CYP	cytochrome P-450
D_5LR	dextrose 5% in lactated Ringer's solution
D_5NS	dextrose 5% in normal saline solution
$D_5/0.2NS$	dextrose 5% in quarter-normal saline solution
$D_5/0.45NS$	dextrose 5% in half-normal saline solution
D_5W	dextrose 5% in water
$D_{10}W$	dextrose 10% in water
$D_{50}W$	dextrose 50% in water
dl	deciliter
DNA	deoxyribonucleic acid

(continued)

ABBREVIATIONS *(continued)*

DS	double-strength
EC	enteric-coated
ECG	electrocardiogram
EEG	electroencephalogram
EENT	eyes, ears, nose, and throat
ENDO	endocrine
E.R.	extended-release
°F	degrees Fahrenheit
FDA	Food and Drug Administration
g	gram
GFR	glomerular filtration rate
GI	gastrointestinal
GU	genitourinary
H_1	histamine$_1$
H_2	histamine$_2$
HDL	high-density lipoprotein
HEME	hematologic
HIV	human immunodeficiency virus
HPV	human papilloma virus
hr	hour
h.s.	at bedtime
HSV	herpes simplex virus
HZV	herpes zoster virus
ICP	intracranial pressure
I.D.	intradermal
IgA	immunoglobulin A
IgE	immunoglobulin E
I.M.	intramuscular
INR	international normalized ratio
I.V.	intravenous
IVPB	intravenous piggyback
kg	kilogram
KIU	kallikrein inactivator unit
L	liter
LA	long-acting
LD	lactate dehydrogenase
LDL	low-density lipoprotein
LOC	level of consciousness
LR	lactated Ringer's solution
M	molar
m^2	square meter
MAO	monoamine oxidase

ABBREVIATIONS (continued)

mcg	microgram
mEq	milliequivalent
mg	milligram
MI	myocardial infarction
min	minute
ml	milliliter
mm	millimeter
mm^3	cubic millimeter
mmol	millimole
mo	month
MS	musculoskeletal
Na	sodium
NaCl	sodium chloride
NG	nasogastric
NPH	human isophane insulin
NPO	nothing by mouth
NS	normal saline solution
0.225NS	quarter-normal saline (0.225%) solution
0.45NS	half-normal saline (0.45%) solution
NSAID	nonsteroidal anti-inflammatory drug
OTC	over the counter
p.c.	after meals
PCA	patient-controlled analgesia
P.O.	by mouth
P.R.	by rectum
p.r.n.	as needed
PSVT	paroxysmal supraventricular tachycardia
PT	prothrombin time
PTCA	percutaneous transluminal coronary angioplasty
PVC	premature ventricular contraction
q	every
q.i.d.	four times a day
RBC	red blood cell
REM	rapid eye movement
RESP	respiratory
RNA	ribonucleic acid
RSV	respiratory syncytial virus
SA	sinoatrial
sec	second
SGOT	serum glutamic oxaloacetic transaminase
S.L.	sublingual

(continued)

ABBREVIATIONS *(continued)*

S.R.	sustained-release
stat	immediately
supp	suppository
tab	tablet
T_3	triiodothyronine
T_4	thyroxine
t.i.d.	three times a day
USP	United States Pharmacopeia
UTI	urinary tract infection
VLDL	very low-density lipoprotein
WBC	white blood cell
wk	week

INDEX

- **Generic and alternate names:** lowercase initial letter
- **Trade names:** uppercase initial letter

A

abacavir sulfate, 1–3, 3–7
abacavir sulfate and lamivudine, 1–3
abacavir sulfate, lamivudine, and zidovudine, 3–7
abbreviations, 827–830
Acanya, 350
AccuHist DM, 662
AccuHist Pediatric Drops, 588
Accuretic, 191
Accuzyme, 381
Aceta with Codeine, 222
acetaminophen, 215–218, 218–222, 222–226, 226–228, 243–248, 303–306, 316–319, 326–329, 339–342, 721–726
acetaminophen and codeine phosphate, 222–226
acetaminophen and hydrocodone bitartrate, 226–228
acetaminophen, caffeine, and butalbital, 215–218
acetaminophen, caffeine, and dihydrocodeine bitartrate, 218–222
acrivastine, 583–585
acrivastine and pseudoephedrine sulfate, 583–585
Activella, 404
Actonel with Calcium, 463
Actoplus Met, 455
adapalene 0.1%, 343–344
adapalene 0.1% and benzoyl peroxide 2.5%, 343–344
Adderall, 229
Adderall XR, 229
adriamycin, 807–809

Advair Diskus 100/50, 694
Advair Diskus 250/50, 694
Advair Diskus 500/50, 694
Advair HFA 45/21, 694
Advair HFA 115/21, 694
Advair HFA 230/21, 694
Advicor, 171
Aggrenox, 108
AH-Chew, 761
AK-Poly Bac Ophthalmic, 481
AK-Spore, 504
AK-Spore HC, 506
AK-Trol, 508
Alacol DM, 659
albuterol sulfate, 750–753
Aldactazide, 195
Aldoril 15, 154
Aldoril 25, 154
Aldoril D30, 154
Aldoril D50, 154
alendronate sodium, 387–390
alendronate sodium and cholecalciferol, 387–390
Alesse, 812
aliskiren, 61–65
aliskiren and hydrochlorothiazide, 61–65
Allay, 226
Allegra-D 12 Hour, 691
Allegra-D 24 Hour, 691
AlleRx, 768
AlleRx-D, 795
Allfen-DM, 681
Americet, 215
Amerifed, 625
amiloride hydrochloride, 65–68
amiloride hydrochloride and hydrochlorothiazide, 65–68

S

Y

Z